MW01008393

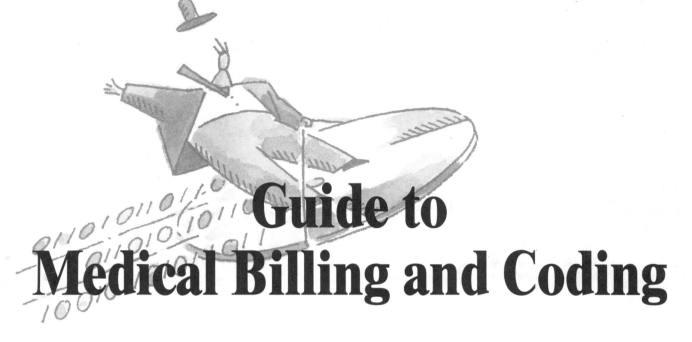

Guide to Medical Billing and Coding

An Honors Certification™ Book

Second Edition

ICDC Publishing, Inc.

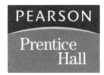

PEARSON

Prentice
Hall

Upper Saddle River, New Jersey 07458

Library of Congress Cataloging-in-Publication Data

Guide to medical billing and coding.—2nd ed.

   p. ; cm.

"An honors certification book."

Rev. ed. of: Guide to medical billing. 6th ed. c2004.

Includes index.

ISBN 0-13-172252-2

1. Medical offices—Management—Handbooks, manuals, etc. 2. Medical fees—Handbooks, manuals, etc. 3. Health insurance claims—Handbooks, manuals, etc. 4. Accounts receivable—Management—Handbooks, manuals, etc. 5. Nosology—Code numbers—Handbooks, manuals, etc.

[DNLM: 1. Practice Management—economics. 2. Forms and Records Control. 3. Patient Credit and Collection. 4. Reimbursement Mechanisms. W 80 G9468 2007] I. Guide to medical billing.

R728.5.G87 2007

651.5'04261—dc22   2006004942

Publisher: Julie Levin Alexander
Publisher's Assistant: Regina Bruno
Executive Editor: Joan Gill
Assistant Editor: Bronwen Glowacki
Director of Marketing: Karen Allman
Senior Marketing Manager: Harper Coles
Marketing Coordinator: Michael Sirinides
Marketing Assistant: Wayne Celia, Jr.
Director of Production and Manufacturing: Bruce Johnson
Managing Production Editor: Patrick Walsh
Production Liaison: Julie Li
Production Editor: Assunta Petrone/Preparé, Inc.
Manufacturing Manager: Ilene Sanford
Manufacturing Buyer: Pat Brown
Senior Design Coordinator: Maria Guglielmo
Interior Designer: Amy Rosen
Cover Designer: Solid State Graphics
Composition: Preparé, Inc.
Printing and Binding: Edwards Brothers, Inc.
Cover Printer: Phoenix Color Corporation

Pearson Education Ltd.
Pearson Education Singapore Pte. Ltd.
Pearson Education Canada, Ltd.
Pearson Education—Japan
Pearson Education Australia Pty. Limited

Pearson Education North Asia Ltd.
Pearson Educación de Mexico, S.A. de C.V.
Pearson Education Malaysia Pte. Ltd.
Pearson Education Inc., Upper Saddle River, New Jersey

10 9 8 7

ISBN 0-13-172252-2

Disclaimer

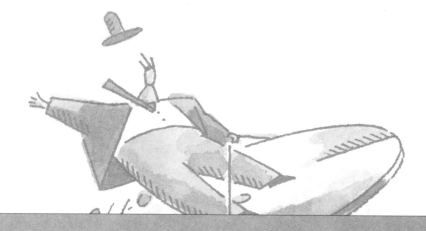

This text is a guide to the medical billing field. Decisions should not be based solely on information within this guide. Decisions impacting the practice of medical billing must be based on individual circumstances including legal/ethical considerations, local conditions, and payer policies.

The information contained in this text is based on experience and research. However, in the complex, rapidly changing medical environment, this information may not always prove correct. Data used are widely variable and can change at any time. Readers should follow current coding regulations outlined by official coding organizations.

Any five-digit numeric *Current Procedural Terminology*, fourth edition (CPT®) codes, services, and descriptions, instructions, and/or guidelines are copyright 2006 (or such other date of publication of CPT® as defined in the federal copyright laws) American Medical Association. All Rights Reserved.

CPT® is a listing of descriptive terms and five-digit numeric identifying codes and modifiers for reporting medical services performed by physicians. This presentation includes only CPT® descriptive terms, numeric identifying codes, and modifiers for reporting medical services and procedures that were selected by ICDC Publishing, Inc. (ICDC) for inclusion

in this publication. The most current CPT® is available from the American Medical Association. No fee schedules, basic unit values, relative value goods conversion factors, or scales or components thereof are included in CPT®.

ICDC has selected certain CPT® codes and service/procedure descriptions and assigned them to various specialty groups. The listing of a CPT® service or procedure description and its code number in this publication does not restrict its use to a particular specialty group. Any procedure or service in this publication may be used to designate the services rendered by any qualified physician.

The American Medical Association assumes no responsibility for the consequences attributable or related to any use or interpretation of any information or views contained in or not contained in this publication.

The publisher and author do not accept responsibility for any adverse outcome from undetected errors, opinion, and analysis contained in this text that may prove inaccurate or incorrect or the reader's misunderstanding of an extremely complex topic. All names used in this book are completely fictitious. Any resemblance to persons or to companies, current or no longer existing, is purely coincidental.

Contents

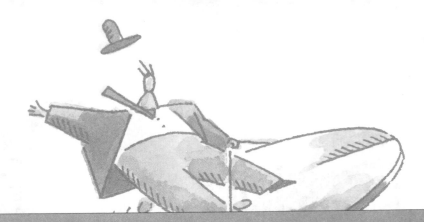

4 Medicare and Medicaid 101

5 Workers' Compensation 140

6 Managed Care 162

SECTION 3
FINANCES AND ACCOUNTING 193

7 Medical Practice Accounting 195

Preface

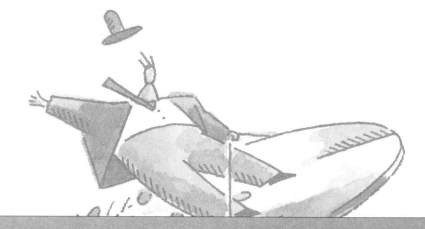

Introduction

Medical billing and coding is the study of medical billing procedures from the time a patient walks into the office to the moment the patient walks out, as well as the final billing and reconciliation of the patient's account.

Medical billing is one of the fastest-growing employment opportunities in the United States today. Insurance companies, medical offices, hospitals, and other healthcare providers are in great need of trained personnel to create and bill medical claims.

The most important ingredient to success is the desire to learn, without which the learning process is ineffective. The desire to learn can lead to a rewarding career in the medical billing field.

Writing Style

The straightforward, easy-to-understand writing style presents information clearly and concisely. Patient and provider names, diagnoses, exercises, and examples in this training material have been designed to incorporate a lighthearted, humorous context. We have found that humorous writing improves the ability to comprehend and retain information.

Text Features

Special features of the text, such as learning objectives, key terms and definitions, end-of-chapter exercises, and Honors Certification™ challenges, enhance understanding and retention of the material.

Learning Objectives Each chapter begins with a bulleted list of learning objectives to help focus the students on the most pertinent topics, key skills, and concepts covered in that chapter.

Key Terms and Definitions Key terms are listed at the beginning of the chapter and defined within the text. Key terms are bolded and defined when initially introduced, thus allowing for quick identification. This structural element allows the students to read the term in context to the related material. In addition, the students can remain focused on reading the material without having to stop and refer to the glossary for a definition.

On the Job Now Exercises These in-text exercises allow the students to immediately practice concepts as they are learned. They are professional practice exercises that will prepare the students for "real-life" job duties.

Practice Pitfalls This special feature provides the students with a professional insider's point of view. These practice pitfalls provide additional information for professional success and ideas, shortcuts, good habits to follow in the office, as well as bad work habits, the outcomes of sloppy work, and common mistakes that the students can avoid.

Summaries Each chapter ends with a bulleted list of key concepts. These summaries are useful study tools that enable the students to assess their level of knowledge and are also useful as a quick study reference.

End-of-Chapter Exercises

Questions for Review located at the end of the chapter help to reinforce key concepts. Answering questions without looking back at the chapter will help students determine if they have grasped the principles within the chapter or if there is a need for further study. The questions also serve to prepare students for examinations. **Vocabulary Word** and **Other Exercises** give students the opportunity to put their knowledge into practice. These hands-on exercises help to ensure competence in medical billing. Answers are contained in the instructor materials for this course.

Honors Certification™ Challenges Our trademarked Honors Certification™ Challenges are presented at the end of every chapter. These challenges provide an opportunity for students to graduate from the program "with honors" by passing a series of additional examinations. These challenges focus on the skills learned in each chapter and give students a chance to prove that they have mastered the material and are capable of performing these skills in the workplace. These requirements are the same skills the students will be asked to perform on the job. Taking and passing these exams will not only earn the students the certification but will also prepare them for the real working world. This extra distinction allows students and schools to certify that the students have achieved mastery of the skills needed to succeed. Employers find this certification useful in recruiting and employing the best students. The Honors Certification™ Challenges are located in the Instructor Resource Guide.

Pedagogy The *Guide to Medical Billing and Coding* will aid the students in learning the skills necessary to become a successful medical biller. The material is designed to be comprehensive yet user friendly. The text follows a logical learning format by beginning with a broad base of information and then, step by step, follows the course for learning the specific medical biller job duties.

Organization of the Text

Guide to Medical Billing and Coding provides students with all the theoretical knowledge and practical skills needed to achieve success as a medical biller. The text introduces the students to the medical practice, before proceeding on to the more in-depth procedures and practices of the medical office and hospital. All aspects of medical billing and coding procedures are covered. Content includes a variety of subjects such as International Classification of Disease (ICD-9-CM) coding, Current

Procedural Terminology (CPT®) coding, stress and time management, the CMS-1500 form and medical procedures, the UB-92 form and hospital procedures, as well as basic office functions and communications.

Ancillary and Program Material

When designing a curriculum and related materials, ICDC does extensive research regarding the skills employers consider essential for job performance. The curriculum and related books and materials are then written to ensure that students learn each of these essential skills. Many schools have gained state and accrediting agency approval with these materials. ICDC's material provide instructors and training institutions with all the materials needed to quickly and easily start and run a new program.

Both *The Practice of Medical Billing and Coding* and the *Guide to Medical Billing and Coding Instructor Resource Guide* are designed to reinforce the concepts learned in the *Guide to Medical Billing and Coding* and also provide the students an opportunity to practice and sharpen their skills.

The Practice of Medical Billing and Coding— *The Practice of Medical Billing and Coding* is a **Real Life™** exercise book that helps the student master skills learned in the *Guide to Medical Billing and Coding*. *The Practice of Medical Billing and Coding* is designed as an exciting, interactive simulated work program and helps the student make the transition from students to actual employee. Medical practice accounting, billing and coding, and related business skills are taught in a simulated medical office environment. These experiential learning activities allow the students to develop critical skills and "work" from the classroom or at home. The exercise book facilitates confidence and skill building by allowing the practicing of skills in a virtual setting which closely mimics being "on-the-job". The exercise book contains simulation exercises, cases, documents, and forms packaged in realistic scenarios.

Guide to Medical Billing and Coding Instructor Resource Guide—This all inclusive combined performance evaluator and curriculum gives the instructors the necessary tools to both run and manage a medical billing program, and assess the student's progress at critical points in the program.

The Instructor Resource Guide includes the following components:

- **Program Overview**—Provides the instructor with general information on the program's structure, and details how to obtain maximum benefits from the program materials.
- **Modularization of the Program**—The program modules are structured to be small, individual, and topic-specific in order to emphasize the importance of learning through participation and practice. The modules also follow the sequence of the *Guide to Medical Billing and Coding* textbook. The flexible modular design allows schools to easily alter the program's length and sequence, and to have concurrent enrollments. The Modularization of the Program includes:
  - Module Objectives.
  - Program Prerequisites.
  - Chapters Covered.
  - Lab and Lecture Hours.
- **Transparency Masters**—Forms and documents for the program are provided for in-class presentations.
- **Program Marketing Materials**—Twenty plus sample marketing letters and brochures are provided for marketing the program including a labor market survey form and medical biller job analysis.
- **Professional Achievement of Certification and Educational Requirements (PACER™) Curriculum**—Provides the instructor with all the necessary materials needed to quickly and easily start a new program. The PACER™ curriculum includes the following:
  - **Daily Lesson Plans**
    - Topics/Lessons Covered.
    - Performance Objectives.
    - Required Materials.
    - Discussion and Investigation Questions.
    - Teaching Methodologies/Evaluation.
- **Performance Evaluators and Answer Keys (PEAK™)**—Provides the instructor with the necessary tools to assess the student's progress at critical stages in the program. The PEAK™ are categorized by chapter and include the following:
  - On the Job Now Exercise Answers.
  - End of Chapter Exercise Answers.
  - Honors Certification™ Challenges.
  - Honors Certification™ Challenges Answers.
- **Test Banks**—The questions and exams are developed from module objectives. Test Banks include the following:
  - Fill-in Exams.
  - Multiple Choice Exams.
  - Test Bank Answer Keys.

To purchase *The Practice of Medical Billing and Coding* or the *Guide to Medical Billing and Coding Instructor Resource Guide,* call Prentice Hall at (800) 526-0485 or visit their website at www.prenhall.com.

Before You Start

Dates Please note that when YY is used in reference to a date, YY indicates the current year (12/01/YY). When PY is used in reference to a date, PY indicates the prior year or last year (12/01/PY). When NY is used in reference to a date, NY indicates the next year (12/01/NY).

Birth Dates Birth dates will be referenced with CCYY-##. This means that the ## should be subtracted from the current year to determine the birth year.

Example: What is the birth date 10/04/CCYY-14, if **CCYY = 2005**?

2005 − 14 = 1991; therefore, the birth date = **10/04/1991**.

Forms Forms to be used to complete the exercises in this text are located in Appendix B. These forms should be copied as needed.

About the Author

ICDC Publishing, Inc. has been writing and creating vocational school materials since 1989. As a training center, Insurance Career Development Center (ICDC) trained students in various vocational occupations. ICDC authors are all professionals who have worked and have extensive training and knowledge in the field of their particular area of study for which they write.

Acknowledgments

Many people have contributed to the development and success of *Guide to Medical Billing and Coding.* We extend our thanks and deep appreciation to the many students and classroom instructors who have provided us with helpful suggestions for this edition of the text.

We would like to express our thanks to the following individuals:

Janet Grossfeld, Adelante Career Institute, Van Nuys, CA; Hollis Anglin and Michael Coffin, Dawn Training Institute, New Castle, DE; Michael Williams, 4-D College, Colton, CA; Anna McCracken and Lynn Russell, American Career College, Los Angeles, CA; Lowell P. Theard, PH.D, MD, Culver Health Associates, Culver City, CA; Tabari Jeffries; Krisia J. Hernandez; Sean Adams; Sydney Adams; Floree Brown; Nathaniel Brown Sr.; Celia R. Luna; Teresa Aguilar; Anita M. Garcia; Sharon E. Brown; Alexandra Fratkin; and CarolAnn Jeffries, PA-C, MHS.

Thanks to the CPA firm of Miller, Kaplan, Arase, and Company, LLP.

We would also like extend our appreciation to the following reviewers for providing valuable feedback throughout the review process:

Kendra Allen, LPN
Ohio Institute of Health Careers
Columbus, OH

Jan West-Boagni, BA
American Career College
Carson, CA

Jennifer M. Donnell
Vatterott College
Springfield, MO

Karen S. Mooney, CPC, CMSCS
Thompson Institute
Harrisburg, PA

Jackee Kaplan, CPC
MedVance Institute, Atlantis, FL
Palm Beach Community College,
Lake Worth, FL

Leslye Danglade, BS
Miami-Dade College
Miami, FL

Jane Carroll, MS
Walla Walla Community College
Clarkston, WA

Ronald W. Deamer
Concorde Career Institute
Portland, OR

Janice Verniglio-Smith
Central Arizona College
Apache Junction, AZ

1

Introduction to
Medical Billing and Coding

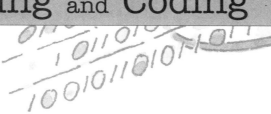

After completion of this chapter
you will be able to:

- List the job responsibilities of a medical biller.
- List the different types of healthcare settings.
- Identify the symptoms of stress.
- List things that can help a person deal with stress.
- Discuss the two main issues covered by HIPAA and the exceptions to the HIPAA privacy guidelines.

- Explain what disclaimers are and how to use them appropriately.
- List and describe the instances in which the patient should be notified and the patient chart notated.
- List the most common causes of fraud.
- Describe how to plan a vacation so that it least impacts fellow co-workers.

Keywords and Concepts
you will learn in this chapter:

- Audits
- Bonding
- Claims Audit
- Embezzlement
- Errors and Omissions Insurance

- External Auditor
- External Audits
- Fraud
- Health Maintenance Organizations (HMOs)
- HIPAA

- Internal Audits
- Job Stress
- Provider
- Respondeat Superior
- Subpoena
- Subpoena Duces Tecum

The medical biller is an important part of the medical environment. As a medical biller, it is your responsibility to properly bill for services received by patients. Because most of the revenues generated by a medical office involve patient care, billing and collecting the revenue generated from patient care is one of the vital functions of the medical biller.

As such, the medical biller is an integral part of the medical team. Their contribution is essential to running the medical office.

Medical billers also may handle filling out claim forms, corresponding with patients, managing office supplies, and handling minor accounting for the office. The scope of a medical biller's duties often will depend on the size of the office. Larger offices may have multiple personnel responsible for running the office, setting appointments and handling the clients. Smaller offices may assign more of these duties to a medical biller/receptionist.

For purposes of this course, we will cover all duties that a medical biller may perform in a smaller practice setting. The main provider of service used throughout this guide for illustrative purposes is Paul Provider, M.D., 5858 Peppermint Place, Anytown, USA 12345. Many other providers of service will be used as well.

Job Roles and Duties

Medical billers play a diversified role in the medical office. The most common duties associated with medical billing include:

- Billing insurance carriers for services performed.
- Billing patients for any amounts not covered by the insurance carrier.
- Doing basic accounting for the practice, including keeping track of incoming and outgoing cash flow.
- Handling collections on overdue accounts.
- Scheduling appointments for patients.
- Greeting patients.

- Maintaining and updating patient files, and filing and retrieving files when needed.
- Answering the office phones.
- Ordering general office supplies.
- Keeping abreast of and utilizing appropriate computer programs for billing, correspondence, and accounting.

Job Titles

Although the main purpose of this course is to teach medical billing and coding, students who successfully pass this course often qualify for other jobs as well. The most common job titles include:

- Medical Coder.
- Medical Coding Specialist.
- Hospital Biller.
- Patient Account Manager.

The Medical Team

In any medical office, there are a number of people who work together to provide complete health care to the patient. A **Provider** is the person or entity that provides healthcare services. This can be a doctor, chiropractor, hospital, emergency facility, x-ray technician, or any certified professional who is licensed to provide healthcare services. Although the doctor may be the main provider, without the ancillary people it would be difficult for the office to function. Each member of the team is vital to providing overall patient care.

In a medical office setting there often are three areas of team members:

- The Physician.
- The Medical Assistant.
- The Biller and Receptionist.

Medical assistants not only assist the provider with the care of the patient, they also handle some minor procedures themselves. For example, they often are responsible for sterilization of equipment, room preparation, setting up the patient, and administering injections.

The medical biller and receptionist also have important duties. These can include ensuring that the provider has patients scheduled in an appropriate manner. Also, without the billing of patients and collecting of revenues, there would not be enough money to continue to run the office.

The office manager supervises the staff and handles the day-to-day organization of the medical office. The office manager also may be responsible for scheduling staff, payroll, and management of office expenses.

In a hospital setting, the same levels of patient care exist with some minor differences. The doctors usually provide the direction of care by giving verbal or written orders to the nursing staff. The nurses and other medical personnel provide most of the direct patient care. The billing department is often separate from the other departments and simply handles the billing of patients and the collecting of revenues. However, in a hospital setting, there are additional administrative, reception, and other departments.

Regardless of the number of departments a medical provider has, each department is a necessary part of the whole operation. Without any one department, the facility could easily cease to exist.

Types of Healthcare Settings

There are several places a medical biller can work, depending on their experience and their preferences. The most common places include those listed here.

Provider's Office

There are many areas in a provider's office that a medical biller may work. In addition to handling the billing, a medical biller may perform all other front office duties, such as greeting clients and handling patient intake. They often will be responsible for scheduling patient appointments and maintaining patient files.

Billing Company

Some medical billers work for independent billing companies. These companies usually perform the billing for a number of doctors. Doctors who only have a small practice may not need a full-time medical biller. If the provider only sees 10 or 15 patients a day, performing the billing for those 10 to 15 patients may only take an hour. Having a full-time medical biller would probably not be cost-effective. In smaller medical offices, the medical assistant may handle the tasks of greeting patients and making appointments. However, the billing information regarding the patients seen and the procedures performed may be sent to a medical billing company for handling.

The medical company will create the claims and often will handle patient accounting. They will load any information regarding payments received onto the account and then bill the patient for any balance remaining. Some billing companies have the capacity to transmit information directly into the provider's computer. Thus, the provider's office has information that is mostly current regarding each patient and their account.

Hospital

Hospitals need billers who can make sure that every item that the patient uses is accounted for and billed. In a hospital setting, billers will have little contact with the patients. The only exception is when a patient or the parent of a patient comes to the billing office to make a payment on their account. Most often, this happens when a portion of the fee is payable before the services are rendered.

Health Maintenance Organization

Health Maintenance Organizations (HMOs) are groups that provide services in exchange for premiums. Unlike traditional insurance, many HMOs act as both the insurance carrier and the provider of services. However, there are always times when an HMO facility sees a patient that is not one of their members. This most often occurs during a medical emergency when the patient is transferred to the nearest facility. If a patient is treated at an HMO facility, but they are not a member of that HMO, the HMO facility will bill the patient or their insurance carrier for the services provided.

An HMO facility may have to bill another insurance carrier when a patient with a work-related injury sees their regular HMO provider for treatment. Because most workers are covered by Workers' Compensation insurance, the HMO will bill the Workers' Compensation carrier for the services.

Pharmacy

More and more insurance plans are covering prescription drugs. Although many pharmacies will rely on the patient to file their own claim, some pharmacies are offering insurance billing as one of their services. This is especially true because Medicare now provides basic benefits for drug coverage.

Medical Equipment Provider

Companies that supply medical equipment for patient use outside the hospital (e.g., a wheelchair) sometimes will have billers on staff. Some of these companies may rely on the patient to file their own insurance claim. However, equipment providers are realizing that it can be a wonderful marketing tool to file insurance claims for the patients.

Other Care Facilities

Numerous other types of facilities need medical billers on staff. These can include nursing homes, convalescent homes, hospices, rehabilitation centers, or any place that provides medical services.

Within each of these settings there are numerous specialties. For example, an individual provider may specialize in general practice, cardiology, pediatric medicine, or any number of other specialties. Medical billers, however, are needed and may find employment at all of these facilities.

Basic Skill Requirements of the Medical Biller

There are some basic initial skills that are required to become a successful medical biller: oral and written communication skills, basic knowledge of anatomy and physiology, a strong medical terminology, basic math skills, basic computer skills, critical reading and comprehension, and an ability to be detail oriented.

Interpersonal Skills

The following interpersonal skills will help you to get along harmoniously with others in the workplace.

Place the company ahead of yourself. Give your absolute best at work. Establish a reputation that shows people they can rely on you to do good work on time.

Be willing to admit when you are wrong. Rather than losing face, people will appreciate your honesty.

Speak well of others whenever possible. Remember to praise people for a job well done, both to them and to their superiors.

Show an interest in what others say. Take the time to listen to others. If you cannot spare the time, politely find a way to postpone the conversation. For example, "Unfortunately I am under a deadline. How about if we discuss this further over lunch?"

Give credit where credit is due. If someone else helps you with a project, even in a small way, do not take the credit for their work. Be sure that the superiors know who actually did the work. If you try to take credit for work that someone else has done, you will eventually be exposed and people will be less willing to help or trust you in the future.

Compromise. Sometimes you may disagree with a co-worker. In such cases, a compromise can work wonders toward keeping the relationship intact and resolving the conflict. Try to find a solution in which each of you gain something. Allow them to win one point, while you win another.

Make others look good, especially your supervisor. If you are asked to help with a project, do your best work. Go the extra mile in finding solutions for a problem, and then allow the responsible person to turn in the project and take credit for their share. If they

take credit for your work, do not refute it. You do not know if something was said at a different time. If you start jumping in and insisting that you helped, you appear to lack confidence in others and yourself.

Introduce yourself to new people. The office environment often will change quickly. Taking the time to learn the names of those you work with lets them know that they are important to you. Take the time to make small talk and find out something about them.

Build networks. Be willing to refer work to others who can do a better job than you. Also, take work from others that they want you to try. Talk to people about non-work-related matters during lunch hours or break times. Get to know them a little better, and let them get to know you.

Smile and be positive. Positive people are more pleasant to be around. No one wants to spend time with someone who brings out the worst in everyone. Maintain a positive attitude. If you are positive, it makes other people positive as well.

Try to keep your personal problems to yourself. Constantly discussing personal problems at work can make others feel uncomfortable and will often strain your relationship, as they may be reluctant to engage in conversation with you.

Keep your mouth shut. If someone passes information on to you, do not share it with others unless you are specifically asked to do so.

Confirm rumors before acting on them. Often things get twisted around in the office grapevine and bear no resemblance to the truth after it has gone through the 20th telling.

Actions to Avoid

There are several actions that should be avoided on the job. These include:

- Having loud phone conversations.
- Not cleaning up after yourself in common areas such as the kitchen or lounge.
- Looking over a co-worker's shoulder.
- Going through a co-worker's desk.
- Neglecting to say please and thank you.
- Wearing too much perfume or cologne.
- Not being clean, especially in your work area: The appearance of a work area reveals a lot about a person.
- Smoking.
- Talking behind someone's back.
- Asking someone else to tell a lie or to be dishonest.

- Blaming someone else when you are at fault.

- Asking someone, especially a subordinate, to do an errand that is not work-related.

- Telling offensive jokes or making sexist or politically incorrect comments.

- Complaining about another person.

- Being condescending toward others.

On the Job Now

Directions: Rate yourself on each of the qualities listed below, and then answer the following questions.
1 = Never, 2 = Almost Never, 3 = Sometimes, 4 = Almost Always, 5 = Always.

Do you:

Embrace innovation?	1	2	3	4	5
Take the initiative?	1	2	3	4	5
Consider everything within your job title?	1	2	3	4	5
Strive for knowledge recognition rather than social recognition?	1	2	3	4	5
Let your work speak for itself or take pride in the quality of your work?	1	2	3	4	5
Like to learn new skills?	1	2	3	4	5
Ally yourself with powerful people?	1	2	3	4	5
Have high morale?	1	2	3	4	5

Are you:

Willing to learn and do someone else's job?	1	2	3	4	5
Logical, not emotional?	1	2	3	4	5
Self-confident?	1	2	3	4	5
Willing to take on more than your responsibilities?	1	2	3	4	5

1. For which assets did you circle a 5? _____

_____

2. For which assets did you circle a 4? _____

_____

3. For which assets did you circle a 1, 2, or 3? _____

_____

4. What can you do to improve each of those assets that you ranked yourself 1, 2, or 3? _____

_____

_____

Stress

Job stress is defined as the harmful physical and emotional responses that occur when the requirements of the job do not match the capabilities, resources, or needs of the worker.

Often people will say, "A little bit of stress is good for you." However, this often depends on your definition of stress, as well as on how much is a "little bit." What people often mean is that a challenge can be good for you.

Challenges energize us psychologically and physically and help motivate us to learn new skills. When a challenge is met, we feel relaxed and satisfied. Thus, challenges can be an important ingredient for healthy and productive work.

Although challenges can be good for you, stress is not. Stress causes negative physiological reactions, such as an increase in adrenaline and heart rate, without the physical ability to expend and use the adrenaline.

Symptoms of Stress

Stress can cause a variety of symptoms that can inhibit your ability to function properly, both at work and in your daily life. The most common symptoms of stress include:

- Headaches.
- Anxiety.
- High blood pressure.
- Trouble falling asleep or other sleep disturbances.
- Difficulty concentrating.
- Short temper.
- Upset stomach.
- Job dissatisfaction.
- Low morale.
- Hyperventilation.
- Clenching or grinding of the teeth.

Pent-up stress also can cause emotional outbursts, ranging from intense anger to tears and self-pity. Chronic stress can cause problems in relationships, heart problems, and immune system deficiencies.

Handling Stress

Although stress is a part of everyday life, it is important to deal with stress appropriately so that it does not accumulate and overwhelm you. Handling stress is an important part of being able to function in the working world.

Quick stress relievers can include:

- Exercising vigorously.
- A massage.
- Deep, slow breathing.
- Getting more sleep.
- Skipping extra caffeine in items such as coffee, cola, and chocolate.
- Eating properly and regularly.

Other means of handling stress may take a bit longer to accomplish a stress-free state but can be more effective. These include:

Finding the humor in life. Learn to laugh at the mistakes you make and things that go wrong. Laughter is a great stress reliever.

Creating a new attitude. Try to see each problem as a challenge. Think of it as a chance for you to go up against an imaginary adversary and come out victorious by conquering the problem. By changing your attitude toward problems you can create an aura of excitement, thus giving yourself the energy to tackle and handle problems.

Giving yourself opportunities to relax. You should spend at least half an hour every day doing something that helps to relax your body and mind. This can be reading a book, exercising, socializing with friends, or whatever helps you work off stress and relax. Remember, these should be activities that give you pleasure, not those that give you stress of a different nature.

Creating a stress barrier. Do not bring your family or life problems to work, and do not take your work problems home with you. Establishing a routine that provides a break between the two environments can help. Some people create this barrier by having a long commute home, others will take a few minutes after arriving home to relax before tackling home activities, and others will stop off on the way home to do something else.

These types of habits can help you keep the troubles of work and home from interfering with each other.

Making a "To Do" list. We often get overwhelmed thinking of all the things we need to accomplish, and sometimes everything we think of leads to something else. Just like trying to remember the names of the seven dwarfs, we suddenly start renaming them until we have ten dwarfs instead of seven. Even then, we keep thinking in the back of our minds that we have forgotten something.

Tasks are like the names of the dwarfs. You can end up naming and renaming lots of things you have to do and still feel like you have not remembered everything. However, if you take the time to write down the tasks you are facing, suddenly many of them seem more manageable. Now you have a goal in mind and a clear direction of what needs to be accomplished. You will feel good knowing what you have to do, and you will feel even better when you start to accomplish some of them and scratch them off the list.

Also remember to do one thing at a time. Multitasking does not mean doing everything at once. Performing the items on your list one at a time allows you to concentrate on each item and be more productive, which gives you the opportunity to complete them more efficiently.

Ask others not to disturb you. If you have a time-sensitive project or a fast-approaching deadline, ask not to be disturbed. Hang a sign on your desk with the words "Please Do Not Disturb, Important Deadline Looming." In some companies, notifying others that you do not want to be disturbed can be easily accomplished by closing your door.

Ask the receptionist to hold your calls, or, if you have voice mail, switch to a greeting that informs people that you are working on a very important project. Include in your message when you will be available and ask them to leave a message or call you back at a later time.

Other people are busy, too, and they understand the need to buckle down and focus on a project. Most people are more than willing to respect your request.

On the Job Now

Directions: Make a sign with the following (or similar) phrase, "Please Do Not Disturb, Important Deadline Looming!" Be creative and make it attractive, but do not take so long that it becomes a major project. Consider making it a trifold sign, one that will stand on your desk or one that you can easily hang from the side of your desk. Use this sign whenever it is necessary.

Prevacation Work Planning

Taking a vacation can be great for you but stressful for your co-workers. Taking a vacation means the rest are left with one less person to carry on the work.

Although many people think only of themselves when planning a vacation, good medical billers also think of their company. Following are some guidelines to use when planning a vacation.

Take your vacation during the company's slow period. Nearly all companies have one or two seasons that are busier than others. Schedule your vacation around these times so that you are there when you are most needed. Co-workers and especially your bosses will appreciate your thoughtfulness. Some people may think that scheduling a vacation during the busy time will reveal how valuable they are. Unfortunately, the

negative impression that they are thinking only of themselves and not of the company will outweigh any thoughts of how important their skills are.

Before leaving, be sure that your desk is in order. All paperwork and folders should be filed appropriately. This allows anyone who needs something to find it when you are away. All work with a due date before your vacation should be completed and turned in. Sometimes, this means working through lunch or working harder to make sure things are accomplished. Others can get a negative impression of you if you leave without completing assignments or without properly filing things away so others can find them.

Let others know two weeks in advance that you are leaving. This gives your supervisors and others enough advance notice for any projects that need your input for completion.

Leave a number with a trusted co-worker for emergencies. Providing a number at which you can be reached in case of emergency shows those in your office that you care. A brief word, such as "So-and-so knows how to reach me if it is an emergency," should be enough to let people know of your whereabouts.

Enjoy your vacation. Ignore what is happening at work. Give your mind and body a break. This will allow you to come back and face work with a fresh outlook because you will be more rested, refreshed, and ready to take on new challenges.

Certification Programs for Medical Billers

Currently, there is no state or federal certification or licensing requirement for medical billers. However, more and more employers are requesting or requiring certification of their medical billing and coding applicants.

Certification offers increased job security, income, prestige, advancement, and recognition, as well as professional affiliation.

There are several different certification programs:

American Academy of Procedural Coders
2144 S. Highland Drive, Suite 100
Salt Lake City, UT 84106
800-626-2633
http://www.aapc.com

Certification as a Certified Procedural Coder (CPC-A) or Certified Procedural Coder (CPC-H)

American Health Information Management
Association
919 N. Michigan Ave., Suite 1400
Chicago, IL 60611-1683
or: P.O. Box 97349
Chicago, IL 60690-7349
800-335-5535
http://www.ahima.org

Certification as Certified Coding Associate (CCA) or Certified Coding Specialist (CCD)

Professional Association of Health Care Office
Managers
461 East Ten Mile Road
Pensacola, FL 32534-9716
800-451-9311
http://www.pahcom.com

Certification as a Certified Medical Manager (CMM).

For further information on coding certification, contact the companies that are listed here.

Legal Issues

There are several legal issues that affect the medical biller on a daily basis. These include privacy regulations, rules and regulations regarding allowable collections procedures, and fraud.

Privacy Guidelines

The very nature of health care requires a great deal of personal information to be gathered and maintained about many individuals. Therefore, the needs of the company must be carefully weighed against the person's right to privacy so as to avoid unwarranted invasions of that right.

In particular, medical information is considered to be privileged and confidential in the context of the physician/patient relationship. Unauthorized disclosure of information may represent a violation of that confidentiality.

The confidentiality of medical records has assumed a new importance for several reasons:

1. People are becoming more litigation-minded.
2. Health plans reimburse for more sensitive services that were excluded in the past, for example, alcohol detoxification, mental health treatment, and AIDS-related illnesses.
3. More employers are self-administering or self-funding their health plans, which means that highly personal medical information is, in some instances, routinely handled by fellow employees.
4. New HIPAA regulations require that all personnel involved in the healthcare process respect the patient's right to privacy and confidentiality.

HIPAA

In 1996, the **Health Insurance Portability and Accountability Act (HIPAA)** was signed into law to set a national standard for electronic transfer of health data. The portability issues refer to persons being covered by insurance when they transfer from one job to another. These issues are most important to the health claims examiner. However, the privacy issues and the health insurance fraud and abuse issues are vitally important for the medical biller to understand.

HIPAA encompasses two main issues:

1. Portability, or the ability to transfer insurance companies and still be covered for preexisting conditions; and

2. Accountability, generally dealing with the patient's right to privacy from the healthcare provider, health insurer, and any other parties required in the healthcare process (e.g., billers, clearinghouses, etc.), and the lack of fraud and abuse when dealing with healthcare.

Regarding the Privacy section of HIPAA, the Department of Health and Human Services states:

The privacy requirements limit the release of patient Protected Health Information (PHI) without the patient's knowledge and consent beyond that required for patient care. Patient's personal information must be more securely guarded and more carefully handled when conducting the business of health care.

Most healthcare entities were required to meet the standards set in the privacy issues section of HIPAA on April 14, 2003. HIPAA calls for severe civil and criminal penalties for noncompliance, including fines up to $25,000 for multiple violations of the same standard in a calendar year; and fines up to $250,000 or imprisonment up to 10 years for knowing misuse of individually identifiable health information.

General Rules

There are several general rules for ensuring that privacy guidelines are met:

1. Always obtain an authorization to release information before releasing any information. Most releases routinely signed in the medical practice only authorize the physician to release information necessary to process a patient's claim. Additional authorization should be obtained to release any information to other parties. These releases should state exactly what information is to be released, the dates of any services provided that fall within the release, the person to whom the information may be released, the signature of the patient, the date of the signature, and the date the release expires.

2. Gather only the information that is necessary and relevant to the billing or processing of the claim.

3. Use only legal and ethical means to collect the information required. Whenever permission is necessary, obtain written authorization from the insured or patient (guardian or parent if the patient is a minor).

4. When requested, and subject to any applicable legal or ethical prohibition or privilege, the insured or patient concerned should be advised of the nature and general uses to be made of the information.

5. Make every reasonable effort to ensure that the information on which an action is based is accurate, relevant, timely, and complete.

6. On request, the patient or insured should be given the opportunity to correct or clarify the information given by or about him or her, and the file should be amended to the extent that it is fair to both the provider and the patient or insured. Requests for review or clarification of medical information will be accepted only from the person from whom the information was obtained.

7. In general, disclosures of information to a third party (other than those described to the insured or patient) should be made only with the written authorization of the patient or insured. This includes disclosure to employers, family members, or former spouses.

8. All practical precautions should be taken to ensure that medical files are physically secure and that access to the use of such files is limited to authorized personnel. This includes not leaving files out, locking all files, and even turning your computer screen away from where it might be seen by other persons. Security passwords and other security measures also may be required, depending on your office situation.

9. All personnel involved in the keeping of medical records should be advised of the need to protect the Right of Privacy in obtaining required information and the need to treat all individually identifiable information as confidential. Willful abuse of the privacy of any insured or patient by the employee may be cause for dismissal.

10. The disclosure of a diagnosis should never be made to an insured or his or her family. If the insured requests this information, refer the insured to the physician. There may be a reason the patient does not know his or her diagnosis.

11. Never release any information to an ex-spouse. This includes the patient's address, phone number, when services were rendered, to whom, and other information. The ex-spouse should be instructed to contact the patient directly.

12. Do not leave files, patients' records, or appointment books open on your desk or in an area where they may be seen by others. This includes patient's files or information that may be displayed on a computer screen. The best way to handle this is to be sure that all files are closed or are turned over on your desk. Computer screens must be placed in such a way that they cannot be seen by anyone passing by. If necessary, use a screen saver or other unrestricted document that can be clicked on to replace the one you are working on instantaneously.

13. If a minor patient has the legal right to authorize treatment or services, disclosure to the parents, legal guardians of the minor, or to other persons may be a violation of HIPAA or the confidentiality of Medical Information Privacy and Security Act (MIPSA).

14. Be cautious about releasing information to a patient's employer, even if an authorization to release information has been obtained.

If in doubt as to whether specific information should be released, check with your supervisor before, not after, releasing it.

These guidelines cover some of the basic aspects of HIPAA privacy regulations. For detailed information regarding HIPAA guidelines, complete rules and regulations regarding HIPAA are printed in the Federal Register.

Faxing

When faxing items, be aware of sensitive information. All faxes should contain a cover sheet that announces to whom the fax is addressed, who it is from, and a note that the enclosed information is personal and confidential. Information regarding diagnosis, treatments, sexually transmitted diseases, HIV, drug or alcohol abuse, or financial data should never be faxed. Following is sample wording for the fax confidentiality statement:

The enclosed information is intended exclusively for the individual or entity to which it is addressed and contains information which is privileged, confidential or exempt from disclosure under federal or state laws. If the reader of this message is not the recipient or the agent or employee responsible for delivering this facsimile transmission to the intended recipient you are hereby notified that any dissemination, distribu-

tion, or copying of the information contained in this facsimile is strictly prohibited. If you have received this facsimile in error, please notify our office immediately by telephone and return the original facsimile to us at the above address.

When faxing other information, consider asking the receiving party for a code number (i.e., the patient's ID number or birth date), then black out all pertinent information on the patient and replace it with the code number.

Items should only be faxed in an emergency. Otherwise, regular or certified mail should be used.

The guidelines listed are just that. The final decisions are up to you. Use common sense and put yourself in the place of the patient or insured.

Exceptions

There are a few exceptions to the privacy laws. In the following instances, the privacy guidelines may be considered less stringent, or the patient may be deemed to have waived their rights to confidentiality:

1. Less stringent guidelines apply for physicians who are employed by insurance companies. Disclosure to their employers of patient records and information is more routine.

2. Cases of gunshot wounds, stabbings resulting from criminal actions, and suspected child abuse that must be reported to the local police department or childcare agency. Some states also require that incidents of spousal abuse be reported.

3. Reports of communicable diseases and some diseases and illnesses of infants and newborns. These are most often used for compiling statistics and attempting to stop the spread of communicable diseases.

4. Information obtained by the Medicare insurance carrier that pertains to a patient may be reported directly to that patient's beneficiary or his representative. The Medicare insurance specialist cannot accept or withhold information they receive regarding a patient, even if the information is marked "confidential."

5. If a patient is seen at the request of a third party who is covering the bill (i.e., workers' compensation cases), limited confidentiality is waived and the information may be provided to the person or company ordering the procedures.

6. If records are subpoenaed or a search warrant is issued, records may be turned over to the court or their representatives.

Fraud

Fraud is defined as intentional misrepresentation of a fact with the intent to deprive a person of property or legal rights. The most common instance of fraud that occurs in the health claims industry is doctors or other providers of service billing for goods or services that were not actually provided.

Because of the high incidence of abuse, all billed services must be documented in the medical record to prove that they were actually provided. The "law of documentation" states that "if it wasn't documented, it didn't happen." Billing for services not provided is a serious offense and constitutes fraud. If a person is convicted, the penalties are extremely stiff. In addition, both the physician and the medical biller can be held liable for the filing of fraudulent claims.

The most common cases of fraud include:

1. Overbilling or billing for services not rendered.
2. Altering records or claims to upgrade the service presented (i.e., billing for a high-complexity office visit when the services provided were for a low-complexity visit).
3. Changing dates on services or splitting procedures (i.e., placing different dates on services that were actually performed on the same date, changing the date to make it appear as if treatment were rendered after the surgery follow-up days, rather than during the follow-up days).
4. Unbundling of charges (i.e., listing lab charges as though a number of separate tests were done when several tests were done simultaneously from the same sample).
5. Allowing a patient to use the medical coverage card of another patient, or billing services under an incorrect patient name (i.e., Sally Smith, 23, not covered under her parents' insurance, is billed as Sandy Smith, her 16-year-old sister, who is covered).
6. Allowing, offering, soliciting, or accepting a kickback or return of monies for a referral or for use of a specific product.
7. Altering the diagnosis to substantiate procedures performed.
8. Billing twice for the same services.

9. Billing group services as if they were individual services (i.e., a psychiatrist visits several patients in a group session but bills as if each patient was seen individually).
10. Ordering or billing for services that were performed but were not medically necessary.
11. Accepting payment in full from insurance carriers. Such practice is considered fraudulent (especially with Medicare) because the insurance is actually paying for 100% of the services, not the 80% (or other coinsurance percentage) which they contracted with the patient to pay. Such a practice often leads physicians to increase their bills to make up the difference, and can lead to patients overutilizing services; as there is no financial incentive to limit visits.

If occasional cases are written off because of hardship, this should be documented in the records, along with an explanation of the hardship circumstances and the reasoning for the dismissal of the debt.

12. Billing different patients at different rates (i.e., one charge for Medicare patients and a different charge for uninsured patients for the same services).
13. Requiring patients to pay balances in excess of Medicare, Medicaid, or HMO limits.
14. Requiring Medicare patients to pay for services that should be covered by Medicare, thus not being limited by the Medicare-approved amount.
15. Failing to refund copayments and deductible charges for Medicare patients whose charges have been deemed by Medicare to be not medically necessary.
16. Submitting claims to two or more insurers without disclosing that more than one insurance may cover the charges.
17. Billing Medicare or other insurance carriers when bills should be submitted to a third party (i.e., workers' compensation coverage, a third party that may be liable in the case of an accident).

If the physician is engaging in such practices and it can be shown that the biller participated, or even if they merely knew about the fraudulent acts and did nothing, the medical biller can be charged as an accomplice, even if they received no money themselves. As a precautionary measure, having billers initial the claims they create or submit for payment can help to track down the guilty party.

Because a physician is considered ultimately responsible for everything that goes on in his or her practice, the physician may be considered guilty of fraud even if he or she had no knowledge of the crime. The physician may be criminally sentenced or may merely have to reimburse the insurance carrier for all fraudulently submitted claims.

If a person, either a physician or a biller, is found guilty of Medicare or Medicaid fraud, they are excluded from ever participating in the program again.

HIPAA and Fraud and Abuse

The new HIPAA fraud statutes have greatly broadened the scope of the federal government for prosecuting fraud and abuse in the healthcare industry. HIPAA defines four new criminal healthcare fraud offenses: Health Care Fraud, Theft or Embezzlement in Connection with Health Care, False Statements Relating to Health Care Matters, and Obstruction of Criminal Investigations of Health Care Offenses.

HIPAA now defines a healthcare benefit program as "any public or private plan or contract, affecting commerce, under which any medical benefit, item, or service is provided to any individual, and includes any individual or entity who is providing a medical benefit, item, or service for which payment may be made under the plan or contract." By including private health benefit plans and any individual or entity, they have effectively given themselves the right to prosecute anyone involved in the healthcare industry for fraud or abuse.

The following four sections further define the HIPAA statutes.

Health care fraud (18 USC 1347): Whoever knowingly and willfully executes, or attempts to execute, a scheme or artifact—

1. to defraud any health care benefit program; or
2. to obtain, by means of false or fraudulent pretenses, representations, or promises, any of the money or property owned by, or under the custody or control of, any health care benefit program,

in connection with the delivery of or payment for health care benefits, items, or services, shall be fined under this title or imprisoned not more than 10 years, or both. If the violation results in serious bodily injury (as defined in section 1365 of the title), such person shall be fined under this title or imprisoned not more

than 20 years, or both; and if the violation results in death, such person shall be fined under this title, or imprisoned for any term of years or for life, or both.

The medical biller needs to keep in mind that if he creates or submits a health claim which he knows to be fraudulent, he may be held liable under this portion of the statute.

Theft or embezzlement in connection with health care (18 USC 669):

a. Whoever knowingly and willfully embezzles, steals, or otherwise without authority converts to the use of any person other than the rightful owner, or intentionally misapplies any of the moneys, funds, securities, premiums, credits, property, or other assets of a health care benefit program, shall be fined under this title or imprisoned not more than 10 years, or both; but if the value of such property does not exceed the sum of $100 the defendant shall be fined under this title or imprisoned not more than one year, or both.

b. As used in this section, the term "health care benefit program" has the meaning given such term in section 24 (b) of this title.

Any medical biller that does any of the following: accepts payment on claims which they know to be fraudulent; misapplies medical payments to the wrong account; takes home office supplies, equipment, or other items with the intent to keep; and drafts unauthorized checks to himself or others, may be held liable under this portion of the statute.

False statements relating to health care matters (18 USC 1035):

a. Whoever, in any matter involving a health care benefit program, knowingly and willfully—
   1. falsifies, conceals, or covers up by any trick, scheme, or device a material fact; or
   2. makes any materially false, fictitious, or fraudulent statements or representations, or makes or uses any materially false writing or document knowing the same to contain any materially false, fictitious, or fraudulent statement or entry,

   in connection with the delivery of or payment for health care benefits, items, or services, shall be fined under this title or imprisoned not more than five years, or both.

b. As used in this section, the term "health care benefit program" has the meaning given such term in section 24 (b) of this title.

A medical biller that creates false claims and/or claim documents, alters and/or falsifies claim information, lies about claims situations, and does not come forward to disclose fraudulent situations that they are aware of, may be held liable under this portion of the statute.

Obstruction of criminal investigations of health care offenses (18 USC 1518):

a. Whoever willfully prevents, obstructs, misleads, delays or attempts to prevent, obstruct, mislead, or delay the communication of information or records relating to a violation of a Federal health care offense to a criminal investigator shall be fined under this title or imprisoned not more than 5 years, or both.

b. As used in this section the term "criminal investigator" means any individual duly authorized by a department, agency, or armed force of the United States to conduct or engage in investigations for prosecutions for violations of health care offenses.

Destroying records, not turning over files or documents when asked, lying to investigators, and generally being uncooperative during an investigation may cause a medical biller to be liable under this portion of the statute.

It is important for the medical biller to be aware of these issues. If you discover a possibly fraudulent claim, it is important to bring it to your supervisor's attention as soon as possible. Additionally, if an investigation is initiated, you should cooperate fully with the investigators. Not doing so could be construed as hindering their investigation, and this can make you liable for fines and imprisonment up to five years. It is important to note that the statutes are written in such a way that you can be found guilty of hindering an investigation even if that investigation later fails to turn up fraud.

Additionally, medical billers need to be cautious about the statements or comments they make regarding a claim, especially written comments that are placed in a file. If those comments turn out to be fraudulent, the medical biller may be held liable.

Embezzlement

Embezzlement is the act of an employee illegally taking funds from a company they work for. Embezzlement can be committed by anyone in a firm, including the receptionist, the biller, or the physician.

To protect against embezzlement:

1. Accurate records must be kept of all transactions. Be sure to issue a receipt for all amounts received and to accurately record these amounts against the patient's account.
2. Any amounts removed should be notated and a receipt given for them. This is not only true for amounts that may have been taken from the cash drawer to pay for office supplies but also for amounts a physician may remove. Even if the physician is the sole owner of the practice, he or she should never be allowed to take money from the cash drawer without issuing a receipt. Such a practice helps keep accurate records for financial accounting purposes, and protects the keeper of the cash drawer from being charged with removing the money.
3. All checks should be immediately stamped FOR DEPOSIT ONLY and the account number should be written or stamped on the check. The bank should be given instructions that they are never to cash a check made payable to the practice and cash should never be given back from a deposit.
4. All monthly bank statements should be matched with the daily and monthly journals for the office. Total deposits should tally with the total of all daily journals. Any discrepancies should be reported immediately to a supervisor.
5. If embezzlement is suspected, the proper person should be notified. In the case of a co-worker, this is usually their supervisor. If a worker knows of embezzlement by a co-worker and says nothing, they are guilty of being an accomplice to the crime.
6. A bond (insurance against embezzlement) should be obtained for each member of the practice who deals directly with the practice's receipts. These bonds can be issued on individual persons, on a job position, or for the entire office staff.
7. If you notice poor bookkeeping or inaccurate records that were kept by a previous employee or a current co-worker, this should be brought to the attention of your supervisor or employer. You should then document the problems in writing and

ask the supervisor or employer to initial a copy for you to keep. This may provide minimal protection in case the problems with the records were found to conceal embezzlement or mismanagement of funds.

As with fraud, a physician is considered ultimately responsible for everything that goes on in his or her practice. If embezzlement is found, the physician may be considered guilty and may be responsible for monies embezzled by their employees.

Employee Bonding and Errors and Omission Insurance

Generally, an employer is liable for harms caused by an employee while that employee is acting within the scope of their employment. This is called **respondeat superior**. However, a court of law may find the employee personally responsible for an incident that occurred as a result of an error, omission, or negligent act committed by the employee. A professional liability policy usually covers errors, omissions, or negligent acts, which may arise as an employee carries out his normal or usual duties. **Errors and omissions** is part of a professional liability insurance policy in most cases. This insurance covers damages caused by mistakes (errors) or damages caused by something an employee failed to do (omissions).

Some employers protect themselves from employee dishonesty by bonding their employees. **Bonding** is the process by which an employer can be indemnified for the loss of money or other property sustained through dishonest acts of a "bonded" employee. Bonding can cover many types of acts including larceny, theft, embezzlement, forgery, misappropriation, wrongful abstraction, willful misapplication, or other fraudulent or dishonest acts committed by an employee, alone or in collusion with others.

Claim Audits

A **claims audit** is an analysis of claims payments made to a healthcare provider to determine whether the claims were allowable and whether the provider was paid the appropriate amount for services rendered. This type of audit usually includes reviewing the medical record to determine if services were documented and medically necessary. An **external auditor** is someone hired by an insurance company or governmental organization such as Medicare or Medicaid to perform an audit. **Audits** are performed to prevent and detect fraud. Fraud means that the provider knew, or reasonably should have known, that a statement or claim submitted was false.

Medical billing personnel are required by law to cooperate with regulatory audits or investigations consistent with their contracts and applicable law. Audits are performed to ensure compliance with the established reimbursement requirements. A provider may be selected for an audit for a variety of reasons including questionable billing practices, a complaint lodged with a referral or enforcement agency, or it could result from random selection.

There are two types of audits: internal audits and external audits. **Internal audits** are considered to be prospective reviews because they are performed before a claim is submitted for payment. **External audits** are considered to be retrospective reviews because they are performed after a claim has been submitted for payment and after the claim has been processed by the insurance carrier.

Once the external auditor completes their audit, they will perform an audit exit with the medical biller or the person overseeing the audit. In addition, the external auditor will issue an audit report to the provider detailing their findings. Penalties for noncompliance with regulations and guideline include:

- Recoupment of funds.
- Reporting to a regulatory agency or relevant law enforcement agency.
- Terminating or suspending the provider's participation or contract.
- Suspending claims for special review.
- Imposing certain corrective actions.
- Suspending payment for a specified period of time.

Medical Ethics

Ethics is defined as the rules or standards governing the conduct of members of a profession. In general, medical ethics defines a right and proper way of treating patients.

The American Medical Association has created a set of standards that all physicians are expected to uphold. These standards include the following:

- Providing competent service with compassion and respect for patients.

Practice

Pitfalls

Examples of abusive billing include:

- Repeatedly submitting duplicate claims for the same service provided to the same member on the same date.
- Billing for services that were not provided.
- Repeatedly billing services at a different level or intensity than that actually provided.
- Repeatedly billing for medically unnecessary services.
- Repeatedly using diagnosis codes that are not consistent with medical records.
- Repeatedly billing certain procedure codes when a global code is more appropriate.
- Repeatedly billing certain procedure codes in addition to a global code that reflects those procedures.
- Billing for services provided by an individual who is not licensed to provide the service.
- Repeatedly failing to follow applicable Medicare and standard industry billing guidelines.
- Submitting false or fraudulent information.

- Dealing honestly with people.
- Being a law-abiding citizen but also working to change those laws that may not be in the best interests of the patient.
- Respecting the rights of others.
- Continuing to study and upgrade skills with the latest in medical advancement.
- Providing emergency medical treatment to anyone who is in need.
- Working to improve the community.

Although the medical biller has not sworn an oath to uphold these principles, he or she should realize that the physician for whom he or she works upholds this oath. As an adjunct to the physician, the medical biller also should do his or her best to uphold these standards and to assist the physician in doing so.

Among other things, ethics guidelines include:

1. Not making critical remarks about your physician, another physician, or any treatment given or not given.

2. If you discover that a patient is being treated by more than one physician for the same ailment, notify your physician immediately. It is not only unethical for two physicians to treat a patient for the same condition, but also it can be potentially dangerous. Prescription overdose or complications between treatment plans could result if one physician is unaware of treatment given by another physician.

3. Respecting the dignity of others. This includes calling patients and co-workers by their appropriate title and last name (i.e., Dr. Smith, Mrs. Hall), not using slang terms in reference to someone (i.e., honey, dear, sweetie); making no references to race, religion, creed, color, sex, or ethnic origin unless it is medically necessary for the treatment of the patient; and refraining from touching a patient or co-worker unless it is medically necessary.

4. Refusing to participate in illegal or unethical acts or to conceal the illegal or unethical acts of others.

Subpoenas

Occasionally, the medical records of a patient may be needed in a court action. In such cases a subpoena is issued requesting the records. A **subpoena** is a court order demanding a person to appear at a certain time and place. A **subpoena duces tecum** or a subpoena for production of evidence requires the person to produce books, records, papers, or other tangible evidence.

One person in the office should be designated in charge of medical records. This person should be the only person to accept a subpoena of medical records. If you are designated to be that person, the subpoena must be served in person. It cannot be laid on a desk or sent through the mail. No one else should accept the subpoena in your absence.

A witness fee or mileage amount may be provided to the witness. You should request any fees payable at the time the subpoena is served.

If the subpoena is only for the records (i.e., not for the recordkeeper as a witness as well), you should call the attorney who sent the subpoena and ask if the records can be sent. If so, send the records by certified mail, return receipt requested.

You will usually be given a specified amount of time to produce the records. Occasionally, the records will need to be turned over at the time of the subpoena. In all cases, consult with the physician before turning over the records. If the physician is unavailable, let the server know that you are unable to turn over the records without proper authorization and let them know when they can come back and serve the subpoena directly on the physician. This will give you time to be sure that the records are complete, accurate, and in good order. Also be sure that all signatures are identifiable and make copies.

In most cases, the original record must be sent. Always keep a copy of all records sent. This allows you to check for changes in the records and protects against loss of information if the records are lost. Number the pages before copying so that you can determine if any pages are missing.

If there is more than one physician in your office, be sure that the subpoena is served on the recordkeeper for that physician or to that physician directly.

If you are unable to accept the subpoena and no one is present who is authorized to accept it, explain the situation to the person serving the subpoena. Suggest a time when they can come back or ask them to contact the doctor's attorney. Then inform the doctor or their attorney of the situation.

Once a subpoena has been served, ask the doctor to check over the medical records to be sure that they are accurate and complete, then number the pages and make a complete copy. The original file should then be sent out immediately (if delivery by certified mail is allowed) or placed under lock and key to avoid tampering. Find out the day of the trial and comply with all orders given by the court. Be sure not to allow anyone to see the records or tamper with them. The records should be turned over to the appropriate party. Be sure to obtain documentation indicating that you delivered the records.

Subpoena Notification

If a subpoena is served to request medical records, many offices will notify the patient in writing that the records have been requested. This allows the patient's attorney to file papers with the court to block the subpoena.

If there is very little time between the date that the subpoena was served and the date that the records have been requested, the letter may be faxed or the patient may be contacted by telephone. In either case, be sure to let the patient know that they do not have the authority to stop you from releasing the records. They must have their attorney file a motion with the court in order to have the subpoena rescinded. A sample of a subpoena notification can be seen in **Figure 1–1**.

Paul Provider, M.D.
5858 Peppermint Place
Anytown, USA 12345
(765) 555-6768

PATIENT NOTIFICATION OF SUBPOENA

Date:
To:
Address: _____

Dear Ms. Patient and Attorney:

Please note that records pertaining to you are being sought by _____; as shown in the subpoena attached to this Notice.

If you object to us furnishing any part of the records described in this action, you must file papers with the court prior to our release of these records. This subpoena requires that we furnish the records on or by _____ (date).

You or your attorney of record may contact the attorney for the party seeking to examine such records and determine whether they are willing to agree to cancel or limit this subpoena. If no such agreement is reached and you are not already represented by an attorney in this action, **you should consult an attorney to advise you of your rights in this matter.**

If we do not have notification in writing regarding the cancellation or limitation of this subpoena at least 24 hours prior to the above date, we will assume you have no objection to us releasing this information.

Signed: _____   Date: _____

■ **Figure 1–1** Subpoena Notification

Instances in Which the Patient Should Be Notified and the File Notated

The following sections include situations that may warrant the sending of a letter to the patient. In each case, the letters are samples and should be modified to fit the individual circumstances.

A copy of the letter should always be placed in the patient's file. The physician may choose to have the patient sign this letter and return it, which serves to acknowledge receipt of the letter and the information it contains. This is a further step to protect the physician against a lawsuit.

If a signature is requested, two copies of the letter should be sent to the patient and a third copy placed in the file. The patient should keep one of the copies, and sign the other and return it. If a letter is not returned with a signature within two weeks of having been mailed, call the patient and discuss the situation with them, then document the phone conversation in the patient's medical file.

Patient Who Fails to Keep an Appointment

If a patient fails to keep an appointment when their condition is serious or needs constant monitoring, a letter should be sent advising the patient of the need for treatment or monitoring **(Figure 1–2)**. The patient may not realize the seriousness of his or her condition, and he or she may hold the doctor liable for this lack of knowledge if consequences arise as a result of lack of treatment.

Patient Left Facility Against Medical Advice

Occasionally, a patient will leave the hospital against medical advice, or will refuse to follow the advice given by the doctor. In such cases, the medical practice needs to be protected against lawsuits resulting from the lack of proper treatment.

In the case of a patient who leaves a treatment facility against the advice of their doctor, the facility often will ask the patient to sign a form stating that

---

Paul Provider, M.D.
5858 Peppermint Place
Anytown, USA 12345
(765) 555-6768

Date:
Dear. Mr./Ms. Patient:

An appointment was scheduled for you on (date) _____ at _____ a.m./p.m. which you failed to keep. Please be advised that I consider your condition to be serious and in need of further medical treatment and/or monitoring.

Please contact my office for another appointment as soon as possible. If you choose to be treated by another physician, I urge you to seek an appointment with him or her without delay. With your authorization, I would be happy to share any test results or medical records with such a physician.

Two copies of this letter are enclosed. One is for your files. Please sign the second copy and return it to our office in the enclosed envelope.

Please understand my purpose in writing this letter is concern for your overall medical health.

Sincerely,

Paul Provider, M.D.

Patient Signature: _____ Date: _____

■ **Figure 1–2** Failed Appointment Letter

PAUL PROVIDER PATIENT TREATMENT CENTER

STATEMENT OF PATIENT LEAVING AGAINST MEDICAL ADVICE

Date:

    This letter is to certify that I, _____(patient name), am leaving the above-named facility at my own insistence and against the advice of my attending physician and other treatment facility authorities. I understand the dangers of my leaving at this time. This letter hereby releases the facility, its employees and officers and any attending physicians from any and all liability which may be caused as a result of my departure.

    This letter may also be construed as an agreement to hold harmless the above facility, its employees and officers and any attending physicians from any and all liability which may be caused as a result of my departure.

Patient Signature: _____   Date: _____

Parent/Guardian Signature: _____   Date: _____

Witness: _____   Date: _____

Witness: _____   Date: _____

    If the patient refuses to sign this form, place an X in the space at left, fill out the form, and have it signed by two treatment center personnel. The words SIGNATURE REFUSED should be placed on the line reserved for the patient signature.

■ **Figure 1–3** Statement of Patient Leaving Against Medical Advice

they are leaving even though they understand the doctor advises against it. A patient cannot be restrained from leaving or forced to sign the waiver. If the patient refuses to sign the waiver, a notation should be made on the form of the refusal to sign and the form should then be signed and dated by two witnesses.

    Most facilities have a standard form to use for this purpose. A copy of a form can be seen in **Figure 1–3**.

Refusal to Follow Treatment

There are some patients who refuse to follow the advice of their physician. This can range from a decision not to give up smoking for improving overall health to a patient refusing to take the prescribed medication that could save their life.

    In all cases, the practice should be protected as much as possible by having the patient sign a letter **(Figure 1–4)**. The letter should state the condition of the patient, the medical advice, and the possible consequences of not following the advice. Having a signed

copy of this letter in the patient's file helps to protect against a lawsuit in which the patient states they were not informed of the consequences of not following the medical advice.

Termination of Treatment

It sometimes becomes necessary for a patient to terminate their care with a physician. This most often happens at the request of the patient and is often a result of circumstances beyond their control (e.g., relocation).

    To protect the practice, it is best to ask the patient to complete a letter of termination of care **(Figure 1–5)**.

When a Physician Terminates Care

Occasionally, a physician will feel the need to terminate the care of a patient when the patient continually refuses to follow medical advice. Termination of treatment should occur only after the patient has been fully advised of the consequences of not following the prescribed medical advice **(Figure 1–6)**.

Paul Provider, M.D.
5858 Peppermint Place
Anytown, USA 12345
(765) 555-6768

Date:

Dear Mr./Ms. Patient:

Two weeks ago you were diagnosed with hypertension (high blood pressure). At that time I prescribed a dosage of 500 mg of Diuril (Chlorothiazide) to be taken twice daily. It has come to our attention that you are not taking your medication as prescribed. I strongly urge you to take your medication as prescribed and return to my office for another checkup in two weeks to monitor your condition. If you choose to seek care from another physician, we will be happy to provide him or her with any test results or records.

Please understand that not taking your medication can result in severe damage to your kidneys, heart, circulatory system and other organs. Not getting your hypertension under control can lead to a heart attack, stroke or even death.

Please sign the bottom of this letter and return it in the enclosed envelope to attest that you have read it and are aware of the consequences that may result from not following the medical advice given to you.

Sincerely,

Paul Provider, M.D.

Patient Signature: _____ Date: _____

Figure 1–4 Refusal to Follow Treatment Letter

Paul Provider, M.D.
5858 Peppermint Place
Anytown, USA 12345
(765) 555-6768

LETTER CONFIRMING TERMINATION OF TREATMENT

Date:

Dear Mr. /Ms. Patient:

This letter is to confirm our understanding that as of _____(date) you wish to discharge Donald Doctor, M.D. as your physician. We will be sorry to see you go.

Please know that we have enjoyed the opportunity to serve you and will be happy to provide your medical records, with your authorization, to any new physician you choose.

Please sign the bottom of this letter to confirm termination of treatment and return it to our office in the enclosed envelope.

Thank you very much.

Sincerely,

Paul Provider, M.D.

I hereby acknowledge receipt of this letter and agree to termination of treatment on the above date.

Patient Signature: _____ Date: _____

Figure 1–5 Letter Confirming Termination of Treatment

Paul Provider, M.D.
5858 Peppermint Place
Anytown, USA 12345
(765) 555-6768

Date:

Dear Mr. /Ms. Patient:

I find it necessary to terminate any further care of your case due to your repeated refusal to follow medical advice. It is my opinion that your condition requires further treatment or serious consequences may develop. I strongly urge you to seek the care of another physician immediately.

I would be happy to provide, upon your authorization, any test results or medical records needed by the new physician.

If you desire, I shall continue to provide your medical care for the next _____ days, until _____. This should give you ample time to secure the services of a new physician.

Please sign one copy of this letter and return it to our office to acknowledge that you have read and understand this information. The second copy is for your records.

Sincerely,

Paul Provider, M.D.

Patient Signature: _____ Date: _____

■ **Figure 1–6** Physician Terminating Care Letter

CHAPTER REVIEW

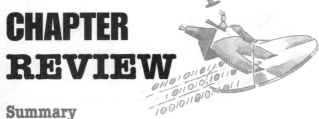

Summary

- Some of the job responsibilities of the medical biller include billing insurance carriers, billing patients, performing basic office accounting, handling collections, scheduling appointments, and handling charts.

- Although stress is a part of everyday life, it is important to deal with stress appropriately.

- The medical biller should be aware of the appropriate legal and ethical issues. These include being aware of the most common causes of fraud as well as understanding HIPAA guidelines.

- Instances or situations in which the patient should be notified and the patient's chart notated include when a patient fails to keep appointments; when a patient leaves a medical facility against medical advice; and when a patient refuses to follow medical advice.

Assignments

Complete the Questions for Review.
Complete Exercises 1–1 through 1–3.

Questions for Review

Directions: Answer the following questions without looking back at the material covered in this chapter. Write your answers in the space provided.

1. List three job responsibilities of the medical biller.

    1. _____ P. 4 _____

    2. _____

    3. _____

2. List six symptoms of stress. ___ P. 8 _____

    _____

    _____

3. List five stress relievers.

    1. _____ P. 8 _____

    2. _____

    3. _____

    4. _____

    5. _____

4. List six types of healthcare settings.

    1. _____ P 5 _____

    2. _____

    3. _____

    4. _____

    5. _____

    6. _____

5. (True or False?) Do not compromise when you have a disagreement with a co-worker, as it only proves that you are wrong and makes you look bad. ___ False _____

6. List the four things to consider before taking a vacation.

   1. _____ *P. 9* _____

   2. _____

   3. _____

   4. _____

7. Discuss two main issues of HIPAA.

   1. _____ *P. 11* _____

   _____

   2. _____

   _____

8. List the most common causes of fraud. _____ *P. 13* _____

   _____

   _____

9. (True or False?) The diagnosis or disclosure of an illness should never be made to the patient, even if he or she asks for this information. _____ *F* _____

10. Name three instances in which the patient should be notified and a notation made in the patient's chart.

   1. _____ *P. 19* _____

   2. _____

   3. _____

   If you are unable to answer any of these questions, refer back to that section in the chapter, and then fill in the answers.

Exercise 1-1

Directions: Find and circle the words listed below. Words can appear horizontally, vertically, diagonally, forward, or backward.

```
J C Y X J A J F R P N I C H Y Z U Q R N W M B U E I M Z O T
X U C K H Y Z Z I X D O M U P H I N S A Y L Y P S W Q A L C
D C L P K H F M J S D F Z P L O J S Q R D H V V Z B O U V P
X Z R Y Q S B J T K W L I O A K K O S U J V T C I N H A B X
Q U W O A J N Z N W I Z Q T G M I Z Q K R W E P A K K C M L
C S T R A T E K T O X C L O U W A I I C Y S X X M W C J D U
V Y J O P S F E M Z M N L L H K X Y L M N U T U T V X W Q A
T F H K I W I Y S K S W T C H G N K W N G U E X V B N W X I
K F Y A H B H Z Q G V I U M J J W Y J Q X R R S X Z X X Y M
T R D X Z Q K U J T X U E M U E I F G F G R N N N B E K B A
X S T I Y Y L R B F W T C Q G Z M N V T X H A T R L G G B T
A A Y R R W B W V N C Y G W M P F K Y I Y R L V Z K H G Y A
D U H D P I I H H Y M A Z N B T S B T A B R A B Z A Q Z Z R
Q F T L M F G N V X L J F H X R P M Q P Q C U Z W R M D J L
M Q N H H M H D S Q C K B I Z U V I Z F V V D K F A Y D H J
H F W G Y O E P N I N Y R U W Z N L O H U H I H F T N O B T
E W P U H V T K K Y O W U Y I L O I E E S C T R T H T S O C
R Y E P M A X U W I V R P B T U Y I R C V O O Y Y I A N Q G
O I D D Z D C O Y V L L Y B F B L N Z H G A J Z A I Q S L S
Y R B J L A Y J V C D P C D L O F T L I D R R W Z Z K U Z S
F S M T Y I J D Z X Z L Q P U F M U M T H S S E R T S B O J
C O U N V I R T S E A C S G R N B Y Q L T L O Q P Y E W Z W
K K W X N Q A F K I S G R U K V D F B L W P H V U V T Z S A
P R F B F U M V M K V T N F X U U O V I N N S Y H U N P V O
G R B S I W R S V Q O E U I O M F F P N C Y R S K O I Q H L
R Z J Z V K A Q Z Q N W N L D J Z P G V Z R G P Q W E T T F
X L Z C Y U N H T L T V V K O N L W Y G T Z N Y R R M D W W
V N U I D E S T C C P J L O V D O Y T K K T B Q J D K L P K
Q U T I Z L G D Q E D G D J Q W D B Z F X B L J C Q K Q I J
E P T W L D Q E P Q I Q T W R T K G A P K U U J G B Y I E Z
```

1. Bonding

2. Claims Audit

3. External Audit

4. HIPAA

5. Job Stress

Exercise 1-2

Directions: Complete the crossword puzzle by filling in a word from the keywords that fits each clue.

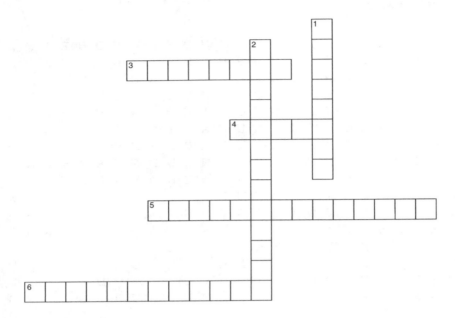

Across

3. A demand to appear at a certain time and place to give testimony on a certain matter.
4. Intentional misrepresentation of a fact with the intent to deprive a person of property or legal rights.
5. Someone hired by an insurance company or governmental organization, such as Medicare or Medicaid, to perform an audit.
6. The act of an employee illegally taking funds from a company for which they work.

Down

1. The person or entity that provides healthcare services. This can be a doctor, chiropractor, hospital, emergency facility, x-ray technician, or any certified professional who is licensed to provide healthcare services.
2. Considered a prospective review because it is performed before a claim is submitted for payment.

Exercise 1-3

Directions: Match the following terms with the proper definition by writing the letter of the correct definition in the space next to the term.

1. ___D___ Errors and Omissions Insurance

2. ___B___ Health Maintenance Organizations (HMOs)

3. ___A___ Respondeat Superior

4. ___C___ Subpoena Duces Tecum

a. An employer that is liable for harms caused by an employee while that employee is acting within the scope of their employment.

b. Organizations or companies that provide both the coverage for care and the care itself. Members pay a set amount every month and the organization or company agrees to provide all their care, or to pay for the covered care they cannot provide.

c. Requires the person to produce books, records, papers, or other tangible evidence.

d. This insurance covers damages caused by mistakes (errors) or damages caused by something an employee failed to do (omissions).

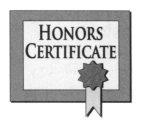

Honors Certification™

The certification challenge for this chapter will be a written test of the information contained in this chapter. Each incorrect answer will result in a deduction of up to 5% from your grade. You must achieve a score of 85% or higher to pass this test. If you fail the test on your first attempt, you may retake the test one additional time. The items included in the second test may be different from those in the first test.

2

Clinical Records and
Medical Documentation

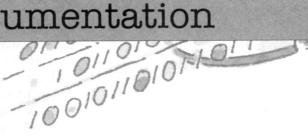

After completion of this chapter
you will be able to:

- Describe how a medical chart is organized.
- Describe how charts for pediatric and emergency patients are different from other medical charts.
- Demonstrate how to file x-rays in a chart.
- Properly file a patient chart.
- List the rules for medical documentation.
- Properly complete a signature card.
- Describe the use of a signature card.
- Explain why and for how long records should be retained.
- Describe the process for storing medical records.
- Describe features available with electronic medical charting.
- Discuss the pros and cons of computerized medical charting.
- Properly complete a records transfer request.
- Discuss the purpose of a Patient Information Sheet.
- Properly complete a Patient Information Sheet with information from a given situation.
- Discuss the purpose of the Authorization to Release Information and the Assignment of Benefits forms.
- Properly complete an Insurance Coverage Form with information from a given situation.
- List the guidelines for facilitating the gathering of information.

Keywords and Concepts
you will learn in this chapter:

- Alphabetical Filing
- Alter
- Assignment of Benefits Form
- Children's Chart
- Claim
- Correction Fluid
- Electronic Prescriptions

- Emancipation
- Encounter Forms
- Guarantor
- Insurance Coverage Form
- Maintaining Records
- Noncompliance
- Patient History Form

- Patient Information Sheet
- Pediatric Charts
- Release of Information Form
- Request for Additional Information Form
- Signature Card
- SOAP Notes

Keeping accurate patient charts is essential to the running of a good medical practice. Without accurate patient charts, the provider may find it difficult to treat the patient's condition properly. Additionally, it can be difficult to bill insurance companies or the patient for treatment that was performed.

Medical charts contain a number of forms. Some of these forms are needed at each visit. Other forms, such as those authorizing treatment, are completed once and merely stored in the patient's file.

Maintaining records means keeping the information in a record updated and filing the chart or record in a manner that makes it easy to locate if you should need it at a later date. In this chapter, we will cover the general practices in maintaining patient charts. The actual forms within a chart will also be covered in this chapter.

Medical Charts

In most medical offices, a separate chart is kept on each and every patient. Although this can often necessitate the repetition of some information, it is necessary to ensure compliance with HIPAA guidelines and to keep the information separate for each patient.

Medical billers often are responsible for creating new patient charts. This means completing or having the patient complete the initial forms and putting them in the charts in the proper order. If the patient has an insurance card or other proof of coverage, a photocopy of this information is included with these forms. Every page in the medical chart must have patient identification information contained on it.

Often the medical biller or receptionist is the first person who sees a new patient. At that time, they may ask the patient (or their parent or guardian in the case of a minor) to complete a number of forms. It helps to have the required forms already placed together on a clipboard so that the patient can complete them easily. These forms then need to be placed in the patient's chart in the proper order. If forms are not in the proper order, a lot of time may be spent searching for the right information.

There are many different types of forms used in the medical office, and the style of the forms varies from provider to provider. There also are a number of companies that create and produce medical forms. The actual creation of the chart will therefore differ from provider to provider.

Additionally, some providers will use a single-fold manila folder for charts, whereas others will use a multipage chart.

The easiest way to determine the order into which the medical office puts patient charts is to look at an existing chart. Below is an example of the types of forms and the order that a medical office might use with a multipage chart.

Page 1 of the Patient Chart:

- Acknowledgment of Receipt of Privacy Practices Notice
- Registration
- Medical History/Physicals

Page 2 of the Patient Chart:

- Examination/Treatment Forms
- Pathology/Laboratory/X-ray Reports
- Operative Reports
- Discharge Summaries

Page 3 of the Patient Chart:

- Billing Forms for Previous Visits

Page 4 of the Patient Chart:

- Consent Form
- Signature on File
- Financial Arrangements
- Correspondence Log
- Letters To/From Provider

Some charts contain a fifth page or a back pocket for other information.

During the course of treatment, the physician may add additional forms to the patient chart, such as a History and Physical Form, Progress Notes, or a Medication Flow Sheet for tracking prescribed medicine. If the patient is a child, a pediatric chart should be assembled.

After the patient has become established and has had several visits, lab and x-ray results and consultation reports may be submitted from other providers. These results should be reviewed by the physician or, in some offices, by a nurse. If reviewed by a nurse, abnormal lab, x-ray, or urgent results or requests will be forwarded directly to the physician for an immediate response. After review, these results should be stamped with the date and signed by the physician before they are filed in the patient chart.

Items should be grouped together (i.e., all pathology reports together, followed by all laboratory reports, etc.). They should then be in order by date, with the most recent one on top. A specific order allows the doctor to find the data he needs quickly and easily.

Items should be placed in the patient's file as soon as they are received from the doctor. If a report comes in from an outside entity (i.e., results of tests from an outside lab), the report should be given to the doctor immediately with the patient's file. The doctor should initial the report to indicate that he has looked at it before the report is placed in the file. Reports should not be placed in a medical record without first being initialed by the provider.

To facilitate finding the forms within the charts quickly and easily, many companies create forms of different lengths. Additionally, the name of the form is printed on the bottom. This allows you to see the bottom of each form, and the name of the form, when the forms are properly stacked in the medical chart.

Some of the charts also may be duplicated on each side. This allows the provider to use the same form for multiple visits without creating excess paper in the chart. Once one side of the form has been completed, the form can be turned over and additional information can be placed on the reverse side.

If you are preparing a chart for a patient's visit, be sure that the provider has space on the necessary forms for recording their examination, treatment plan, and progress notes. If necessary, add additional forms to the chart. Most medical offices add additional forms on top of the existing forms rather than underneath them. This places the most current information on the top where it can be found easily.

Under no circumstances should you remove the old information from a chart, no matter how full the chart has become. Medical treatment plans can extend over a length of time. At any point in the treatment plan, the provider may need to refer back to the initial examination or treatment plan to understand the patient's situation fully.

Pediatric Charts

Some medical offices use a different type of chart for children. These are called **children's charts** or **pediatric charts**. Pediatric charts may have additional or different forms. For example, a Children's Medical History form would eliminate information that is not appropriate for children, such as pregnancy history.

Pediatric charts also require additional forms, such as an Immunization Record, to track immunizations and forms for hearing and vision exams. These records often are needed by a parent before they are allowed to enroll their child in a public school.

Some medical offices also may use restraints on young children to prevent them from moving and causing themselves injury during medical treatment. The use of these restraints must be authorized by a parent or guardian.

Emergency Patients

Medical offices may see patients on a one-time, emergency basis. These may be people from out of town who have a medical emergency or patients who need a procedure done and are unable or unwilling to see their normal provider for treatment. They may also be a patient seeking a second opinion on the treatment plan suggested by their normal provider.

Many medical offices have a separate chart for these patients. Because these patients will not be receiving extended treatment, many of the documents in a normal chart such as callback and telephone records will not be needed. However, even these patients need to give the provider information regarding their medical history.

The forms that are normally included in an emergency patient record include:

- Registration.
- Medical History.
- Doctor's Notes (or Treatment Plan).
- Release and Consent Forms.

Because there are far fewer forms for emergency or one-time patients, many medical offices will use a simple manila folder for these patients rather than a multipage chart.

Radiology

Many offices also take radiological films (x-rays) of patients. Because x-rays often are the same size as the body part being x-rayed, they can be rather large. Because of this, x-rays are often stored separately from the patient files.

X-rays are often placed in a large envelope and labeled with the name of the patient, the date that the x-ray was taken, and the specific body part shown on the x-ray (i.e., right wrist). Many offices also label the x-ray itself with this information. Additionally, many medical offices include a birth date, an account number, or other identifying number to ensure that the x-rays for two people with similar names are not mixed up.

Once the x-ray has been properly labeled, be sure to add the information to the patient chart. By documenting all the x-rays that have been taken in the patient chart, a provider can easily see if there was an earlier x-ray taken of a body part that he is treating. This can help to show changes in the patient or in their condition or disease.

X-rays often are kept in a back office and are filed alphabetically by the last name of the patient. It is important to remember not to place other items in the same pocket with the medical x-rays, as these items may scratch the x-ray.

Some providers also take pictures of a patient to document conditions or situations. These pictures may be needed to verify the need for treatment to an insurance carrier or for explanations provided to the patient. These pictures should be labeled and treated in the same manner as the x-rays. However, some medical offices will file pictures directly in the patient chart, as they often are small enough to fit in the chart.

Practice
Pitfalls

If you are writing on the envelope, write on it before placing the x-ray inside. This will prevent damage to the x-ray from pressing too hard on it.

Over time, labels placed on x-rays or charts may lose their adhesion and become loose. If you notice any labels beginning to peel away from an x-ray or chart, they should be reaffixed as soon as possible, or new labels applied.

To make labeling easier, some medical offices use x-ray film that has a white covering in one corner for labeling the x-ray. This is put on by the manufacturer and usually solves the problem of missing labels.

Filing the Chart

Once the chart has been completed, it will need to be filed so that it can be easily located. Medical offices are run in many different ways, and because of this there are several different filing methods. It will take time to determine which filing system is right for your situation.

Because of HIPAA regulations, the name of the patient should not appear on the outside of the chart. This is especially true if the charts are kept in a place that is visible to other patients or to anyone entering the office. If at all possible, all patient charts should be placed in a locked room that is inaccessible to anyone who is not authorized to enter. If this is not possible, charts should only contain information that is considered to be nonpersonal on the outside. Thus, charts should be identified with a number rather than with the patient's name. Some medical offices will use an account number that is alphanumeric (a combination of numbers and letters). In such cases, care must be taken to preserve the patient's identity. The letters used should not be those that could indicate the patient's name.

A numeric or alphanumeric filing system often will necessitate having a master list with the patients' names in alphabetical order. This will allow you to quickly and easily find the correct patient chart.

When creating a new chart for a patient, be sure to label the chart as soon as it is put together. If the practice uses a numeric or alphanumeric filing system, the chart information should be added to the master list immediately.

Many times, a master list is computerized. Even when the list is on the computer, a printed list always should be kept available. This will allow you to access patient charts when the computer is down or in use by another person.

Adding a file to a computerized master list can be quick and easy. If the master list is not computerized, or if you are unable to add the information to the master list immediately, you can write the information on the printed master list.

Alphabetical Filing

If a practice keeps its charts in an area that is not accessible or viewable by unauthorized personnel, then an alphabetical filing system may be used. **Alphabetical filing** simply means filing the charts alphabetically by the first letter of the patient's last name.

Many medical offices use color coded tabs for alphabetical filing. Depending on the number of patients or files, the color coding may be broken down into the first letter of the last name, or the first two letters of the last name.

Many medical supply companies sell labels with letters in a multitude of colors. It is not uncommon to have nine or 10 colors used, for example: A is red, B is orange, C is yellow, D is green, and so on.

By placing the proper label or labels on the outside of the chart, you can easily see any charts that are out of order. Additionally, it is much easier to find a chart because you have only a few to look through rather than a large number of them.

Each practice will have a specific area for the letter to be placed on the outside of the chart. Keeping the letters in the proper area also will help you to spot charts that may be out of order.

Medical Documentation Rules

Regardless of the type of medical practitioner you work for, there are some important factors to include when documenting in a medical chart.

A patient's chart often will include notations from three or more different people within the medical office:

- Medical biller/receptionist.
- Medical assistant (or nurse in a hospital).
- Medical provider (physician, surgeon, anesthesiologist, etc.).

There is much more litigation in the world today. Because of this, everyone who touches a medical chart needs to think about what they are writing in the chart before a lawsuit is filed.

The following rules are important to remember when performing medical charting:

Document only in your area of responsibility. You are not the provider or medical assistant. Therefore, your notations on the chart should be limited to those areas that are your responsibility for the patient. This can include appointment setting, follow-up phone calls, and encounters in the reception area. Under no circumstances should you make any notations regarding the patient's treatment, even when asked to do so by the provider.

Never use correction fluid on a chart or obscure any writing. Correction fluid, "Wite-Out" or any liquid that covers over the writing on paper should never be used. If you make a mistake, draw a single line through the error in such a way that the original entry can still be read. Then write the correction directly next to the crossed out entry and initial it. If a malpractice lawsuit is ever filed, correction fluid will make people wonder what was removed. By drawing a single line through the entry, there is no question about what was there before.

Use standard abbreviations and terms. Each office should have a set of standard abbreviations and terms to be used in medical documentation. Using different abbreviations and terms can cause confusion in the records. These confusions can be detrimental to the treatment of a patient, or can lead to confusion during a lawsuit, which may mean a higher damage award. A chart of standard abbreviations and terms should be available to all office staff.

Do not write in the margins. If most material written in the chart falls within the margins, but one sentence is outside the margins, it can appear as though that sentence was added at a later time and inserted into the available space. If you run out of room, write on the next line. If there is no next line, use an additional form and continue writing on it. Paying for an additional form is much less costly than having a lawyer argue that the material was on the chart from the beginning.

Never alter the information on a chart. To **alter** means to change or amend (add to) the information contained in a record or chart. If there is information in a chart that has changed or needs to be corrected, the information should be documented on the next available line, with the date of documentation.

Never write information in a patient chart that you do not want them to see. Patient charts legally belong to both the patient and the provider. However, the provider is considered to be the legal custodian of the records. Thus, a patient is allowed to see their records any time they wish to do so. However, they may not remove the records from the provider's office.

Document anything the patient says with quotation marks. Juries tend to believe that anything that is put in quotation marks was a direct quote. This can work to the provider's advantage if the patient had originally said something good; then later sues. This is especially true when you are listing the details of a follow-up phone call. Because there is no face to face contact in which observations can be made, words can carry a greater impact.

Take the time to document noncompliance. Noncompliance means not following the instructions given by the provider. If the provider has suggested that the patient perform a certain action (i.e., physical therapy exercises twice a day, etc.), ask if the patient is performing such actions during a follow-up call. If the patient indicates that they are not doing so, make sure that this is recorded in the chart. This will protect the provider in case the patient sues. Juries will wonder if the patient's outcome would have been different if the patient had followed the provider's advice.

Be specific when documenting. The more specific you can be in a reasonable period of time, the better. For example, instead of saying "Patient was referred to a specialist," include the name, title, and address of the specialist and for what the patient was referred. This person may be able to testify for the provider if the patient never followed up on the referral.

If you see something in the chart that could be a potential problem, bring it to the attention of the provider. The provider is ultimately responsible for the information contained in a patient chart. Although the provider should not alter the record, they can add additional information that can help counter something that should not have been said.

Document in ink. Many states require that information contained in the patient chart be documented in ink. Pencil is not acceptable. If you have difficulty expressing yourself without reworking the wording, write the information on a piece of scratch paper first, then write it into the patient's chart.

Be sure that any change to a patient's appointment is documented. If the patient calls and says that they will be late, be sure it is noted on the patient's chart. If the patient calls to cancel or reschedule the appointment, be sure it is notated. If the patient later sues the provider, you can show documentation that the patient repeatedly changed or canceled appointments. The argument can then be made that the patient's condition could have been better taken care of if they had sought treatment for the problem earlier. Documenting changes to an appointment also can fend off accusations of sloppy documentation if the patient chart no longer matches the appointment book. For example, if the patient postponed an appointment for a week, the chart may have one date and the appointment book a different date.

When documenting an appointment, include the reason for the appointment. If the patient indicates that they are having a problem, this should be notated on both the appointment calendar and the patient's chart. This not only helps the provider know what to look for but also helps to protect the provider if the patient then cancels an appointment. The provider

will have a better understanding of how urgently the patient may need care.

Make detailed notes of follow-up calls. If the proper follow-up call is not performed, the provider may be considered guilty of "patient abandonment." This can carry a high price tag in the event of a lawsuit. Many providers have the medical biller or receptionist make follow-up calls. This is completely legal. However, if the procedure was extraordinarily difficult or the results were not those anticipated, it might be better if the provider herself made the follow-up call. This will show more concern for the patient.

Update the patient's medical history at each visit. This is not as complicated as it might sound. Simply asking the patient if there have been any changes to their medical history or to their drug/medication use is sufficient. If the patient indicates that there has been no change, note the date on the chart and "No Change in Medical History" (sometimes abbreviated as NCMH).

SOAP Notes

Many medical offices use the SOAP note format to standardize medical evaluation entries made in clinical records. **SOAP** stands for Subjective, Objective, Assessment, and Plan. Medical documentation of patient complaint(s) and treatment must be consistent, concise, and comprehensive. SOAP notes should be documented in such a way as to know everything there is to know about the current status of the patient. The four parts of a SOAP note are:

1. The first part of the format is the Subjective portion of the SOAP note, which consists of subjective observations. These are symptoms that the patient or the patient's representative verbally expresses. These subjective observations include the patient's descriptions of pain or discomfort, the presence of nausea or dizziness, and a multitude of other descriptions of dysfunction, discomfort, or illness.
2. The next part of the format is the Objective observation. These objective observations include symptoms that the medical provider actually can see, hear, touch, feel, or smell. Included in objective observations are measurements such as temperature, pulse, respiration, skin color, swelling, and the results of tests.
3. Assessment follows the objective observations. Assessment is the diagnosis of the patient's

condition. In some cases, the diagnosis may be clear; however, in other cases, an assessment may not be clear and could include several diagnosis possibilities.

4. The last part of the SOAP note is the Plan. The plan may include laboratory tests, x-rays, or medications ordered for the patient; treatments performed; patient referrals; patient disposition, such as being sent home or to the hospital; patient directions for care; and any follow-up directions.

Signature Cards

It is important that all pertinent data regarding a patient's condition and treatment be added to the medical record. This record not only helps the doctor to track the patient's progress and determine what treatment is best but also helps to verify the services that were done and the need for those services.

Because of the importance of maintaining proper records, only certain authorized persons should ever be allowed to make notations or changes to a patient's medical records. Each change or notation should be initialed or signed and dated. If reports or other data are received from outside entities (i.e., a lab report from an outside lab), the report should be presented to the doctor along with the patient's chart. The doctor should then initial the report, indicating that he has seen it before it is placed in the patient's medical record.

The appropriate people will be different for each office, and for the jobs within an office. For example, a biller may be allowed to make changes to a patient's insurance information or account but not to any of their medical data. The best way to track those authorized to make notations or changes is by use of signature cards.

A **signature card** shows the person authorized to make changes, the dates they are authorized for, and the scope of the changes they are allowed to make (**see Figure 2–1**). These cards should be kept in the billing office.

If a change is to be made to a person's authority or scope of the records they may change, an ending date should be placed in the "Authorized date . . . to:" space. A new signature card should be completed with the new data. The old signature card should be kept on file. Then, if an auditor or other person is looking through older medical records and needs to know whose signature was signed on a certain date with the authority, the old signature card can be pulled.

Some medical offices choose to have a signature log on file. A signature log contains the information from several signature cards on a single sheet of paper. The disadvantage of signature logs is that some data on a signature log can be outdated, whereas other data is still current. Because several people are listed on a single paper, if one person leaves the practice, then their name is no longer valid but the other signatures still are. Such a system makes it much more difficult to track authority. You may need to go through any number of signature logs to find the signature that you are looking for.

Signature cards have the advantage of allowing each authorized person to be listed on a separate card. This can be neater in an office that has a high turnover rate or in which the job status and authority for notations often changes. The current cards are kept in a card file in front of a divider in alphabetical order by last name. The outdated cards are kept behind the divider in alphabetical order.

If an authorized person's initials are different than their full name (i.e., full name Charles Smith-Lyton, M.D., but they go by Charles Lyton and sign their initials CL, MD), then a notation should be placed under the letter "S" and the card placed under the letter "L." This allows you to find the card quickly and easily.

Retention of Records

Storing medical charts can become a huge undertaking for a medical practice, especially if it is large and has been in operation for a number of years. However, it is important to maintain patients' medical charts for an extended period of time.

All records should be kept as long as they are needed. However, because many conditions are linked to previous episodes of care, records may be needed on patients long after they have been treated for a condition. For example:

1. Pediatric records may be needed for a 30-year-old pregnant woman to determine if she had measles as a child.

2. Scarlet fever in a young child can cause damage to the heart that may not show up until the patient is 50 or 60 years old.

3. Hereditary links are being found in numerous conditions, providing a need for the doctors of children and even grandchildren to see the medical records of a patient.

For these reasons, many medical offices put their medical records on microfiche, microfilm, or computer files, and keep them indefinitely.

Paul Provider, M.D.
5858 Peppermint Place
Anytown, USA 12345
(765) 555-6768

SIGNATURE CARD   Date Created _____

A copy of this card shall be maintained on file at all times and updated as needed. The following person
is authorized to make notations and/or changes to the patient medical records as indicated.

Name _____ Title _____

Authorized From _____ to _____

Signature: _____ Initials: Printed _____ Signed _____

Scope of authorization (i.e., all records and files, insurance data only, etc.) _____

_____

_____

■ **Figure 2–1** Signature Card

The laws vary from state to state; however, many states require medical offices to keep records for several years after the patient has died. This essentially can mean keeping medical records forever, especially if the practice treats a number of young patients.

One of the main reasons for keeping records so long is the way the laws are written. Many states allow patients to sue a provider five or even 10 years after the patient discovers a problem. If they do not discover a problem until 30 years after treatment has ended, they still have the right to sue for five more years. In effect, you cannot be certain that a patient will not sue, and that the records will not be needed, until five to 10 years after the patient is dead.

This means that there is a tremendous amount of paperwork that a medical office must maintain. To make it easier, records of patients who are no longer seen by the medical office will often be placed in storage.

Additionally, federal regulations mandate that records on Medicare and Medicaid patients be retained for at least seven years after treatment. At any time during this seven-year period, the medical practice can be audited and must provide substantiation for their charges and receipts.

For tax purposes, records should be kept for at least four years after the tax return is filed.

Practice Pitfalls

It is better to err on the side of keeping files a little longer than sending them to the shredder as soon as the time limit expires. As luck would have it, you will not need information from the file until after it is shredded.

Storing Medical Records

When storing medical records, it is important to keep them in a manageable order in order to locate the records if you should need them at a later date. This often means creating lists of the items that are included in the storage boxes and properly labeling these boxes.

Many companies use numerical or alphabetical labels on their boxes. For example, the labeling on a box might be shown as "Medical Charts, 2000, A–K." This could mean that charts for all patients who terminated care in the year 2000 whose last names began with A–K would be found in this box. However, a master list would still be needed to easily find a chart, as it may be difficult to determine in which year a patient terminated treatment.

Box: Medical Charts 1999, A–L	
Adams, Sean	10/01/68
Adams, Sydney	12/14/70
Adams, Thomas	06/05/56
Adamson, Kirk	05/10/63
Alexander, Betty	08/21/35
Alexander, Karen	11/03/60

■ **Figure 2–2** Sample Master List for Box Contents

Labeling boxes with clearly defined content indicators can allow them to be stored in a logical sequence. This makes these boxes, and the files that they contain, much easier to locate.

Because many patients may have the same or similar names, it is important to create a master list that will give you the detail you need to locate the correct medical chart. This is often done by listing the name of the box at the top of the master list page (**see Figure 2–2**). The medical charts included in that box are then listed in alphabetical order by the patient's last name. Another piece of identifying information also can be included, such as the patient's birth date.

If the medical office has been around for a while, there may be a large number of boxes in storage (**see Figure 2–3**). In this case, listing the contents in each box may not be practical. These medical offices often will create a single list of all charts that are in storage. This list includes the name of the patient on the chart, the identifying information (i.e., birth date or account number), and the name of the box in which the chart can be found.

Many medical providers use a storage service to help with file management and storage. The medical provider's files will be placed in specified storage

boxes and placed in a specific location at the storage company. The storage company will usually pick up the boxes to be stored and take them to the facility and place them in the designated location.

Electronic Medical Charting

More and more computer programs are including electronic medical charting. Previous computer programs used by the medical office were often limited to billing software. Those that were considered "high-tech" may have included the opportunity to submit the claims electronically rather than just print them on paper and mail them to the insurance carrier.

However, new software programs include a much wider variety of features. Following are some of the most common features, as well as information about how these features could impact the job of the medical biller.

Patient Identification. In addition to the standard patient information included in software programs (i.e., name, address, employer, and insurance information, etc.), many new programs include the addition of a patient photograph. This photo allows the medical staff to ensure they are working on the proper patient before services are rendered. It has the added benefit of

Patient Name	Birth Date	Box
Adams, Amy	03/15/48	Med Charts 2000 A–L
Adams, Sean	10/01/68	Med Charts 1999 A–L
Adams, Sydney	12/14/70	Med Charts 1999 A–L
Adams, Thomas	06/05/56	Med Charts 1999 A–L
Adamson, Kirk	05/10/63	Med Charts 2001 A–L
Alexander, Betty	08/21/35	Med Charts 1999 A–L
Alexander, Karen	11/03/60	Med Charts 1999 A–L

■ **Figure 2–3** Sample Master Storage List for Practice

decreasing fraud caused by one person seeking treatment under a different person's Medicaid or insurance coverage. Additionally, it can increase customer satisfaction as medical staff will be able to recognize more patients.

If this type of software is used in the medical office, it will often fall to the medical biller or the receptionist to take a quick snapshot of the patient and download it into the computer program. Additionally, the patient's information will need to be added into the program.

Prescription Control. Some software programs allow the creation of electronic prescriptions. **Electronic prescriptions** are prescriptions that are entered into the provider's computer, and then electronically sent to the computer at the patient's pharmacy.

There are many advantages of electronic prescriptions over paper prescriptions. These include:

- Prescriptions can be sent immediately, without the patient having to carry a paper prescription to the pharmacist.
- There is no danger of the patient losing the prescription, as there is with a paper prescription.
- The prescription is typed rather than handwritten, preventing errors from misinterpreting a provider's handwriting.
- There are fewer errors resulting from pharmacists entering the prescriptions into their computer.
- Provider computers can be tied to the patient's chart, thus alerting the provider if there is a possible complication with a patient's medical condition or other medications.

Although electronic charting programs can provide enhancement to the medical practice, they do not take the place of the paper chart. It is still important to ensure that the patient's chart is completely updated at all times. If the chart is subpoenaed by the courts, printing out and sending a computerized chart not only takes more time but may be unacceptable as a court document.

Computerized Files

More and more medical offices are utilizing computerized files. In fact, there are now computer programs that allow a medical office to keep all their patient records, including x-rays, in a computerized file.

The provider is also able to display a patient's record from anywhere in the office. This can allow them to have the patient's records right next to them as they are treating the patient. They, or the medical assistant, can make notations on the medical record as the treatment is taking place. This can prevent problems caused by providers having to remember what treatment was provided. Sometimes providers will work on several patients at the same time. It is easy to become confused regarding which patient had which treatment.

However, even when sophisticated computer records exist, it is important that the practice still maintains a full set of paper files. This is because of the complexity of medical records and for legal considerations. In a written record, it is easier to determine when changes have been made to a document. The handwriting or ink color may be different.

Additionally, most states require that any documentation in a medical record includes the signature or initials of the person making the notation, as well as the date. Many states also carry the provision that medical records must be written on paper or printed. Some states go so far as to say that medical records must be "written in ink" or that a "signature is required on each page." For example, Florida law says that the "caregiver's signature (not stamp or facsimile)" must be included on each page. In such cases, the entire record would need to be printed out and signed each time a change was made to the record.

An additional problem with computer files is the issue of vulnerability. Computers, and the records on them, can be hacked into by outsiders. Allowing this information to be shared with anyone without the patient's approval is a violation of HIPAA laws.

Additionally, computers get viruses and hard drives can become inoperable. If all files are stored on the computer, this allows the medical office to be vulnerable. If a computer crashes in the middle of treating a patient, written records will still leave the provider with a clear picture of the work that needs to be done.

Because much of the patient information is stored in electronic files, it is important to ensure the privacy of these files. This includes making sure that all files require a login and password to access them. Security levels also need to be in place to ensure that people do not have access to records they do not need to do their job.

Everyone in the office must be made aware of the need to maintain the secrecy of their login name and password. To share this information with anyone, even inadvertently, could be considered a violation of HIPAA regulations.

Paul Provider, M.D.
5858 Peppermint Place
Anytown, USA 12345
(765) 555-6768

I,_____(Patient's Name)_____, request and authorize Paul Provider, M.D., to release the following medical information from the medical records of _____

_____ (myself or patient name) to the physician of facility listed below.

Information to be released _____

_____

_____

_____

Dates of treatment: From: _____ To: _____ Information should be sent to:
Person: _____
Facility: _____
Adress: _____
Street, City, Zip: _____
Phone: _____
Date information is to be sent: _____

I release you from all legal responsibility or liability that may arise from this authorization.

Signed _____ Date _____

■ **Figure 2–4** Sample Record Tranfer Form

Record Transfers

At times, it may be necessary for a doctor to transfer records or medical information to another doctor. This is often the case when a patient transfers their care to a specialist, moves to another area, or begins treatment with another physician. In order to avoid legal complications, written permission should be obtained from the patient regarding the right to transfer information, specifically what information should be transferred, and when the transfer is to take place. Often a letter such as the one in **Figure 2–4** is used.

When transferring records or data, do not send the original record or file. Instead, make a copy of all the data to be transferred. The envelope containing the records should be marked "Personal and Confidential." To ensure security, most medical offices will send the information via courier, or via registered mail, return receipt requested. The receipt can specify, if necessary, that the information be delivered only to the person to whom it is addressed (i.e., the doctor). This ensures that it is not opened by others in the office and handled carelessly. A cover page should be included with the information that states that the information contained should be considered confidential and is for the express use of and dissemination to only the person to whom it is addressed.

Be sure that you transfer only that data that the patient has authorized. If data that has not been authorized is on the same page (i.e., information regarding two separate diagnoses), cover the nonpertinent information and make a copy. If it is not possible to cover the data, make a copy of the record, black out the nonpertinent information, and then copy the page again. This prevents the information from being revealed by holding the page up to the light or by other means.

Under no circumstances should a patient be allowed to take their records, or any data from their records, to the doctor themselves. Doing so can allow the patient to alter the records, falsify the information, or remove data from the records. Such actions could put both the patient and the provider at risk. For example, a patient may remove the evidence that a certain drug was prescribed in order to get an additional supply of the drug. However, the new provider may prescribe a drug which is counteractive or could produce an adverse reaction when mixed with the first drug.

Medical Documentation Forms

Whether the patient has insurance coverage or will be responsible for payment of the services themselves, a **claim** or bill for the services rendered by a provider will be prepared. In the following sections we will walk you through the basic forms needed in a medical chart in order to properly bill the patient.

When a patient walks into a provider's office for the first time, a patient file must be established and several forms must be filled out. These forms provide all the information needed to treat and bill the patient. The most commonly used forms include the following:

* The Patient Information Sheet.
* The Release of Information Form.
* The Assignment of Benefits Form.
* The Patient History Form.

Each form has a distinct purpose and, in one style or another, will be present in nearly every provider's office. However, sometimes two or more items are combined on a single form. This is most often true of the Release of Information Form, the Assignment of Benefits Form, and the Patient Information Sheet.

Filling out these forms is relatively simple, as the information called for is self-explanatory. Let's look at each of the forms in greater detail.

Patient Information Sheet

The **Patient Information Sheet** is used to collect general information regarding the patient **(see Figure 2–5)**. The medical biller should always ensure that the information obtained on the Patient Information Sheet is complete and accurate, as this information will be used for billing and collection and for notifying family members in case of emergency. The Patient Information Sheet should be updated periodically to ensure its accuracy.

There are various versions of this form, but they all usually request the following basic information:

* Name: first, middle, and last.
* Address and telephone number.
* Business address, telephone number, and occupation.
* Date of birth.
* Social Security number.
* Person responsible for payment, or insured's name.
* Spouse's name and occupation.

On the Job Now

Directions: Complete a Patient Information Sheet and create patient charts for Dr. Paul Provider's office for the following five patients. Individual folders may be used to keep information for each patient. Refer to the Patient Data Table and Provider Data Table in Appendix C for information. (These five patients will be used throughout this guide for illustrative purposes. Other patients may be used as well.)

1. Abby Addison
2. Bobby Bumble
3. Cathy Crenshaw
4. Daisy Doolittle
5. Edward Edmunds

Paul Provider, M.D.
5858 Peppermint Place
Anytown, USA 12345
(765) 555-6768

PATIENT INFORMATION SHEET

INSURED'S INFORMATION

Patient Account No.: _____ Assigned Provider: _____ Birth Date: _____

Name: (Last, First, Middle) _____ Gender: _____

Address: _____

Home Phone: _____ Marital Status: _____ Social Security #: _____

Employer Name: _____ Work Phone: _____

Employer Address: _____

Employment Status: _____ Referred By: _____

Allergies/Medical Conditions: _____ Email Address: _____

Primary Ins Policy: _____ Address: _____

Member's ID #: _____ Group #: _____ Insured's Name: _____

Secondary Ins Policy: _____ Address: _____

Member's ID #: _____ Group #: _____ Insured's Name: _____

SPOUSE'S INFORMATION

Patient Account No.: _____ Assigned Provider: _____ Birth Date: _____

Name: (Last, First, Middle) _____ Gender: _____

Social Security #: _____ Employment Status: _____

Employer Name: _____ Work Phone: _____

Employer Address: _____

Allergies/Medical Conditions: _____ Student Status: _____

Primary Ins Policy: _____ Address: _____

Member's ID #: _____ Group #: _____ Insured's Name: _____

Secondary Ins Policy: _____ Address: _____

Member's ID #: _____ Group #: _____ Insured's Name: _____

CHILD #1

Patient Account No.: _____ Assigned Provider: _____ Birth Date: _____

Name of Minor Child: _____ Social Security #: _____

Gender: _____ Marital Status: _____ Relationship to Insured: _____

Allergies/Medical Conditions: _____ Student Status: _____

Primary Ins Policy: _____ Insured's Name: _____

Secondary Ins Policy: _____ Insured's Name: _____

CHILD #2

Patient Account No.: _____ Assigned Provider: _____ Birth Date: _____

Name of Minor Child: _____ Social Security #: _____

Gender: _____ Marital Status: _____ Relationship to Insured: _____

Allergies/Medical Conditions: _____ Student Status: _____

Primary Ins Policy: _____ Insured's Name: _____

Secondary Ins Policy: _____ Insured's Name: _____

CHILD #3

Patient Account No.: _____ Assigned Provider: _____ Birth Date:_____

Name of Minor Child: _____ Social Security #: _____

Gender: _____ Marital Status: _____ Relationship to Insured: _____

Allergies/Medical Conditions: _____ Student Status: _____

Primary Ins Name: _____ Insured's Insured: _____

Secondary Ins Name: _____ Insured's Insured: _____

CHILD #4

Patient Account No.: _____ Assigned Provider: _____ Birth Date: _____

Name of Minor Child: _____ Social Security #: _____

Gender: _____ Marital Status: _____ Relationship to Insured: _____

Allergies/Medical Conditions: _____ Student Status: _____

Primary Ins Name: _____ Insured's Insured: _____

Secondary Ins Name: _____ Insured's Insured: _____

<u>EMERGENCY CONTACT</u>

Name: _____ Home Phone: _____ Other Phone: _____

Address: (City, State, Zip) _____

ACKNOWLEDGMENT AND AUTHORITY FOR TREATMENT AND PAYMENT

Initial

_____ I consent to treatment as necessary or desirable to the care of the patient(s) named above, including but not restricted to whatever drugs, medicine, performance of operations and conduct of laboratory, x-ray, or other studies that may be used by the attending doctor, his/her nurse or qualified designate:

_____ I also acknowledge full responsibility for the payment of such services and agree to pay for them upon demand, in full, AT THE TIME OF SERVICE. If the physician must use a collection agency/attorney or court to collect its charges, then I will pay reasonable attorney fees and costs incurred in collecting same, regardless of insurance coverage.

_____ I hereby authorize payment directly to Paul Provider, M.D. of the medical expense benefits otherwise payable to me but not to exceed my indebtedness to said physician on account of the enclosed charge.

_____ I hereby authorize any medical practitioner, medical or medically related facility, insurance or reinsuring company, consumer reporting agency, or employer having information with respect to any physical or mental condition and/or treatment of me or my minor children and any other non-medical information of me and my minor children to give to the group policyholder, my employer, or its legal representative, any and all such information.

_____ I understand the information obtained by the use of the Authorization will be used to determine eligibility for insurance, and eligibility for benefits under any existing policy. Any information obtained will not be released by/to any organization EXCEPT to the group policyholder, my employer, reinsuring companies, the Medical Information Bureau, Inc., or other persons or organizations performing business or legal services in connection with my application, claim, or as may be otherwise lawfully required or as I may further authorize.

_____ I further agree that a photographic copy of this Authorization shall be valid as the original. This Authorization shall be valid for one year from the date shown below.

Signature of Insured: _____ Date: _____

Signature of Spouse: _____ Date: _____

■ **Figure 2–5** Patient Information Sheet

Practice Pitfalls

The patients should be asked to present their insurance card and a valid form of identification. This is done to ensure that the person seeking treatment is actually the person to whom the insurance card has been issued. A copy of both the insurance card and identification should be made and placed in the patient's chart.

- Information about patient referral.
- Driver's license number.
- Close relative or friend to contact in case of emergency.
- Insurance billing information.

Obtain the names, addresses, and policy and group numbers of all carriers insuring the patient. This is important because of coordination of benefits clauses included in most health insurance policies. If the patient has an insurance card, make a copy of the card to keep in the patient's file. Insurance coverage should be verified before rendering services. The insurance information should be rechecked every six months, as this information may change.

Guarantor

A **guarantor** is a person that undertakes the responsibility for payment of a debt. This situation is most commonly presented in a medical practice when services are rendered for care of a child. The parent or guardian of that child is legally obligated for payment of the child's medical services. A form should be signed indicating that the guarantor will be responsible for the payment fees for medical services rendered. This signature requirement is usually located on the Patient Information Sheet. An anticipated insurance payment does not replace the guarantor's obligation to pay any outstanding balance.

Emancipated Minor

Emancipation is a legal process whereby a child assumes responsibility for himself, and the child's parent or legal guardian is no longer legally responsible for the child. A child can become emancipated in several ways. In some states, a minor can become emancipated just by claiming himself so; in other states, court approval is required. However, regardless of the process used to attain emancipation, once a minor is considered emancipated he is entitled to make his own medical decisions and also is responsible for payment of any medical services received.

Encounter Form

Encounter Forms are used to record both clinical and financial information about the patient, and frequently are used as billing and routing documents. These forms also are referred to as charge tickets, fee slips, and superbills in the physician's office and as a chargemaster in the hospital. The Encounter Form should be filled out and attached to the front of the patient's medical chart when a patient comes for a visit. These forms should be sequentially numbered so that they may all be accounted for.

In order to fully capture revenue, the encounter form submitted to the insurance carrier must reflect the services rendered with the correct diagnosis code. An example of an encounter form is shown in **Figure 2–6**.

Hospital Admission Form

Hospital Admission Forms are used to record both clinical and financial information about the patient when they are admitted into a facility. They are very similar to encounter forms. The information obtained on the form in used by the billing personnel to properly bill the patient. An example of a hospital admission form is shown in **Figure 2–7**.

Release of Information Form

The **Release of Information Form** is used to allow the provider to request additional information from other providers of service or to share information with an insurance carrier (**see Figure 2–8**). If the doctor submits an insurance claim for the patient, the patient must sign a Release of Information Form before information may be given to an insurance company, attorney, or other third party. According to the Privacy Act, it is illegal to release any information regarding a patient without the patient's knowledge and written consent. Without this signature, the provider's office is not allowed to submit a claim to the insurance carrier because disclosing the patient's diagnosis and other medical information to the insurance carrier would be a breach of the privacy laws.

The patient's signature is usually good for one year from the date the release is signed. If the patient is a child, the parent or guardian must sign the release. Often a release of information statement is included on the actual claim form describing treatment. This brief statement does not take the place of having a completed and signed release of information statement in the patient's file.

The **Request for Additional Information Form** is a form designed to ask for information or records from various sources. The medical biller will usually use the Request for Additional Information form (**see Figure 2–9**) to request additional information needed to bill for services rendered. All information needed from a particular source should be requested at the same time.

Encounter Form

Date:

Paul Provider, M.D.
5858 Peppermint Place ● Anytown, USA 12345 ● (765) 555-6768

Provider Information

Name:	
Address:	
City:	State:	Zip Code:
Telephone#:	
Fax#:	
Tax ID #:	
Medicaid ID #:	
Medicare ID #:	

Provider's Signature: _____ Date: _____

Patient Information

Name:	
Address:	
City:	State:	Zip Code:
Telephone#:	
Patient Account #:	
Date of Birth:	
Gender:	
Relationship to Guarantor:	
Marital Status:	
SSN #:	

Insurance Type: ☐ Private   ☐ Medicare   ☐ Medicaid   ☐ Workers' Compensation   ☐ Other _____

Appointment Information

Appt. Date:		Time:	
Request Next Appt. Date:		Time:	
Date of First Visit:			
Date of Injury:			
Referring Physician:			

Guarantor Information

Name:	
Insurance ID#:	
Insurance Plan Name:	
Insurance Plan Group#:	
Employer Name:	
Employer Address:	
City:	State:	Zip Code:
SSN #:	

Authorization

☐ Authorization to Release Information
☐ Authorization for Assignment of Benefits
☐ Authorization for Consent for Treatment
☐ I understand that my insurance will be billed as a courtesy to me but that there may be a patient responsibility remaining on account.

Signature: _____ Date: _____

Clinical Information

	Date of Service	Place of Service	CPT Code/Description	ICD-9 Code/ Description	Fee
1.					
2.					
3.					
4.					
5.					
6.					
7.					
8.					

Billing Instructions

Notes:

Special Instructions:

Statement of Account Information

Previous Balance:	$	Payment:	$
Today's Fee:	$	Received by:	
Copay:	$	☐ Cash	
Adjustment:	$	☐ Check	
		☐ Credit Card	
New Balance:	$	☐ Other	

■ **Figure 2–6** Sample Encounter Form

Hospital Admission Form

Provider Information					Admission Information			
Name:					Admission Date:		Time:	
Address:					Discharge Date:		Time:	
City:		State:		Zip Code:	Attending Phy's ID#:		Date of Injury:	
Telephone#:		Fax#:			Attending Physician:			
Medicare ID#:		UPIN#:			**Guarantor Information**			
Tax ID #:		Accepts Medicare Assignment:	☐		Name:			
Provider Rep:		Date:			Address:			

Patient Information								
					City:	State:	Zip Code:	
Name:					Insurance ID #:		SSN:	
Address:					Insurance Name:			
City:		State:		Zip Code:	Insurance Group #:			
Telephone#:		Patient Control #:			Employer Name:			
Date of Birth:		Gender:			**Authorization**			
Marital Status:		Relationship to Guarantor:			☐ Authorization to Release Information			
Student Status:	☐ Full-time	☐ Part-time			☐ Authorization for Assignment of Benefits			
Insurance Type:	☐ Pvt ☐ M/care ☐ M/caid ☐ WC ☐ Other _____				☐ Authorization for Consent for Treatment			
					☐ My insurance will be billed but there may be a balance due.			
					Signature:_____ Date:_____			

Clinical Information					
Principal Diagnosis:					
Other Diagnosis:					
Surgical Procedure:					
Other Procedures:					
Remarks:					
Previous Balance:	Today's Fee:	Payment:	Adjustment:	New Balance:	

Figure 2–7 Sample Hospital Admission Form

PAUL PROVIDER, M.D.
5858 PEPPERMINT PLACE
ANYTOWN, USA 12345
(765) 555-6768

RELEASE OF INFORMATION FORM

I AUTHORIZE any physician, medical practitioner, hospital, clinic, or other medical or medically related facility, insurance or reinsurance company, the Medical Information Bureau, Inc., consumer reporting agency, or employer having information available as to diagnosis, treatment and prognosis with respect to any physical or mental condition and/or treatment of me or my minor children and any other non-medical information of me and my minor children to give to the group policyholder, my employer, or its legal representative, any and all such information.

I UNDERSTAND the information obtained by the use of this Authorization will be used to determine eligibility for insurance, and eligibility for benefits under any existing policy. Any information obtained will not be released by/to any person or organization EXCEPT to the group policyholder, my employer, reinsuring companies, or other persons or organizations performing business or legal services in connection with my application, claim, or as may be otherwise lawfully required or as I may further authorize.

I KNOW that I may request to receive a copy of this Authorization.

I AGREE that a photographic copy of this Authorization shall be as valid as the original.

I AGREE this Authorization shall be valid for one year from the date shown below.

Signature of Insured and/or Spouse _____ Date _____

Name(s) of minor child(ren) _____

Figure 2–8 Release of Information Form

PAUL PROVIDER, M.D.
Medical Billing Office
5858 Peppermint Place
Anytown, USA 12345
(765) 555-6768

Date: _____

Re: Policyholder:_____

Patient Account #: _____

Employee: _____

Dependent: _____

Dear _____ :

We need additional information from you.

We are writing to_____

_____

_____

_____

_____

_____

Please respond on the reverse of this letter or attach additional information or documentation. Thank you.

Sincerely yours,

Serving all your medical needs for 17 years!

■ **Figure 2–9** Request for Additional Information

PAUL PROVIDER, M.D.
5858 PEPPERMINT PLACE
ANYTOWN, USA 12345
(765) 555-6768

ASSIGNMENT OF BENEFITS

I authorize payment directly to the above named provider of medical expense benefits otherwise payable to me but not to exceed my indebtedness to said provider for any services furnished to me by that provider.

The signature on this form or a photocopy is valid for one year from the date indicated.

Signature _____ Date _____

■ **Figure 2–10** Assignment of Benefits Form

Assignment of Benefits Form

The **Assignment of Benefits Form** is a request for all insurance payments to be directed to the provider holding the assignment (**see Figure 2–10**). Most providers consider this a necessity for those patients who have insurance, because the assignment ensures that monies paid for services provided are issued directly to the provider and not to the patient or subscriber. Assignment of benefits indicates that the payer is authorized to send payment directly to the provider of services. The Assignment of Benefits Form should be signed, dated (preferably date stamped), and attached to the insurance verification form. If the patient has signed an Assignment of Benefits, you would type "Signature on File" in the signature field on the claims form or other document to indicate that payment is to be made to the provider.

Patient History Form

The Patient History Form is important to the physician (**see Figure 2–11**). The **Patient History Form** helps in identifying previous incidents of illness that may be important in treating the patient's present condition. This is usually a detailed form with basic health questions requiring only yes or no answers (an actual Patient History Form is more detailed and extensive than the one that we have provided, which is for sample purposes only). The provider will give the patient a complete history and physical in the exam room. The provider will then complete a physical exam and include his findings. Some physicians may dictate a medical history report (see the Medical Reports chapter).

The Patient Information Sheet, Release of Information Form, Assignment of Benefits Form, and Patient History Form should all be completed by the patient at the time of the first visit. However, it is the job of the person receiving the forms from the patient to ensure that these forms are complete. If the answer to a question is "no," the patient should write the word "no" in the field. If the information is not applicable, the patient should write "N/A" in the field. This ensures that the patient has looked at each of the fields and responded to them. This can prevent problems when a patient mistakenly skips over a question, when the answer could be important for their proper care.

Insurance Verification

An **Insurance Coverage Form** is a form used to verify and document insurance coverage information. The patient's portion of the charges will usually be collected at the time service is rendered. Each office has a standard form for verification of coverage. **Figure 2–12** shows a sample Insurance Coverage Form.

This form covers much of the pertinent information needed to determine the patient's portion of the claim, and assists in gaining the maximum reimbursement for the patient. Maximum reimbursement may be obtained by following any requirements set forth in the contract, such as obtaining preauthorization for certain services or taking advantage of benefits which might be paid at a higher percentage (i.e., preadmit testing, outpatient instead of inpatient surgeries, etc.).

Some forms will have room for information on other family members so that family deductible and coinsurance maximum amounts can be tracked.

Paul Provider, M.D.
5858 Peppermint Place
Anytown, USA 12345
(765) 555-6768

Patient History

Date: _____

Patient Name _____ Age _____

Any allergies to food or medicine?   No   Yes
If yes: Allergic to: _____

Have you ever been hospitalized?   No   Yes
If yes: Indicate date and reason: _____

Have you ever been diagnosed or experienced:

Bladder Infections	_____	Underweight	_____	Anemia	_____
Ear Infections	_____	Epilepsy	_____	Overweight	_____
Sinus Infections	_____	Seizures	_____	Hay Fever	_____
Vision Problems	_____	Mumps	_____	Chickenpox	_____
Frequent Headaches	_____	Sickle Cell Anemia	_____	Heart Murmur	_____

Other _____

Are you currently taking any medication(s)?
If yes: Name of medication(s): _____

Date of last Tuberculosis and/or Tetanus shot: _____

Check any of the following that any blood relative has or has had:

Anemia	_____	Heart Disease	_____	Thyroid Problems	_____
Sickle Cell Anemia	_____	Heart Attack	_____	Diabetes	_____
Stroke	_____	Birth Defects	_____	Asthma	_____
Cancer	_____	Mental Retardation	_____	Kidney Disease	_____
Tuberculosis	_____	Alcoholism	_____	High Blood Pressure	_____

Patient Signature: _____ Date: _____

■ **Figure 2–11** Sample Patient History Form

Paul Provider, M.D.
5858 Peppermint Place
Anytown, USA 12345
(765) 555-6768

Insurance Coverage Form

INSURED: _____ BIRTH DATE: _____

SSN: _____ EFFECTIVE DATE: _____

INSURANCE POLICY: _____

ADDRESS: _____

ID/MEMBER #: _____ GROUP #: _____

DEPENDENT AGE LIMIT: _____

_____

INDIV. DEDUCTIBLE AMOUNT: _____ 3 MO CARRYOVER:_____

FAMILY DEDUCTIBLE: _____ AGGREGATE/NONAGGREGATE

STANDARD COINSURANCE _____LIFETIME MAXIMUM_____

COINSURANCE LIMIT _____

_____

BENEFITS PAID AT OTHER THAN THE STANDARD COINSURANCE % [Including benefit, coinsurance amount and special circumstances, (i.e., SSO allowed at 100%, required for hysterectomy, coronary bypass, etc.)]:

_____

_____

PREAUTHORIZATION REQUIRED FOR: _____

_____

_____

ACCIDENT BENEFIT AMOUNT: _____ TREATMENT TO BE RECEIVED WITHIN _____ DAYS

OTHER NOTES/COMMENTS: _____

_____

TOTAL PAYMENTS (CCYY)

Indicate below the names of the insured and their dependents. When any of the following information is received, write it in pencil followed by the date. This will help you to realize when a patient's deductible has been met and if they are nearing any maximum benefit.

	INSURED	DEPENDENT	DEPENDENT	DEPENDENT	DEPENDENT
NAME:	_____	_____	_____	_____	_____
DEDUCTIBLE:	_____	_____	_____	_____	_____
COINS PD:	_____	_____	_____	_____	_____
LIFETIME:	_____	_____	_____	_____	_____

■ **Figure 2–12** Insurance Coverage Form

Practice
Pitfalls

Make sure that you get preauthorization or preapproval of benefits for services specifically indicated in the contract that require such. Otherwise, there may be a payment penalty imposed, which significantly reduces the benefits paid, or there may be a complete denial of benefits.

You will need to contact the insurance carrier to complete this form accurately. Provide the insurance carrier with the name of the patient, the name of the insured, and the policy name/number. The carrier can then provide you with the information needed to complete each field.

Some carriers may prefer to have you fax the Insurance Coverage Sheet to them rather than spend time with you on the phone. If this is the case, also fax the Release of Information Form with the patient's signature on it.

On the Job Now

Directions: Using the contracts in the following chapter, complete an Insurance Coverage Form for Abby Addison, Bobby Bumble, Cathy Crenshaw, Daisy Doolittle, and Edward Edmunds. Refer to the Patient Data Table in Appendix C for additional information.

Additional Suggestions

There are a number of things to keep in mind when dealing with patients. Of course, client service should always be your first and foremost concern, but at the same time you need to have regard for the medical office. It is important to obtain all necessary information from the patient. Remember that one of the primary objectives of the medical biller is to minimize the amount of time between the physician's service and the complete payment of the bill. The information that can facilitate this process may include the following:

1. Ask the patient to fill out all necessary forms for setting up the patient file. Give the patient sufficient time to fill out the forms and check that they are complete before accepting them. Many offices mail the forms to the patient before their first visit to ensure their completeness.

2. Be sure you understand the policies of the office for which you work regarding the completion of forms and payment for bills. This way you can explain them accurately to the patient at the time of their first visit.

3. Use the office forms consistently and accurately so that the tracking of information runs smoothly, regardless of who enters the information.

4. Secure all the details of the insurance information. If the patient or insured has a card, make a copy of it for your files. Make sure the information contains the subscriber's name, the policy number, the effective date, the company that holds the policy or the name of the policy, and the insurance carrier's address.

5. Make sure the patient understands the provider's policy regarding any amounts that the insurance carrier does not pay or does not cover.

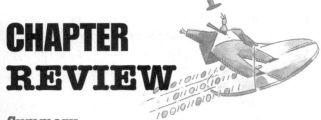

CHAPTER REVIEW

Summary

- Maintaining patient files in a proper manner is one of a medical biller's most important jobs.
- The medical biller/receptionist, medical assistant, and the physician are the individuals most likely responsible for maintenance of the patient chart.
- It is important that everyone who makes notations in a patient chart follows the rules of proper medical charting.

- It is important for the medical biller to know how to properly store charts and how to retrieve stored charts.
- SOAP notes may be useful in abstracting information for billing purposes.
- There are several forms that need to be included in all medical charts. These forms include the Patient Information Sheet, the Assignment of Benefits form, the Authorization to Release Information form, and the Patient History Form. Many of these forms will need to be completed by the patient at the time of their first visit.

Assignments

Complete the Questions for Review.
Complete Exercises 2–1 through 2–3.

Questions for Review

Directions: Answer the following questions without looking back into the material just covered. Write your answers in the space provided.

1. What are 10 of the 15 medical documentation rules?

  1. _____

  2. _____

  3. _____

  4. _____

  5. _____

  6. _____

  7. _____

  8. _____

  9. _____

  10. _____

2. What information do you need on a master list when storing patient records? _____

_____

_____

3. What does alphabetical filing mean? _____

_____

4. How long should you keep medical records, and why? _____

_____

_____

5. What three people often will be involved in documenting a patient chart?

    1. _____

    2. _____

    3. _____

6. List five of the items that should be included on the Patient Information Sheet.

    1. _____

    2. _____

    3. _____

    4. _____

    5. _____

7. What is the purpose of the Patient Information Sheet? _____

_____

8. Define Noncompliance. _____

_____

_____

9. What is the purpose of the Insurance Coverage Sheet? _____

_____

10. What is an Assignment of Benefits Form? _____

_____

_____

If you are unable to answer any of these questions, refer back to that section in the chapter, and then fill in the answers.

Exercise **2-1**

Directions: Find and circle the words listed below. Words can appear horizontally, vertically, diagonally, forward, or backward.

```
F D S T G H S Z B I D T K T F
Z G A Q C B I L D O W R R O N
H D Q Q D G G N L M D A G V L
P X Q V L S N L P Q H H U L M
S E T O N P A O S C W C T V S
F Y Y J M E T H C J A S B O G
C J J I S O U I O Q T N C U N
H M A M M O R R Z A L E A Y I
S L I C N T E P E F F R Q T R
C L T K A W C M D F A D Q T E
Q A N I D O A K I N R L O P T
O S D Y I B R W T T G I V P L
Q E T E I N D O B Q W H K F A
P C E R A S R J H X D C Y A O
E N C O U N T E R F O R M D H
```

1. Alter
2. Children's Chart
3. Claim
4. Encounter Form

5. Guarantor
6. Pediatric Chart
7. Signature Card
8. SOAP Notes

Exercise **2-2**

Directions: Complete the crossword puzzle by filling in a word from the keywords that fits each clue.

Across

5. A legal process whereby a child assumes responsibility for himself, and the child's parent or legal guardian is no longer legally responsible for the child.

Down

1. Keeping the information in a record updated and filing the chart or record in a manner that makes it easy to locate if you should need it at a later date.
2. Filing medical charts alphabetically by the first letter of the patient's last name.
3. Not following the instructions given by the provider.
4. A liquid that covers over the writing on paper.
6. A form that helps identify previous incidents of illness that may be important in treating a patient's present condition.

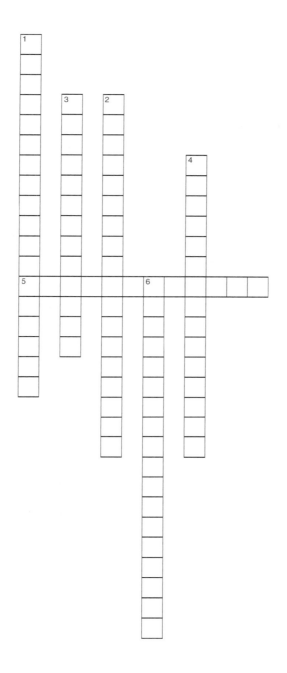

Exercise 2-3

Directions: Match the following terms with the proper definition by writing the letter of the correct definition in the space next to the term.

1. _____ Assignment of Benefits Form

2. _____ Electronic Prescriptions

3. _____ Insurance Coverage Form

4. _____ Patient Information Sheet

5. _____ Release of Information Form

6. _____ Request for Additional Information Form

a. A form used to allow the provider to request additional information from other providers of service or to share information with an insurance carrier.

b. A form used to collect general information regarding the patient.

c. A form designed to ask for information or records from various sources.

d. A form used by many practices to verify insurance coverage and document this information.

e. A form requesting all insurance payments to be directed to the provider holding the assignment.

f. Prescriptions that are entered into the provider's computer, then electronically sent to the computer at the patient's pharmacy.

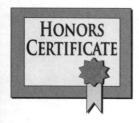

Honors Certification™

You will be given a written test of the information contained in this chapter. Each incorrect answer will result in a deduction of up to 5% from your grade. You must achieve a score of 85% or higher to pass this test. If you fail the test on your first attempt, you may retake the test one additional time. The items included in the second test may be different from those in the first test.

SECTION 2
HEALTH INSURANCE PROGRAMS

3

Health Insurance
Contract Interpretation

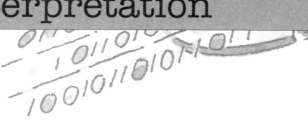

After completion of this chapter
you will be able to:

- Describe how Blue Cross/Blue Shield and other indemnity plans share expenses.
- Define the basic terms used in an insurance contract.
- Explain how the various elements of a contract can affect billing.
- Properly complete a Treatment Authorization Request form.
- Describe the common basic benefits that are included in a contract.
- Accurately calculate deductible amounts given a contract and scenario.
- Describe how major medical limits (i.e., coinsurance limits, lifetime maximums, etc.) can affect the insurance carrier's payment on a claim.
- Explain what COBRA is and how it affects coverage for preexisting conditions.

- Explain how exclusions and allowed amounts can affect payment on a claim.
- Describe the precertification process.
- Describe what utilization review is and how it can affect benefit payments.
- List situations in which a surgery may be considered unnecessary.
- State the purposes of Second Surgical Opinions and how they can affect claim payments.
- Describe the two types of second surgical opinion programs.
- Properly define the terms used in coordination of Benefits.
- List the 13 Order of Benefit Determination rules.
- Use the OBD rules to determine the proper primary, secondary, and tertiary payers on a given claim.

Keywords and Concepts
you will learn in this chapter:

- Accident
- Actively-at-Work
- Aggregate Deductible
- Allowed Amount

- Authorized Treatment Record Form
- Basic Benefits
- Carryover Provision

- Coinsurance
- Concurrent Review
- Conversion Factor
- Coordination of Benefits (COB)

- Copayment
- Deductible
- Eligibility
- Exclusions
- Explanation of Benefits (EOB)
- Family Deductible
- Fee Schedule
- Group Plan
- Indemnity Insurance Plans
- Lifetime Maximum

- Mandatory Program
- Mental and Nervous Expenses
- Nonaggregate Deductible
- Order of Benefit Determinations (OBD)
- Preadmission Testing
- Preauthorization
- Precertify
- Preexisting Conditions

- Primary Plan
- Prospective Review
- Retrospective Review
- Second Surgical Opinion Consultation
- Secondary Plan
- Unnecessary Surgery
- Usual, Customary, and Reasonable (UCR)
- Voluntary Program

Interpreting and understanding contracts is one of the most important aspects of being a medical biller. The healthcare contract is the one document that is used to determine the benefits that the insurance carrier will pay for services rendered.

The wording and terminology of health insurance contracts can often be confusing to someone who is not well versed in the insurance field. For this reason, medical billers often will be called on to interpret the provisions of a contract for billing purposes or to explain benefits to a patient.

Also, many medical practices prefer to collect the patient's portion of the bill (that portion not covered by insurance) at the time services are rendered. In order to properly calculate the amount due from the patient, it is important that medical billers are able to interpret the benefits covered in the contract.

Additionally, an astute medical biller can often suggest options to a patient or provider that will provide greater coverage under the terms of the contract. For example, a contract may provide 100% coverage for certain services that are performed on an outpatient basis. If a patient has inpatient surgery scheduled for a listed procedure, it can be beneficial for the medical biller to inform the provider of the increased payment for outpatient surgery. It is then up to the provider and the patient to determine if the increased coverage is benefi-

cial to the patient in their particular circumstance or situation.

Blue Cross/Blue Shield

There are many insurance carriers doing business within the United States. One of the largest of these is the Blue Cross/Blue Shield group. Although many people consider Blue Cross/Blue Shield to be separate or different from many other companies, in truth their contracts cover many of the same procedures and have many of the same benefits as other indemnity plans.

Indemnity insurance plans, also called fee-for-service, have been the traditional form of commercial health insurance. Indemnity insurance is a principle of insurance that provides medical coverage when a loss occurs, and restores the insured party to their approximate financial condition before the loss occurred. Under an indemnity plan, the covered person chooses his or her own physician, specialist, hospital, or other provider. Indemnity plans require that the insured person pay a predetermined portion of annual medical expenses out-of-pocket, called the "deductible." These plans also require the covered person to pay a predetermined percentage of additional annual expenses up to a preset maximum; that share is called the "coinsurance" requirement.

These plans often pay benefits at a set amount, such as 80% of the covered services. The patient is responsible for the remaining 20%, as well as any amounts not covered by the insurance carrier.

The concepts discussed in this chapter apply to all types of contracts, including Blue Cross/Blue Shield, managed care contracts (discussed more fully in Chapter 6) and preferred provider plans.

Contract Provisions

If a biller is familiar with the provisions of a specific contract, they may be able to provide added benefits due to the scheduling of a patient, or the manner in which a claim is filed.

We have provided you with three contracts at the end of this chapter: Ball Insurance Carrier (Blue Corporation), Rover Insurers, Inc. (Red Corporation), and Winter Insurance Company (White Corporation). Each contract is different. Throughout this chapter, we will refer to these contracts to help familiarize you with the provisions in each contract.

Eligibility

The first item that is considered on the contract is **eligibility**, or the qualifications that make the person eligible for coverage. To be eligible for benefits under most group insurance policies the member must be a full-time employee at the company. For example, in the Winter Insurance Company contract, an employee must work a minimum of 30 hours per week to be covered by this contract. The contract also covers who is considered a dependent of the employee.

Of course, if a person has purchased individual coverage and is not covered by their place of work, there would be no minimum work requirements. However, there would still be qualifications to have coverage as a dependent under this plan.

Dependent eligibility is usually defined by the relationship to the employee and the age of the dependent. For example, in the Winter contract, a child is covered until age 19, or to age 23 if they are a full-time student. If an eligible dependent becomes disabled before age 19, or before age 23 if a full-time student, dependent coverage would continue until age 23. Children include unmarried natural children, legally adopted children, foster children, and those for whom the employee is considered the legal guardian.

Some contracts have provisions that state that if a husband and wife (or parent and child) work for the same employer and are covered under the same contract, the spouse or child cannot be covered as a dependent on the employee's policy. Also, some contracts state that if both spouses are working at the same company and are covered under the same contract, the children may be covered by one parent or the other but not both. This prevents the insurance carrier from having to pay twice for the same patient and services rendered.

On the Job Now

Directions: Review the contracts at the end of this chapter and complete the following questions.

What are the eligibility requirements for:

Winter Insurance Company/White Corporation _____

_____

_____

Rover Insurers, Inc./Red Corporation _____

_____

_____

Ball Insurance Carrier/Blue Corporation _____

_____

_____

Effective Date

The next item to be considered is whether or not the contract was in force at the time the services were rendered. This often is dependent on a minimum length of time an employee must have worked for a company.

There also is an **"actively-at-work"** stipulation that is included in many contracts. The actively-at-work provision states that a person must be at work (or actively engaged in their normal activities, if a dependent) on the date coverage becomes effective. If he or she is not at work or actively engaged in their normal activities, the contract does not become effective until the employee or dependent returns to work.

As a medical biller, it is important that you are sure that a patient is eligible and is covered under an insurance policy in order to receive benefits. Many providers contact the insurance company prior to performing a procedure to be sure that the patient is covered. This is especially important when a patient is covered under an individual policy and pays a monthly premium for coverage.

Termination of Coverage

This section of a contract provides information regarding when coverage will terminate for both the employee and their dependents. It is important to note when coverage ceases as the insurance carrier will not pay benefits after this date. You should be aware that coverage will often continue until the end of the month in which an employee terminates. Knowing this, it is important to schedule any follow-up visits before the end of the month if you know that a patient's insurance is being terminated.

Preauthorization

A number of insurance carriers will require that certain benefits be preauthorized before the services are received. **Preauthorization** means to gain approval of the services that are to be performed, as well as to obtain an understanding of whether or not the insurance carrier will provide coverage for these services.

Many insurance carriers have a standard preauthorization form (**see Figure 3–1**). This form is used to request information regarding the patient, the diagnosis, and the procedures to be performed.

To complete a Preauthorization Request Form, you must enter the following information:

Name of Patient: Enter the name of the patient who will receive the services.

Address: Enter the patient's address.

City, State, Zip: Enter the city, state, and zip code of the patient.

Sex: Enter 'M' for Male or 'F' for female.

Marital Status: Enter the patient's marital status. This is especially important when the patient is a dependent of the insured.

Date of Birth: Enter the patient's date of birth.

Insurance Policy Name/Group Number: Enter the insurance policy name or number that the patient is insured under.

Name of Insured: Enter the name of the insured. This may be a spouse or parent of the patient. In rare instances it may be a different relation to the insured (i.e., the patient is a grandchild of the insured and the insured has custody).

Relationship to Insured: Check the appropriate relationship box.

Diagnosis Description: Enter the English-Language description of the patient's illness, injury, or condition.

ICD-9-CM Code: Enter the ICD-9-CM code(s) associated with the patient's condition. These codes indicate the patient's diagnosis.

Reason for Services: Describe the reason or the medical justification for the services that will be rendered. If necessary, include any laboratory reports, x-rays, pictures, or other documentation to justify the need for services.

Specific Services: Enter the specific services for which the provider is seeking authorization. These should be identified by specific CPT® or HCPCS procedure codes (which identify service or item). Each service or item should be listed on a separate line.

Units: Enter the number of units or the number of times the provider feels this service should be performed (i.e., 10 for requesting 10 psychiatric visits).

Charges: Enter the charges for each service or item. This should be the charge for a single unit of service, not the total amount for all the units you are requesting.

Signature: The provider must sign the Treatment Authorization Request.

Paul Provider, M.D.
5858 Peppermint Place
Anytown, USA 12345

PREAUTHORIZATION REQUEST

Name of Patient: _____

Address: _____

City, State, Zip: _____

Sex: _____   Marital Status: _____   Date of Birth: _____

Insurance Policy Name/Group Number: _____

Name of Insured: _____

Treatment authorized by: _____

Treatment authorization number: _____

Diagnosis Description: _____

_____

ICD-9 Code(s): _____

Reason for Services: _____

_____

_____

_____

_____

Specific services you are requesting authorization for: _____

___ CPT Code: _____   Units: _____   Charges: _____

_____

_____

_____

_____

_____

I hereby certify that the above information is true and correct to the best of my knowledge.

Signature: _____   Date: _____

■ **Figure 3–1** Preauthorization Request Form

PAUL PROVIDER, M.D.
5858 Peppermint Place
Anytown, USA 12345
(765) 555-6768

Authorized Treatment Record Form

Patient Name: _____

Policy Name: _____

Above patient has been authorized for the following treatment(s):

Diagnosis: _____

Authorized Procedure(s): _____

Allowed Number of Treatments: _____

Treatment Authorized by: _____

Treatment Authorization Number: _____

TREATMENT RECORD

Visit	Date	Procedure(s)	Provider
1	_____	_____	_____
2	_____	_____	_____
3	_____	_____	_____
4	_____	_____	_____
5	_____	_____	_____
6	_____	_____	_____
7	_____	_____	_____
8	_____	_____	_____
9	_____	_____	_____
10	_____	_____	_____
11	_____	_____	_____
12	_____	_____	_____
13	_____	_____	_____
14	_____	_____	_____
15	_____	_____	_____
16	_____	_____	_____
17	_____	_____	_____
18	_____	_____	_____
19	_____	_____	_____
20	_____	_____	_____

■ **Figure 3–2** Authorized Treatment Record Form

Authorized Treatment Record Form

An **Authorized Treatment Record Form (see Figure 3–2)** is a form used to track the usage of preauthorized services rendered by a provider's office. Once the medical office receives the preauthorization request back from the insurance carrier, the treatments provided for those particular services should be tracked using the Authorized Treatment Record Form.

Contract Benefits

The next section of the contract usually details the benefits that the contract covers. These can include basic benefits and major medical benefits. Premiums are based on the number and amount of benefits that a contract covers. The greater the coverage, the higher the cost of the premiums. For example, a contract that covers charges at 90% of the allowed amount (allowed amounts will be discussed later) and has a $100 deductible, usually will cost more than a comparative contract that covers charges at 70% of the allowed amount and has a $250 deductible.

Basic Benefits

Basic benefits are those benefits usually paid at 100%, and are paid before major medical benefits are paid. Therefore, it is possible for the insurance plan to pay basic benefits even when the patient has not yet met their deductible. Not all contracts will have basic benefits. Most basic benefit plans have been replaced with managed care plans.

Some contracts have a basic benefit that is based on the unit value (a number based on the difficulty of a procedure and the overhead needed; see Allowed Amount) being multiplied by a basic conversion factor (see Ball Insurance Carrier contract). This allows a small portion of most services to be paid at 100% with the remaining portion paid at the normal coinsurance percentage. These types of basic benefits do not cover all procedures.

Accident Benefits

One of the most common basic benefits is an accident benefit. An **accident** is defined as an unintentional injury that has a specific time, date, and place. Under the Winter Insurance Company contract, the first $300 of services that are a result of an accident occurrence are paid at 100%. After that, the remaining charges are paid at 90%. This benefit is for the first $300 of charges that are incurred within 120 days of the date of the accident, so follow-up care should be scheduled within that 120-day period in order to get the higher rate. Also, be aware that if other providers charge for the same accident, it is the first $300 of *all* charges that receives the 100% benefit. Therefore, if Tommy Tucker gets hit by a car, remember that there may be ambulance charges, hospital charges, physician's charges, x-ray technician charges, and other charges. It is important to get your claim in as quickly as possible to ensure that the provider you work for is reimbursed at 100% and not at 90%.

Additionally, be sure to indicate on the bill that services are a result of an accident. On the CMS-1500 claim form, this is box 10b and 10c, and the date of the accident is indicated in box 14. (The CMS-1500 claim form will be explained in detail in the chapter titled CMS-1500.) If your office does not use the CMS-1500, be sure that there is a place to indicate that this was an accident, or type it on the bottom of the bill. This data also should be noted in the patient chart so that when the Explanation of Benefits (EOB) is received from the insurance carrier, you can determine if the correct benefits were applied (i.e., the bill was paid at 100%).

On the Job Now

Directions: Study the contracts at the end of this chapter and complete the following questions.

What are the terms of the accident benefit for:

Winter Insurance Company/White Corporation _____

_____

_____

Rover Insurers, Inc./Red Corporation _____

_____

_____

Ball Insurance Carrier/Blue Corporation _____

_____

_____

Preadmission Testing

In the past, a patient would enter the hospital the day before surgery for routine tests such as a chest x-ray and a blood test. The hospital would then admit the patient and watch over them to ensure that they had nothing to eat or drink in the 24 hours before the surgery. Insurance carriers realized there would be a great savings if the patient were to visit the hospital for the tests, return home, and then return the next day for the surgery. This eliminated the charges for an overnight stay in the hospital.

To encourage this practice, some insurance companies began offering an extra incentive for **preadmission testing**, or testing done before the patient enters the hospital for surgery. Some insurance carriers now cover these charges at 100% rather than at their normal coinsurance percentage.

Tests performed at the facility where the patient will be admitted, and performed within 24 hours of admittance, are usually allowed under this benefit. If it is appropriate for the patient's condition, consider scheduling this option, or at least make the patient aware of it.

Second Surgical Opinions

Some insurance carriers cover a second surgical opinion at 100%. This originally started out as a cost-cutting measure. The hope was that only those surgeries that were necessary would be confirmed, with some patients receiving alternative (and less expensive) treatments, or with treatment being considered completely unnecessary.

Second surgical opinions have become less popular among insurance carriers because the cost savings seems to be minimal, if any. Many doctors are reluctant to go against the word or prescribed treatments of another physician. They do not want to contradict their peers, and also do not want to open themselves up to a lawsuit by suggesting a less radical treatment that may eventually prove less effective. Therefore, they often will simply confirm the diagnosis and the prescribed treatment of the original physician.

If you are billing for second surgical opinion services, be sure to use one of the second surgical opinion or consultation CPT® codes. These codes will be explained in detail in the chapter on Reference Books.

Outpatient Facility Charges

Some surgeries are simple or routine enough to be performed on an outpatient basis. This means that the patient enters the facility in the morning, has surgery, and, after a brief recovery period, returns home the same day. There are no overnight or room and board charges. To encourage outpatient surgery when and where possible, some insurance carriers will cover such charges at 100%.

On the Job Now

Directions: Study the contracts at the end of this chapter and complete the following questions.

What basic benefits does each contract have?

Winter Insurance Company/White Corporation _____

_____

_____

Rover Insurers, Inc./Red Corporation _____

_____

_____

Ball Insurance Carrier/Blue Corporation _____

_____

_____

Major Medical Benefits

This section of the contract lists the particular benefits and stipulations that a contract provides.

Deductible

The first item usually listed is the amount of the **deductible**. The deductible is the amount that the individual patient must pay before benefits are paid by the insurance carrier. Deductibles are usually accumulated according to a calendar year. Thus, each January 1st, the amount the patient has paid toward their deductible returns to zero and the patient must start paying again.

The exception to this is in contracts which have a "**carryover provision.**" A deductible carryover provision means that any amounts that the patient pays toward their deductible in the last three months of the year will carry over and will be applied toward the next year's deductible. Remember, the patient pays their deductible before the insurance is required to pay any benefits. Therefore, if the patient is still paying a deductible in the last three months of the year, the insurance carrier has not had to pay any major medical benefits on this patient up to that time.

If you are in the month of September and it is appropriate for the patient's condition, ask the patient if they would like to schedule services for after October 1. The deductible payments will then apply not only for this year but also for the following year, if their plan has a carryover provision.

Family Deductible

Family deductibles work the same way individual deductibles do in that once a certain limit is reached, no more deductible is taken. For a **family deductible**, a specified number of family members must satisfy their individual deductible. Once the required number of family members meets their individual deductible, the family deductible is then considered met for the remaining family members. There are two types of family deductibles: aggregate and nonaggregate.

An **aggregate deductible** requires all major medical deductibles applied for all family members be added together to attain the family limit.

A **nonaggregate** deductible requires a specified number of individual deductibles be satisfied before the family limit is met.

On the Job Now

Directions: Indicate the individual and family deductible amount for the following contracts.

Winter Insurance Company/White Corporation _____

_____

Rover Insurers, Inc./Red Corporation _____

_____

Ball Insurance Carrier/Blue Corporation _____

_____

Directions: Fill in the deductible amount that should be paid on this claim.

The Barton family is covered under the Winter Insurance contract. The following is an accumulation of their deductible amounts:

Family Member	Deductible Met
Billy	$25
Barry	$45
Bobby	$85
Betty	$0
Family Deductible Met Total to date	$155

Betty now submits a claim for $500 in services. She need only pay $_____ toward her deductible as, when added to the family total, the $200 family deductible limit is met. Even though none of the family members have met their individual limit, the family limit has been satisfied. Therefore, no more deductible will be taken on any member of this family.

In nonaggregate family deductible limits, the added sum of what each family member has paid is not important. Rather, a specified number of individuals in the family must meet their individual deductible limit in order for the family limit to be met. Nonaggregate family limits often require that the family pay more money toward the deductible.

On the Job Now

Directions: Fill in the deductible amount that should be paid on this claim.

The Barton family is now covered under the Ball Insurance Carrier contract. The following is an accumulation of their deductible amounts:

Family Member	Deductible Met
Billy	$25
Barry	$45
Bobby	$85
Betty	$0
Family Deductible Met Total to date	$155

Betty now submits a claim for $500 in services. She must pay the $_____ toward her deductible. Even then, the family deductible has still not been satisfied.

If the next claim is for Billy for $75, the full $75 amount would be considered part of the deductible, thus bringing the amount Billy has paid toward his deductible to $100. However, the family deductible still has not been met because only one family member (Betty), not two, have reached their individual family limit.

Only when Billy, Barry, or Bobby has paid $125 toward their deductible will the family deductible be considered to be met. At that time, no more deductible would be taken on any member of the family.

Practice Pitfalls

As a biller, try to be aware of where each member of a family stands in relation to their deductible payments. This can be done fairly simply by looking at the patient ledger for each family member. The patient with the most charges during the year has probably gone the farthest toward meeting their deductible. Also, if the insurance carrier has previously made several payments, the deductible has usually (although not always) been satisfied.

If more than one member of a family is being treated, consider submitting the bill for the member(s) with the highest payments on their deductible. Then submit the claims for the other family members at a later date.

Let's assume that the entire Barton family came down with an illness and had to come in for office visits. The whole family comes in and is treated on the same day. You check their charts and discover that they are covered by the Ball contract and:

Family Member	Deductible Met
Billy	$25
Barry	$45
Bobby	$85
Betty	$0
Family Deductible Met Total to date	$155

As a biller, it would be best to submit the claims for Bobby and Barry first, and then submit the claims for the remaining family members about a week later. This would ensure that only an additional $120 in deductible ($40 on Bobby and $80 on Barry) would have to be covered by the family. If all the bills were submitted at once, the claims examiner may choose to process the claims for Betty and Billy first, thus taking a deductible of $225 ($125 on Betty and $100 on Billy).

Coinsurance and Copayments

Coinsurance is an agreement to share expenses between the member and the insurance carrier. This is usually expressed in percentages (i.e., the insurance covers 80% of the approved amount of a bill, and the patient covers 20%). A **copayment** is a fixed amount a member must pay for a covered service.

It is important for the biller to know the coinsurance percentage on a patient's insurance in order to collect the proper payment from the patient at the time services are rendered. Let's say you are visited by a patient who is covered under the Ball Contract and has not yet met their deductible. If the services totaled $500, you should collect $200 from the patient. First collect the $125 deductible for which the patient will be responsible, then collect 20% of the remaining $375 ($75).

Collecting the patient's portion of the payment before the patient leaves the office is one way to ensure that most of the bill will be paid. If a medical biller overcharges the patient, the insurance carrier will pay benefits to the provider only up to the amount of their bill. If additional monies are due, the insurance carrier will reimburse the patient.

Coinsurance Limit or Out-of-Pocket Limit

Many insurance companies are aware that the costs of a catastrophic illness can ruin a family financially. Because insurance carriers want to keep people enrolled, they must leave them with enough resources to consistently pay premiums. For this reason, many insurance carriers have a coinsurance limit, also called an out-of-pocket limit. This limit stipulates that if the coinsurance portion of a patient's bills reaches a certain amount, all subsequent claims will be paid at 100% of the allowed amount. For example, the Ball Contract has a coinsurance limit of $400. Because the coinsurance amount is based on 20% of the allowed amount (with the insurance covering 80% of the allowed amount), the patient must have bills with approved amounts totaling over $2,125 in a calendar year ($125 is applied toward the deductible, $2,000 multiplied by 20% equals the $400 limit).

As a medical biller, if your patient has an illness that generates numerous claims totaling large amounts, you should attempt to schedule as many of the visits in the same year as possible. This will allow bills that are over the coinsurance limit to be paid at a higher percentage than those under it, thus decreasing the burden on the family and allowing the doctor a greater possibility of collecting the full amount.

On the Job Now

Directions: Study the contracts on the following pages and complete the following questions. Write your answers in the space provided.

What is the coinsurance limit for:

Winter Insurance Company/White Corporation _____

_____

Rover Insurers, Inc./Red Corporation _____

_____

Ball Insurance Carriers/Blue Corporation _____

_____

Mental/Nervous Expenses

Mental and Nervous expenses include claims submitted for psychiatric services, marriage and family counseling services, and drug and alcohol treatment. Often there are different limits and coinsurance percentages for mental and nervous expenses.

Many contracts have a calendar year maximum or a maximum number of visits for these types of services.

It is important for the biller to understand any limits on the number of treatments or amounts covered by insurance. Make the doctor aware of these limits so that the doctor can suggest or schedule treatments accordingly.

Lifetime Maximum

There is a **lifetime maximum** payment amount for most contracts. Once the patient reaches the lifetime maximum amount, the insurance carrier will not cover any additional expenses. The lifetime maximum is the total dollar payments the insurance carrier will make toward the lifetime care of this patient. However, this amount is so high that it is seldom reached, except in extreme cases.

Billers should be aware of this maximum amount, especially for patients with high medical expenses or those who have been with the same insurance carrier (and under the same policy) for an extended period of time.

If the patient is about to reach their lifetime maximum (or may reach it within the next year) suggest to the patient that they may want to consider switching their insurance coverage. This is especially relevant if the patient is covered under a policy provided by their employer. If the employer offers more than one plan, the employee may be able to switch plans during the open enrollment period when they are sure to get coverage. Proof of good health is not required during an open enrollment period.

Preexisting Limitations

Many contracts will not cover conditions that existed before a patient was covered under a contract (called **preexisting conditions**). This prevents a patient from not paying for insurance coverage, then discovering that they have a serious illness and seeking insurance to cover that illness.

The term preexisting has a different meaning for each contract. Most often, it is defined as a condition for which the patient has sought treatment within a given time period before insurance coverage has begun. If the patient has sought treatment for such a

condition before coverage, benefits for treatment may not be covered or may be limited to a certain dollar amount. Usually, the restrictions for benefits will cease once the patient has been covered under a contract for 12 months or longer. A few contracts allow coverage after six months.

Some contracts also have a "treatment-free" period. With this provision, if the patient can go without treatment for a specified period of time (often 90 days), then the insurance carrier will no longer consider the condition to be preexisting and will cover the illness or condition under the normal terms of the contract.

Remember that treatment includes any kind of contact in relationship with the illness, including the office visit or testing that was used to diagnose the illness. It also includes treatment of the condition, tests or office visits to monitor the condition, and filling of prescriptions relating to the condition.

If you become aware that a preexisting situation may exist, discuss the options with the doctor. It may be possible to schedule treatments in such a way that benefits will not be cut too drastically. Also, be sure to note when coverage for the condition will begin, usually after the person has been covered by the contract for 12 months. This may allow for better scheduling of treatments near that date so that the procedures are covered.

HIPAA/Health Insurance Portability

On August 26, 1996, a new law regarding health insurance was signed by President Clinton. This law is called the Health Insurance Portability and Accountability Act of 1996 (HIPAA). The most important changes include preexisting limitations, prior coverage certification, and privacy issues.

Under the new law, preexisting exclusions are limited to six months, and credit must be given for prior coverage. Therefore, if a person is covered by insurance, and then transfers insurance coverage to a new company within 63 days of ceasing coverage at the old company, the new insurance carrier may not apply preexisting provisions. If there was a break of more than 63 days between the termination of the old coverage and the available date of new coverage, preexisting exclusions are limited to six months.

Preexisting limitations are also not allowed for pregnancy or newborns. Therefore, if a woman transfers coverage when she is pregnant, then the new insurance carrier must cover the costs associated with the pregnancy.

If a person declines coverage under a new plan because they are covered under a previously existing plan, and then they lose their benefits under the old plan, they may then enroll under the new plan without preexisting limitations. Preexisting limitations may not be applied to those who transfer from one plan to another during a company's open-enrollment period.

Companies also are now required to provide written certification of all prior coverage. They must provide this information upon termination of coverage.

Consolidated Omnibus Budget Reconciliation Act (COBRA)

Congress passed the landmark Consolidation Omnibus Budget Reconciliation Act health benefit provisions in 1986. The law amends the Employee Retirement Income Security Act (ERISA), the Internal Revenue Code, and the Public Health Services Act to provide continuation of group health coverage that otherwise would be terminated.

COBRA contains provisions giving certain former employees, retirees, spouses, and dependent children the right to temporary continuation of health coverage at group rates. This coverage, however, is only available in specific instances. Group health coverage for COBRA participants is usually more expensive than health coverage for active employees, as usually the employer formerly paid a part of the premium. It is ordinarily less expensive, however, than individual health coverage.

Employees are no longer allowed to continue COBRA coverage on a policy if they are covered under a new policy. In the past, many employees would continue coverage on an old policy until the preexisting limitation had been satisfied on the new insurance. Because the new insurance is no longer allowed to apply preexisting limitations, the need for this coverage has been eliminated. Many people may still elect to continue coverage on the old policy until they have satisfied any length of employment requirements (i.e., must be employed for 90 days). However, the waiting period is not considered a break in coverage for purposes of the 63-day break in coverage. Therefore, if an employee terminates at one company (and ceases coverage), and is hired at a second company within 63 days, they are considered continuously covered even if they must satisfy a 90-day waiting period before coverage begins with their new employer.

When hiring, employers are not allowed to discriminate against those with higher medical costs. This is true even though the higher costs will eventually show an increase in the company's insurance premiums.

For those who do not satisfy the continuous coverage requirements, preexisting exclusions are limited to conditions for which treatment was received within six months before coverage. Exclusions are only allowed to remain in effect for 12 months. Therefore, after 12 months the carrier must cover the condition, whether it was preexisting or not. If a person did not enroll when they first became eligible, then preexisting exclusions are allowed to continue for up to 18 months. This is because some people will not apply for coverage until they have a condition that they know is going to require extensive treatment. They will then attempt to get coverage on that condition.

A new insurance carrier may choose to enact the preexisting limitations on certain items that were not included in previous medical coverage. This allowance is limited to coverage for mental health, substance abuse treatment, prescriptions, dental care, and vision care. For example, if a participant's old plan did not include coverage for mental health benefits, then the new plan may elect to enact a preexisting limit only on the mental health benefits which it normally offers in the plan.

Practice Pitfalls

When a patient transfers insurance, changes employers, or loses eligibility under their insurance (i.e., a child reaches maximum dependent age), they should be issued a certificate that details their previous coverage. Because this is a new situation, many patients may not be aware of the significance of this certificate.

Ask patients to provide a copy of this certificate and file this copy in the patient's chart. If the patient then receives treatment for a condition that would be considered preexisting, include a copy of the certificate with the patient's claim. This will help to prevent denial of the claim.

On the Job Now

Directions: Read each scenario below and determine whether or not the certificate of prior insurance should be included with the claim, and why or why not. (PY = prior year; CY = current year.)

1. Jennifer received treatment for a chronic ulcer on 7/1/PY and again on 8/1/PY. On 10/1/PY she quit her old job and began working for a new employer on 10/15/PY. She immediately signed up for insurance and her coverage became effective after a 30-day waiting period, on 11/15/PY. On 1/15/CY she was seen by a doctor for additional ulcer treatment. Should you send in a copy of her coverage certificate with the 1/15/CY claim? _____

   _____

   _____

2. Mary received treatment for diabetes on 7/1/PY and again on 8/1/PY. On 10/1/PY she quit her old job and began working for a new employer two weeks later, on 10/15/PY. She immediately signed up for insurance and her coverage became effective after a 90-day waiting period, on 1/15/CY. On 10/15/CY she was seen by a doctor for additional diabetes treatment. Should you send in a copy of her coverage certificate with the 10/15/CY claim? _____

   _____

   _____

3. Tom received treatment for kidney disease 2/1/CY and again on 3/1/CY. On 10/1/CY he quit his old job and began working for a new employer two weeks later, on 10/15/CY. He immediately signed up for insurance and his coverage became effective after a 30-day waiting period, on 11/15/CY. On 12/15/CY he was seen by a doctor for additional kidney disease treatment. Should you send in a copy of his coverage certificate with the 12/15/CY claim? _____

   _____

   _____

4. Betty received a routine visit for pregnancy on 7/1/PY and again on 8/1/PY. On 10/1/PY she began working for a new employer. She immediately signed up for insurance and her coverage became effective after a 30-day waiting period, on 12/15/PY. She did not have prior coverage. On 1/15/CY she was seen by a doctor for an additional routine visit. Should you send in a copy of her coverage certificate with the 1/15/CY claim? _____

   _____

   _____

5. Jessie received treatment for anorexia on 7/1/PY and again on 8/1/PY. On 10/1/PY she quit her old job and chose not to continue coverage under COBRA rules. On 12/15/PY she began working for a new employer. She immediately signed up for insurance and her coverage became effective after a 30-day waiting period, on 1/15/CY. On 10/25/PY she was seen by a doctor for additional anorexia treatment. Should you send in a copy of her coverage certificate with the 10/25/PY claim? _____

   _____

   _____

Exclusions

Every contract will have a list of **exclusions**. These are items that the insurance carrier does not cover. It is important to check the list of exclusions before scheduling surgery or other expensive treatments for a patient. If the procedures or treatments are not covered, the patient will be responsible for the entire amount of the bill. Many doctors who routinely perform procedures that are not covered (i.e., cosmetic surgeons) often will require payment in full before scheduling the surgery.

Allowed Amounts

Insurance carriers limit payment to a specified amount. The **allowed amount** is what the insurance company considers to be a reasonable charge for the procedure performed, and is often less than the amount that the doctor bills.

A nationwide listing of allowable amounts is not really equitable because it costs a lot more to do business in Los Angeles (higher nurse and secretary salaries, rents, costs of supplies, etc.) than it does in a rural medical clinic in Louisiana. Because of this, a system called **Usual, Customary, and Reasonable (UCR)** was established.

Under UCR, each procedure that is performed has been given a number value (called a relative unit value) based on how difficult the procedure is to perform, the overhead involved, and the chance of incurring a malpractice lawsuit. For example, it takes a lot more skill, time, and medical supplies to perform brain surgery than it does to clean a skinned knee and put a bandage on it. Therefore, brain surgery is given a much higher unit value than cleaning and bandaging a skinned knee. Because each procedure has a different unit value, there are often several codes for the same type of procedure. For example, there are five different codes for an office visit of a new patient. The code used depends on how difficult the patient's condition is to treat and the skill level involved in this treatment. Because different unit values are assigned to each code, it is important that the biller code the procedures correctly.

This unit value is multiplied by a conversion factor. A **conversion factor** is a numerical factor used to multiply or divide to arrive at a sum. The conversion factor is determined by the first three digits of the zip code in which the services were performed and what type of services they were.

The type of service is broken out into four groups:

- Medical Services (office visits).
- Surgical Services (procedures which invade the body).
- X-ray and Laboratory Procedures (x-rays taken and lab tests performed).
- Anesthesia Services.

Although the unit value for a procedure would remain the same no matter where in the nation it was performed, the conversion factor would change depending on the cost of doing business in a given area. Thus, the factors for Louisiana would be far less than those for Los Angeles.

Multiplying the conversion factor by the unit value gives you the allowed amount. Applicable deductible and coinsurance amounts are subtracted from the allowed amount before the insurance carrier makes payment.

Some insurance plans do not use allowed amounts or usual and customary charges in determining claim payments but instead base payment on a fee schedule. A **fee schedule** is a list of predetermined charges for medical services and supplies. Reimbursement for services rendered to patients under a fee schedule based plan is limited to the maximum charge allowed by the fee schedule at the time of the service or the provider's fee, whichever is lower.

Practice Pitfalls

If the claim is for $125 but the allowed amount of the procedure(s) is $75, the insurance carrier will only apply that $75 toward the deductible. Thus, even though the patient is paying $125 for the services, only $75 of their deductible limit has been met. The patient would still need another $50 (under the Ball Insurance Carriers contract) of allowed charges to meet their deductible.

Likewise, if the claim is for $500 and the allowed amount is $350, the patient could be responsible for quite a large a bill. Under the Ball contract, the $125 deductible would be subtracted from the allowed amount, leaving $225. This would then be multiplied by the 80% coinsurance rate and the insurance carrier would send a check for $180. The patient would be responsible for the remaining $320.

Not all insurance carriers use the same list of relative value units. Therefore, the allowed amount for one insurance carrier will be different from the allowed amount of a different insurance carrier.

Additionally, the insurance carrier will never consider more than the billed amount. Therefore, if the allowed amount for a bill is $200, but the doctor only charged $150, the insurance carrier will consider the billed amount to be the allowed amount of $150. The carrier will then subtract any remaining deductible to be paid, and multiply the remainder by the coinsurance percent.

As a biller, if you notice that the doctor's charges for a particular procedure are always the same as the allowed amount, it may mean that the doctor is charging less than what the insurance carriers consider to be reasonable for that procedure. Discuss this with the doctor and consider raising the billed amount for this procedure.

Likewise, if the allowed amount is always significantly lower than the billed amount, you may wish to discuss lowering the fee with the doctor. Be aware that allowed amounts are nearly always lower than billed amounts, so lowering of fees should not be done without serious consideration.

Precertification of Inpatient Admissions

To **precertify** means to get preapproval for admission on elective, nonemergency hospitalization. Contact is made either with the plan administrator or another entity sanctioned to determine the necessity of the admission. Most often, these entities are composed of a specialized group of nurses working under the direction of a physician. The nurses deal directly with the physician's office and the facility to determine whether the admission is necessary and whether the number of days of care is medically necessary. If the patient stays longer than the approved number of days, the additional days of care

may not be paid for or the usual payment may be reduced by a percentage specified by the plan. The objective in this program is to prevent unnecessary admissions and to get the patient out of the hospital as soon as is medically appropriate.

For these reasons, it is important that all medical billers check the terms of the contract if possible. Often information on precertification is included directly on the patient's insurance card. This information will say something like:

> *All voluntary inpatient admissions must be precertified 48 hours prior to admission. In case of emergency admission, please contact the carrier within 24 hours of admission or benefits may be reduced or services not covered.*

Some programs provide for precertification only before or on the day of hospitalization. Other programs provide for a complete approach to managing the care, which entails a utilization review program.

As part of HIPAA, the Federal Government has mandated that no precertification can be required on maternity confinements. The law stipulates a confinement for a normal delivery cannot be limited to less than 48 hours (two days) or in the case of a Cesarean section 96 hours (four days). The law, however, does not state that a concurrent review could not be done. Therefore, if the patient stays hospital confined beyond the two days for a normal delivery or four days for a C-section and the plan has concurrent review and extended stay provisions, applicable penalties can be imposed on those extra days.

Utilization Review

As previously indicated, precertification or a **prospective review** determines the need and appropriateness of the recommended care. **Utilization Review** is the process for monitoring the use and delivery of medical services. Utilization Review (UR) programs contain the following three components:

1. Precertification (before) or prospective review.

2. Concurrent review (during the confinement).

3. Retrospective review (after termination of confinement).

Concurrent review determines whether the estimated length of time and scope of the inpatient stay is justified by the diagnosis and symptoms. This review is conducted periodically during the projected length of time the patient is in the hospital. If the length of stay exceeds the criteria or if there is a change in treatment, the matter is referred to the medical consultant for review.

At no time does the consultant dictate the method of treatment or the length of stay. These decisions are left entirely to the patient and the attending physician. However, the consultant is entitled to inform the patient, physician, and facility that the continued stay exceeds the approved number of days and may not be covered by the plan as medically necessary. It is then the patient's responsibility to decide what course to take.

Retrospective review is used to determine after discharge whether the hospitalization and treatment were medically necessary and covered by the terms of the benefit program. This type of review may be used as a substitute for admission and concurrent reviews when the failure to notify the UR program of an admission prevents the regular review procedures. However, the main drawback to the retrospective review is that the patient and providers are not notified about the services that will not be covered until after they have been provided. The best programs always work most effectively when the patient is notified beforehand that he or she will be primarily responsible for payment of services. This approach deters the member from incurring unnecessary expenses.

Second Surgical Opinion Consultations

Surgical claims represent the second highest categorical cost to carriers (hospitalization ranks first). The United States has the world's highest rate of surgical treatment because neither the physician nor the patient has much financial incentive to consider less expensive alternatives.

About 80% of all surgeries can be considered "elective." That is, they are not required because of a life-threatening situation. The objective of a **Second Surgical Opinion Consultation (SSO)** is to eliminate elective surgical procedures that are classified as unnecessary.

Unnecessary surgery is that which is recommended as an elective procedure when an alternative method of treatment may be preferable for a number of reasons, including:

- The surgery itself may be premature, taking into consideration all pathologic indications.

- The risk to the patient may not justify the benefits of surgery.

- An alternative medical treatment may be superior for both medical and cost-effective reasons.

- A less severe surgical procedure may be preferable under the circumstances; or no medical or surgical procedure may be necessary at all.

In this program, the patient consults an independent specialist to determine whether the recommended elective surgical procedure is advisable. This process is not intended to interfere with the patient–physician relationship or to prevent the patient from receiving necessary elective operations.

This program may be administered in one of two ways:

1. A **mandatory program** requires the patient to obtain an SSO for special procedures, or there is an automatic reduction or denial of benefits. For an example of this type of program, see the Rover Insurers, Inc. contract.

2. A **voluntary program** encourages participants to have an SSO, but there is no automatic reduction of benefits if the patient does not comply. In both approaches, the SSO and related tests are usually paid at 100% so that the patient will not have any out-of-pocket expenses for conforming to the program.

The SSO program has met with much criticism because it has not effectively reduced the number of elective surgeries. One of the main reasons for this ineffectiveness is that physicians may be reluctant to tell a patient that a surgery is not necessary. This attitude stems from the growing number of malpractice lawsuits. For example, if a physician states that a patient does not need surgery and a sudden emergency situation arises that is related to the original need for surgery, the physician may be held liable under a malpractice suit. Consequently, many plans are abandoning the SSO plan provision.

On the Job Now

Directions: Review the contracts at the end of this chapter and indicate which contracts have a second surgical benefit provision.

_____

_____

Coordination of Benefits

Coordination of benefits (COB) is a process that occurs when two or more plans provide coverage on the same person. Coordination between the two plans is necessary to allow for payment of 100% of the allowable expense.

Before standardized coordination rules were adopted by the benefits industry, a person covered under two policies could collect full benefits from both. Thus, the member could actually make a profit by being sick or injured. Because each plan would prefer to pay as the secondary payer, it became necessary to develop rules to determine when a plan should pay as primary, secondary, or tertiary.

The 13 rules determining the order of payment are referred to as the **Order of Benefit Determinations (OBD)** (see Appendix C).

Definitions

Words commonly found in COB provisions are defined as follows:

Allowable Expense—Any necessary, reasonable, and customary item of medical or dental expense, at least partly covered under at least one of the plans covering the patient. Items excluded by the secondary plan, such as dental services and vision care services, would not be considered allowable. Conversely, amounts limited under the secondary plan would be considered allowable (the entire charge). For example:

1. Each plan provides a limit of $35 per visit for outpatient psychiatric care. The psychiatrist charges $50 per visit. As long as the $50 is within the UCR guidelines of one of the two plans, the entire $50 would be considered an allowable expense under COB.

2. Based on the primary plan's UCR guidelines, the amount allowed for a surgery is $1,200. The secondary plan's UCR for the same surgery is $1,000. When coordinating benefits, the secondary plan would allow the greatest amount allowed by at least one of the plans. Therefore, the allowable amount when coordinating would be $1,200.

Claim Determination Period—Usually means a calendar year. It does not include any part of a year before the effective date of duplicate coverage under the secondary plan.

Explanation of Benefits (EOB)—A letter from a payer indicating how a member's benefits have been applied in response to the submission of a claim. The EOB indicates deductibles, coinsurance amounts, nonallowed amounts, UCR limitations, and other variable items. An EOB is required by law to be generated on each claim submission showing the disposition of the claim (how it was paid, denied, or pended for additional information).

Group Plan—A form of coverage with which coordination of benefits is allowed. A plan may include:

- Group, blanket, or franchise insurance policy or plan if not individually underwritten.
- Health maintenance organization or hospital or medical service prepayment policy available through an employer, union, or association.
- Trustee policy or plan, union welfare policy or plan, multiple employer policy or plan, or employee benefit policy or plan.
- Governmental programs (Medicare) or policies or plans required by a statute, except Medicaid.
- "No fault" auto policy or plan. (Applies to some plans only. The plan must specify whether or not this is applicable.)

Primary Plan—Benefit plan that determines and pays its benefits first without regard to the existence of any other coverage.

Secondary Plan—Plan that pays after the primary plan has paid its benefits. The benefits of the secondary plan take into consideration the benefits of the primary plan and may reduce its payment so that only 100% of allowable expenses is paid.

On the Job Now

Directions: Assume that all of the adults in the following questions have active coverage. For each scenario, indicate which party would be primary, secondary, tertiary, and so on, by writing 1, 2, 3, or 4 in the blank space next to the person. If the person is not responsible for the dependent(s) at all, write N/A.

1. A remarried mother has custody of her children six months of the year. Her coverage was effective 6/1/1999 and her date of birth (DOB) is 10/15/CCYY-35. The natural father's coverage was effective 5/1/2000 and his date of birth is 8/10/CCYY-41. The mother's husband's coverage was effective 5/1/1998 and his date of birth is 9/1/CCYY-32. The father's wife's coverage was effective 6/15/1999 and her date of birth is 7/4/CCYY-44.

   _____ Mother _____ Father _____ Stepfather _____ Stepmother

2. A remarried mother has custody of her children. However, by court decree, the father has financial responsibility for their healthcare costs. The mother's DOB is 4/1/CCYY-34 and her coverage was effective 2/15/2000. The father's DOB is 3/15/CCYY-37 and his coverage was effective 3/1/1997. The stepfather's DOB is 12/15/CCYY-37 and his coverage was effective 3/1/1996. The stepmother's DOB is 8/17/CCYY-35 and her coverage was effective 6/1/1999.

   _____ Mother _____ Father _____ Stepfather _____ Stepmother

3. Two natural parents are married. The mother's DOB is 7/1/CCYY-28. The father's DOB is 7/1/CCYY-29. The mother's effective date of coverage is 6/1/1998. The father's effective date of coverage is 6/1/1999.

   _____ Mother _____ Father _____ Stepfather _____ Stepmother

4. Two natural parents are married. The mother's DOB is 7/1/CCYY-28. The father's DOB is 7/1/CCYY-29. The mother's effective date of coverage is 6/1/1998. The father's effective date of coverage is 6/1/1999. The mother's plan does not have a COB provision.

   _____ Mother _____ Father _____ Stepfather _____ Stepmother

5. Two natural parents are divorced and neither has remarried. By court decree, the grandparents have legal custody of the children. Also by court decree, the father has financial responsibility for the children's medical care. The mother's DOB is 4/1/CCYY-34 and her coverage was effective 2/15/2000. The father's DOB is 3/15/CCYY-37 and his coverage was effective 3/1/1997. The grandmother's DOB is 12/15/CCYY-60 and her coverage was effective 3/15/1986. The grandfather's DOB is 8/17/CCYY-65 and his coverage was effective 6/1/1989.

   _____ Mother _____ Father _____ Grandfather _____ Grandmother

CHAPTER REVIEW

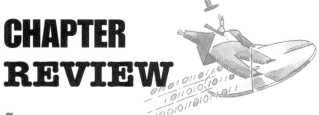

Summary

- It is vital that medical billers understand how to properly interpret the basic and major medical benefits of a contract.

- It will take practice to accurately understand the coverages provided under contracts, and to suggest treatment options that will provide the greatest benefits.

- Medical billers must understand important provisions in a contract such as preauthorization and precertification that can impact payment on a patient's claim.

Assignments

Complete the Questions for Review.
Complete Exercises 3–1 through 3–6.

Questions for Review

Directions: Answer the following questions without looking back into the material just covered. Write your answers in the space provided.

1. What is eligibility? _____

_____

2. Basic benefits are usually paid at 100% and are _____

_____

3. Define accident. _____

_____

4. What is preadmission testing? _____

_____

5. What is outpatient surgery? _____

_____

6. What is a deductible? _____

_____

7. Define aggregate family deductible. _____

_____

8. What is coinsurance? _____

_____

9. What happens when a patient reaches their coinsurance limit? _____

_____

10. What are mental/nervous expenses? _____

_____

11. What happens when a patient reaches their lifetime maximum? _____

12. What is a preexisting condition? _____

_____

13. What is an exclusion? _____

14. What is an allowed amount? _____

_____

15. How do you get the allowed amount? _____

16. The _____ is the benefit plan that determines and pays its benefits first without regard to the existence of any other coverage?

17. The _____ is the plan that pays after the primary plan has paid its benefits.

18. What is a Group Plan? _____

_____

19. What is an EOB? _____

_____

20. What does it mean to be Actively-at-Work? _____

_____

If you are unable to answer any of these questions, refer back to that section in the chapter, and then fill in the answers.

Exercise 3-1

Directions: Calculate the amount of deductible that will be taken and answer the following questions.

The Apple family is covered under the Winter Insurance Company/White Corporation contract. Their previous deductible payments are as follows:

200 Agg.

	Annie	Adam	April	August	Ashley
Carryover paid	0.00	5.00	10.00	55.00	0.00
Deductible paid	10.00	0.00	5.00	5.00	0.00
		55	*15*	*60*	

1. What is the individual deductible limit on this contract? 1. _100._

2. What is the family deductible limit on this contract? 2. _200_

3. Is the family limit aggregate or nonaggregate? 3. _Ag_

4. How much has been paid toward the family deductible? 4. _20_

5. Annie incurs allowed charges of $35. How much will be applied to the deductible? 5. _35_

6. How much has Annie now met on her deductible? 6. _45_

7. How much has now been paid toward the family deductible? 7. _55_

8. August incurs allowed charges of $55. How much will be applied to the deductible? 8. _40._

Pd 5 toward Ded + 55 last yr so 60 Applied

9. How much has August now met on his deductible? 9. _100._

10. How much has now been paid toward the family deductible? 10. _95_

11. April incurs allowed charges of $55. How much will be applied to the deductible? 11. _55_

12. How much has April now met on her deductible? 12. _70_

13. How much has now been paid toward the family deductible? 13. _150._

14. Adam incurs allowed charges of $60. How much will be applied to the deductible? 14. _50_

15. How much has Adam now met on his deductible? 15. _55_

16. How much has now been paid toward the family deductible? 16. _200_

17. Annie incurs allowed charges of $35. How much will be applied to the deductible? 17. _0_

18. How much has Annie now met on her deductible? 18. _45_

19. How much has now been paid toward the family deductible? 19. _200_

Exercise 3-2

Directions: Calculate the amount of deductible that will be taken and answer the following questions.

The Bear family is covered under the Rover Insurers, Inc./Red Corporation contract. Their previous deductible payments are as follows:

	Brad	**Bonnie**	**Barbra**	**Brian**
Carryover paid	0.00	5.00	10.00	55.00
Deductible paid	10.00	0.00	5.00	5.00

1. What is the individual deductible limit on this contract?   1. _150_

2. What is the family deductible limit on this contract?   2. _300_

3. Is the family limit aggregate or nonaggregate?   3. _Non-Ag_

4. How many people are needed to meet the family deductible for this year?   4. _2_

5. Bonnie incurs allowed charges of $55. How much will be applied to the deductible?   5. _55_

6. How much has Bonnie now met on her deductible?   6. _60_

7. How many people are now needed to meet the family deductible?   7. _2_

8. Brian incurs allowed charges of $85. How much will be applied to the deductible?   8. _85_

9. How much has Brian now met on his deductible?   9. _145_

10. How many people are now needed to meet the family deductible?   10. _2_

11. Barbra incurs allowed charges of $105. How much will be applied to the deductible?   11. _105_

12. How much has Barbra now met on her deductible?   12. _120_

13. How many people are now needed to meet the family deductible?   13. _2_

14. Brad incurs allowed charges of $60. How much will be applied to the deductible?   14. _60_

15. How much has Brad now met on his deductible?   15. _70_

16. How many people are now needed to meet the family deductible?   16. _2_

17. Bonnie incurs allowed charges of $35. How much will be applied to the deductible?   17. _35_

18. How much has Bonnie now met on her deductible?   18. _95_

19. How many people are now needed to meet the family deductible?   19. _2_

20. Brian incurs allowed charges of $35. How much will be applied to the deductible?   20. _5_

21. How much has Brian now met on his deductible? 21. _150_

22. How many people are now needed to meet the family deductible? 22. _2_

Carry over from last yr only
95 counts

23. Barbra incurs allowed charges of $55. How much will be applied to the deductible? 23. _36_

24. How much has Barbra now met on her deductible? 24. _150_

25. How many people are now needed to meet the family deductible? 25. _2_

26. Brad incurs allowed charges of $60. How much will be applied to the deductible? 26. _60_

27. How much has Brad now met on his deductible? 27. _130_

28. How many people are now needed to meet the family deductible? 28. _2_

29. Bonnie incurs allowed charges of $35. How much will be applied to the deductible? 29. _35_

30. How much has Bonnie now met on her deductible? 30. _130_

31. How many people are now needed to meet the family deductible? 31. _2_

3/4 had carry overs from previous yr.

Exercise 3-3

Directions: Calculate the amount of deductible that will be taken and answer the following questions.

The Carpenter family is covered under the Ball Insurance Carriers/Blue Corporation contract. Their previous deductible payments are as follows:

	Carry	Connie	Cathy	Chris
Carryover paid	0.00	5.00	10.00	55.00
Deductible paid	10.00	0.00	5.00	5.00

1. What is the individual deductible limit on this contract? 1. _125_

2. What is the family deductible limit on this contract? 2. _250_

3. Is the family limit aggregate or nonaggregate? 3. _NON AG_

4. How many people are needed to meet the family deductible? 4. _2_

5. Connie incurs allowed charges of $35. How much will be applied to the deductible? 5. _35_

6. How much has Connie now met on her deductible? 6. _40_

7. How many people are now needed to meet the family deductible? 7. _2_

8. Carry incurs allowed charges of $55. How much will be applied to the deductible? 8. _55_

9. How much has Carry now met on her deductible? 9. _65_

10. How many people are now needed to meet the family deductible?

11. Chris incurs allowed charges of $60. How much will be applied to the deductible?

12. How much has Chris now met on his deductible?

13. How many people are now needed to meet the family deductible?

14. Chris incurs allowed charges of $35. How much will be applied to the deductible? *Met*

15. How much has Chris now met on his deductible?

16. How many people are now needed to meet the family deductible?

17. Connie incurs allowed charges of $95. How much will be applied to the deductible?

18. How much has Connie now met on her deductible?

19. How many people are now needed to meet the family deductible?

20. Carry incurs allowed charges of $45. How much will be applied to the deductible?

21. How much has Carry now met on her deductible?

22. How many people are now needed to meet the family deductible?

23. Cathy incurs allowed charges of $105. How much will be applied to the deductible?

24. How much has Cathy now met on her deductible?

25. How many people are now needed to meet the family deductible?

26. Carry incurs allowed charges of $85. How much will be applied to the deductible?

27. How much has Carry now met on her deductible?

28. How many people are now needed to meet the family deductible? *Carry met current yr*

29. Chris incurs allowed charges of $85. How much will be applied to the deductible?

30. How much has Chris now met on his deductible?

31. How many people are now needed to meet the family deductible?

32. Cathy incurs allowed charges of $90. How much will be applied to the deductible?

33. How much has Cathy now met on her deductible?

34. How many people are now needed to meet the family deductible?

10. 2
11. 60
12. 120
13. 2
14. 5
15. 125
16. 2
17. 85
18. 125
19. 2
20. 45
21. 110
22. 2
23. 105
24. 120
25. 2
26. 15
27. 120
28. 1
29. 0
30. 125
31. 1
32. 5
33. 125
34. 1

Exercise **3-4**

Directions: Find and circle the words listed below. Words can appear horizontally, vertically, diagonally, forward, or backward.

```
P S J D S K Q T T S U B W L V R Z O P I X G
B M A O B L S M C M N V S A B F G R J I P W
C J A S E A T F L J N O E C E Y E K B H Y R
O F R R I F S C L B F W I X N A M J U D R A
I P S P G L A I L V U T Z S D Z G A S R E X
N H O I K K R W C I K L N M U U Y M P C G K
S R J V B D D J E B R G I B E L S Z O B R J
U P E W C I T G S B E S S V V M C V D O U Y
R F K H A P V Y S X S N A Z Y R U X W Z S K
A W E I V E R E V I T C E P S O R T E R Y Z
N Q B J S H Y I O T I G B F N N A M F C R G
C T R Z O F L N N P F V Y G I Y Z E Y T A T
E C X B X W T E E M D B B P L T E Q F B S Z
A L L O W E D A M O U N T E K S S I Q S D
R Z U B S I B Q S S C B V D C N R Q T T E Y
R U A T C G V K D G X I H H L R Z D R S C O
H N I C E A X D G B T Z E P D Y D B E A E M
C N A M A P T F T C L D L S Y A M K C L N W
G K S U N N I F A T U Q U Q Y S X K E Q N D
L Q N W G M O E J L F H I T Q R V X R U U R
M W A S J Q C W E F L P N W V U K J P I J M
E L B I T C U D E D R Z X P K T B A X I K F
```

1. Accident
2. Actively-at-Work
3. Allowed Amount
4. Basic Benefits
5. Coinsurance
6. Deductible

7. Exclusions
8. Fee Schedule
9. Preadmission Testing
10. Precertify
11. Retrospective Review
12. Unnecessary Surgery

Exercise 3-5

Directions: Complete the crossword puzzle by filling in a word from the keywords that fits each clue.

Across

2. An amount that the member pays at each visit.

8. A deductible that requires that a specified number of family members must satisfy their individual deductible.

10. The total dollar payments the insurance carrier will make toward the lifetime care of a patient.

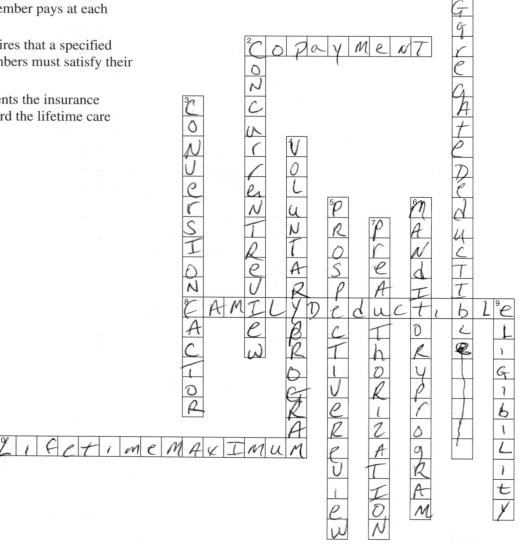

Down

1. A deductible that requires all major medical deductibles applied for all family members be added together to attain the family limit.

2. The process for monitoring the use and delivery of medical services.

3. A numerical factor used to multiply or divide to arrive at a sum.

4. Encourages participants to have an SSO, but there is no automatic reduction of benefits if the patient does not comply.

5. Determines the need and appropriateness of the recommended care.

6. Requires the patient to obtain an SSO for special procedures, or there is an automatic reduction or denial of benefits.

7. To gain approval of the services that are to be performed, and often to obtain an understanding of whether or not the insurance carrier will provide coverage for those services.

9. The qualifications that make a person eligible for coverage.

Exercise 3-6

Directions: Match the following terms with the proper definition by writing the letter of the correct definition in the space next to the term.

1. __F__ Authorized Treatment Record Form

2. __H__ Carryover Provisions

3. __J__ Coordination of Benefits

4. __I__ Indemnity Insurance Plans

5. __A__ Mental and Nervous Expenses

6. __C__ Nonaggregate Deductible

7. __E__ Order of Benefit Determinations

8. __G__ Preexisting Conditions

9. __B__ Second Surgical Opinion Consultation

10. __D__ Usual, Customary, and Reasonable (UCR)

a. Claims submitted for psychiatric services, marriage and family counseling, and drug and alcohol treatment.

b. Used to eliminate elective surgical procedures that are classified as unnecessary.

c. A deductible that requires a specified number of individual deductibles be satisfied before the family limit is met.

d. Under this system, each procedure that is performed has been given a number value (called a relative unit value) based on how difficult the procedure is to perform, the overhead involved, and the chance of incurring a malpractice lawsuit.

e. The 13 rules determining the order of insurance benefit payment.

f. A form used to track the usage of preauthorized services rendered by a provider's office.

g. Conditions that existed before a patient was covered under a contract.

h. Any amounts that the patient pays toward their deductible in the last three months of the year will carry over and will be applied toward the next year's deductible.

i. A principle of insurance that provides medical coverage when a loss occurs, and restores the insured party to their approximate financial condition that they had before the loss occurred.

j. A process that occurs when two or more plans provide coverage on the same person. Coordination between the two plans is necessary to allow for payment of 100% of the allowable expense.

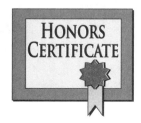

Honors Certification™

The certification challenge for this chapter will be a written test of the information contained in this chapter. Each incorrect answer will result in a deduction of up to 5% from your grade. You must achieve a score of 85% or higher to pass this test. If you fail the test on your first attempt, you may retake the test one additional time. The items included in the second test may be different from those in the first test.

BALL INSURANCE CARRIERS   *(800) 555-5432*

3895 Bubble Blvd. Ste. 283, Boxwood, CO 85926   (970) 555-5432

INSURANCE CONTACT: __Betty Bell__   PHONE NUMBER: __(970) 555-9876__

Policy: Blue Corporation, 9817 Bobcat Blvd., Bastion, CO 81319
Insurance Group # and Suffix: 98135/BLUE

Basic/Major Medical Plan   Effective 09/1/93

ELIGIBILITY EMPLOYEE: Must work a minimum of 30 hours per week. Is eligible for coverage the first of the month following three consecutive months of continuous employment.
DEPENDENTS: Are eligible for coverage from birth to age 19 or to age 23 if a full-time student or handicapped prior to age 19/23 (proof of disability must be furnished within 31 days after dependent reaches limiting age). Not eligible as a dependent if eligible as an employee. Unmarried natural children, legally adopted and foster children are included (includes legal guardianship). If both parents are covered by the plan, children may be covered by one employee only.

EFFECTIVE DATE EMPLOYEE: If written application is made prior to eligibility date, coverage becomes effective the first of the month following three months of continuous employment.
DEPENDENTS: The date acquired by the covered employee becomes the effective date if written application is made within 31 days of eligibility date. If confined in a hospital on date of eligibility, coverage will not start until the first of the month following the date the confinement ends. Newborns are automatically covered for the first 30 days following birth. Coverage will be terminated after 30 days unless written application for coverage is submitted by the employee within 31 days of birth.

TERMINATION OF COVERAGE EMPLOYEE: Coverage terminates the last day of the month following termination of employment, or when the employee ceases to qualify as an eligible employee, or following request for termination of coverage.
DEPENDENTS: Coverage terminates the date the employee's coverage terminates or the last day of the month during which the dependent no longer qualifies as an eligible dependent.

BASIC BENEFITS

PREADMISSION TESTING - Outpatient diagnostic tests performed prior to inpatient admissions; paid at 100% of UCR.

SUPPLEMENTAL ACCIDENT EXPENSE - 100% of the first $300 for services incurred within 90 days of accident.
INPATIENT HOSPITAL EXPENSE
  DEDUCTIBLE: $50.
  ROOM AND BOARD: 100% Up to semi-private room charge. ICU up to $600 per day.
  MISCELLANEOUS FEES: 100% Unlimited.
  MAXIMUM PERIOD: Ten days per period of disability.
SURGERY
  CONVERSION FACTOR: $8.50.
  CALENDAR YEAR MAXIMUM: $1,600 per person.
  REMARKS: Voluntary sterilizations covered.
ASSISTANT SURGERY
  CONVERSION FACTOR: $8.50.
  CALENDAR YEAR MAXIMUM ALLOWANCE: $320 per person. Maximum of 20% of surgeon's allowance or billed charge, whichever is less.
  REMARKS: Voluntary sterilizations covered for women only.
IN-HOSPITAL PHYSICIANS
  DAILY MAXIMUM: $21 for the first day; $8 per day thereafter.
  MAXIMUM PERIOD: Ten days per period of disability.
  REMARKS: Only one doctor can be paid per day.

ANESTHESIA
CONVERSION FACTOR: $7.50.
CALENDAR YEAR MAXIMUM: $300 per person.
REMARKS: Voluntary sterilizations covered.

OUTPATIENT PHYSICIANS VISITS
CONVERSION FACTOR: $7.50.
CALENDAR YEAR MAXIMUM: $300 per person.
REMARKS: Chiropractors, M.D.s, D.O.s and acupuncturists allowed.

X-RAY AND LABORATORY
CONVERSION FACTOR: $7.
CALENDAR YEAR MAXIMUM: $200 per person.
REMARKS: Professional component charges covered at 40% of UCR allowance for procedure. Routine procedures are not covered.

MAJOR MEDICAL EXPENSES

INDIVIDUAL CALENDAR YEAR DEDUCTIBLE: $125; three month carryover provision.

FAMILY MAXIMUM DEDUCTIBLE: Two family members must satisfy their individual calendar year deductible in order to satisfy the family deductible.

STANDARD COINSURANCE: 80%.

COINSURANCE LIMIT: $400 out-of-pocket per individual; $800 out-of-pocket per family (not to include deductible); aggregate.

APPLICATION OF COINSURANCE LIMIT: Coinsurance limit applies in the calendar year in which the limit is met and the following calendar year.

OUTPATIENT MENTAL/NERVOUS EXPENSE: 50% coinsurance while not a hospital inpatient.

LIFETIME MAXIMUM: $1,000,000 per person.

ROOM LIMIT: Semi-private room rate.

HOSPITAL DEDUCTIBLE: Not covered.

HOME HEALTH CARE: 120 visits per calendar year. Prior hospital confinement required.

PREEXISTING LIMITATION: If treatment received within six months prior to effective date, $2,000 maximum payment until patient has been covered continuously under the plan for 12 months.

ANESTHESIA: Calculated using actual time.

MEDICARE
TYPE: Coordination of Benefits.
REMARKS: Assume all Medicare benefits whether or not individual actually enrolled. Subject to all other plan provisions.

EXCLUSIONS
1. Expenses resulting from self-inflicted injuries.
2. Work-related injuries or illnesses.
3. Services for which there is no charge in the absence of insurance.
4. Charges or services in excess of UCR or not medically necessary.
5. Charges for completion of claim forms and failure to keep appointments.
6. Routine or preventative or experimental services.
7. Eye refractions; contacts or glasses; orthotics (eye exercises); radial keratotomy or other procedures for surgical correction of refractive errors.
8. Custodial care.
9. Cosmetic surgery unless for repair of an injury or surgery incurred while covered or result of mastectomy.
10. Dental care of teeth, gums or alveolar process (TMJ) except: a) reduction of fractures of the jaw or facial bones; b) surgical correction of harelip, cleft palate or prognathism; c) removal of salivary duct stones; d) removal of bony cysts of jaw, torus palatinus, leukoplakia, or malignant tissues.
11. Reversal of voluntary sterilization.
12. Diagnosis or treatment of infertility including artificial insemination, in vitro fertilization, etc.
13. Contraceptive materials or devices.
14. Non-therapeutic abortions except where the life of the mother is endangered.

15. Expenses for obesity, weight reduction, or diet control unless at least 100 lbs. overweight.
16. Vitamins, food supplements and/or protein supplements.
17. Sex-altering treatments or surgeries or related studies.
18. Orthopedic shoes or other devices for support or treatment of feet except as medically necessary following foot surgery.
19. Bio-feedback related services or treatment.
20. Experimental transplants.
21. EDTA Chelation therapy.

COMPREHENSIVE DENTAL BENEFITS

DEDUCTIBLE: $50.
FAMILY DEDUCTIBLE LIMIT: $150; nonaggregate. COINSURANCE: 80%.
MAXIMUM: No lifetime maximum. $1,000 per calendar year maximum.
SPACE MAINTAINER ELIGIBILITY: Employees and dependents.
FLUORIDE ELIGIBILITY: Dependents up to age 18 only.
ORTHODONTIA: No coverage.
CLAIM COST CONTROL: Predetermination of benefits and alternate course of treatment based on customarily employed methods.
PROSTHETIC REPLACEMENTS: Five-year replacement rule applies to replacements of any previously installed prosthetics.
ORDERED AND UNDELIVERED: Excludes expenses for any devices installed or delivered after 30 days following termination of insurance.
ORAL SURGERY: Covered at regular coinsurance rate, subject to calendar year maximum.
EXTENSION OF BENEFITS: 12 months.
MISSING AND UNREPLACED: Applies.

ROVER INSURERS INC.
5931 ROLLING ROAD
RONSON, CO 81369
(970) 555-1369

INSURANCE CONTACT: Ravyn Ranger   **PHONE NUMBER:** (970) 555-0863
POLICY: RED CORPORATION, 1234 Nockout Road, Newton, NM 88012   **EFFECTIVE 01/01/01**
INSURANCE GROUP # AND SUFFIX: 41935/RED

ELIGIBILITY EMPLOYEES must work a minimum of 30 hours per week. They are eligible for coverage the first of the month following one consecutive month of continuous employment. DEPENDENTS are eligible for coverage from birth to age 19, or to age 25 if a full-time student or handicapped prior to age 19/25. Is not eligible as a dependent if eligible as an employee. Unmarried natural children, legally adopted children, foster children, and legal guardianship children are included. If both parents are covered by the plan, children may be covered by one parent only.

EFFECTIVE DATE - EMPLOYEE becomes effective, if written application is made prior to eligibility date, on the first of the month following 30 days of continuous employment. If employee is absent from work due to disability on the date of eligibility, coverage will not start until the first of the month following the date of return to active work.
DEPENDENTS become effective on the date the covered employee becomes effective, if written application is made within 31 days of eligibility date. If confined in a hospital on the date of eligibility, coverage will not start until the first of the month following the date the confinement ends. Newborns are automatically covered for the first 14 days following birth. Coverage terminates after 14 days unless written application for coverage is submitted by the employee within 31 days of birth.

TERMINATION OF COVERAGE - EMPLOYEE'S coverage terminates the last day of the month following termination of employment or when the employee ceases to qualify as an eligible employee, or following request for termination of coverage. DEPENDENTS' coverage terminates the date the employee's coverage terminates, or the last day of the month during which the dependent no longer qualifies as an eligible dependent.

EXTENSION OF BENEFITS - If covered under the plan when disabled, may continue coverage in accordance with COBRA. No other extension available.

COMPREHENSIVE MEDICAL BENEFITS

PREADMISSION TESTING - Outpatient diagnostic tests performed prior to inpatient admissions are paid at 100% whether through a network provider or not.

PRECERTIFICATION - Voluntary, nonemergency inpatient admissions must be approved at least five days prior to admission. Emergency admissions must be precertified within 48 hrs. of admission. Benefits are reduced to 50% if not performed as required.

SECOND SURGICAL OPINION - The SSO is paid at 100% of UCR. It is required for the following: bunionectomy, cataract extraction, chemonucleolysis, cholecystectomy, coronary bypass, hemorrhoidectomy, hysterectomy, inguinal herniorrhaphy, laparotomy, laminectomy, mastectomy, meniscectomy, oophorectomy, prostatectomy, salpingectomy, submucous resection, total joint replacement (hip or knee), tenotomy, varicose veins (all procedures). **IF SSO NOT PERFORMED, ALL RELATED EXPENSES PAYABLE AT 50%.**

SUPPLEMENTAL ACCIDENT EXPENSE - 100% is paid on the first $500 for services incurred within 90 days of the date of accident. Subject to $20 copayment. After $500, payments are subject to calendar year deductible. Provider does not have to be a network member to receive 100% benefit. Common accident provision applies.

OUTPATIENT FACILITY CHARGES PAYABLE AT 100% - Network outpatient facility expenses for following procedures paid 100%. Does not include professional charges: arthroscopy, breast biopsy, cataract removal, bronchoscopy, deviated nasal septum, pilonidal cyst, myringotomy w/tubes, esophagoscopy, colonoscopy, herniorrhaphy (umbilical, to five years old), skin and subsequent lesions, benign and malignant (2cms+).

INDIVIDUAL CALENDAR YEAR DEDUCTIBLE - $150; three month carryover provision. All plan services subject to deductible unless otherwise indicated.

FAMILY MAXIMUM DEDUCTIBLE - $300, nonaggregate. Two family members must meet individual deductible limit.

STANDARD COINSURANCE - 80% for Network providers; 60% for Non-network providers.

COINSURANCE LIMIT - $1,250 out-of-pocket per individual; $2,500 out-of-pocket per family. Two individuals must meet their individual out-of-pocket limit to satisfy the family limit. Limits not to include deductible, surgery expenses reduced because SSO not performed, or hospital benefits reduced because precertification not performed. 100% of allowed amount paid thereafter for network providers; 80% for non-network providers.

LIFETIME MAXIMUM - $1,000,000 per person.

PREEXISTING LIMITATION - If treatment is received within 90 days prior to effective date, no coverage on that condition for six months from the effective date (continuously covered for six consecutive months) unless treatment free for three consecutive months which ends after the effective date of coverage.

INPATIENT HOSPITAL EXPENSE IF NO PRECERTIFICATION, ADMISSION PAID AT 50%
DEDUCTIBLE - $200, waived for network facilities, applies to non-network. Inpatient hospital expenses not subject to regular Major Medical deductible.
ROOM AND BOARD - Network providers: 80% of semi-private/ICU; Non-network providers: 60% of semi-private/ICU.
MISCELLANEOUS FEES - Network: 80%; Non-network: 60%.
EXCLUSIONS - Well baby care. Automatic coverage for first seven days if baby is ill. Otherwise, no coverage.

MENTAL/NERVOUS/PSYCHONEUROTIC - Includes substance abuse and alcoholism.
OUTPATIENT MENTAL AND NERVOUS TREATMENT
PAYABLE - $60 per visit for first 5 visits; $30 per visit for next 21 visits.
COINSURANCE - 80% for first five visits (maximum payable: $60 per visit), 50% per visit for next 21 visits (maximum payable: $30 per visit).
CALENDAR YEAR MAXIMUM - 26 visits.
INPATIENT MENTAL AND NERVOUS TREATMENT
PHYSICIAN SERVICES - 70% applies to network and non-network providers.
HOSPITAL SERVICES - 70% network and non-network providers.

MAMMOGRAMS
COINSURANCE - 80% Network providers; 60% Non-network providers.
REQUIREMENTS - Baseline mammogram for women age 35–39; for ages 40–49, one allowed every two years; for ages 50+, one allowed every year.

X-RAY AND LABORATORY - PROFESSIONAL COMPONENTS - Professional charges paid at 25% of UCR.

DURABLE MEDICAL EQUIPMENT
COINSURANCE - 50%.
REQUIREMENTS - Prescribed by M.D.; must not be primarily necessary for exercise, environmental control, convenience, comfort or hygiene. Must be an article only useful for the prescribed patient. Covered up to purchase price only.

ANESTHESIA: Use actual time.

MEDICARE
TYPE - Maintenance of benefits.
REMARKS - Assume all Medicare benefits whether or not individual actually enrolled. Subject to all other plan provisions.

EXCLUSIONS
1. Expenses resulting from self-inflicted injuries.
2. Work-related injuries or illnesses.
3. Services for which there is no charge in the absence of insurance.
4. Charges or services in excess of UCR or not medically necessary.
5. Preexisting conditions.
6. Charges for completion of claim forms and failure to keep appointments.
7. Routine or preventative or experimental services.
8. Eye refractions; contacts or glasses; orthotics (eye exercises); radial keratotomy or other procedures for surgical correction of refractive errors.
9. Custodial care.
10. Cosmetic surgery unless for repair of an injury or surgery incurred while covered or result of mastectomy.
11. Biofeedback related services or treatment.
12. Dental care of teeth, gums or alveolar process (TMJ) except: a) reduction of fractures of the jaw or facial bones; b) surgical correction of harelip, cleft palate or prognathism; c) removal of salivary duct stones; d) removal of bony cysts of jaw, torus palatinus, leukoplakia, or malignant tissues.
13. Reversal of voluntary sterilization.
14. Diagnosis or treatment of infertility including artificial insemination, in vitro fertilization, etc.
15. Contraceptive materials or devices.
16. Pregnancy; pregnancy-related expenses of dependent children for the delivery including Caesarian section. Related illnesses may be covered such as pre-eclampsia, vaginal bleeding, etc.
17. Non-therapeutic abortions except where the life of the mother is endangered.
18. Vitamins.

WINTER INSURANCE CO, 9763 WESTERN WAY, WHITTIER, CO 82963, (970) 555-2963
POLICY: WHITE CORPORATION, 1234 Whitaker Lane, Colter, CO 81222   EFFECTIVE DATE: 06/01/02
INSURANCE GROUP # and SUFFIX: 54321/WHI
INSURANCE CONTACT: Wilma Williams   PHONE NUMBER: (970) 555-1234

ELIGIBILITY EMPLOYEE: Must work a minimum of 35 hours per week. Is eligible for coverage the first of the month following 60 consecutive days of continuous employment.
DEPENDENTS: Are eligible for coverage from birth to age 19, or to age 24 if a full-time student or handicapped prior to age 19/24 (proof of disability must be furnished within 31 days after dependent reaches limiting age). Dependent is not eligible as a dependent if eligible as an employee. Unmarried natural children, legally adopted and foster children are included (also includes legal guardianship). If both parents are covered by the plan, children may be covered by one employee only.

EFFECTIVE DATE EMPLOYEE: If written application is made prior to the eligibility date, coverage becomes effective the first of the month following 60 days of employment.
DEPENDENTS: The date acquired by the covered employee becomes the effective date if written application is made within 31 days of the eligibility date. Newborns are automatically covered for the first seven days following birth; well-baby charges excluded. Coverage will terminate after seven days unless written application for coverage is submitted by the employee within 31 days of birth.

TERMINATION OF COVERAGE EMPLOYEE: Coverage terminates the last day of the month following termination of employment or when the employee ceases to qualify as an eligible employee, or following request for termination of coverage.
DEPENDENTS: Coverage terminates the date the employee's coverage terminates, or the last day of the month during which the dependent no longer qualifies as an eligible dependent.

EXTENSION OF BENEFITS - If covered under the plan when disabled, employee may continue coverage for 12 months following the date of termination or until no longer disabled, whichever is less.

COMPREHENSIVE MEDICAL BENEFITS

SUPPLEMENTAL ACCIDENT EXPENSE - 100% of first $300 for services incurred within 120 days of date of accident. Not subject to deductible.

PLAN BENEFITS INDIVIDUAL CALENDAR YEAR DEDUCTIBLE: $100; three month carry-over provision.
FAMILY MAXIMUM DEDUCTIBLE: $200, aggregate.
STANDARD COINSURANCE: 90% except 100% of hospital room and board expenses for 365 days per lifetime.
COINSURANCE LIMIT: $750 out-of-pocket per individual; $1,500 out-of-pocket per family. Two separate members must satisfy the individual limit, not to include deductible. Applies only in the calendar year in which the limit is met.
LIFETIME MAXIMUM: $300,000 per person.
PREEXISTING LIMITATION: On 6/1/02 no restriction. After 6/1/02, if treatment received within 90 days prior to effective date, no coverage for that condition for 12 months from the effective date (continuously covered for 12 months) unless treatment free for three consecutive months ending after the effective date of coverage.

X-RAY AND LABORATORY REMARKS: Professional component charges covered at 40% of UCR allowance for procedure. Routine procedures are not covered.

INPATIENT HOSPITAL EXPENSE Room and board payable at 100% of semi-private room rate. Miscellaneous expenses covered at 90%. Nonmedically necessary, well baby care and cosmetic services excluded. Personal comfort items not covered.

MENTAL/NERVOUS/PSYCHONEUROTIC INCLUDES SUBSTANCE ABUSE AND ALCOHOLISM.
OUTPATIENT MENTAL/NERVOUS TREATMENT
COINSURANCE: 50% while not hospital confined.
CALENDAR YEAR MAXIMUM: None.
INPATIENT MENTAL/NERVOUS TREATMENT
PHYSICIAN SERVICES: Covered at 90%.
HOSPITAL SERVICES: Covered at 90%.
ALLOWED PROVIDERS: Psychiatrists and clinical psychologists. Marriage and Family Child Counselor and Licensed Clinical Social Worker allowed with referral from M.D.

EXTENDED CARE FACILITY LIFETIME MAXIMUM: 60 days.
HOSPITAL SERVICES: 80% of billed room and board charge.
REQUIREMENTS: Stay must begin within 14 days of acute hospital stay of at least three days. Extended care must be due to same disability that caused hospitalization and continued hospital care would otherwise be required.

DURABLE MEDICAL EQUIPMENT COINSURANCE: Covered at 90%.
REQUIREMENTS: Must be prescribed by M.D. Must not be primarily necessary for exercise, environmental control, convenience, comfort, or hygiene. Must only be useful for the prescribed patient. Covered up to purchase price only.

ANESTHESIA Computed using block time.

REMARKS Covered expenses include charges for the initial set of contact lenses which are necessary due to cataract surgery. Handicapped children are limited to a $15,000 lifetime maximum after attainment of age 19. Coordination of Benefits according to National Association of Insurance Carriers (NAIC) guidelines. Subject to Third Party Liability and subrogation.

MEDICARE INTEGRATION TYPE: Nonduplication of benefits applies.
REMARKS: Assume all Medicare benefits whether or not individual actually enrolled.

EXCLUSIONS
1. Expenses resulting from self-inflicted injuries, work related injuries, or illnesses.
2. Charges or services: in excess of UCR, not medically necessary, for completion of claim forms, for failure to keep appointments; for routine, preventative or experimental services.
3. Eye refractions; contacts or glasses; orthotics (eye exercises); radial keratotomy or other procedures for surgical correction of refractive errors.
4. Custodial care and/or convalescent facility coverage.
5. Cosmetic surgery unless for repair of an injury or surgery incurred while covered or result of mastectomy.
6. Diagnosis or treatment of infertility including artificial insemination, in vitro fertilization, etc., contraceptive materials or devices, non-therapeutic abortions except where the life of the mother is endangered, reversal of voluntary sterilization.
7. Pregnancy-related expenses for dependent children.
8. Expenses for obesity, weight reduction, or diet control unless at least 100 lbs. overweight.
9. Vitamins, food supplements, and/or protein supplements.
10. Sex altering treatments or surgeries or related studies.
11. Orthopedic shoes or other devices for support or treatment of feet except as medically necessary following foot surgery.
12. Bio-feedback related services or treatment, EDTA chelation therapy.

COMPREHENSIVE DENTAL BENEFITS

INTEGRATED: Deductible provisions, lifetime maximum and coinsurance limit combined with comprehensive Major Medical.

CALENDAR YEAR DEDUCTIBLE: $100.

DEDUCTIBLE CARRYOVER: No carryover.

FAMILY DEDUCTIBLE LIMIT: $200, aggregate.

COINSURANCE: 90%.

COINSURANCE LIMIT: $500 (Patient responsibility, not to include disallowed amounts or the deductible.)

APPLICATION OF COINSURANCE LIMIT: Applies only in the calendar year in which the limit is met.

FAMILY COINSURANCE LIMIT: $1,000.

MAXIMUM: $300,000 lifetime.

MAXIMUM PER CALENDAR YEAR: $1,500.

ORTHODONTIA ELIGIBILITY: Dependents only.

SPACE MAINTAINER ELIGIBILITY: Dependents only.

FLUORIDE ELIGIBILITY: Employees and dependents.

ORTHODONTIC: 90% coinsurance.

ORTHODONTIC MAXIMUM: $800 lifetime; not subject to the $1,500 calendar year maximum.

CLAIM COST CONTROL OPTIONS: Predetermination of benefits required on claims over $500; alternate course of treatment based on customarily employed method. Benefits cut to 50% if no predetermination done.

PROSTHETIC REPLACEMENTS: Five-year rule applies to replacement of any previously installed prosthetics.

ORDERED AND UNDELIVERED: Excludes expenses for any devices installed or delivered after 30 days following termination date of insurance.

MISSING AND UNREPLACED EXCLUSION: Applies.

REMARKS: Orthodontic benefits are payable as incurred, rather than amortized over the period of time during which work is performed.

SMALL GROUP HMO CONTRACT

[Carrier] Summer Insurance Company
18932 Spring Road, Autumn, CO 82974
(970) 555-9631

CONTRACT HOLDER: Rocky Corporation
1234 Ribbon Road, Rudolph, CO 81208
Effective Date of Contract: January 1, 1998
Insurance Group # and Suffix: 67980/ROC

INSURANCE CONTACT: Sammy Rock

PHONE NUMBER: (970) 555-0846

ELIGIBILITY

Employees: Actively at work for a minimum of 35 hours per week. Is eligible after 30 continuous work days. Employees who enroll more than 30 days after their employment date are considered Late Enrollees. Late Enrollees are subject to this Contract's Preexisting Conditions limitation.

Coverage terminates the date an Employee ceases to be an Actively at Work, Full-Time Employee for any reason.

Dependents: Dependents include the Employee's legal spouse, the Employee's unmarried Dependent children who are under age 19, and the Employee's unmarried Dependent children, from age 19 until their 23rd birthday, who are enrolled as full-time students at accredited schools. Exception: Any dependent who does not reside in the Service Area is not an eligible Dependent. Eligible Dependents will not include any Dependent who is covered by this Contract as an Employee or on active duty in the armed forces of any country.

"Unmarried Dependent children" include legally adopted children, step-children if they depend on the Employee for most of their support and maintenance and children under a court appointed guardianship.

THE ROLE OF A MEMBER'S PRIMARY CARE PHYSICIAN (PCP)

A Member's PCP provides basic health maintenance services and coordinates a Member's overall health care. Anytime a Member needs medical care, the Member should contact his or her Primary Care Physician. In a Medical Emergency, a Member may go directly to the emergency room. If a Member does, then the Member must call his or her Primary Care Physician or the Care Manager and Member Services within 48 hours, or We will provide services under this HMO Plan only if We determine that notice was given as soon as was reasonably possible.

REFERRAL FORMS

A Member can be referred for Specialist Services by a Member's PCP. Except in the case of a Medical Emergency, a Member will not be eligible for any services provided by anyone other than a Member's PCP (including but not limited to Specialist Services) if a Member has not been referred by his or her PCP. Referrals must be obtained prior to receiving services and supplies from any Practitioner other than the Member's PCP.

MEDICAL NECESSITY

Members will receive designated benefits only when Medically Necessary and Appropriate. We or the Care Manager may determine whether any benefit was Medically Necessary and Appropriate, and We have the option to select the appropriate Participating Hospital to render services if hospitalization is necessary. Decisions as to what is Medically Necessary and Appropriate are subject to review by our quality assessment committee or its physician designee.

LIMITATION ON SERVICES

Except in cases of Medical Emergency, services are available only from Participating Providers. We shall have no liability or obligation to cover any service or benefit sought or received by a Member from any Physician, Hospital, other Provider unless prior arrangements are made by Us.

SCHEDULE OF SERVICES AND SUPPLIES

The services or supplies covered under the contract are subject to all copayments and are determined per calendar year per Member, unless otherwise stated. Maximums apply only to the specific services provided.

SERVICES COPAYMENTS: Copayment $15, unless otherwise stated

Emergency Room Copayment $50, credited toward Inpatient admission if admitted within 24 hours

Coinsurance 0% except as stated on the Schedule of Services and Supplies for Prescription Drugs

MAXIMUM LIFETIME BENEFITS Unlimited, **except** as otherwise stated

HOSPITAL SERVICES:

Inpatient $150 Copayment/day for a maximum of 5 days/admission. Maximum Copayment $1,500/Calendar Year. Unlimited days.

Outpatient $15 Copayment/visit

PRACTITIONER SERVICES RECEIVED AT A

HOSPITAL:

Inpatient Visit $0 Copayment

Outpatient Visit $15 Copayment/visit; no Copayment if any other Copayment applies.

Emergency Room $50 Copayment/visit/Member (credited toward Inpatient Admission if Admission occurs within 24 hours)

SURGERY:

Inpatient $0 Copayment

Outpatient $15 Copayment/visit

HOME HEALTH CARE Unlimited days, if preapproved; $0 Copayment.

HOSPICE SERVICES Unlimited days, if preapproved; $0 Copayment.

MATERNITY/PRENATAL CARE $25 Copayment for initial visit only; $0 Copayment thereafter.

MENTAL NERVOUS CONDITIONS AND SUBSTANCE ABUSE:

Outpatient $15 Copayment/visit maximum 20 visits/Calendar Year.

Inpatient $150 Copayment/day for a maximum of 5 days per admission. Maximum Copayment: $1,500/ Calendar Year. Maximum of 30 days inpatient care/ Calendar Year. One Inpatient day may be exchanged for two Outpatient visits.

THERAPEUTIC MANIPULATION $15 Copayment/visit; maximum 30 visits/Calendar Year

PODIATRIC $15 Copayment/visit (excludes Routine Foot Care).

PREADMISSION TESTING $15 Copayment/visit.

PRESCRIPTION DRUG 50% Coinsurance [May be substituted by Carrier with $15 Copayment.]

PRIMARY CARE PHYSICIAN $15 Copayment/visit.

OR CARE MANAGER SERVICES (OUTSIDE HOSPITAL)

PRIMARY CARE SERVICES $15 Copayment/visit.

REHABILITATION SERVICES Subject to the Inpatient Hospital Services Copayment above. The Copayment does not apply if Admission is immediately preceded by a Hospital Inpatient Stay.

SECOND SURGICAL OPINION $15 Copayment/visit.

SPECIALIST SERVICES $15 Copayment/visit.

SKILLED NURSING CENTER Unlimited days, if preapproved; $0 Copayment.

THERAPY SERVICES $15 Copayment/visit.

DIAGNOSTIC SERVICES.

INPATIENT $0 Copayment

OUTPATIENT $15 Copayment/visit

NOTE: No services or supplies will be provided if a Member fails to obtain preauthorization of care through his or her primary care physician or health center or care manager. Read the Member provisions carefully before obtaining medical care, services or supplies. Refer to the section of this contract called "Noncovered Services and Supplies" for a list of the services and supplies for which a Member is not eligible for coverage under this contract.

COVERED SERVICES & SUPPLIES

Under this HMO Plan, Members are entitled to receive the benefits in the following sections when Medically Necessary and Appropriate, subject to the payment by Members of applicable copayments as stated in the applicable Schedule of Services and Supplies.

(a) **OUTPATIENT SERVICES.** The following services are covered only at the PCP's office, or elsewhere upon prior written Referral by a Member's PCP:

1. **Office visits** during office hours, and during non-office hours when Medically Necessary.
2. **Home visits** by a Member's PCP.
3. **Periodic health examinations** to include:
   a. Well child care from birth including immunizations;
   b. Routine physical examinations, including eye examinations;
   c. Routine gynecologic exams and related services;
   d. Routine ear and hearing examination; and
   e. Routine allergy injections and immunizations (but not if solely for the purpose of travel or as a requirement of a Member's employment).
4. **Diagnostic Services.**
5. **Casts and dressings.**
6. **Ambulance Service** when certified in writing as Medically Necessary by a Member's PCP and approved in advance by Us.
7. **Procedures and prescription drugs to enhance fertility,** except where specifically excluded in this Contract.
8. **Prosthetic Devices** when We arrange for them. We cover only the initial fitting and purchase of artificial limbs and eyes, and other prosthetic devices. We do not cover replacements, repairs, wigs.
9. **Durable Medical Equipment** when ordered by a Member's PCP and arranged through Us.
10. **Prescription Drugs and contraceptives which require a Practitioner's prescription,** insulin syringes and needles, glucose test strips and lancets, colostomy bags, belts and irrigators when obtained through a Participating Provider. A prescription or refill will not include more than:
    a. the greater of a 30 day supply or 100 unit doses for each prescription or refill; or
    b. the amount usually prescribed by the Member's Participating Provider.
11. **Nutritional Counseling** for the management of disease.
12. **Dental x-rays** when related to Covered Services.
13. **Oral surgery** in connection with bone fractures, removal of tumors and orthodontogenic cysts, and other surgical procedures, as We approve.
14. **Food and Food Products for Inherited Metabolic Diseases:** We cover charges incurred for the therapeutic treatment of inherited metabolic diseases, including the purchase of medical foods (enteral formula) and low protein modified food products. For the purpose of this benefit: "inherited metabolic disease" means a disease caused by an inherited abnormality of body chemistry for which testing is mandated by law.

(b) **INPATIENT HOSPICE, HOSPITAL, REHABILITA-
TION CENTER & SKILLED NURSING CENTER BENE-
FITS.** The following services are covered when
hospitalized by a Participating Provider at Participating
Hospitals (or at Nonparticipating facilities upon prior
written authorization by Us):

1. Semi-private room and board accommodations Except as stated below, We provide coverage for Inpatient care for:
   a. a minimum of 72 hours following a modified radi-
      cal mastectomy; and
   b. a minimum of 48 hours following a simple mas-
      tectomy.

   We also provide coverage for the mother and newly
   born child for:
   a. up to 48 hours of inpatient care following a vagi-
      nal delivery; and
   b. a minimum of 96 hours of inpatient care
      following a cesarean section.

   We provide such coverage subject to the following:
   a. the attending Practitioner must determine that in-
      patient care is medically necessary; or
   b. the mother must request the inpatient care.
2. Private accommodations will be provided only when
   approved in advance by Us. If a Member occupies a
   private room without such certification Member
   shall be liable for the difference between payment
   by Us to the Provider and the private room rate.
3. General nursing care.
4. Use of intensive or special care facilities.
5. X-ray examinations including CAT scans but not
   dental x-rays.
6. Use of operating room and related facilities.
7. Magnetic resonance imaging "MRI".
8. Drugs, medications, biologicals.
9. Cardiography/Encephalography.
10. Laboratory testing and services.
11. Pre- and postoperative care.
12. Special tests.
13. Nuclear medicine.
14. Therapy Services.
15. Oxygen and oxygen therapy.
16. Anesthesia and anesthesia services.
17. Blood, blood products and blood processing.
18. Intravenous injections and solutions.
19. Surgical, medical and obstetrical services; We also
    cover reconstructive breast Surgery, Surgery to re-
    store and achieve symmetry between the two
    breasts and the cost of prostheses following a mas-
    tectomy on one breast or both breasts.
20. Private duty nursing only when approved in ad-
    vance by Us.
21. The following transplants: Cornea, Kidney, Lung,
    Liver, Heart and Pancreas.
22. Allogeneic bone marrow transplants.
23. Autologous bone marrow transplants and associat-

ed dose intensive chemotherapy: only for treatment
of Leukemia, Lymphoma, Neuroblastoma, Aplastic
Anemia, Genetic Disorders (SCID and WISCOT
Alldrich) and Breast Cancer, when approved in advance by Us, if the Member is participating in a clinical trial.

24. Peripheral Blood Stem Cell Transplants.

(c) **BENEFITS FOR SUBSTANCE ABUSE AND NON-
BIOLOGICALLY-BASED MENTAL ILLNESSES.** The following Services are covered when rendered by a
Participating Provider at Provider's office or at a Participating Substance Abuse Center or Health Center upon
prior written referral by a Member's PCP. This section
does *not* address coverage for a Biologically-based
Mental Illness.

1. **Outpatient.** Members are entitled to receive up to
   twenty (20) outpatient visits per Calendar Year. Benefits include diagnosis, medical, psychiatric and
   psychological treatment and medical referral services by a Member's PCP or the Care Manager for
   the abuse of or addiction to drugs and Non-Biologi-
   cally-based Mental Illnesses. Payment for nonmedical ancillary services (such as vocational
   rehabilitation or employment counseling) is not provided. Members are additionally eligible, upon referral by a Member's PCP or the Care Manager, for up
   to sixty (60) more outpatient visits by exchanging
   one or more of the inpatient hospital days described
   below where each exchanged inpatient day provides two outpatient visits.
2. **Inpatient Hospital Care.** Members are entitled to receive up to thirty (30) days of inpatient care benefits
   for detoxification, medical treatment for medical conditions resulting from the substance abuse, referral
   services for substance abuse or addiction, and Non-
   Biologically-based Mental Illnesses.

(d) **BENEFITS FOR BIOLOGICALLY-BASED MENTAL
ILLNESS OR ALCOHOL ABUSE.** We cover treatment of
a Biologically-based Mental Illness or Alcohol Abuse the
same way We would for any other illness. We do not pay
for Custodial care, education or training.

(e) **EMERGENCY CARE BENEFITS - WITHIN AND
OUTSIDE OUR SERVICE AREA.** The following Services
are covered under this HMO Plan without prior written
referral by a Member's PCP in the event of a Medical
Emergency as Determined by Us.

1. A Member's PCP is required to provide or arrange
   for on-call coverage twenty-four (24) hours a day,
   seven (7) days a week. Unless a delay would be
   detrimental to a Member's health, Member shall call
   a Member's PCP or Health Center or Us or the Care
   Manager prior to seeking emergency treatment.
2. In the event Members are hospitalized in a Nonparticipating Facility, coverage will only be provided
   until Members are medically able to travel or be
   transported to a Participating Facility. If Members

elect to continue treatment with Nonparticipating Providers, We shall have no responsibility for payment beyond the date Members are Determined to be medically able to be transported. If transportation is Medically Necessary, We will cover the reasonable and customary cost. Members will be subject to all Copayments which would have been required had similar benefits been provided upon prior written referral to a Participating Provider.

3. The Copayment for an emergency room visit will be credited toward the Hospital Inpatient Copayment if Members are admitted as an Inpatient to the Hospital as a result of the Medical Emergency.

(f)   **THERAPY SERVICES.** The following Services are covered.

1. Speech, Physical, Occupational, and Cognitive Therapies are covered for non-chronic conditions and acute Illnesses and Injuries. This benefit consists of treatment for a 60 day period per incident of Illness or Injury, beginning with the first day of treatment, provided that a Member's PCP certifies in writing that the treatment will result in a significant improvement of a Member's condition within this time period and treatment is approved in writing by us.

2. Chelation Therapy, Chemotherapy treatment, Dialysis Treatment, Infusion Therapy, Radiation Therapy, and Respiration Therapy.

(g)   **HOME HEALTH SERVICES.** The following Services are covered.

1. **Skilled nursing services**, provided by or under the supervision of a registered professional nurse.

2. Services of a **home health aide**, under the supervision of a registered professional nurse, or if appropriate, a qualified speech or physical therapist.

3. **Medical Social Services** by or under the supervision of a qualified medical or psychiatric social worker, in conjunction with other Home Health Services, if the PCP certifies that such services are essential for the effective treatment of a Member's medical condition.

4. **Therapy Services** as set forth above.

5. **Hospice Care** if Members are terminally Ill or terminally Injured with life expectancy of six months or less, as certified by the Member's PCP. Services may include home and hospital visits by nurses and social workers; pain management and symptom control; instruction and supervision of family Members, inpatient care; counseling and emotional support; and other Home Health benefits listed above.

Nothing in this section shall require Us to provide Home Health Benefits when in Our Determination the treatment setting is not appropriate, or when there is a more cost effective setting in which to provide Medically Necessary and Appropriate care.

(h)   **DENTAL CARE AND TREATMENT.** The following services are covered when rendered by a Participating Practitioner upon prior Referral by a Member's PCP. We cover:

1. the diagnosis and treatment of oral tumors and cysts; and

2. the surgical removal of bony impacted teeth.

We also cover treatment of an Injury to natural teeth or the jaw, but only if:

1. the Injury occurs while the Member is covered under any health benefit plan;

2. the Injury was not caused, directly or indirectly by biting or chewing; and

3. all treatment is finished within 6 months of the date of the Injury.

Treatment includes replacing natural teeth lost due to such Injury. But in no event do we cover orthodontic treatment.

For a Member who is severely disabled or who is a child under age 6, We cover:

a. general anesthesia and Hospitalization for dental services; and

b. dental services rendered by a dentist regardless of where the dental services are provided for a medical condition covered by this Contract which requires Hospitalization or general anesthesia.

(i)   **TREATMENT FOR TEMPOROMANDIBULAR JOINT DISORDER (TMJ)** Not covered. We do not cover any services or supplies for orthodontia, crowns or bridgework.

(j)   **THERAPEUTIC MANIPULATION** Limited to 30 visits per Calendar Year, and no more than two modalities per visit.

NONCOVERED SERVICES AND SUPPLIES THE FOLLOWING ARE NOT COVERED SERVICES UNDER THIS CONTRACT.

Acupuncture except when used as a substitute for other forms of anesthesia.

Ambulance services for transportation from a Hospital or other health care Facility, unless Member is being transferred to another Inpatient health care Facility.

Broken Appointments (Charges for)

Blood or blood plasma which is replaced by or for a Member.

Care and/or treatment by a **Christian Science Practitioner**.

Completion of claim forms.

Cosmetic Surgery, except as otherwise stated in this Contract; complications of Cosmetic Surgery; drugs prescribed for cosmetic purposes.

Custodial or **domiciliary** care.

Dental care or treatment, including appliances, except as otherwise stated in this Contract.

Dose intensive chemotherapy, except as otherwise stated in this Contract.

Educational services and supplies providing: training in the activities of daily living; instruction in scholastic skills such as reading and writing; preparation for an occupation; or treatment for learning disabilities.

Experimental or Investigational treatments, procedures, hospitalizations, drugs, biological products or medical devices, except as otherwise stated in this Contract.

Extraction of teeth, except for bony impacted teeth. Services or supplies for or in connection with:

a. except as otherwise stated in this Contract, exams to determine the need for (or changes of) **eyeglasses** or lenses of any type;

b. eyeglasses or lenses of any type except initial replacements for loss of the natural lens; or

c. eye surgery such as radial keratotomy, when the primary purpose is to correct myopia (nearsightedness), hyperopia (farsightedness) or astigmatism (blurring).

Services or supplies provided by Members of the Employee's **family**.

Fertility treatments including harvesting, storage and / or manipulation of eggs and sperm. This includes, but is not limited to: in vitro fertilization; embryo transfer; embryo freezing; and Gamete intra-fallopian Transfer (GIFT) and Zygote Intrafallopian Transfer (ZIFT), drugs and drug therapy.

Hearing aids and hearing examinations to determine the need for hearing aids or the need to adjust them.

Herbal medicine.

Hypnotism.

Illegal occupations or activities.

Work-related Illness or Injury, including a condition which is the result of disease or bodily infirmity, which occurred on the job and which is covered or could have been covered for benefits provided under workers' compensation.

Local anesthesia charges.

Membership costs for health clubs, weight loss clinics and similar programs.

Marriage, career or financial counseling, sex therapy or family therapy, and related services.

Methadone maintenance.

Nonprescription drugs or supplies, except;

a. insulin needles and syringes and glucose test strips and lancets;

b. colostomy bags, belts, and irrigators; and

c. as stated in this Contract for food and food products for inherited metabolic diseases.

Pastoral counseling services.

Personal convenience or comfort items.

Any service provided without prior written Referral by the Member's **PCP**, except as specified in this Contract. In the event of a Medical Emergency, any amount which is greater than the amount We Determine to be the **reasonable and customary charge**.

Rest or convalescent cures.

Room and board charges for any period of time during which the member was not physically present overnight in the Facility.

Routine Foot Care, except:

a. an open cutting operation to treat weak, strained, flat, unstable or unbalanced feet, metatarsalgia or bunions;

b. the removal of nail roots; and

c. treatment or removal of corns, calluses or toenails in conjunction with the treatment of metabolic or peripheral vascular disease.

Self-administered services such as: biofeedback, patient-controlled analgesia on an Outpatient basis, related diagnostic testing, self-care and self-help training.

Services or supplies:

a. eligible for payment under either federal or state programs (except Medicaid and Medicare);

b. for which a charge is not usually made;

c. for which a Member would not have been charged if he or she did not have health care coverage;

d. provided by or in a Government Hospital unless the services are for treatment:
- of a nonservice Medical Emergency; or
- by a Veterans' Administration Hospital of a nonservice related Illness or Injury;

Sterilization reversal.

Sex-alteration treatment, including surgery, sex hormones, and related medical, psychological and psychiatric services; services and supplies arising from complications of sex transformation.

Telephone consultations.

Transplants, except as otherwise listed in the Contract.

Transportation.

Vision therapy.

Vitamins and dietary supplements.

Services or supplies received as a result of a **war**, declared or undeclared; police actions; services in the armed forces; or riots or insurrection.

Weight reduction or control, unless there is a diagnosis of morbid obesity; special foods, food supplements, liquid diets, diet plans or any related products.

Wigs, toupees, hair transplants, hair weaving or any drug if such drug is used in connection with baldness.

COORDINATION OF BENEFITS AND SERVICES:
OBD rules apply for coordination of benefits.

Covered Services	MEDICARE		COMMERCIAL						
	Standard	Medi-Medi	AMG	Rocky	CAT	MIPC	CAIT	SBA	RICE
Hospital visits (99221-99239)	G	G	G	G	G	G	G	G	G
Office visits (99201-99215)	-	G	G	G	G	G	G	G	G
Emergency department visits (99281-99285)	G	G	P	G	G	P	G	P	G
X-rays & Ultrasounds	G	G	G	G	G	G	G	G	G
Magnetic resonance imaging services	P	P	G	G	P	G	P	G	P
Lab fees (8001-89999)	G	G	G	G	G	G	G	G	G
Inpatient surgery									
Facility charges	P	P	P	P	P	P	P	P	P
Physician visits	G	G	G	G	G	G	G	G	G
Surgeon	P	P	G	G	P	G	G	G	G
Assistant surgeon	P	P	G	G	P	G	G	G	G
Anesthesiologist	P	P	P	P	P	P	P	P	P
X-ray technician	P	P	P	P	P	P	P	P	P
Outpatient surgery									
Facility charges	P	P	P	P	P	P	P	P	P
Physician visits	G	G	G	G	G	G	G	G	G
Surgeon	P	P	G	G	P	G	G	G	G
Assistant surgeon	P	P	G	G	P	G	G	G	G
Anesthesiologist	P	P	P	P	P	P	P	P	P
X-ray technician	P	P	P	P	P	P	P	P	P

Legend: G = Medical Group Responsibility; P = Plan/HMO Responsibility; G/P = Shared Responsibility; - = Not Covered

This chart shows a sampling of CPT® codes and the party that bears responsibility for covering costs for each procedure under numerous different plans. It is important to check the correct column for the plan being processed to determine if services are covered or not.

4

Medicare and
Medicaid

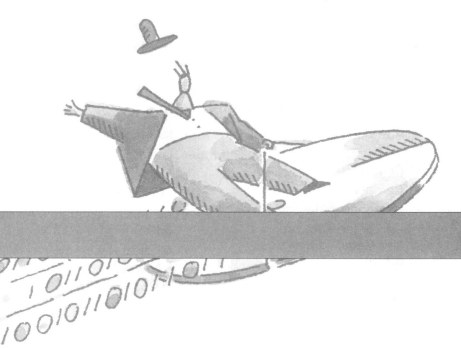

After completion of this chapter you will be able to:

- State the eligibility requirements for Medicare.
- Describe the types of Medicare coverage and the benefits for each.
- State the exceptions when patients may submit a Medicare bill themselves.
- State the guidelines for collecting the patient portion of a Medicare claim.
- List the claims that require acceptance of assignment.
- Describe how to post Medicare payments.
- Describe "Assignment of Benefits" and how it can affect the amount collected on a Medicare claim.
- Properly "balance bill" a Medicare claim.
- State the most common reasons for a "not medically necessary" denial and describe how this affects the amount collected from the patient.
- Describe how to submit claims when Medicare is coordinated with other insurance.

- Properly complete an Advance Beneficiary Notice and describe when it would be used.
- Describe the five levels in the Medicare appeals process.
- Describe what a Medicare HMO is.
- Describe the purpose of the Medicaid program.
- Explain how to verify a patient's eligibility for Medicaid coverage.
- List the benefits covered under the Medicaid program.
- Define and describe the EPSDT program.
- State the rule for time limits for Medicaid claims and the exceptions to this rule.
- List the services that require a Treatment Authorization Request.
- Properly complete a Treatment Authorization Request.
- State the guidelines for submitting Medicaid claims.

Keywords and Concepts
you will learn in this chapter:

- Advance Beneficiary Notice (ABN)
- Benefit Period
- Carriers
- Categorically Needy
- Center for Medicare and Medicaid Services (CMS)
- Clean Claims
- Diagnosis-Related Group (DRG)
- Downcoding
- Durable Medical Equipment (DME)
- Durable Medical Equipment Regional Carriers (DMERCs)
- Early and Periodic Screening, Diagnosis and Treatment (EPSDT)
- Eligibility Card
- End-Stage Renal Disease (ESRD)

- Intermediaries
- Limiting Charges
- Medically Needy
- Medicaid
- Medicaid Remittance Advice (MRA)
- Medical Necessity Denials
- Medicare
- Medicare Abuse
- Medicare Fraud
- Medicare Health Insurance Claim Number (HICN)
- Medicare HMO
- Medicare Redetermination Notice (MRN)
- Medicare Remittance Notice (MRN)
- Medicare Secondary Payer (MSP)
- Medicare Supplements

- Medicare Summary Notice (MSN)
- Medigap
- National Provider Identifiers (NPI)
- Nonparticipating Providers
- Notice of Non-Coverage
- Payer of Last Resort
- Part A
- Part B
- Part C
- Part D
- Participating Providers
- Provider Identification Number (PIN)
- Resource-Based Relative Value Scale (RBRVS)
- Share of Cost
- Unique Physician Identification Number (UPIN)

Medicare

Medicare is the Federal Health Insurance Benefit Plan for the Aged and Disabled, enacted under Title XVIII of the Social Security Act. This program is for people 65 years of age or older and also for certain people who are totally disabled. The **Center for Medicare and Medicaid Services (CMS)** is the organization that oversees the Medicare program. CMS was formerly known as the Health Care Financing Administration (HCFA).

Social Security Administration offices throughout the United States take applications for Medicare, determine eligibility, and provide general information about the program. Many different insurance companies, usually one or two within each state, administer the actual processing of the claims.

Medicare Eligibility

Following are some of the guidelines governing Medicare eligibility.

Based on Age

An individual is eligible for Medicare coverage on the first day of the month in which she reaches age 65. People born on the first day of the month are eligible on the first day of the month preceding their birth date.

Example:

Birthday: June 25, eligible for Medicare June 1

Birthday: June 1, eligible for Medicare May 1

Based on Disability

Medicare coverage for totally disabled persons begins on the first day of the 25th month from the date approved for Social Security Disability or Railroad Retirement benefits. Those covered include disabled workers of any age, disabled widows between the ages of 50 and 65, disabled beneficiaries age 18 and over who receive Social Security benefits because of disability before age 22, the blind, and Railroad Retirement annuitants.

Based on ESRD

End-stage renal disease (ESRD) occurs when a person's kidneys fail to function. As a result, the patient usually begins dialysis treatments or has a kidney transplant operation. Because of the multiple problems associated with this disease, patients are considered to be totally disabled, even though some individuals with this disease continue to work. Eligibility for Medicare ESRD is dependent upon the type of treatment the patient is receiving. As a result, the following special rules apply to ESRD patients.

The employer's group health plan is the primary payer for the first 30 months after a patient (under age 65) with ESRD becomes eligible for Medicare. This 30-month period begins based on the earlier of (1) the month in which a regular course of renal dialysis is initiated, or (2) the month the patient is hospitalized for a kidney transplant.

Medicare is the secondary payer during this 30-month period but will revert to the primary status beginning with the 31st month. As a general rule, all services under a dialysis program are Medicare-assigned (defined later in this section).

Medicare coverage is also available for ESRD beginning the fourth month if the patient does not have insurance coverage and is receiving hemodialysis. Medicare effective dates for home/self dialysis and transplants vary depending on the type of treatment and where the treatment is performed.

The Parts of Medicare

There are four parts to the Medicare program: Part A, Part B, Part C, and Part D. The services covered under the four parts of Medicare are as follows:

1. **Part A** is considered the basic plan or hospital insurance. This part covers facility charges for acute inpatient hospital care, skilled nursing, home health care, and hospice care.
2. **Part B** is the medical (supplementary, voluntary) insurance that covers physician services, outpatient hospital services, home health care, outpatient speech and physical therapy, and durable medical equipment.
3. **Part C** is the Medicare advantage portion and includes coverage in an HMO, PPO, and so on.
4. **Part D** is the prescription drug component (effective 2006).

Part A

Part A, the hospital coverage portion of Medicare, is automatic on enrollment for the following individuals:

- All people age 65 and over, if entitled to (a) monthly Social Security benefits, or (b) pensions under the Railroad Retirement Act,

- All people who reached the age of 65 before 1968, whether or not under the Social Security or Railroad Retirement Programs, and
- Workers who reach 65 in 1975 or after need 20 quarters of Social Security work credits if female, or 24 quarters of Social Security work credits if male, to be fully insured.
- Some spouses may receive Medicare benefits derived strictly from their eligible spouse's work credits. Using the eligible spouse's social security number with the appropriate letter behind it designates benefits are based on the eligible spouse.

Effective July 1, 1973, all people age 65 years and over who are not otherwise eligible for Part A may enroll by paying the full cost of such coverage, provided they also enroll in Part B. Aliens may be eligible for coverage in the Medicare program if they have been U.S. residents for five years.

Benefits

There is a Part A deductible amount that is taken from the first inpatient hospital admission. The use of Medicare benefits for an inpatient is measured by benefit periods. A **benefit period** begins with the first day of admission to the hospital. A benefit period ends after the patient has been discharged from the hospital or skilled nursing facility for a period of 60 consecutive days (including the day of discharge). A new benefit period begins and another inpatient deductible would be taken if the patient were readmitted. For 2006, the Part A deductible is $952 per benefit period. $ 1184

If a member remains in the hospital for an extended period of time, additional copayments are required. Medicare deducts the copay amount from the billed amount and then pays the amount in excess of the copay.

The 2006–inpatient hospital copayments are as follows:

- 1st day–60th day = Deductible only, no additional copayment.
- 61st day–90th day = $238 copaymen⁺
- 91st day–150th day = $476 c⌐

These days are known as the 6ᴸ
These copayments are not renew
For skilled nursing facilities (⌐
arate copayment schedule and re

eligible for this benefit, a doctor must certify the necessity of skilled nursing and rehabilitative care on a daily basis. Custodial care is not covered nor is it available for occasional rehabilitative care. In addition, the Medicare intermediary approves the stay.

The 2006 SNF copayments are as follows:

- 1st day–20th day = No copayment. Because admission is usually from an acute care facility, during which time the deductible was met, 100% of the allowable is generally paid by Medicare.
- 21st day–100th day = $119 copayment per day.

Multiple admissions can occur during a calendar year. However, the maximum number of allowable days is 100 per benefit period.

Part A claims are processed by private insurance companies called **intermediaries**.

Part B

Part B is the supplementary medical insurance, which covers physician and outpatient hospital services. It is considered a supplemental plan because each participant must pay a stipulated amount each month for the benefits. Private insurance companies, called **carriers**, process Part B claims.

The rules, limits, and maximums under this coverage are subject to change annually.

Benefits

The 2006 deductible is $124 per calendar year. After the deductible has been satisfied, generally 80% of the approved charge will be paid.

Beginning January 1, 2006, the Medicare Part B deductible will be indexed to the increase in the average cost of Part B services for Medicare beneficiaries. In other words, the amount charged for the Part B deductible will depend on the amount spent by Medicare for payments for services.

Part C

Medicare beneficiaries may choose to have covered items and services furnished to them through a Medicare Health Maintenance Organization. If a Medicare beneficiary selects this coverage, they are required to receive services according to the selected carrier's arrangements. When patients are enrolled in a Medicare HMO, claims for these patients must be submitted to the HMO.

Practice Pitfalls

Beneficiaries may enroll, disenroll, or change their Medicare HMO. For this reason, frequent verification of patient eligibility is important. To determine if the patient is enrolled in a Medicare HMO, ask the patient at the initial interview, or see if there is a sticker attached to the Medicare identification card indicating that the beneficiary has coverage through a Medicare HMO.

Part D

In an effort to provide better health coverage for Medicare beneficiaries, starting in the year 2006 Medicare beneficiaries will receive limited coverage for prescription drug benefits.

Allowable Charges

In 1992 the federal government established a standardized physician payment schedule based on a **resource-based relative value scale (RBRVS)**. The RBRVS was designed to address the soaring cost of physician health care in the United States; the imbalance between practicing in high-cost or low-cost geographic areas; and physician specialties.

Payments for services in the RBRVS system are determined by the resource costs required to provide the particular service. There basically are three components of the RBRVS: the physician's total work, relative specialty practice cost, and professional liability insurance. Payments are calculated by multiplying the combined costs of a service by a conversion factor (a monetary amount that is determined by the CMS). Payments also are adjusted for geographical differences in resource costs.

A RBRVS for a particular procedure is comprised of a physician's total work (50%); practice costs (45%); and malpractice costs (5%). Total work is defined by six factors: time; technical skill; mental effort; physical effort; judgment, and stress. These factors are measured before, during, and after the specific service or procedure. Practice costs are defined as overhead costs including office rent, nonphysician salaries, equipment and supplies.

On the Job Now

Directions: Name the four parts of Medicare and the benefits provided under each part.

P 103

1. _____
   _____

2. _____
   _____

3. _____
   _____

4. _____
   _____

Medicare Health Insurance Card (HIC)

A Medicare health insurance card is issued to every person who is entitled to Medicare benefits and may be identified by its red, white, and blue coloring. When billing for a patient who is a Medicare recipient, al-ways request the patient's Medicare health insurance card. This card indicates whether the patient has Part A (hospital); Part B (medical, physician services); Part C (HMO, PPO); or Part D (prescription drug) coverage, and when each became effective. A copy of this card should be made and placed in the patient's chart (**see Figure 4–1**).

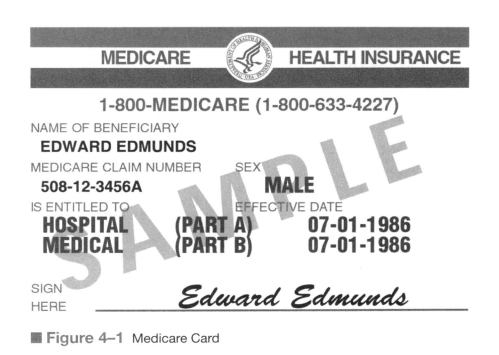

■ Figure 4–1 Medicare Card

The card identifies the Medicare beneficiary and includes the following information:

- Name as it appears on the Social Security records.
- Medicare Health Insurance Claim Number (HICN).
- Beginning date of Medicare entitlement for particular services.
- Sex.
- Place for beneficiary signature.

The patient's **Medicare health insurance claim number (HICN)** is a unique identification number assigned to Medicare beneficiaries, which normally consists of a Social Security number followed by a letter of the alphabet and possibly another letter or number (i.e., 123-45-6789A). The alpha character at the end of the number indicates how the beneficiary became entitled but does not indicate the type of coverage that the patient has. The beneficiary or provider must include the HICN on all claims submitted to Medicare for payment, as well as on all related bills or documents.

The Medicare card also has a letter code indicating the recipient's status. The letter codes are as follows:

- A—Wage earner.
- B—Spouse.
- C#—Disabled child (the C is always followed by a number).
- D—Widow.
- HDA—Disabled adult.
- J#, K#—Special monthly benefits, for an individual or spouse who has not contributed enough quarters into the Social Security Administration to automatically qualify for Medicare.
- T—Individual with end-stage renal disease.
- W—Disabled widow or widower.

Medicare entitlement extends to Railroad Retirement Beneficiaries. The HICN assigned to these individuals usually begins with an alphabetical prefix and is followed by six or nine digits (i.e., A 123-45-6789). Railroad retirees are indicated by the following letters preceding the patient's identification number:

- MA
- A
- WA
- A
- WA

Practice Pitfalls

The Medicare card should be checked at least once every year, as Medicare HICN can change according to the beneficiary's record of entitlement. This is especially true in the case of female beneficiaries, as their name, HICN, and suffix can change according to marital status. Also, a copy of the Medicare card should be made and placed in the patient's chart.

Medicare Physician Identification Numbers

Unique Physician Identification Numbers (UPINs) and Provider Identification Numbers (PINs) are assigned to providers when they enroll in Medicare. Although a provider should have only one UPIN number, he or she may have several PIN numbers. A different PIN number is assigned for each practice setting (location, specialty, and group affiliation) in which the provider participates.

UPINs

Medicare has established a **Unique Physician Identification Number (UPIN)** for identifying the physician ordering or referring services. This is a national number used to identify the physician. UPINs also are assigned to enrolling group practices, nurse practitioners, physician assistants, clinical social workers, physical and occupational therapists, and respiratory therapists.

UPINs are six digits in length and consist of a letter followed by five numbers. The numeric portion is randomly assigned. The initial letter of the UPIN indicates the type of provider as follows:

Initial Letter	Type of Practitioner
A–M	Medical doctors (medical doctors and doctors of osteopathy)
T–V	Other doctors (such as chiropractors, dentists, podiatrists, and optometrists)
R–S	Nonphysician practitioners (such as physician assistants, nurse practitioners, and certified registered nurse anesthetists)
W–Z	Group UPINs

PINs

In addition to UPIN numbers, physicians and healthcare providers who wish to bill Medicare also are assigned **Provider Identification Numbers (PINs)**.

These numbers also are known as Medicare billing numbers, Physician Profiling Numbers, and Medicare Provider Numbers. For Medicare carrier claims submitted by providers, this number identifies the provider that performed the services for the beneficiary.

Because PINs are assigned by the local carriers, they vary in structure and format from carrier to carrier.

National Provider Identifiers (NPI)

Providers must use multiple identifiers for programs and organizations with which they do business because, currently, there is no universally accepted national identification number for healthcare providers. As mandated by the Health Insurance Portability and Accountability Act of 1996 (HIPAA), the Center for Medicare and Medicaid Services (CMS) has devised a provider identification system called **national provider identifiers (NPIs)**. The objective of the National Provider Identifier system is to assign a unique national identifier number to each and every provider of Medicare healthcare services. The number would be used by all health plans and would eliminate the current system of multiple numbers for a single provider.

The NPI will be a standard unique health identifier for providers, and it will consist of nine numbers plus a check-digit in the tenth position. All covered entities must use the NPI for all claims or payers on May 23, 2007.

NPI numbers will eventually replace UPINs and PIN numbers for providers.

Medicare Billing Notices

The **Medicare Remittance Notice (MRN)** is an explanation of benefits issued to providers (who accept Medicare assignment) for claims submitted to Medicare for a certain period of time. This document is sent to a provider by the Medicare carrier or intermediary and lists all the claims submitted by the provider that were paid for a specified time period **(see Figure 4–2)**. MRNs provide a report of claim determination, check for the payable amount, and provide an explanation of how or why a claim was processed as it was. Each carrier/intermediary has variations in this format.

The MRN will list the patient's name, the date services were rendered, the services that were rendered, the billed amount, and the Medicare approved amount. It also shows the part of the approved amount that was applied toward the patient's deductible, the patient's coinsurance amount, and the amount Medicare is paying.

The **Medicare Summary Notice (MSN)** is an explanation of benefits sent to the Medicare beneficiary, detailing the processing of claims submitted for payment **(see Figure 4–3)**.

Following is an explanation of the MSN:

1. **Date:** Date MSN was sent.
2. **Customer Service Information:** Who to contact with questions about the MSN. Provide your Medicare number (3), the date of the MSN (1), and the date of the service you have a question about (7).
3. **Medicare Number:** The number on the Medicare Card.
4. **Name and Address:** Lists the Medicare beneficiary's address.
5. **Be Informed:** Message regarding Medicare fraud and abuse.
6. *(Part A)* **Hospital Insurance—Inpatient Claims;** or *(Part B)* **Medical Insurance—Outpatient Facility Claims;** or *(Part B)* **Medical Insurance—Assigned Claims;** or *(Part B)* **Medical Insurance—Unassigned Claims:** Indicates type of service provided.
7. **Dates of Service:** Dates service was provided.
8. **Claim Number:** Number that identifies this specific claim.
9. **Benefit Days Used** *(Part A)*: Shows the number of days used in the benefit period. **Amount Charged** *(Part B)*: Amount the provider billed Medicare.
10. **Non-Covered Charges** *(Part A)*: Shows the charges for services denied or excluded by the Medicare program for which the patient may be billed. **Medicare Approved** *(Part B)*: Amount Medicare approved for this service or supply.
11. **Deductible and Coinsurance** *(Part A)*: The amount applied to the patient's deductible and coinsurance. **Medicare Paid Provider** *(Part B)*: Amount Medicare paid the provider. For unassigned claims this section is called "Medicare Paid You."
12. **You May Be Billed:** The amount the provider may bill the patient.
13. **See Notes Section:** If letter appears, refer to (15) for explanation.
14. **Provider's Name and Address:** Provider's name and billing address.
15. **Services Provided** *(Part B)*: Brief description of the service or supply received.
16. **Notes Section:** Explains letters in (13) for more detailed information about this claim.
17. **Deductible Information:** How much of the deductible the patient has met.
18. **General Information:** Important Medicare news and information.
19. **Appeals Information:** How and when to request an appeal.

CARRIER NAME
ADDRESS 1
ADDRESS 2
CITY, STATE ZIP
(909) 111-2222

**MEDICARE
REMITTANCE
NOTICE**

PROVIDER NAME	PROVIDER #:	1111111111
ADDRESS 1	PAGE #:	1 OF 1
ADDRESS 2	CHECK/EFT #:	00001111111
CITY, STATE ZIP	STATEMENT #:	F21103AA0101SYS

IMPORTANT INFORMATION FOR SUPPLIERS

PERF PROV	SERV DATE	POS	NOS	PROC	MODS	BILLED	ALLOWED	DEDUCT	COINS	GRP/RC-AMT		PROV PD
NAME EDMUNDS, EDWARD		HIC 508123456A		ACNT 34567890			ICN 02105104002000			ASG Y MOA MA01		
1111111111	0315 031502	12	1	L0310	GZ	500.00	0.00	0.00	0.00	OA-50	250.00	0.00
REM: M25										CO-50	250.00	
1111111111	0315 031502	12	1	L0317	GAGK	250.00	250.00	0.00	50.00	OA-100	0.00	200.00
PT RESP 50.00				CLAIM TOTALS		750.00	250.00	0.00	50.00		500.00	200.00
ADJ TO TOTALS: PREV PD		0.00		INTEREST	.19	LATE FILING CHARGE			0.00	NET		200.19
NAME EDMUNDS, EDWARD		HIC 508123456A		ACNT 123456789			ICN 02105104012200			ASG Y MOA MA130 MA13		
1111111111	0301 030102	12	1	K0010		50.00	0.00	0.00	0.00	CO-16	50.00	0.00
PT RESP 0.00				CLAIM TOTALS		50.00	0.00	0.00	0.00		50.00	0.00
ADJ TO TOTALS: PREV PD		0.00		INTEREST	0.00	LATE FILING CHARGE			0.00	NET		0.00

SUMMARY OF NON-ASSIGNED CLAIMS

NAME EDMUNDS, EDWARD		HIC 508123456A		ACNT 123456789			ICN 02102104012100			ASG Y MOA MA15 MA18 MA01		
1111111111	0303 030302	12	1	E0143	NU	150.00	111.97	0.00	22.39	OA-100	89.58	0.00
REM: M3 M25										PR-42	38.03	
PT RESP 150.00				CLAIM TOTALS		150.00	111.97	0.00	22.39	127.61	0.00	
ADJ TO TOTALS: PREV PD		0.00		INTEREST	0.00	LATE FILING CHARGE			0.00	NET		0.00

CLAIM INFORMATION FORWRDED TO: ACE INS

TOTALS:	# OF CLAIMS	BILLED AMT	ALLOWED AMT	DEDUCT AMT	COINS AMT	TOTAL RC-AMT	PROV PD AMT	PROV ADJ AMT	CHECK AMT
	3	950.00	361.97	0.00	72.39	677.61	200.00	0.19-	200.19

PROVIDER ADJ DETAILS:	PLB REASON CODE	FCN	HIC	AMOUNT
	L6			0.19-

GLOSSARY: GROUP, REASON, MOA, REMARK AND REASON CODES

CO   Contractual obligation. The patient may not be billed for this amount.
OA   Other adjustment
PR   Patient responsibility
16   Claim/service lacks information which is needed for adjudication. Additional information is supplied using remittance advice remark codes whenever appropriate.
42   Charges exceed our fee schedule or maximum allowable amount.
50   These are non-covered services because this is not deemed a "medical necessity" by the payer.
100   Payment made to patient/insured/responsible party.
M3   Equipment is the same or similar to equipment already being used.
M25   Payment has been (denied for the/made only for a less extensive) service because the information furnished does not substantiate the need for the (more extensive) service. If you believe the service should have been fully covered as billed, or if you did not know and could not reasonably have been expected to know that we would not pay for this (more extensive) service, or if you notified the patient in writing in advance that we would not pay for this (more extensive) service and he/she agreed in writing to pay, ask us to review your claim within 120 days of the date of this notice. If you do not request review, we will, upon application from the patient, reimburse him/her for the amount you have collected from him/her (for the/in excess of any deductible and coinsurance amounts applicable to the less extensive) service. We will recover the reimbursement from you as an overpayment.
MA01 If you do not agree with what we approved for these services, you may appeal our decision. To make sure that we are fair to you, we require another individual that did not process our initial claim to conduct the review. However, in order to be eligible for a review, you must write to us within 120 days of the date of this notice, unless you have a good reason for being late.

An institutional provider, e.g., hospital, Skilled Nursing Facility (SNF), Home Health Agency (HHA) or hospice may appeal only if the claim involves a reasonable and necessary denial, a SNF recertified bed denial, or a home health denial because the patient was not homebound or was not in need of intermittent skilled nursing services, or a hospice care denial because the patient was not terminally ill, and either the patient or the provider is liable under Section 1879 of the Social Security Act, and the patient chooses not to appeal.

If your carrier issues telephone review decisions, a professional provider should phone the carrier's office for a telephone review if the criteria for a telephone review are met.

MA13 You may be subject to penalties if you bill the beneficiary for amounts not reported with the PR (patient responsibility) group code.
MA15 Your claim has been separated to expedite handling. You will receive a separate notice for the other services reported.
MA18 The claim information is also being forwarded to the patient's supplemental insurer. Send any questions regarding supplemental benefits to them.
MA130 Your claim contains incomplete and/or invalid information, and no appeal rights are afforded because the claim is unprocessable. Please submit a new claim with the correct/complete information.
L6   Interest.

■ **Figure 4–2** Sample Medicare Remittance Notice

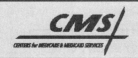

Medicare Summary Notice

*1   July 1, CCYY

*4 EDWARD EDMUNDS
8888 EVERY LANE
ANYTOWN, USA 12345

*2   CUSTOMER SERVICE INFORMATION

*3   Your Medicare Number: 508-12-3456A

If you have questions, write or call:
Medicare
555 Medicare Blvd., Suite 200
Medicare Building
Medicare, US XXXXX-XXXX

*5   BE INFORMED: Beware of "free" medical
services or products. If it sounds too good to
be true, it probably is.

Local: (XXX) XXX-XXXX
Toll-free: 1-800-XXX-XXXX
TTY for Hearing Impaired: 1-800-XXX-XXXX

This is a summary of claims processed from 05/10/CCYY through 06/10/CCYY.

*6   PART A HOSPITAL INSURANCE – INPATIENT CLAIMS

Dates of Service	Benefit Days Used	Non- Covered Charges	Deductible and Coinsurance	You May Be Billed	See Notes Section
Claim Number: 12435-84956-84556-45621 ***8**					a
Cure Hospital, 213 Sick Lane, ***14**					
Evansville, CA 90012					
Referred by: Paul Jones, M.D.					
04/25/YY – 05/09/YY ***7**	***9** 14 days	***10** $0.00	***11** $912.00	***12** $912.00	***13** b
Claim Number: 12435-84956-845556-45622					
Continued Care Hospital, 124 Sick Lane,					
Evansville, CA 90012					
Referred by: Paul Jones, M.D.					
05/09/YY – 06/20/YY	11 days	$0.00	$0.00	$0.00	

*6   PART B MEDICAL INSURANCE – ASSIGNED CLAIMS

Dates of Service	Services Provided	***9** Amount Charged	Medicare Approved	Medicare Paid Provider	You May Be Billed	See Notes Section
Claim Number: 12435-84956-84556-45623			***10**	***11**		
Paul Jones, M.D., 123 West Street,						
Evansville, CA 90012						
Referred by: Scott Wilson, M.D.						
04/19/YY	1 Influenza immunization (90724)	$5.00	$3.88	$3.88	$0.00	c
04/19/YY	1 Admin. flu vac (G0008) ***15**	5.00	3.43	3.43	0.00	c
	Claim Total	**$10.00**	**$7.31**	**$7.31**	**$0.00**	

THIS IS NOT A BILL – Keep this notice for your records.

■ **Figure 4–3** Medicare Summary Notice

(continued on next page)

Your Medicare Number: 508-12-3456A

---

*16   Notes Section A:

a The amount Medicare paid the provider for this claim is $XXXX.XX.

b $912.00 was applied to your inpatient deductible.

c This service is paid at 100% of the Medicare approved amount.

---

*17   Deductible Information:

You have met the Part A deductible for this benefit period.

You have met the Part B deductible for CCYY.

*18   General Information:

You have the right to make a request in writing for an itemized statement which details each Medicare item or service which you have received from your physician, hospital, or any other health supplier or health professional. Please contact them directly, in writing, if you would like an itemized statement.

Compare the services you receive with those that appear on your Medicare Summary Notice. If you have questions, call your doctor or provider. If you feel further investigation is needed due to possible fraud and abuse, call the phone number in the Customer Service Information Box.

*19   Appeals Information – Part A and Part B

If you disagree with any claims decision on either Part A or Part B of this notice, you can request an appeal by November 1, CCYY. Follow the instructions below:

1) Circle the item(s) you disagree with and explain why you disagree.

2) Send this notice, or a copy, to the address in the "Customer Service Information" box on
   Page 1. (You may also send any additional information you may have about your
   appeal.)

3) Sign here _____   Phone number _____

Revised 02/04

On the Job Now

Directions: Answer the following questions. Refer to the text if necessary. *P107*

What is an MRN and to whom is it sent? _____

_____

_____

What is an MSN and to whom is it sent? _____

_____

_____

Collecting Amounts Due from the Patient

You must bill the patient for any amounts that Medicare lists as the patient's responsibility (after any other coverage has been billed) and honestly attempt to collect these amounts. This means billing the patient at least three times before writing off any portion of the patient's amount. Additionally, you must use the same collection attempts for Medicare patients as you do for non-Medicare patients.

If the patient's portion of the bill is written off, there should be documentation as to why this has happened. Hardship conditions should be fully documented, as well as bankruptcies or other conditions. The patient should be asked to sign a statement verifying this information.

Two cases may be allowed for noncollection attempts: hardship of the patient, and amounts that are too minimal to be cost-effective for established collection procedures. Hardship will usually only be accepted if the medical office can show that patients' portions were waived in only a limited number of cases. In cases of cost-effectiveness, the provider should have a cost analysis performed that determines all the costs involved in collecting on an account. Amounts below this level can be considered not cost-effective. The cost analysis should be updated periodically and kept on file. Failure to bill Medicare patients for their part of the fee can result in fines and penalties, exclusion from the Medicare program, and possible criminal charges.

Billing Deceased Patients

Because Medicare pays for health care for the aged, some patients may die. Before claims are processed, you should have an Assignment of Benefits form signed by the patient in the patient file. There are two ways to handle unpaid bills for such patients. If assignment is accepted, Medicare will process. If assignment is not accepted, Medicare may wait until the patient's estate is settled before making payment.

If the family of the deceased pays the bill, they should complete form CMS-1660 showing that they have paid it and attach the receipt. Medicare will then send payment to the person who paid the bill.

Posting Medicare Payments

Payments received from Medicare may be lower than the physician's billed charge. If the provider accepts Medicare's assignment, it is important that the medical biller knows how to post payments to the patient's ledger and make adjustments.

On receipt of the MRN, the patient(s) chart(s) indicated on the MRN should be pulled. Post each payment individually to each patient ledger card (in today's world, most patient account programs are computerized; however, the premise of our program is manually based) and to the daily journal. Separate entries should be made for each patient on the daily journal (not in a lump sum).

If the Medicare allowed amount is less than the billed charge, an adjustment or write-off will need to be made on the ledger card. After the payment has been posted, the next entry on the ledger card should be the adjustment to the charges. Enter the difference between the billed amount and the Medicare approved amount. This amount will be entered on the ledger card in the adjustment column and will be subtracted from the remaining balance. This entry will ensure that Medicare recipients are not being billed for charges that exceed the Medicare approved amount.

Assignment of Benefits

To be a participating provider, the provider must agree to accept assignment on all Medicare claims. By doing this, the provider receives payment directly from Medicare rather than the payment going to the beneficiary. In addition, the provider has agreed to accept the amount approved by the Medicare carrier for the covered services. The patient is not responsible for any amount in excess of the approved amount.

Physicians Who Accept Assignment

When a provider agrees to accept Medicare assignment for a bill, Medicare will pay the provider directly for that bill. The physician may bill the patient only for any deductibles or coinsurance amounts not paid by Medicare on the assigned bill. As a result, the total fee that providers may receive from Medicare and from beneficiaries for an assigned bill is limited to what Medicare deems to be an appropriate fee for the particular service or procedure (the Medicare "allowance").

To encourage providers to accept assignment, the Medicare allowance is higher for physicians who agree to accept assignment for all bills for Medicare-eligible persons. These providers are called "**participating providers**." Thus, participating providers agree not to practice "balance billing," or charging patients for more than the Medicare allowed amount.

Providers who treat Medicare patients but who decide whether to accept assignment on a case-by-case basis are called "**nonparticipating providers**." If assignment is accepted on a claim, the rules for participating providers apply. If assignment is not accepted, the Medicare payment is made directly to the beneficiary.

Mandatory Assignment

Providers may usually accept or not accept Medicare assignment. However, there are some services that require acceptance of assignment. These include:

Practice Pitfalls

Providers may collect reimbursement for excluded services, unmet deductibles, and coinsurance from the beneficiary.

To accept or not accept assignment of Medicare benefits for a claim, the provider must enter an X in the square for either Yes or No in block 27 of the CMS-1500 form.

- Clinical diagnostic laboratory services.
- Medicare patients who also are eligible for Medicaid.
- Ambulatory surgery centers.
- Method II home dialysis supplies and equipment.
- Physician's assistant, nurse midwives, nurse specialists, nonphysician anesthetists, clinical psychologists, and clinical social workers services.
- Effective February 1, 2001, all physicians, nonphysician practitioners, and suppliers must take assignment on all claims for drugs and biologicals furnished to any patient enrolled in Medicare Part B.

Limiting Charges

Federal law prohibits a doctor who does not accept assignment from charging more than 15% above Medicare's approved amount. This is called **limiting charges**. Balance billing by nonparticipating physicians is strictly limited to this amount. Participating physicians are not affected because they are not allowed to balance bill Medicare patients for any services. The limiting charge applies only to physicians' services. Ambulance companies and other nonphysician providers are not subject to limiting charge regulations.

Following are two examples of how this rule affects the payment of claims.

Example 1. Provider accepts assignment.

Billed Charge	Medicare Approved Amount	Medicare Pays	Member Pays
$42	$35 (2006 Part B deductible amount = $124)	$35 to ded = 0 pd	$35
$90	$75	$75 to ded = 0 pd	$75
$480	$400	$400 − $14 to ded = $386 × 80% = $308.80 pd	$14 + $77.20 (20%) = $91.20

Example 2. Provider does not accept assignment.

Billed Charge	Medicare Approved Amount	115% Medicare Approved Amount	Medicare Pays	Member Pays
$42	$35 (2006 Part B deductible amount = $124)	$40.25	$40.25 to ded = 0 pd	$40.25
$90	$75	$86.25	$86.25 − $83.75 to ded = $2.50 × 80% = $2.00 pd	$83.75 + $ .50 (20%) = $84.25
$480	$400	$460.00	$460 × 80% = $368.00 pd	$92.00

Some providers routinely write off any amounts not covered by Medicare. This practice is prohibited by law, as it means that Medicare covers 100% of the bill. Thus, there is no monetary incentive to the patient not to overuse services.

Surgery Disclosure Notice

Specific requirements must be followed for nonparticipating providers who perform elective surgeries over $500. For surgeries that are elective (i.e., surgery scheduled in advance, not an emergency, when delay would not result in impairment or death), are not assigned, and for which a charge greater than $500 is expected, the provider must notify the patient of certain information in writing. This information includes the following:

- Name and description of the procedure.
- Fact that the surgery is elective.
- Expected charge for the surgery.
- Approximate Medicare allowable.
- Amount by which the physician's charge exceeds the allowable.
- The amounts of the patient's responsibility.

Failure to provide this information could result in penalties being assessed. Medicare carriers may contact providers and request a signed copy of the notification. See **Figure 4–4** for a sample of a Surgery Disclosure Notice.

Paul Provider, M.D.
5858 Peppermint Place
Anytown, USA 12345
(765) 555-6768

Date: (MM DD CCYY)

Dear (Beneficiary's Name):

I do not plan on accepting Medicare assignment for your surgery. The law requires that when assignment is not taken, and the charge is $500 or more, or when performing elective surgery, the following information must be provided prior to surgery. These estimates assume that you have met your annual Medicare Part B deductible.

Type of surgery _____
Estimated charge _____
Medicare estimated payment _____
Expected amount charges exceeds Medicare allowable _____
Your actual payment (includes your Medicare coinsurance) _____

Sincerely,
(Physician's Signature)
Paul Provider, M.D.

■ **Figure 4–4** Surgery Disclosure Notice

On the Job Now

Directions: Calculate the adjustment and the amount that you may bill the patient in the following examples. Assume in all cases that the patient has fully met their deductible for the year and that the provider is a nonparticipating provider.

	Billed Amount	Medicare Approved	Medicare Paid	Collectible Amount	Adjustment	Balance Due From Patient
1.	175.00	115.40	92.32	132.71	59.60	40.39
2.	35.00	3.00	2.40	3.45	32.00	1.05
3.	375.00	323.60	258.88	372.14	113.26 51.40	113.26
4.	45.00	40.00	32.00	46	5.00	14.00
5.	1,500.00	1225.60	980.48	1409.44	274.40	428.96
6.	950.00	138.05	110.44	158.76	811.95	48.32
7.	20.00	4.72	3.78	5.43	15.28	1.65
8.	95.00	86.86	69.49	99.89	8.14	13.03 30.40
9.	175.00	135.70	108.56	156.06	39.30	47.50
10.	75.00	50.30	40.24	57.85	24.70	17.61
11.	260.00	250.00	200.00	287.50	10	87.50
12.	545.00	295.95	236.76	340.34	249.05	44.39
13.	1,200.00	968.53	774.82	1113.81	231.47	338.99
14.	450.00	445.00	356.00	511.75	5	155.75
15.	750.00	560.15	48.12	644.14	189.85	596.02

Medical Necessity Denials

Medical necessity denials are the most common reason for denial of claims by Medicare; these are services that are considered not medically necessary. In Medicare claim processing, this phrase has a wide variety of meanings. The three most common situations that are given for a "not medically necessary" denial are:

1. The diagnosis does not match the service. If no clear connection can be made between the diagnosis and the related services, additional information should be provided to justify the medical necessity of services.

2. Frequency of services is greater than allowed. Medicare has specific limits for the number of times a specific service can be performed. For example, a patient age 65 and over is allowed one mammography screening every two years. If the second mammogram is done before the two-year limit is up, it will be denied as not medically necessary.

3. Level of service does not match diagnosis. This denial is most often used with office visit codes. For example, if the diagnosis for a patient were a simple fracture of the arm, a Level V office visit would be denied. Some Medicare agencies will down-code the level to the appropriate Level II code, but others will simply deny the visit as not medically necessary. **Downcoding** occurs when an insurance carrier changes a code to a similar code that has a lower level of service.

If a claim is denied as not medically necessary, any amounts paid by the patient must be refunded within 30 days of the notification of denial. If you wish to appeal the denial, send in the claim and any related documentation to the Medicare carrier and request a formal review. Be sure to detail exactly which services you are appealing

Practice
Pitfalls

Claims with incidental services may list that certain procedures are not medically necessary. In such cases, Medicare is not stating that the service is not medically necessary, but that the second procedure is incidental to or an integral part of the first procedure. For example, a laparoscopy is an integral part of removal of a lesion. The removal procedure would be allowed and paid; however, the laparoscopy procedure would be denied. Therefore, the second procedure would be denied as not medically necessary. In essence, this is a form of downcoding, but the use of the "not medically necessary" denial can lead to confusion and concerns among your patients. It is important to check the CPT® and HCPCS codes carefully in order to be sure that a single code does not cover both procedures.

(instead of asking the carrier to review the entire claim), and include documentation to support the medical necessity of services. The information will be reviewed to make a new determination regarding medical necessity.

If the claim is denied, you may request that the Medicare carrier provide you with all the information they used to make the denial determination. The request must be made in writing and should list the patient's name, the date of services, the services that were denied, and the reasons Medicare indicated on the forms for the denial. You also should state that you are requesting the information under the Freedom of Information Act. Any information sent by the carrier should be studied and retained for future reference.

Medicare Secondary Payer

Some individuals covered by Medicare also have other insurance to pay their medical bills. Medicare pays secondary (**Medicare Secondary Payer (MSP)**) to employer-sponsored group insurance, individual policies carried by the employee, workers' compensation insurance, beneficiary entitled to Black Lung benefits, automobile or no-fault insurance, and third-party liability. Medicare pays primary to Medicare supplemental plans (Medigap insurance), Medicaid, and after 30 months of end-stage renal disease.

The patient should be questioned during their first visit to determine all insurance coverage(s) that could affect payment of a claim.

Certain diagnoses have been identified as being workers' compensation–related. If the patient is diagnosed with one of these conditions, the Medicare carrier will probably request additional information, or deny the claim as covered by workers' compensation. This list of diagnoses can be obtained from the Department of Labor.

When submitting a claim for secondary payments to Medicare, a copy of the claim as originally submitted to the primary carrier should be submitted. The primary insurance EOB should be attached, along with any necessary evidence to support services. No changes should be made on the claim, including altering the "amount paid" and "amount now due" boxes to reflect the payment made by the primary carrier.

If a Medicare patient is covered by primary insurance and receives a payment from the primary insurance that is greater than the Medicare allowed amount, the provider cannot charge the patient for any amounts (including the 20% coinsurance normally collected). The full allowed amount has been collected from the primary insurance carrier. The provider is allowed to keep any amounts paid by the primary insurance that are over the Medicare-allowed amount without violating his agreement with Medicare. If the patient's insurance pays less than the amount Medicare determines to be the patient's responsibility (deductible and coinsurance amounts), the provider is allowed to bill the patient for the difference between the amount collected from the primary insurance and the patient's responsibility as determined by Medicare.

If a third party is determined to be liable for expenses (i.e., auto or other accident), that carrier should be billed first. If the carrier denies payment, a copy of the EOB should be filed with the Medicare claim. If the patient later sues and is granted monetary compensation, Medicare will demand a repayment of the benefits they have paid. The patient may be asked to sign a form that states that they will inform Medicare of the court's decision or a settlement. If the patient receives payment without informing Medicare, they are responsible for repaying Medicare. See *Medicare Secondary Payer Table* in Appendix C.

Medicare and Veterans

Veterans may be eligible for benefits with the Veterans Health Administration (VHA), and at the same time be eligible for Medicare coverage. In these cases, the patient is required to make a choice between being covered by VHA benefits or by Medicare.

Once a patient has chosen and completed the proper enrollment forms, claims for services rendered should be sent to the appropriate office. Medicare may pay for services when the services provided are Medicare-covered services and are not covered by the VHA.

Diagnosis-Related Group Billing

Effective October 1, 1983, Medicare instituted **Diagnosis-Related Group (DRG)** payments for inpatient hospital claims.

Under DRG, a flat-rate payment is made based on the patient's diagnosis instead of the hospital's itemized billing. If the hospital can treat the patient for less, it retains the savings. If treatment costs more, the hospital must absorb the loss. Neither Medicare nor the patient is responsible for the excess amount for hospital claims only, and this does not involve billing from provider offices. It is very important to code diagnoses accurately (to the fifth digit, if warranted), as payments are based on diagnosis coding.

Provisions have been made for cases atypically expensive (based on the diagnosis) because of complications or an abnormally long confinement. Known as Outliers, these cases will be reimbursed on an itemized or cost percentage basis instead of DRG. The bill from the hospital must indicate that it is an Outlier.

Excluded from DRG are long-term care, children's care, and psychiatric or rehabilitative hospitals. Also, several states have obtained waivers from DRG.

DRG Benefit Payment Calculations

As shown in the following examples, the maximum liability under a plan includes only the expenses that are covered by the plan and that the insured is legally obligated to pay.

Example 1. Itemized hospital bill exceeds Medicare DRG allowance.

Hospital Bill	$ 8,700
DRG Allowance	$ 7,000
Medicare Payment	$ 6,048 5816
(Medicare Payment = DRG allowance - $952 -1184 Medicare Part A Deductible)	
Patient's Responsibility	$ 952 1184
Hospital Write-off	$ 1,700

Although the Medicare DRG allowance is less than the itemized hospital bill, the insured is legally obligated to pay only the $952 Part A 2006 deductible.

Example 2. Medicare DRG allowance exceeds itemized billed amount.

Hospital Bill	$ 8,700
DRG Allowance	$10,000
Medicare Payment	$ 9,048 8816
Patient's Responsibility	$ 952 1184

Even though the Medicare payment exceeds the itemized hospital bill, the insured is still legally obligated to pay the $952 Part A 2006 deductible.

On the Job Now

Directions: Compute the hospital write-off amount for the following scenario.

Hospital Bill	$ 9,500
DRG Allowance	$ 7,500
Medicare Payment	$ 6,548 6316
(Medicare Payment = DRG allowance - $952 Medicare Part A 2006 Deductible)	
Patient's Responsibility	$ 952 1184
Hospital Write-off	$ 2,000

Directions: Compute the patient's responsibility amount for the following scenario.

Hospital Bill	$	5,000
DRG Allowance	$	7,500
Medicare Payment	$	6,548 *6316*
Patient's Responsibility	$	___*952*___ *1184*

Durable Medical Equipment

Durable Medical Equipment (DME) is equipment that meets all of the following requirements:

- Can withstand repeated use.
- Is primarily and customarily used to serve a medical purpose.
- Is generally not useful to a person in the absence of an illness or injury.
- Is appropriate for use in the home.

Often a provider will prescribe special equipment for use by a beneficiary in his home. The equipment may provide therapeutic benefits or enable the beneficiary to perform certain tasks that he is unable to undertake because of certain medical conditions or illnesses. DME includes, but is not limited to:

- Diabetic supplies.
- Canes, crutches, walkers.
- Commode chairs.
- Home oxygen equipment.
- Hospital beds.
- Wheelchairs.

The Center for Medicare and Medicaid Services has four carriers that process Durable Medical Equipment, Prosthetics, Orthotics, and Supplies (DMEPOS) claims. These carriers are referred to as **Durable Medical Equipment Regional Carriers, or DMERCs**. Each DMERC covers a specific geographic region of the country.

Medicare Denials

Medicare may deny claims for numerous reasons. If a claim is denied, the reason for the denial will appear on the MRN. This will often be a code, which refers to an in-depth explanation.

One of the most common denials is because of "incorrect patient information." The information actually may not be incorrect, it may just be different from what Medicare's computer has. For example, if a patient is listed on the Medicare records as Sam S. Smith, and you list him as Samuel S. Smith, or Sam Simpson Smith, or Sam

Smith, the Medicare computer may reject the claim. To prevent this from happening, copy the patient's data exactly as it appears on the Medicare card. This is the information you should have in your records and in the computer data banks, even if Mr. Smith completes his Patient Information Sheet differently.

Another message commonly found on Medicare claims is the following:

We understand that you may not have known that Medicare would not pay for this service. If you believe this service should have been covered, or if you did not know or could not have been expected to know that Medicare would not pay for this service, or if you notified the beneficiary in writing in advance that Medicare would not pay for this service and he/she agreed to pay, ask us to review your claim.

This indicates that the physician has provided a service that Medicare considers "medically unnecessary." If the physician could not be expected to know that this service would be considered medically unnecessary (i.e., Medicare never informed the physician either on a previous MRN or through a newsletter or personal letter), then Medicare is obligated to pay the physician if the claim is submitted for review. For this reason, you should submit all denied Medicare claims for review.

Advance Beneficiary Notice (ABN)

The provider is responsible for knowing the Medicare policies for their state and for informing a patient in writing when Medicare is likely to deny payment for a planned procedure. If a provider fails to provide a proper **Advance Beneficiary Notice (ABN)** in situations that require one, the provider can be held liable under the provisions of Limitation of Liability (LOL) laws (Title XVIII, section 1879). An ABN is a written notice a provider gives a Medicare beneficiary before rendering services, which informs a patient that a particular procedure may not be considered medically necessary by Medicare, and that if payment is denied by Medicare, the patient will be responsible for paying for the procedure. LOL provisions require only that the beneficiary be notified and the beneficiary's signature indicating receipt can, and very likely will, result in the beneficiary's financial liability.

The provider must have reasonable cause to believe the procedure will be denied as not medically necessary. Reasonable cause can include a procedure that is listed as not covered under Medicare guidelines

Patient's Name: Edmunds, Edward
Medicare # (HICN): 508-12-3456A

Paul Provider, M.D.
5858 Peppermint Place, Anytown, USA 12345

Advance Beneficiary Notice (ABN)

NOTE: You need to make a choice about receiving these health care items or services.

We expect that Medicare will not pay for the laboratory test(s) that are described below. Medicare does not pay for all of your health care costs. Medicare only pays for covered items and services when Medicare rules are met. The fact that Medicare may not pay for a particular item or service does not mean that you should not receive it. There may be a good reason your doctor recommended it. Right now, in your case, Medicare probably will not pay for -

Items or Services:
Insurance Physical
Because:
Routine service; not covered under Medicare benefits.

The purpose of this form is to help you make an informed choice about whether or not you want to receive these items or services, knowing that you might have to pay for them yourself. Before you make a decision about your options, you should read this entire notice carefully.

Ask us to explain, if you don't understand why Medicare probably won't pay.
Ask us how much these items or services will cost you (Estimated Cost: $ 90.00),
in case you have to pay for them yourself or through other insurance.

PLEASE CHOOSE ONE OPTION. CHECK ONE BOX. SIGN & DATE YOUR CHOICE.

☐ **Option 1. YES**   I want to receive these items or services.

I understand that Medicare will not decide whether to pay unless I receive these items or services. Please submit my claim to Medicare. I understand that you may bill me for items or services and that I may have to pay while Medicare is making its decision. If Medicare does pay, you will refund me any payments I made to you that are due to me. If Medicare denies payment, I agree to be personally and fully responsible for payment. That is, I will pay personally, either out of my pocket or through any other insurance that I have. I understand I can appeal Medicare's decision.

☐ **Option 2. NO.**   I have decided not to receive these items or services.

I will not receive these items or services. I understand that you will not be able to submit a claim to Medicare and that I will not be able to appeal your opinion that Medicare won't pay.

_____
Date

_____
Signature of patient or person acting on patient's behalf

Note: Your health information will be kept confidential.   Any information that we collect about you on this form will be kept confidential in our offices. If a claim is submitted to Medicare, your health information on this form may be shared with Medicare. Your health information, which Medicare sees, will be kept confidential by Medicare.

OMB Approval No. 0938-0566 Form No. CMS-R-131-L (June 2002)

■ Figure 4–5 Advance Beneficiary Notice (ABN) for General Use (i.e., cosmetic surgery), or a procedure that has been previously denied under similar circumstances.

Medicare has set forth strict guidelines as to the content of this form. To be acceptable, an ABN must be on the approved Form CMS-R-131-G, or on CMS-R-131-L for laboratory tests. The forms in **Figures 4–5** and **4–6**, when completed, meet all ABN requirements.

Patient's Name: Edmunds, Edward
Medicare # (HICN): 508-12-3456A

Laboratory Provider
5859 Peppermint Place, Anytown, USA 12345

ADVANCE BENEFICIARY NOTICE (ABN)

NOTE: You need to make a choice about receiving these laboratory tests.

We expect that Medicare will not pay for the laboratory test(s) that are described below. Medicare does not pay for all of your health care costs. Medicare only pays for covered items and services when Medicare rules are met. The fact that Medicare may not pay for a particular item or service does not mean that you should not receive it. There may be a good reason your doctor recommended it. Right now, in your case, **Medicare probably will not pay for the laboratory test(s) indicated below for the following reasons:**

Medicare does not pay for these tests for your condition	Medicare does not pay for these test as often as this (denied as too frequent)	Medicare does not pay for experimental or research use tests
1. Complete Blood Cell Count (CBC)		

The purpose of this form is to help you make an informed choice about whether or not you want to receive these laboratory tests, knowing that you might have to pay for them yourself. Before you make a decision about your options, you should **read this entire notice carefully.**

Ask us to explain, if you don't understand why Medicare probably won't pay.

Ask us how much these laboratory tests will cost you (**Estimated Cost: $25.00**), in case you have to pay for them yourself or through other insurance.

PLEASE CHOOSE **ONE** OPTION. CHECK **ONE** BOX. **SIGN & DATE** YOUR CHOICE.

☐ **Option 1. YES.**   **I want to receive these laboratory tests.**

I understand that Medicare will not decide whether to pay unless I receive these laboratory tests. Please submit my claim to Medicare. I understand that you may bill me for laboratory tests and that I may have to pay while Medicare is making its decision. If Medicare does pay, you will refund me any payments I made to you that are due to me. If Medicare denies payment, I agree to be personally and fully responsible for payment. That is, I will pay personally, either out of my pocket or through any other insurance that I have. I understand I can appeal Medicare's decision.

☐ **Option 2. NO.**   **I have decided not to receive these laboratory tests.**

I will not receive these laboratory tests. I understand that you will not be able to submit a claim to Medicare and that I will not be able to appeal your opinion that Medicare won't pay. I will notify my doctor who ordered these laboratory test that I did not receive them.

_____
Date

_____
Signature of patient or person acting on patient's behalf

Note: Your health information will be kept confidential. Any information that we collect about you on this form will be kept confidential in our offices. If a claim is submitted to Medicare, your health information on this form may be shared with Medicare. Your health information, which Medicare sees, will be kept confidential by Medicare.

OMB Approval No. 0938-0566   Form No. CMS-R-131-L (June 2002)

■ **Figure 4–6** Advance Beneficiary Notice (ABN) for Laboratory Tests

Practice Pitfalls

Medicare rules state that the providers may not ask all patients to sign an ABN for all service(s) rendered. Generally, these types of generic or blanket notices are not effective. Giving ABNs to beneficiaries where there is no specific, identifiable reason to believe Medicare will not pay is not an acceptable practice. These types of blanket or generic notices may be considered defective and not protect the provider from liability.

Provider should hand-deliver (when reasonable) the ABN to the Medicare beneficiary. This type of delivery ensures receipt of the ABN.

The Medicare Appeals Process

Before requesting a Medicare appeal, first determine if the denial was a result of an error or an omission on your part. If so, resubmit the claim with the errors corrected. If you need further clarification regarding the reason a claim was denied, telephone your Medicare carrier or intermediary. If an appeal goes beyond the initial request for review, the provider of the services should be involved in most cases.

There are five levels to the Medicare appeals process:

1. Redetermination.
2. Reconsideration.
3. Administrative Law Judge.
4. Medicare Appeals Council Review.
5. Judicial Review.

You should go through each level before moving on to the next level. The goal is to improve your reimbursement at the lowest appeal level possible.

Redetermination

You have the right to a review if you are dissatisfied with the settlement of a claim. You must request a review within six months from the date of the original claim determination, and there is no minimum amount in controversy for this level of review. This request must be in writing. Simply submit a statement that explains why you are dissatisfied with the reimbursement on the claim.

When submitting a statement, be sure to include the following:

1. A copy of the original claim, including any reports or attachments.
2. A copy of the MRN.
3. Any additional information to support your position or to justify the medical necessity of the services.
4. If you are appealing an unassigned claim, you must have a written authorization from the beneficiary that you are acting on his or her behalf.

End the request with a thank you. Have the provider sign it. Some Medicare carriers require submission of a specific form to request a review. If this is the case in your area, obtain a copy of the form and complete and submit it.

Medicare should respond within 45 days. If you do not hear from the claims reviewer by this time, call and ask about the status of the review. If the claim was assigned, the provider can be informed of the results of the review. If the claim was unassigned, the patient will be informed.

When requesting a redetermination, do not use previous payments as justification for why a payment should be made. Medicare may decide that all payments were in error and that you owe them a refund.

The redetermination letter issued by the Appeals Department is called the **Medicare Redetermination Notice (MRN)**. It will contain all the information necessary to request the next level of appeal.

Practice Pitfalls

It is very helpful to submit an explanation as to why the service(s) should be paid. It is especially helpful to include any documentation that would support this explanation. Supporting documentation may include but is not limited to:

- Operative reports.
- X-ray reports.
- Test results.
- Consultation reports.
- Progress notes.
- Office notes.
- A letter from the provider of service(s).

Reconsideration

If you are not satisfied with the results of the redetermination, you can request a Fair Hearing. To proceed to this level, the amount in controversy must usually be at least $100 and the hearing must be requested within six months of the review determination. If a single claim is not above $100, you can combine several claims for the same patient together to reach the $100 limit.

The Fair Hearing request form **(see Figure 4–7)** is usually sent to a different office from that of the

DEPARTMENT OF HEALTH AND HUMAN SERVICES
CENTERS FOR MEDICARE & MEDICAID SERVICES

REQUEST FOR HEARING
PART B MEDICARE CLAIM
Medical Insurance Benefits - Social Security Act

NOTICE—Anyone who misrepresents or falsifies essential information requested by this form may upon conviction be subject to fine and imprisonment under Federal Law.

CARRIER'S NAME AND ADDRESS

1 NAME OF PATIENT

2 HEALTH INSURANCE CLAIM NUMBER

3 I disagree with the review determination on my claim, and request a hearing before a hearing officer of the insurance carrier named above.
MY REASONS ARE: (Attach a copy of the Review Notice. NOTE: If the review decision was made more than 6 months ago, include your reason for not making this request earlier.)

4 CHECK ONE OF THE FOLLOWING

☐ I have additional evidence to submit. (Attach such evidence to this form or forward it to the carrier within 10 days.)

☐ I do not have additional evidence.

CHECK **ONLY ONE** OF THE STATEMENTS BELOW:

☐ I wish to appear in person before the Hearing Officer.

☐ I do not wish to appear and hereby request a decision on the evidence before the Hearing Officer.

5 **EITHER THE CLAIMANT OR REPRESENTATIVE SHOULD SIGN IN THE APPROPRIATE SPACE BELOW**

SIGNATURE OR NAME OF CLAIMANT'S REPRESENTATIVE		CLAIMANT'S SIGNATURE	
ADDRESS		ADDRESS	
CITY, STATE, AND ZIP CODE		CITY, STATE, AND ZIP CODE	
TELEPHONE NUMBER	DATE	TELEPHONE NUMBER	DATE

(Claimant should not write below this line)

ACKNOWLEDGMENT OF REQUEST FOR HEARING

Your request for a hearing was received on ______________________. You will be notified of the time and place of the hearing at least 10 days before the date of the hearing.

SIGNED	DATE

Form CMS-1965 (05/03)

Figure 4–7 Request for Medicare Hearing Form

Review, and the people who process these requests are typically more experienced than those at the lower levels. There are three types of hearings:

1. **On the record**—based on the written material and data, which you have already submitted to Medicare, and any additional data you provide.
2. **Telephone Hearing**—allows you to introduce new information over the telephone and speak directly with the reviewer. You may be required to substantiate your phone information with additional written records. The physician should always be available for the telephone hearing so that he or she may answer any questions regarding treatment.
3. **In person**—the patient, the physician, and other parties meet in person. The proceedings are typed or recorded and the tape or transcript is usually available on request.

A decision should be made within 120 days, unless there are extenuating circumstances. You should receive a written explanation of the findings from the hearing. You may receive further reimbursement, or you may again be denied.

Administrative Law Judge (ALJ)

This request must be made within 60 days of the Fair Hearing decision and involve at least $500 in controversy. It can take up to 18 months to receive an ALJ assignment. To succeed at this level, you must prove that yours is an unusual case and that it deserves special consideration. Disagreement with Medicare policies will not be addressed at this level.

Your file will be looked at again. It may be immediately reversed (and payment made) or it may be forwarded to a non-Medicare employee. At this point, you will be contacted regarding details for proceeding with the ALJ Hearing.

The Medicare carrier will usually not have a representative present at the ALJ Hearing. An authorized representative from the provider's office will need to be present to answer questions. You may submit additional data, which shows special complication or situations that made your case unusual.

Medicare Appeals Council Review

An Appeals Council Review request must be made within 60 days of the ALJ decision and the amount in controversy must be at least $500. The Council may, on its own, review the ALJ decision if there is a question that the ALJ decision was not made in accordance with the law.

Federal District Court Hearing

If a provider is still dissatisfied following consideration by the Medicare Appeals Council, and the amount in controversy is at least $1,000, the provider may file an appeal in the federal district court where the provider is located, or in the District of Columbia.

At least $1,000 must be in controversy at this level, and an attorney must represent your case. You must appeal within 60 days of the Appeals Council decision. The provider's attorney will handle the case. The provider may want to contact his medical society for attorneys experienced in this level of the appeals process.

Reviews or Hearings After the Deadline

A review or hearing request must be filed within six months. You may file after the six-month deadline if you can show "good cause" for not doing so sooner. Attach a letter to the request for Review or Hearing explaining the good cause. Medicare defines good cause as:

- There were circumstances beyond your control or significant communication difficulties.
- The delay resulted from your efforts to obtain documentation, which you did not realize could have been provided after filing for the Review or Hearing.
- Your records were destroyed or damaged, delaying the filing of the request.

It may be difficult to convince your carrier to provide an extension of time to request a review or hearing. You may need to consider if the benefits are worth the time and effort.

Medicare Fraud and Abuse

It is important to understand the rules and regulations regarding Medicare reimbursement. Penalties are assessed for not complying with these rules. For minor violations, if the provider accepts assignment, the claim may be returned for correction of the problem and may be subject to postpayment review by Medicare. If the provider does not accept Medicare assignment, the provider may be subject to a penalty per claim. Unintentional errors or mistakes that anyone is likely to make do not constitute a charge of fraud. Other violations, or repeated violations, can subject the provider to audits, stiff fines, dismissal from the Medicare program, and—in some cases—criminal penalties and jail sentences.

On the Job Now

Directions: List the five levels of the Medicare Appeals process.

P. 120

1. _____ ALJ _____
2. _____ Medicare Appeals Council Review _____
3. _____
4. _____
5. _____

Medicare Fraud

Medicare fraud is the intentional misrepresentation of information that could result in an unauthorized benefit. The regulations are very specific about the activities that are allowed and not allowed under the Medicare rules and regulations. Examples of fraudulent practices include:

- Billing for services or supplies not rendered, including billing patients for not showing up to an appointment (because the patient never showed, no services were actually rendered).
- Altering the diagnosis to justify services.
- Altering claim forms to misrepresent or falsify data.
- Duplicate billing.
- Billing Medicare and an additional insurance both as the primary payer.
- Soliciting, offering, or receiving a bribe, kickback, rebate, or finder's fee for any services. This includes fees offered for referring a patient to a specific facility for additional tests or services. It also includes automatically writing off that portion of the bill that is the patient's responsibility, as this is considered a kickback or bribe to the patient to induce them to obtain services from one provider over another.
- Unbundling or exploding charges, or billing for multiple services when one procedure code adequately describes the services provided. Many Medicare carriers provide a list of codes that are often unbundled. The computer is set up to look for these codes and automatically pays

only the major procedure, denying the additional procedures.
- Providers who complete certificates of medical necessity or write prescriptions for patients they have not actually seen.
- Altering amounts charged for services, dates of services, identity of patients, or misrepresenting the services provided to obtain reimbursement. This includes upcoding of services (i.e., billing for a level IV visit when a level II visit was performed).
- Altering the code or description of noncovered services to identify them as covered services.
- Any collusion between the provider and an additional party (i.e., patient, lawyer, etc.) to misrepresent charges or services to obtain reimbursement.
- Altering claims history or medical records to substantiate services that were upcoded or misrepresented.
- Using or allowing the use of an incorrect or additional person's Medicare card to obtain coverage for services.
- Billing inappropriately for "gang visits." For example, heading a group psychotherapy session but billing for each patient as if they had an individual visit.
- Not disclosing or providing false data regarding physician ownership of a clinical laboratory, medical supplier, or other related entity. Physicians are not allowed to refer patients to a lab or medical supplier in which they have a financial interest.

- Split billing, or billing supplies and services as if they were provided over a series of dates rather than during a single visit.
- Collusion with an employee of the insurance carrier to generate false payments.
- Repeated violations of Medicare regulations when warning and instruction have been provided.

Medicare Abuse

Unlike Medicare fraud, **Medicare abuse** does not require the proof of intent to defraud the Medicare system in order to be assessed. Many times, abuse can appear to be similar to fraud, except that it is not possible to establish that abusive acts were committed knowingly, willfully, and intentionally. Abuse includes any item or procedure that is inconsistent with accepted norms or practices:

- Excessive charges for procedures or supplies, or billing over the limiting charge.
- Billing for services that are considered not medically necessary. This includes ordering more tests than necessary for diagnosis or ordering services that are of no great benefit to the patient.
- Billing at different rates for Medicare and for other insurance (unless a lower amount is charged to Medicare in order to comply with fee schedules or limiting charges). There are some exceptions to this rule regarding service fees set by a contractual agreement with a Health Maintenance Organization. This violation includes accepting another insurance carrier's payment as payment in full for services (thus waiving coinsurance amounts). Such a practice results in charging non-Medicare patients 20% less than Medicare patients.
- Improper billing of Medicare when another carrier should be billed, or billing Medicare first when they should be the secondary payer.
- Violation of any of the provisions of the Medicare participation agreement.
- Unintentional unbundling, upcoding, or violations of rules.

Medicare may accept "I didn't know" as an excuse for a single violation of any of the Medicare rules and regulations. However, repeated abuses, especially after a provider has been warned, will result in the upgrading of a violation from an abuse to intentional fraud.

If the carrier identifies overpayments or abuses, they may contact the provider and request documentation to substantiate the claims, or will simply send a request for repayment of an overpaid amount. Do not ignore letters requesting a refund of overpayment. If the provider disagrees with the request, you should file additional documentation to substantiate the services and request a review. If the provider agrees with the overpayment, the Medicare carrier should be reimbursed as soon as possible, along with any fines levied by the carrier. Because a decline in service results in a lower allowed amount, often repayments also must be made to the patient for excessive payment of coinsurance amounts.

Medicare often will audit claims using a peer review system. This is a group of physicians who review documentation regarding the services provided. If they find medical or documentation errors, points will be counted against the provider. When a provider receives a certain number of points, he may be subject to forfeiture of his license. Because of this, it is important that proper care is rendered and all evidence supporting the care and the justification of services be fully documented.

Sanctions and Penalties

Different levels of penalties and sanctions have been included in the Medicare provisions. The most common sanctions include:

1. **Educational contact or warning.** If Medicare determines that you are improperly billing, you may be contacted and instructed of the proper procedures and the necessary steps to rectify the situation. Such a contact may or may not include a formal warning, which is placed in the provider's file.

2. **Recoupment of overpayments.** A letter may be sent requesting repayment of any amounts they feel have been overpaid. If payment is not received (and no review is requested), the carrier may withhold future payments to recoup the losses.

3. **Fines.** Many penalties include the assessment of fines for failure to follow regulations. Fines can vary per incident. Penalties of up to twice the overpayment amount also may be levied. Additional fines may be levied for not repaying overpayments in a timely manner.

4. **Criminal prosecution.** Providers or billers may be criminally prosecuted for fraudulent actions against the Medicare system. Penalties include

conviction of a misdemeanor or felony, and may include additional fines and even jail time.

5. **Suspension or dismissal from the Medicare program.** Repeated or severe abuses can cause a provider (or a biller) to be excluded from the Medicare program. This sanction may be imposed for a limited time (suspension, often for up to five years), or permanently (dismissal). In such a case, announcements are made to all patients and in the press that the provider is no longer allowed to accept Medicare patients. If a patient submits a claim after the provider has been dismissed, they will be informed that the provider is not allowed to provide Medicare services and no coverage exists. A provider who is excluded from participating in the Medicare program may also be excluded from participating in Medicaid; Maternal and Child Health Services (EPSDT program); and Social Service Block Grants.

6. **Referral to licensing agencies and professional societies.** Extremely severe cases, especially those involving fraud, mismanagement of patient care, improper or unprofessional conduct, or unethical practices, may be referred to a state licensing agency or a professional society for possible revocation of licensure.

If the Medicare carrier determines that a penalty or sanction has not solved the problem, they may proceed to the next level of penalty or sanction. Because the provider is responsible for what happens in his office, he will be held responsible for abuses and fraudulent actions committed by his employees or an independent billing service contracted by him.

Medicare Supplemental Insurance

Medicare Supplements (also known as **Medigap** policies) are separate plans written exclusively for Medicare participants that pay for amounts that Medicare does not pay. These policies are specifically designed to supplement Medicare's benefits and are regulated by federal and state law. Supplemental programs offered by most insurance companies have many variations within them. Also, the benefit structures of these programs are formulated by what level of a Medicare approved contract the patient may choose to buy to go with their Medicare. A supplement plan may

be written with any optional benefits that the policy-holder wants. Three common supplement options are:

1. Physicians' services—Covers Part B deductible and 20% coinsurance for reasonable charges.
2. Hospital services—Covers Part A deductible and may or may not cover the various copays not covered by Medicare.
3. Nursing care, prescriptions, and the nonreplaced fees on the first three pints of blood.

With the changes in Medicare, supplemental plans have become much more flexible. Therefore, the benefits can be very complex and comprehensive or very basic.

Medicare and Managed Care

In the mid-1980s, Medicare began looking at the managed care market as a way to save costs.

A **Medicare HMO** is an HMO that has contracted with the federal government under the Medicare Advantage program (formerly called Medicare+ Choice) to provide health benefits to persons eligible for Medicare that choose to enroll in the HMO, instead of receiving their benefits and care through the traditional fee for service Medicare program.

Medicare Notice of Non-Coverage

A **Notice of Non-Coverage** must be provided to all Medicare HMO members at the time of discharge from an inpatient facility. This is a letter that advises them of their right to an immediate professional review on a proposed discharge. This allows patients who feel they are being discharged too early to appeal the decision.

Additionally, all providers and groups must provide Medicare members with a copy of "An Important Message From Medicare" at the time of admission to any inpatient facility. This letter informs patients of their rights with regard to treatment. Inpatient facilities include hospitals, skilled nursing facilities, convalescent hospitals, psychiatric hospitals, and any other facility where the patient will be staying overnight or receiving 24-hour care.

When filling in the variable fields on the letter, make sure the entries are easily understood. The notice should be hand-delivered to the member, and the member's signature should be obtained acknowledging receipt of the notice. A copy of the notice, signed by the member, must be placed in the patient chart.

If a Medicare member disagrees with a plan for discharge from an inpatient medical facility, he/she has the right to request an immediate review of the proposed discharge. If the review is requested by noon of the day following receipt of the notice, the member is not financially liable for the inpatient services until they receive notification that the review board has agreed with the discharge. If the patient does not file the request for review within the specified time period, they may still request a review. However, they will be financially responsible for treatment after the proposed discharge date if their request is denied.

Complete a 1500

Medicare Billing Guidelines

When billing Medicare, the provider must complete the appropriate billing forms. Most Medicare charges are billed on the CMS-1500 form. The CMS-1500 should be used to bill for Medicare services performed outside a hospital setting. The CMS-1500 is the uniform claim form for billing provider services. Detailed instructions for completing the CMS-1500 are covered in a later chapter.

Special requirements on the CMS-1500 for Medicare claims include:

- Block 1a—enter the Medicare HICN, complete with any prefixes and suffixes.
- Blocks 4 and 7—enter the primary insurance policyholder's name and address (if different than the patient).
- Blocks 9–9d—enter the Medigap or other policy information. If the patient and insured are the same, enter "SAME" in block 9. If Medicare is the primary insurer leave 9–9d empty.
- Block 11—enter "NONE" unless the claim is for Medicare as the secondary payer. If so, then list the requested information in blocks 11–11c.
- Block 13—enter "SOF" or "Signature on File" if a participating provider.
- Block 17 and 17a—enter the full name and credentials of the referring, ordering or other source in 17 and enter their UPIN or NPI number in 17a.
- Block 24K—enter the UPIN or PIN number of the performing provider of service or supplier if a group name is entered in block 33.
- Block 30—enter amount.

Mandatory Claims Submission

Federal law makes it mandatory for providers to submit claims for Medicare patients. It is also mandatory that providers submit claims to Medicare electronically. The law and regulation permit a number of exceptions to the electronic billing requirement under special circumstances. Providers are not allowed to charge for the service of billing Medicare. Providers who do not submit a claim or who impose a charge for completing the claim are subject to sanctions. The patient may not submit the claim for payment themselves, except in the following situations:

1. If the patient has other insurance, which should pay as primary, the patient may submit the claim and attach a copy of the other carrier's EOB.
2. If the services are not covered by Medicare, but the patient wishes a formal coverage determination for their records.
3. If the provider refuses to submit the claim (which is a violation of law and the provider may be penalized for such actions).
4. If services are provided outside the United States.
5. When the patient has purchased durable medical equipment from a private source.

Claim Filing Time Limit

Medicare providers have at least 15 months from the date of the service to submit a claim to Medicare. For services rendered between October 1 and September 30, claims must be submitted by December 31 of the following year. However, if documentation is submitted that shows that the delay was a result of an administrative error on the part of the Social Security Administration or the Medicare carrier or intermediary, the time limit may be waived. However, claim payment for assigned claims will be reduced by 10% if the claim is not filed within one year of the date of service. Providers may not bill the patient for this reduction.

Medicaid

Medicaid is not a health insurance program. The Federal Medicaid program was established under Title XIX of the Social Security Act of 1965. The purpose of this program is to provide the needy with access to medical care. The Medicaid program is administered by each individual state, using Federal and state funding.

Practice
Pitfalls

The following suggestions will help with properly completing the billing forms, and complying with Medicare guidelines.

1. It is important that the proper ICD-9-CM code be used to denote the diagnosis. All diagnoses must be coded to the highest digit possible. If a five-digit code exists, it should be used rather than a four-digit code. Additionally, an appropriate ICD-9-CM code should be cross-referenced from block 21 to block 24E for each service indicated in block 24D of the CMS-1500.

2. Keep for reference a fee schedule, list of unbundled services, list of denied services, list of procedures with limits on the number of services, and a list of those procedures that require preauthorization from the carrier. Having these items readily available will assist the physician in making informed decisions regarding the care and treatment of the patient, while still receiving the maximum possible reimbursement for services rendered.

3. If modifiers are not self-explanatory, be sure to include any necessary documentation that substantiates the services rendered.

4. If you have a claim that has numerous procedures or confusing information, send a cover letter that clarifies the services performed and the documentation for the necessity of services.

5. Document everything. If you have received information over the phone, document the full name, title, and department of the person who gave you the information, as well as the date and time of the contact. Sending a follow-up letter which thanks them for their help and puts in writing your understanding of the important points of the conversation is also a wise practice. At the bottom of the letter include a note as follows: "If I misunderstood the information, please contact me at the above number or address to clarify." This letter provides proof of the contact should you need it in an audit. If a contact is received stating that you misunderstood the information, be sure to document it, then notate it on the original letter.

6. Read and retain your Medicare bulletins. They are considered legal notification that you have been made aware of Medicare rules and regulations.

7. Providers may collect any deductible and coinsurance from the patient at the time of service. However, it may be best to wait until after receiving the Medicare Remittance Notice. This prevents the medical office from having to return any amounts that were for services that Medicare deemed were not medically necessary, and allows a more accurate calculation of the amount the patient owes.

8. Medicare rules state that the carrier must pay claims within 30 days for "clean claims." **Clean Claims** are claims that can be paid as soon as they are received because the claims are complete in all aspects and do not need additional investigation. Claims for nonparticipating physicians are not processed as quickly as those for participating physicians. Also, claims submitted electronically are processed faster than those submitted on paper and often contain fewer errors, as reentry of the data is not required.

9. Be courteous and kind when dealing with Medicare representatives.

10. If the amounts listed on the Medicare Remittance Notice (MRN) do not match your data regarding allowed amounts or benefits, contact the carrier for clarification.

11. If a check is received from Medicare that contains an overpayment, first check the records to be sure the payment is incorrect. If an overpayment has occurred, deposit the check and write to Medicare regarding the overpayment. Include in the letter copies of the (MRN), the check, and the claim, along with an explanation of the amount that is overpaid. If an overpayment has occurred, Medicare will deduct the overpayment from the provider's next check.

Each state administers their own Medicaid program, and the name of the program may vary from state to state. Medi-Cal is the name of California's Medicaid healthcare program. This program pays for a variety of medical services for those eligible and enrolled in the program.

Medicaid Eligibility

The regulations governing eligibility under this program are extremely complex. Individuals may be entitled to coverage because of medical, family, or financial situations. The fact that the individual has private insurance does not preclude him from being eligible for Medicaid benefits.

Most Medicaid recipients belong to one of two classes; the categorically needy and the medically needy. **Categorically needy** recipients usually make less than the poverty level every month. They may or may not be working, and may or may not have other health insurance. Coverage for some programs may be limited to pregnant women or their children.

Medically needy recipients are those whose high medical expenses and inadequate healthcare coverage (often a result of catastrophic illnesses) have left them at risk of being indigent. Many disabled and elderly persons fall into this category.

For a claimant's services to be covered under Medicaid, the claimant must be a Medicaid beneficiary and the provider must be an approved Medicaid provider. To be an approved provider, the provider of services must agree to accept Medicaid's determination of approved amounts as binding. That is, similar to Medicare's approved amount on assigned claims, the provider is not allowed to bill the patient for any amount not approved by Medicaid. In recent years, many providers have dropped out of the Medicaid program because their allowances and payments are extremely low, even lower than those provided by Medicare.

Medicaid Covered Services

Medicaid providers must accept the Medicaid allowance as payment in full for service(s) rendered. Providers are forbidden to balance bill patients for amount not paid by Medicaid. In most states Medicaid eligibility is determined by a state-designated organization. Covered benefits under Medicaid include:

- Inpatient hospital care.
- Outpatient hospital services.
- Physician services.
- Laboratory and x-ray services.

- Screening, diagnosis, and treatment of children under age 21.
- Immunizations.
- Home healthcare services.
- Family planning services.
- Outpatient hospital services.
- EPSDT services.

Early and Periodic Screening, Diagnosis and Treatment (EPSDT)

Early and Periodic Screening, Diagnosis and Treatment (EPSDT) services are a preventive screening program designed for the early detection and treatment of medical problems in welfare children (known in California as the Child Health and Disability Prevention (CHDP) program).

The EPSDT program includes such things as medical histories and physical examinations of children, immunizations, developmental assessments, and screening for dental problems, hearing loss, vision problems, and lead poisoning. If problems are found, states may be required to provide services and treatment. To indicate that EPSDT services were rendered, use block 24H on the CMS-1500 form. If billing for EPSDT services, indicate an E in block 24H, and if billing for family planning services, indicate an F in block 24H.

Additional benefits may be offered in various states, including:

- Ambulance charges.
- Emergency room care.
- Podiatry services.
- Psychiatric services.
- Dental services.
- Chiropractic services.
- Private duty nursing.
- Optometric services (eye care).
- Eyeglasses and eye refractions.
- Intermediate care.
- Care in a clinic setting.
- Prosthetic devices.
- Diagnostic and screening services.
- Preventive and rehabilitative services (i.e., physical therapy).
- Treatment for allergies.
- Dermatologic treatments.
- Some medical cosmetic procedures (often reconstructive).
- Prescription drugs.

You can obtain further information from your state's Medicaid agency.

Medicaid Eligibility Verification

When billing for services for Medicaid recipients, you must have a copy of the Medicaid eligibility card for the month the services are rendered. Medicaid recipients will have an **eligibility card** to show that they are eligible for Medicaid.

The guidelines for determining eligibility for Medicaid recipients differ from state to state. It is important that you become familiar with these guidelines by reviewing the manuals that are provided by your state.

Some Medicaid covered services require the Medicaid beneficiary to pay a small fee for services, called a copayment. The services that require copayments vary from state to state.

In most states, Medicaid claims must be submitted within 60 days of the end of the month for which services were rendered. Some of the general exceptions to this rule (these services must be billed within one year of the date of service):

1. Dental bills.
2. Obstetric care.
3. Treatment plan completion.
4. When the patient has other insurance coverage.
5. Retroactive eligibility.
6. In the event that the patient did not inform the provider that there was Medicaid coverage.

Reimbursement from Medicaid

By law, Medicaid is always secondary to private group healthcare plans. Therefore, if the patient has other coverage through their employer or through any other insurance carrier, that carrier should be billed first. Once payment has been received, Medicaid should be billed, and a copy of the EOB from the other carrier attached to the claim.

If Medicaid inadvertently pays primary, it will exercise its right of recovery and seek reimbursement from the private plan. The private plan is required to process Medicaid's request for reimbursement and pay Medicaid back the monies it paid the provider of services.

The Medicaid program does not process its own claims. Medicaid contracts with an organization to act as the fiscal intermediary, similar to Medicare. The intermediary processes the claims according to specifications set forth by the Medicaid program.

The rates under this program are based on the results of reimbursement studies conducted by the Department of Health Services. Reimbursement for hospital inpatient services is based on each facility's "reasonable cost" of services as determined from audit cost reports and annual limitations on reimbursable increases in cost.

Providers are not allowed to bill or submit a claim to the Medicaid beneficiary for any service included in the program's scope of benefits except to collect money from a patient's private healthcare coverage prior to billing Medicaid, or to collect the patient's "share of cost."

Some Medicaid systems collect a small **share of cost** payment or fixed copayment from the patient. A share of cost payment or copayment is the amount the patient is responsible for paying for services rendered. This amount will not be printed on the Medicaid recipient's eligibility card. The amount collected should be indicated in block 10d of the CMS-1500 form. You should always ask about any share of cost when you contact Medicaid to verify the patient's eligibility.

Medicaid Remittance Advice

A **Medicaid Remittance Advice (MRA)** is issued to providers for claims submitted to Medicad for a certain period of time. Payment for claims submitted during this time period is made in a lump sum payment. The MRA provides information about claims that were paid, adjusted, voided, and denied. Some intermediaries send the MRA separate from the claims payment; others combine the claims payment with the MRA. The Medicaid Remittance Advice is very similar to the Medicare Remittance Notice.

Posting Medicaid Payments

As with Medicare, Medicaid payment will probably be lower than the actual billed charges. Because Medicaid recipients are not financially responsible for the balance, an adjustment to the patient's account will have to be made. When the remittance advice is received from Medicaid, each patient ledger will need to be pulled and the payments recorded. The adjustments should be made on the next corresponding entry line on the ledger card if using a manual system. The payment amount should be subtracted from the billed amount and the difference should be written off. If the patient's eligibility for Medicaid is terminated at the time services are rendered, the patient becomes financially responsible for the charges. At that time, the patient should be billed directly.

Appeals

If a Medicaid claim payment is not satisfactory to the provider of services, the provider has the option to file an appeal. An appeal must be made to the fiscal intermediary within 90 days of the action causing the grievance. The appeal must be submitted in writing. Copies of the appeal letter, claim, and any additional documentation should be included with the submission.

The Medicaid Claim Form

Medicaid Claim Forms are required to be filled out when submitting claims to Medicaid. Many states now use the CMS-1500 form for billing, but with the mandatory requirement of most states of electronic billing, this form may soon become obsolete. Additional information on completing the CMS-1500 is covered in a later chapter.

Practice
Pitfalls

The following suggestions will help with properly completing the billing forms, and complying with Medicaid guidelines:

1. Type the claim rather than write it.
2. Use capital letters only when typing claims.
3. Do not strike over to correct errors.
4. Do not use N/A; leave space blank.
5. Be as complete and accurate as possible.
6. Code accurately and to the greatest possible number of digits, using the ICD-9-CM and CPT®.
7. Use all appropriate modifiers and list them in order of importance.
8. Be sure diagnosis codes substantiate the services provided.
9. If a claim is unusual, it may be better to send it manually rather than electronically, if you are permitted to do so. Electronic claims do not allow for the addition of medical reports or additional data to substantiate services.
10. Because Medicaid pays secondary to Medicare, claims for patients who are eligible for both programs should first be billed to Medicare. Medicare will automatically forward the claim to the Medicaid carrier after payment. Medicare often pays more than the Medicaid-allowed amount, and no payment will be forthcoming unless the patient has a deductible that has not been met.
11. If the patient is over age 65 but is not eligible for Medicare, this should be indicated on the claim in the Remarks section, along with the reason. For example, if the patient is an alien, "over 65 and not eligible for Medicare—ALIEN."

Many states' Medicaid forms are read by computer, so it is important to complete them correctly. It is important to use the proper Medicaid billing requirements for your state in order to receive reimbursement from Medicaid.

Medicaid as Secondary Payer

Federal regulations require Medicaid to be the "**payer of last resort**." This means that all third parties, including Medicare, TRICARE, Workers' Compensation, and private insurance carriers, must pay before Medicaid pays. Additionally, providers must report any such payments from third parties on claims filed for Medicaid payment.

If the Medicaid-allowed amount is more than the third-party payment, Medicaid will pay the difference up to the Medicaid-allowed amount. If the insurance payment is more than the Medicaid-allowed amount, Medicaid will not pay an additional amount.

Medicaid is not responsible for any amount for which the recipient is not responsible. Therefore, a provider cannot bill Medicaid for any amount greater than what the provider agreed to accept from the recipient's private plan. If the recipient is not responsible for payment, then Medicaid is not responsible for payment.

Certain Medicaid programs are considered "primary payers." When a Medicaid recipient is entitled to one or more of the following programs or services, Medicaid pays first (this is not an all-inclusive list):

- Vocational Rehabilitation Services.
- Division of Health Services for the Blind.
- Maternal and Child Health Delivery Funds.

Treatment Authorization Request

In many cases, prior authorization is required before services are rendered. A Treatment Authorization Request (TAR) form is completed to obtain authorization for specific services (see **Figure 4–8**, form may vary by state). This form must be completed and sent to the

Verbal Control No. *1	Type of Service Requested *2 □ □ Drug Other	Is Request Retroactive? □ □ YES NO *3	Is Patient Medicare Eligible? □ □*4 YES NO	Provider Phone No. *5	Patient's Authorized Representative (IF ANY) Enter name and address: *6

Provider Name and Address *7		Provider Number *8	FOR STATE USE Provider your request is: *9

- Name and Address of Patient — Patient Name (Last, First, MI) *10 — Medicaid Identification Number *11
- Street Address — Sex *12 — Age *13 — Date of Birth | *14 |
- City, State, Zip Code — Patient Status *15 — □ Home □ Board & Care
- Phone Number *16 — □ SNF/ICF □ Acute
- Diagnosis Description *17 — ICD-9 CM *18 Diagnosis Code
- Medical Justification *19
- *20

FOR STATE USE: □ Approved as Requested □ Approved as Modified (items marked below as authorized may be claimed) □ Denied □ Deferred — By: _____ Medi-Cal Consultant — Comments/Explanation

Line No.	Authorized Yes | No	Approved Units	Specific Services Requested	Units of Service	NDC/UPC or Procedure Code	Quantity	Charges
1	□ □	*21	*22	*23	*24	*25	*26
2	□ □						
3	□ □						
4	□ □						
5	□ □						
6	□ □						

To the best of my knowledge, the above information is true, accurate and complete and the requested services are medically indicated and necessary to the health of the patient.

*27

Signature of Physician or Provider   Title   Date

Authorization is valid for services provided *28 — From Date | | To Date | | — Office — Sequence Number *29

Figure 4–8 State Treatment Authorization Request Form

appropriate agency for authorization to be given before services can be rendered. The prior authorization number should be indicated in block 23 of the CMS-1500 form. Please check with your state's Medicaid fiscal intermediary for prior treatment authorization guidelines. Some of the services that require TARs are:

- Inpatient hospital services.
- Home health agency services.
- Hearing aids.
- Chronic hemodialysis services.
- Some surgical procedures.

Instructions for Completing the TAR

Each state Medicaid agency will have a form for requesting authorization for treatment of Medicaid patients. This form must be completed before the rendering of services. An explanation of how to complete the sample form is provided here.

1. **Verbal Control Number**—This number is given when there is insufficient time to request a Treatment Authorization Number for the services provided. Once a Verbal Control Number is given, you must complete and submit a TAR immediately.

2. **Type of Service Requested**—Place an "X" in the appropriate box.

3. **Request Is Retroactive**—Place an "X" in the appropriate box.

4. **Is Patient Medicare Eligible?**—Place an "X" in the appropriate box.

5. **Provider Phone Number**—Enter the area code and phone number for the provider.

6. **Patient's Authorized Representative (If Any) Enter Name and Address**—If the patient has an authorized representative, enter the name and address of that representative here.

7. **Provider Name and Address**—Enter the name and address of the provider.

8. **Provider Number**—Enter the provider's Medicaid-assigned number.

9. **For State Use**—Leave this area blank. This is where the Medicaid consultant will indicate if the services requested are approved, approved but modified, denied, or deferred. If the TAR is approved but modified, denied, or deferred, the consultant will give an explanation in the Comments/Explanation section. The reviewing consultant must sign and date the TAR, or it is not valid.

10. **Name and Address of Patient**—Enter the patient's last name, first name, and middle initial.

Enter the patient's address and telephone number on the following lines.

11. **Medicaid Identification Number**—Enter the patient's Medicaid identification number as it appears on the eligibility label or ID card.

12. **Sex**—Enter "M" for male or "F" for female.

13. **Age**—Enter the age of the patient.

14. **Date of Birth**—Enter the patient's date of birth in an eight-digit format (i.e., 01/01/CCYY).

15. **Patient Status**—Place an "X" in the appropriate box.

16. **Phone Number**—Enter the patient's telephone number.

17. **Diagnosis Description**—Enter the description of the diagnosis.

18. **ICD-9-CM Diagnosis Code**—Enter the ICD-9-CM Diagnosis code for these services. Diagnosis descriptions and codes must relate to the services requested in the section below.

19. **Medical Justification**—Enter the medical justification (attach consultation report or other medical documentation if necessary) for the Medical Consultant to determine medical necessity. Enter the hospital name and address on the first line on the Medical Justification section. If the patient is inpatient in a SNF/ICF, enter the name and address of the facility in the Medical Justification section.

20. **Authorized Yes/No**—Leave blank. The Medicaid consultant will check these boxes if some services are approved, but others are denied.

21. **Approved Units**—Leave blank. The Medicaid consultant will enter the approved number of units.

22. **Specific Services Requested**—Enter the name of the procedure or service requested. Up to six services may be requested on each TAR.

23. **Units of Service**—Enter the means for determining units of service (i.e., 15 minutes for treatments that are calculated per 15-minute blocks).

24. **NDC/UPC or Procedure Code**—Enter the procedure (CPT) code or the drug code for the procedure or drug you are requesting authorization for. The code on the claim submitted and the TAR must be the same.

25. **Quantity**—Enter the number of times the service or procedure is to be performed.

26. **Charges**—Enter the usual and customary fee for the requested services.

27. **Signature of Physician or Provider**—The signature of the provider of services or authorized

representative must appear in this space. Enter the title of the person signing the TAR and the date.

28. **Authorization Is Valid for Services Provided**— This section will be completed by the state agency reviewing the TAR. The authorized services must be completed within the dates specified. If the TAR is for a hospitalization, the claim submitted cannot have a date of service earlier than the "From Date" on the TAR.

29. **Sequence Number**—The TAR control number is preprinted on the form at the time of production. The consultant may add additional numbers or letters. This number must be entered as the TAR control number on the claim when submitted to Medicaid.

Practice Pitfalls

Because Medicaid eligibility is usually determined periodically, eligibility must be verified monthly to ensure that the patient is eligible for coverage. A provider rendering services to a Medicaid patient must accept the Medicaid payment as payment in full, and cannot balance bill the patient. Medicaid claims are paid directly to the provider of services; therefore, no assignment of benefits is necessary.

Medicaid Billing Guidelines

When billing Medicaid, the provider must complete the appropriate billing forms. Most Medicaid charges are billed on the CMS-1500 form. Special requirements on the CMS-1500 for Medicaid claims are as follows:

- Blocks 4 and 7—enter the primary insurance policyholder's name and address (if different than the patient).
- Blocks 9–9d—enter information if Medicaid is the secondary payer. If Medicaid is the primary insurer leave 9–9d empty.
- Block 10d—enter the share of cost as follows "SOC 2249"—no sign or decimal points are used.
- Block 12—leave blank.
- Block 13—leave blank.
- Block 20—enter an X in the "No" box. Medicaid law forbids billing for services rendered by another provider.
- Block 23—enter the prior authorization number if applicable.
- Block 24A—enter the date in the MM DD YY format in the "From" column. Do not enter a date in the "To" column (no date ranging allowed on Medicaid claims).
- Block 24H for EPSDT—if EPSDT service is provided, indicate with a capital "E"; if family planning services are provided, indicate with a capital "F."
- Block 24I (EMG)—if services rendered are for emergency hospital services provided at the hospital, indicate by marking an X.
- Block 24J (COB)—enter an X if the patient has other insurance, also attach the EOB.
- Block 27—enter an X in the "Yes" box.
- Block 29—enter the amount paid by the other carrier if Medicaid is the secondary payer; otherwise leave blank.
- Block 30—enter the balance due if Medicaid is the secondary payer; otherwise leave blank.

CHAPTER REVIEW

Summary

- Medicare and Medicaid billing guidelines change frequently. It is essential for the medical biller to keep abreast of all the changes that occur.

- Medicare intermediaries send out bulletins on a regular basis. The medical biller should read through these bulletins as soon as possible to become familiar with any updates or changes in the billing procedures.

- Medicaid was established under Title XIX of the Social Security Act of 1965 to provide the needy with access to medical care. The Medicaid card must be used when billing for Medicaid services.

- It is important to remember that providers who accept Medicare patients are not allowed to bill the patient for any amounts that Medicare does not cover. If the patient is covered by other insurance, the other insurance carrier is primary to Medicaid and should be billed first.
- Each state's Medicaid program dictates the appropriate guidelines to use for billing. The correct guidelines must be used or Medicaid may not accept the claim for payment.

Assignments

Complete the Questions for Review.
Complete Exercises 4–1 through 4–3.

Questions for Review

Directions: Answer the following questions without looking back into the material just covered. Write your answers in the space provided.

1. What is Medicare? _____

_____

2. On what three criteria is Medicare eligibility based? _____

_____

_____

3. Medicare _____ is considered the basic plan or hospital insurance and Medicare _____ is the medical insurance that covers physicians' services.

4. Briefly explain how to file an appeal on a Medicare claim. _____

_____

_____

_____

_____

5. What does it mean if a provider accepts assignment of benefits with regard to Medicare? _____

_____

_____

_____

_____

6. What is the purpose of the Medicaid program? _____

_____

7. (True or False?) By law, Medicaid is always primary to private group health insurance plans. _____

8. In what situation are providers allowed to bill or submit a claim to the Medicaid beneficiary? _____

_____

9. Once Medicaid pays, is the doctor allowed to balance bill the patient for any amount Medicaid did not cover?

_____

10. In order for a claimant's services to be covered under Medicaid, the claimant must be a _____

and the provider must be an _____.

If you are unable to answer any of these questions, refer back to that section in the chapter, and then fill in the answers.

Exercise **4-1**

Directions: Find and circle the words listed below. Words can appear horizontally, vertically, diagonally, forward, or backward.

1. Carrier
2. Clean Claim
3. Downcoding
4. Medicaid
5. Medicare
6. Medicare Fraud
7. Medicare HMO
8. Medigap
9. Part B
10. Part D
11. Share of Cost

```
D S C G C R V W P N E K Y
U U H A N Y E M M R A R D
A P M A R I D H A D A A I
R P E L R R D C P I R A A
F L D U Z E I O D X P S C
E E I U X D O E C A L I I
R M G Q E N M F R N J Q D
A E A M T R B T C C W K E
C N P W E A B Q T O V O M
I T D T R A P E B H S B D
D S N M E D I M E D I T Q
E I M E D I C A R E H M O
M I A L C N A E L C J D R
```

Exercise 4-2

Directions: Complete the crossword puzzle by filling in a word from the keywords that fits each clue.

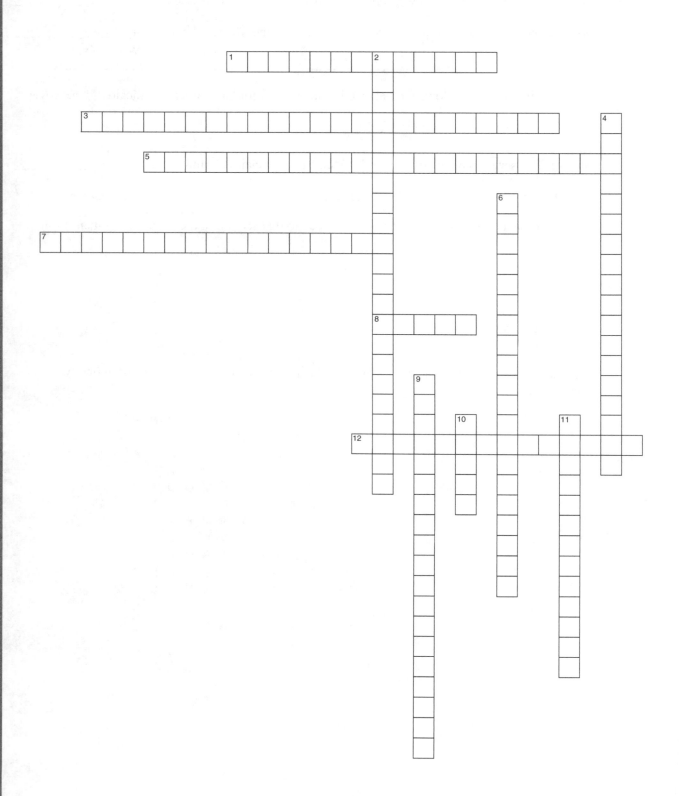

Across

1. A period that begins with the first day of admission to the hospital and ends after the patient has been discharged from the hospital or skilled nursing facility for a period of 60 consecutive days (including the day of discharge).

3. The most common reason for denial of claims by Medicare for services that are considered not medically necessary.

5. Equipment that can withstand repeated use, is primarily and customarily used to serve a medical purpose, is generally not useful to a person in the absence of an illness or injury, and is appropriate for use in the home.

7. Means that all third parties, including Medicare, TRICARE, Workers' Compensation and private insurance carriers, must pay before Medicaid pays.

8. Medicare's basic plan or hospital insurance.

12. A patient whose high medical expenses and inadequate healthcare coverage (often a result of catastrophic illnesses) have left them at risk of being indigent.

Down

2. Providers who agree not to practice "balance billing," or charging patients for more than the Medicare allowed amount.

4. People who usually make less than the poverty level every month.

6. A condition that occurs when a person's kidneys fail to function.

9. Separate plans written exclusively for Medicare participants that pay for amounts that Medicare does not pay.

10. Medicare's advantage portion and includes coverage in an HMO, PPO, and so on.

11. Unlike fraud, this does not require the proof of intent to defraud the Medicare system in order to be assessed. It is quite similar to fraud except that it is not possible to establish that these acts were committed knowingly, willfully, and intentionally.

Exercise 4-3

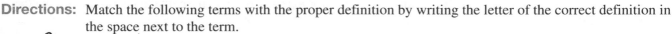

Directions: Match the following terms with the proper definition by writing the letter of the correct definition in the space next to the term.

1. __P__ Advance Beneficiary Notice

2. __e__ Medicaid Remittance Advice

3. __h__ Medicare Summary Notice

4. __N__ Nonparticipating Providers

5. __A__ Provider Identification Number

6. __O__ Resource-Based Relative Value Scale

7. __K__ Center for Medicare and Medicaid Services

8. __M__ Early and Periodic Screening, Diagnosis and Treatment

9. __L__ Medicare Remittance Notice

10. __C__ National Provider Identifiers

11. __F__ Unique Physician Identification Number

12. __B__ Medicare Secondary Payer

13. __J__ Diagnosis-Related Group

a. A number assigned to providers/suppliers in Medicare Part B for the practice location(s) where they provide services to beneficiaries.

b. Medicare pays secondary to employer-sponsored group insurance, individual policies carried by the employee, workers' compensation insurance, beneficiary entitled to Black Lung benefits, automobile or no-fault insurance, and third-party liability.

c. A standard unique health identifier for providers and it will consist of nine numbers plus a check digit in the 10th position.

d. The redetermination letter issued by the Appeals Department that contains all the information necessary to request the next level of appeal.

e. Provides information about claims that were paid, adjusted, voided, and denied.

f. A number for identifying the physician ordering or referring services.

g. One of four regional Medicare carriers responsible for the processing of Durable Medical Equipment claims.

h. An explanation of benefits sent to the Medicare beneficiary, detailing the processing of claims submitted for payment.

i. A unique identification number assigned to Medicare beneficiaries that normally consists of a Social Security number followed by a letter of the alphabet and possibly another letter or number.

j. Under this system, a flat-rate payment is made based on the patient's diagnosis instead of the hospital's itemized billing.

k. The organization that oversees the Medicare and Medicaid programs.

l. An explanation of benefits issued to providers (who accept Medicare assignment) for claims submitted to Medicare for a certain period of time.

m. A preventive screening program designed for the early detection and treatment of medical problems in welfare children.

14. ___I___ Medicare Health Insurance Claim Number

15. ___∅ G___ Durable Medical Equipment Regional Carriers

16. ___∅ D___ Medicare Redetermination Notice

n. Providers who treat Medicare patients but who decide whether to accept assignment on a case-by-case basis.

o. Is a standardized physician's payment schedule. Payments for services are determined by the resource costs needed to provide them.

p. A written notice a provider gives a Medicare beneficiary before rendering services, which informs a patient that a particular procedure may not be considered medically necessary by Medicare, and that if payment is denied by Medicare, the patient will be responsible for paying for the procedure.

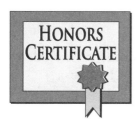

Honors Certification™

The certification challenge for this chapter will be a written test of the information contained in this chapter. Each incorrect answer will result in a deduction of up to 5% from your grade. You must achieve a score of 85% or higher to pass this test. If you fail the test on your first attempt, you may retake the test one additional time. The items included in the second test may be different from those in the first test.

5 Workers' Compensation

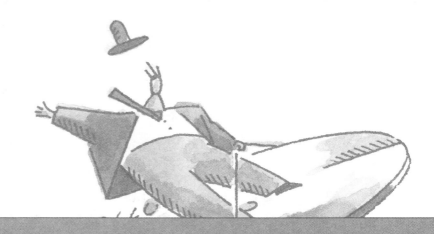

After completion of this chapter
you will be able to:

- Describe the eligibility and basic benefits of workers' compensation.
- List situations or places that would be covered by workers' compensation if an accident were to occur.
- List the types of claims for which workers' compensation provides coverage.
- Describe the three disability levels for workers' compensation claims.
- Describe the benefits provided by workers' compensation coverage.
- Describe what a medical service order is and what it is for.
- Describe how to handle patient records for workers' compensation cases.
- Describe the Doctor's First Report and how it is used.

- State the information that should be included in a Doctor's First Report and Progress Reports.
- List the factors that may delay the close of a workers' compensation case.
- State the guidelines for billing for workers' compensation related services.
- Explain how to handle delinquent claims.
- List signs to look for that may indicate fraud or abuse of a workers' compensation case.
- Describe how third-party liability on a workers' compensation case can affect the medical biller.
- Properly complete lien documents.
- Explain how to handle a claim that is reversed or denied by the workers' compensation board.

Keywords and Concepts
you will learn in this chapter:

- Death Benefits
- Doctor's First Report of Injury/Illness
- Lien
- Medical-Legal Evaluation

- Medical Service Order
- Nondisability
- Permanent Disability
- Physician's Final Report
- Rehabilitation Benefit

- Subjective Findings
- Temporary Disability
- Treating Physicians (TP)
- Vocational Rehabilitation
- Workers' Compensation (WC)

Workers' Compensation (WC) is a separate medical and disability reimbursement program that provides 100% coverage for job-related injuries, illnesses, or conditions arising out of and in the course of employment. The employer, by law, is responsible for the benefits due to an injured employee for work-related injuries and illnesses. WC insurance includes benefits for medical care expenses, disability income, and death benefits.

When a patient first enters the office for treatment of an accident, it is important to obtain a statement of exactly what happened so that you can determine if a claim is covered by WC or by the patient's regular insurance. Job-related injuries include any injuries which happen during the performance of work-related duties, whether they are in or out of the office. Occupational illnesses are considered to be any disorders, illnesses, or conditions that arise at work or from exposure to factors at work. Occupational illnesses may be caused by inhaling, directly contacting, absorbing, or ingesting the hazardous agent. Some occupational illnesses may take years to develop, or remain latent for a number of years before flaring up. For this reason, some states have WC laws that cover employees for years after they cease active employment in a field. For example, construction workers who dealt repeatedly with asbestos may develop asbestosis years after exposure.

Federal WC programs cover federal employees, coal miners (black lung program), longshoremen, and harbor workers. State WC laws cover everyone else. States set up their own guidelines, with the federal government mandating a minimum level of benefits.

Each state's WC Appeals Board has the sole authority to oversee the rights and benefits of an injured or ill employee. It is through this Appeals Board that an applicant (injured employee) will file their WC application.

As a general limitation, most insurance plans specify that the claimant will not be entitled to payment for "bodily injury or disease resulting from and arising out of any employment or occupation for compensation or profit."

Most insurance plans will investigate and then provide benefits for medical care if they suspect that a claim(s) is work-related. Because the resolution of a WC case usually takes one to two years, private plans are obligated to pay the benefits for which the member is entitled and then file a lien with the member and the WC Board to recover their losses when the case is settled.

Once the WC carrier has accepted liability for the claim(s), the plan will discontinue providing benefits for medical care. At that point, the claim would be denied on the basis that it is work-related.

Intent of the Workers' Compensation System

Before WC, injured employees were responsible for their own care, regardless of whether they were hurt on the job or at home. Injured employees would have to seek and pay for their own medical care, and then attempt to collect from their employer if they felt the company was at least partially responsible for their injury. Many times, the only way to collect was by bringing a lawsuit against the employer, thus creating hard feelings between the employer and the injured employee.

If the employer accepted the blame for the accident and agreed to cover medical expenses, they would often choose the medical provider based on price rather than quality of service.

Additionally, employers were not encouraged to stress safety in the workplace, as the damages awarded in an accident often had more to do with the injured employee's injury than with the amount of negligence on the part of the employer.

With the implementation of WC and the inclusion of the WC insurer, both the employer and the injured employee have a third party to address grievances to and to assist with the rehabilitation of the injured worker. WC has the following benefits:

1. It allows injured employees to seek the best available care without irritating their employer, as the WC insurance carrier will be covering the bills.

2. It allows injured employees and employers to understand the rights and responsibilities of injured employees injured on the job. This eliminates many of the lawsuits and the animosity they entail. It also allows the injured employee to be reimbursed quickly, without waiting for the lawsuit to settle, and to gain a higher portion of the award since there are no attorney's fees and court costs involved.

3. It allows the injured employee to continue to receive income during their disability.

4. It relieves the employer of liability for workplace injuries, except in cases of gross negligence.

5. It relieves hospitals, providers, and public charities of the obligation to cover the costs of those injured employees who are unable to pay for services, especially in the case of an accident that causes permanent disability.

6. It allows for compilation of reports that allow studies of workplace accidents. This provides additional information for reducing preventable accidents and for assisting employers with upgrading workplace safety.

7. It allows special provisions for coverage of minors under age 18 (or age 21 in some states).

8. It allows coverage for all injured employees, regardless of the wealth of the employer or the business engaged in. Most states require WC for all businesses with one or more injured employees; however, a few states require a minimum of three to five injured employees.

Employee Activities

The following section contains some general guidelines as to what constitutes an injury or illness as recognized by a WC Board in most states based on the type of activity, not injury.

Company Activities

Company activities can be defined as the following:

1. An injury sustained while attending an activity sponsored by an employer for the purpose of obtaining some business gain (i.e., company party for morale purposes; sporting activity for which the injured employee is provided transportation or the company gains advertisement by virtue of having the injured employee wear a company "athletic shirt").

2. An injury sustained during an activity for which the company provides remuneration.

3. An injury sustained while in the course of a person's occupation.

Use of Company Vehicles

Most WC laws provide coverage for an injury sustained while driving or as an authorized passenger in a company vehicle. This is true whether the injury is incurred in the course of the person's occupation, or if the vehicle is provided as a part of the injured employee's benefits to use to and from work.

The law's interpretation of "in the course of employment" is very different from most laymen's interpretation. For instance, someone injured while eating lunch at a company-sponsored event may be considered covered by WC. Therefore, always undertake investigations and let the Board handle the final determination. An investigation also should be undertaken to determine if benefits may be payable under automobile insurance coverage.

Business Trips

Most WC laws provide coverage for a person who is on a business trip. This coverage is applicable as long as the person is engaged in employment duties. Of course, there are always exceptions to this rule.

Company Parking Lot

Most WC laws provide that if an injured employee is injured in a parking lot that is owned or maintained by his employer and furnished to the injured employee free of charge, he may be covered under WC. In addition, coverage would extend, in some instances, to an injury sustained by the injured employee while on neutral ground between the parking lot and the place of employment. An exception would be if such incidents were specifically excluded in the WC law, or if the injuries were sustained from willful or negligent actions on the part of the injured employee.

Usually, WC is not liable for injuries sustained in a parking lot that is owned by the employer and for which a rental fee is charged for the parking space. In such instances, the injured worker has a free choice to park elsewhere, which would relieve the employer of any and all responsibility.

Occupational Disease

Most of the time, coverage will extend to injured employees who contract a disease that develops by working within a certain industry. For instance, most states provide compensation for individuals working with asbestos material over a period of years who then develop asbestosis or silicosis. Likewise, individuals can develop dermatitis from working with certain chemicals, such as in the exterminating industry.

Sometimes, a claimant may have an occupational illness claim that is submitted to the WC Board, and a concurrent nonoccupational illness claim for which he may be reimbursed under the plan. In such instances, a separate billing should be completed by the provider indicating those charges that were solely for the treatment of the nonoccupational disability.

Time Limits

Injured employees must report their injury or illness to their employer within a reasonable period of time, generally two years. What is considered reasonable will often vary from state to state. However, many states require that the injured employee report an injury within 24 hours.

If a patient indicates that they are being treated for a work-related injury, be sure that they have notified the employer of the injury. If they have not, encourage them to do so immediately. Let them know that their WC benefits may be denied if they do not report the injury within a specified period of time. Also, let them know that many states will refuse to pay anything for claims if the injury is not reported in a timely manner.

Fraud and Abuse

Unfortunately, fraud and abuse occur frequently in the WC system. Many injured employees, employers, providers, and insurance carriers find it easy to defraud the system and reap significant financial rewards.

In the past, there has been little deterrent to abusing the system. It frequently was possible to find a doctor who was willing to testify that injuries were more serious than was first thought. Likewise, numerous lawyers stepped in and set up relationships with doctors to produce claims where no actual injury or illness existed. This is especially true when work-related stress became a popular diagnosis for any one of a number of ailments. Many of these lawyers would locate people in the unemployment office and convince them that they could get better reimbursement through WC than they could through unemployment.

It is important for the medical biller to realize that committing fraud or abuse of the WC system is a felony in most states. Additionally, not reporting suspected or known cases of fraud or abuse is also illegal in many states. Atlthough most claims are legitimate, the medical biller should recognize what constitutes fraud. Following are some signs of fraud or abuse to look out for:

- An injured employee who cannot clearly describe the pain or injury, or whose description changes each time details of the incident are related.
- An injured employee who is overly dramatic regarding their injury.
- An injured employee who complains of an injury that cannot be substantiated by medical evidence. This may include soft tissue injuries which cannot be seen on an x-ray, or a patient who insists that there is a serious injury even when there is medical evidence to the contrary.
- An injured employee who delays the reporting of an injury, especially an injury that is reported on a Monday when the injured employee claims it happened on Friday.
- An injured employee who reports the injury to an attorney or regulatory agency before reporting the injury to their employer.
- An injured employee who changes physicians frequently, or shows up for a first treatment, but seems unhappy with the diagnosis and changes physicians. Patient may be seeking a physician who will grant additional time off work or will testify to a greater degree of injury.
- An injured employee who is a short-term employee, or who was scheduled to terminate employment just after the injury occurred.
- An injured employee who has a history of curious or an excessive amount of WC claims.
- An injured employee who complains of a severe injury and an inability to perform certain tasks but is seen having used the injured limb or body part while in the waiting room.
- An employer who refuses to accept that an injury occurred on the job when there is evidence to the contrary.
- An employer who refuses to complete the necessary paperwork and instead attempts to pay for medical services through the company.
- A medical provider who orders or performs unnecessary procedures or tests.
- A medical provider who inflates the severity of the injury to qualify for higher reimbursement (i.e., lists a fracture as open rather than closed, bills for a high complexity exam rather than a moderate complexity exam).

- A medical provider who charges for services that were never performed, or adds additional procedures onto existing claims.
- A medical provider who makes multiple referrals to a lab, clinic, or hospital and receives a referral fee from these organizations.
- A medical provider who states that an injury exists and needs treatment when no injury is actually present.
- A medical provider who sends in duplicate billings with information changed (i.e., dates) to make it appear that services were performed more than once.
- A medical provider who files many claims with subjective injuries (i.e., pain, strain, emotional disturbance, inability to perform certain functions).
- A medical provider who files claims for several injured employees of the same company that show similar injuries (i.e., injuries for which reports or x-rays may be duplicated).
- An attorney who pressures a provider to provide additional treatment or to increase the severity of the diagnosis.
- An attorney who encourages a provider to charge for services not rendered, stating that the insurance carrier will cover it.
- An attorney who refers numerous clients to a specific provider, which suggests they may be in collusion with each other.

These examples suggest signs that a medical biller should look for. If a biller suspects fraud, it should be reported to the appropriate authority immediately. If a biller becomes aware of fraud by the provider for whom they work, they should seek the help of an attorney. A biller can be considered guilty of fraud if they knew of the fraud and did nothing to prevent it. This is true even if the biller receives no money from the fraud.

Types of Workers' Compensation Benefits

WC provides the following five types of benefits to injured workers:

Nondisability Claims

Nondisability claims are for minor injuries that will not require the patient to be kept from his job. The patient is able to continue working throughout the extent of the injury. On the first visit to the physician the physician should complete a "Doctor's First Report of Occupational Injury or Illness (First Report)." This form and a copy of the bill should be submitted to the WC carrier. These types of claims include medical expenses, including medical services, hospital treatment, surgery, medications and prosthetics or appliances, and durable medical equipment.

Temporary Disability Claims

Temporary disability claims are when the patient is not able to perform his or her job requirements until he or she recovers from the injury involved. When a physician sees a patient in this situation, a first report will be submitted and ongoing reports will be issued every two to three weeks until the patient is discharged to return to work.

Each state has a waiting period before temporary disability becomes effective, usually three to seven days (except in the Virgin Islands, where the waiting period is one day). During temporary disability the injured employee is paid a portion of their salary as a tax-free benefit. Temporary disability ends when the patient is able to return to work, even with limitations or to a different department, or when the patient's condition ceases to improve and the patient is left with a permanent disability.

Temporary disability allows payments to continue to the injured employee even though they are not currently working. Payments are based on the injured employee's salary and the length of the disability. Payments are usually not taxable as income.

Permanent Disability Claims

Permanent disability usually commences after temporary disability when it is determined that the patient will not be able to return to work. The physician will prepare a discharge report stating that the patient is "permanent and stationary." This means that nothing more can be done and the patient will have the disability for the rest of his or her life. The case will be reviewed by the WC Board and, if determined to be permanent, a compromise and release will be issued. This is a settlement from the insurance carrier for a payment to the injured party.

The amount of the settlement is based on the age of the disabled employee, the amount of money they were making at the time of the injury, and the severity of the injury. The older an employee is, the higher the disability rating. This is because of the idea that a younger patient has a better chance of finding other employment or of being retrained for another job than an older employee would. Additionally, death benefits and rehabilitation benefits may be provided.

Permanent disability payments, either in the form of weekly or monthly payments or as a lump sum distribution, are made to the injured employee.

Death Benefits

Death Benefits compensate the family of a deceased employee for the loss of income which the employee would have provided to the family. Some states also provide a burial benefit to assist with the funeral and burial expenses for the employee.

Rehabilitation Benefits

If an injured employee is found to have a permanent disability, some states allow for a **rehabilitation benefit**. A rehabilitation benefit is a benefit provided to retrain the injured employee in a physical ability that will help them to seek future employment (i.e., proper use of a wheelchair, use of the left hand when a person loses their right).

Some states participate in a "work hardening" program, wherein an injured employee is assigned therapy similar to their work in an attempt to strengthen them and build up their endurance toward a full day's work. Often,

injured employees in such a program will be returned to work on a limited or restricted basis. Physicians, therapists, employers, insurance carriers, and all others concerned with the injured employee's case must keep in constant communication to ensure that the patient is not returned to work either sooner or later than possible, and that the injured employee will continue to receive adequate benefits that do not encourage them to cease work.

Many states also allow for **vocational rehabilitation** or retraining in a different job field when the injured employee is unable to return to their former position. This can include courses in colleges and vocational schools, or on-the-job training programs. Often, injured employees are paid a weekly allowance (as in the case of temporary disability) while they are attending school and for a limited time after graduation. The time after graduation is to allow them time to locate a job. The injured employee is then considered to be off temporary disability and having returned to work. Vocational rehabilitation can also include job guidance, résumé preparation, and placement services.

Insurance carriers will often attempt to get the injured employee retrained and back to work as soon as possible, especially as the longer a person is off work, the higher the likelihood that they may never return to full-time employment.

On the Job Now

Directions: List and define the five types of workers' compensation benefits.

1. _____
   _____

2. _____
   _____

3. _____
   _____

4. _____
   _____

5. _____
   _____

Treating Physicians

Treating physicians (TP) are used to initially establish the employee's eligibility for workers' compensation benefits. The role of the TP is to provide care and treatment to the injured employee. Treating physicians share the same physician–patient relationship as any other patient. The TP may be an employer-selected physician or may be selected by the injured employee depending on the circumstances.

Medical-Legal Evaluations

Within the workers' compensation system, medical determinations trigger eligibility for benefits. However, when there are disputed issues over treatment, disability, or for other reasons, a physician other than the TP may be called on to perform a **medical-legal evaluation**.

The term medical-legal means that the evaluation provides medical evidence for the purpose of proving or disproving medical issues in a contested workers' compensation claim. An evaluating physician (also referred to as an Independent Medical Examiner, Qualified Medical Evaluator or Agreed Medical Evaluator) may be called in when a party objects to the TP's report.

Medical Service Order

The first indication that a patient is being treated for a work-related injury is usually when the injured employee enters the provider's office for treatment with a medical service order. Many employers have a standard **medical service order**. A medical service order is a form that states that the patient is being referred to the provider in regards to a work-related injury and that the employer is responsible for coverage of services. A sample of a medical service order is shown below **(see Figure 5–1, form may vary depending on the state)**.

If the patient does not arrive with a medical service order, the biller should contact the company immediately and request that one be faxed over. If the employer does not have a medical service order, the provider should fax one to the employer, and ask the company representative to complete it and fax it back immediately. This form can assist with the collection of a claim in case of a dispute, and a copy should be attached to any claims when they are submitted for payment.

In order to preserve the original signatures for your records, a photocopy should be made of the medical service order before the doctor completes it. The original should be kept for your records. The copy should be signed by the doctor, if necessary, and a photocopy

EMPLOYER
MEDICAL SERVICE ORDER

ON LETTERHEAD

To Dr./Hospital/Clinic _____
Address _____

We are requesting treatment for_____(name)_____,
 in accordance with the workers' compensation statutes for the state of XX. Please submit any necessary reports to the State Compensation Insurance Fund as soon as possible. Compensation cannot be paid without the completion of the proper reports.

Thank you,

Employer Representative_____
Title _____

If the injured employee is unable to return to work immediately, please so indicate by signing and dating this form below. If the injured employee is able to return to work with limitations or restrictions, please describe any limitations on the reverse of this form. This form should be returned to the injured employee for forwarding to the employer.

Dr. _____
Signature_____
Date/Time_____

■ **Figure 5–1** Sample Medical Service Order

made of the front and back for the records. The copy that was signed by the doctor should then be returned to the patient.

If the patient must be referred to an additional facility for testing or treatment, authorization should be obtained from the employer before transferring the patient. The medical biller should call the employer and give the reason for the transfer or referral, the name and address of the facility to which the patient is being transferred, and the treatment needed at the facility. Ask the employer to fax an authorization for transfer or referral. If verbal authorization is given, be sure to record the date and time, and the name and title of the person giving the authorization. The authorization (whether by faxed copy or the verbal information) should be placed directly on or attached to the transfer or referral order and a copy retained for your records.

Patient Records

If a patient is being treated for a work-related injury, all records relating to the injury and treatment should be kept separate from the patient's regular medical records. Because employers are covering the costs of treatment, privacy guidelines are somewhat different than the normal privacy agreement between patient and provider. In WC cases, the agreement is actually between the provider and the employer, not the injured employee. The employer may request to see records regarding the injury, and these records may be subpoenaed. No information pertaining to the injured employee's non-work-related treatment should be made a part of this file, so that confidentiality between the provider and the patient is not breached for non-work-related treatments and conditions.

Many providers place work-related injury records in a colored file so that it can be clearly identified as different from the patient's normal file.

If the physician finds a non-work-related condition during their injury-related examination (i.e., during the exam the physician discovers the patient has a heart condition), the WC agreement would be in force for all treatment relating to the injury, and the patient and his normal insurance carrier would be responsible for treatment of the non-work-related condition. It is important to clarify this with the patient and, if possible, treat the two conditions at separate times. At no time should the doctor bill twice for the same examination. The examination should be charged according to the main activity of treatment (i.e., was most treatment re-

lated to the work-related injury or the non-work-related injury).

Doctor's First Report of Injury/Illness

Regardless of the type of workers' compensation claim or benefits, the doctor must file a **Doctor's First Report of Injury/Illness (see Figure 5–2, form may vary depending on the state)**. This form requests basic information on the date, time, and location of the injury/illness and treatment, the patient's subjective complaints and objective findings, the diagnosis and the treatment rendered. The description of how the accident or exposure happened should be supplied by the patient if possible. **Subjective findings** are those that cannot be discerned by anyone other than the patient (i.e., pain, discomfort). The physician should give an opinion as to the extent of pain, description of activities that produce pain and any other findings. A treatment plan should also be indicated.

If the provider chooses to send a narrative report along with the standard report, the following information should be included:

* A history of the accident, injury or illness.
* Diagnosis.
* Any connection between the primary injury and any subsequent injuries, especially if the interrelating factors between the primary and secondary injuries are not immediately discernable.
* Subjective and objective findings.

Physicians must make a report of injury, disability, or death within a specified time period. This varies from immediately on knowledge of the incident to within 30 days. Different states set different time limits and different requirements for reporting. There also may be different limits for different levels of injury (i.e., injury, disability, death).

The original form should be submitted to the WC agency and a copy of the form sent to the insurance carrier. One copy is retained in the patient's records, and many providers also send a copy to the employer.

The Doctor's First Report of Injury/Illness is an extremely important document. It may be a major factor in the employer's or insurance company's decision to accept or contest the workers' compensation claim. Care should be taken to complete this form properly.

STATE OF CONFUSION

DOCTOR'S FIRST REPORT OF OCCUPATIONAL INJURY OR ILLNESS

Within 5 days of your initial examination, for every occupational injury or illness, send two copies of this report to the employer's workers' compensation insurance carrier or the insured employer. Failure to file a timely doctor's report may result in assessment of a civil penalty. In the case of diagnosed or suspected pesticide poisoning, send a copy of the report to Division of Labor Statistics and Research, P.O. Box 555555, Anytown, USA 12345-6789, and notify your local health officer by telephone within 24 hours.

	PLEASE DO NOT USE THIS COLUMN
1. **INSURER NAME AND ADDRESS**	
2. **EMPLOYER NAME**	Case No.
3. Address: No. and Street City Zip	Industry
4. Nature of business (e.g., food manufacturing, building construction, retailer of women's clothes)	County

5. **PATIENT NAME** (first name, middle initial, last name)	6. Sex ☐Male ☐ Female	7. Date of Mo. Day Yr. Birth:	Age
8. Address: No. and Street City Zip		9. Telephone number ( )	Hazard
10. Occupation (Specific job title)		11. Social Security Number - -	Disease
12. Injured at: No. and Street City County			Hospitalization
13. Date and hour of injury Mo. Day Yr. Hour or onset of illness _____ a.m. _____ p.m.		14. Date last worked Mo. Day Yr.	Occupation
15. Date and hour of first Mo. Day Yr. Hour examination or treatment _____ a.m. _____ p.m.		16. Have you (or your office) previously treated patient? ☐Yes ☐No	Return Date/Code

Patient please complete this portion, if able to do so. Otherwise, doctor please complete immediately; inability or failure of a patient to complete this portion shall not affect his/her rights to workers' compensation under the California Labor Code.

17. **DESCRIBE HOW THE ACCIDENT OR EXPOSURE HAPPENED.** (Give specific object, machinery or chemical. Use reverse side if more space is required.)

18. **SUBJECTIVE COMPLAINTS** (Describe fully. Use reverse side if more space is required.)

19. **OBJECTIVE FINDINGS** (Use reverse side if more space is required.) A. Physical examination B. X-ray and laboratory results (State if non or pending.)

20. **DIAGNOSIS** (If occupational illness specify etiologic agent and duration of exposure.) Chemical or toxic compounds involved? ☐ Yes ☐ No
ICD-9 Code ___ ___ ___ - ___ ___

21. Are your findings and diagnosis consistent with patient's account of injury or onset of illness?   ☐Yes ☐No   If "no," please explain.

22. Is there any other current condition that will impede or delay patient's recovery?   ☐Yes ☐No   If "yes," please explain.

23. **TREATMENT RENDERED** (Use reverse side if more space is required.)

24. If further treatment required, specify treatment plan/estimated duration.

25. If hospitalized as inpatient, give hospital name and location.   Date   Mo.   Day   Yr. Estimated stay
admitted

26. WORK STATUS -- Is patient able to perform usual work?   ☐Yes ☐No
If "no," date when patient can return to: Regular work ____/____/____
Modified work ____/____/____   Specify restrictions _____

Doctor's Signature _____   License Number _____
Doctor Name and Degree (please type) _____   IRS Number _____
Address _____   Telephone Number _____

FORM 5021 (Rev. 4)

Any person who makes or causes to be made any knowingly false or fraudulent material statement or material representation for the purpose of obtaining or denying workers' compensation benefits or payments is guilty of a felony.

■ **Figure 5–2** Sample of a Doctor's First Report of Injury/Illness

Many First Report forms have a space for the occupation of the patient. It is important to list the patient's actual job, so the insurance carrier can determine if the injured employee was engaged in a normal work activity. This also allows the carrier to ensure that the employer listed job titles and normal work activities accurately. Some employers attempt to list employees in less hazardous jobs (i.e., office worker rather than cutting machine operator), as insurance premiums are based on the hazards the injured employee may encounter in the job.

If the First Report requests the time the patient was examined, it is important to list the date and time of the examination as well as the date and time of the injury.

This allows the insurance carrier to know how much time elapsed between the injury and the patient seeking treatment for the injury.

Be sure to indicate the provider's complete address and telephone number on the bottom of the form. This is the address to which payment will be sent. The provider's title (i.e., M.D., D.C.) should be included, as well as their complete license number.

Copy the required number of forms before signing them, and then have the physician sign each copy in ink. Stamped signatures are not acceptable. Additionally, the preparer should place their initials in the lower left-hand corner.

On the Job Now

Directions: Complete a Doctor's First Report of Injury/Illness for the following case. Refer to the Patient Data Table in Appendix C for additional information.

Patient: Bobby Bumble
Job Title: Waiter/Host
Physician: Joanne Jones, M.D.
                1029 Jonathan Lane
                Anytown, USA 12345
                (765) 555-0987
License #:   A1234567
EIN: 11-0987654

Incident: Patient states that at 5:10 p.m. on 10/16/CCYY, he was carrying a dessert tray. He slipped on some soda that was spilled on the floor and landed on his back, striking his head on the floor. The dessert tray turned upside down and landed on him. The patient is complaining of headache and difficulty breathing through his nose.

Injuries: Concussion (no fracture, no apparent brain damage), foreign matter (chocolate mousse) in both eyes, foreign body (cherry) lodged in nose. Patient treated at Provider Medical Center from 10/16/CCYY to 10/19/CCYY.

Procedures Performed: Physical examination and history, new patient, moderate complexity ($70), x-ray of the skull, 2 views ($45), removal of foreign body from nose ($85), irrigation of eyes ($18).

Treatment Plan: Bed rest for two days, wake patient every hour during first 24 hours to ensure no LOC, limited activity for two weeks, re-check in 10 days. Patient estimated able to return to work 10/30/CCYY.

Signed: Joanne Jones, M.D., 10/16/CCYY 6:05 p.m.

Additional pages attached ☐

STATE OF CONFUSION
Division of Workers' Compensation

PRIMARY TREATING PHYSICIAN'S PROGRESS REPORT (PR-2)

Check the box (es) which indicate why you are submitting a report at this time. If the patient is "Permanent and Stationary"

(i.e., has reached maximum medical improvement), do not use this form. You may use DWC Form PR-3.

☐ Periodic Report (required 45 days after last report) ☐ Change in treatment plan ☐ Released from care

☐ Change in work status   ☐ Need for referral or consultation ☐ Response to request for information

☐ Change in patient's condition ☐ Need for surgery or hospitalization   ☐ Request for authorization ☐ Other:

Patient:

Last_____First_____M.I. _____Sex _____

Address_____City_____State_____Zip _____

Date of Injury_____ Date of Birth_____

Occupation _____SS # _____-_____-_____ Phone (_____)_____

Claims Administrator:

Name_____ Claim Number _____

Address_____ City_____ State_____Zip _____

Phone (_____)_____ FAX(_____) _____

Employer name: _____ **Employer Phone** (   ) _____

The information below must be provided. You may use this form or you may substitute or append a narrative report.

Subjective complaints:

Objective findings: (Include significant physical examination, laboratory, imaging, or other diagnostic findings.)

Diagnoses:

1. _____ICD-9-CM _____

2. _____ICD-9-CM _____

3. _____ICD-9-CM _____

■ **Figure 5–3** Sample Progress Report

Treatment Plan: (Include treatment rendered to date. List methods, frequency and duration of planned treatment(s). Specify consultation/referral, surgery, and hospitalization. Identify each physician and non-physician provider. Specify type, frequency and duration of physical medicine services (e.g., physical therapy, manipulation, acupuncture). Use of CPT® codes is encouraged. Have there been any changes in treatment plan? If so, why?

Work Status: This patient has been instructed to:

☐ Remain off-work until _____.

☐ Return to *modified* work on _____ with the following limitations or restrictions.

  (List all specific restrictions re: standing, sitting, bending, use of hands, etc.)

☐ Return to full duty on _____ with no limitations.

Primary Treating Physician: (original signature, do not stamp)   Date of exam: _____

I declare under penalty of perjury that this report is true and correct to the best of my knowledge and that I have not violated Labor Code § 139.3.

Signature: _____   Lic. _____

Executed at: _____   Date: _____

Name: _____   Specialty: _____

Address: _____   Phone: _____

■ Figure 5–3 *(continued)*

Progress Reports

Following the Doctor's First Report of Injury/Illness, the physician should follow up with progress reports (sometimes called supplemental reports) every two or three weeks (**see Figure 5–3**, form may vary depending on the state). Many states have forms for subsequent progress reports; however, they also may allow a narrative report to be filed, rather than the completion of the specified form. Retain a copy for the files and provide the insurance carrier with their required number of copies (usually three or four). Subsequent reports also should be sent at the end of a hospitalization, even if the patient is expected to be readmitted later. This report serves as both a report on the patient's condition, and as a bill.

If the patient's condition changes significantly, a Reexamination Report, or a detailed progress report, should be filed with the insurance carrier.

Physician's Final Report

The WC carrier often will wait until the physician indicates that the patient's condition is permanent and stationary before finalizing a claim. The physician should then notify the WC carrier that no further treatment is needed (or that no further treatment will significantly alter the patient's condition) and that the patient has been discharged. This is called the **Physician's Final Report**. Some states require the final report be submitted on a

Practice Pitfalls

If the physician chooses to send in a narrative report, the following information should be included:

- Complete identification of the patient, including WC case, number, name, and address of the patient.
- Date and description of all examinations and treatment procedures performed since the last report was submitted.
- Progress of the condition since the last report.
- Any proposed changes in the treatment plan.
- Any lab tests, function tests, or other items that show any change in the patient's condition.
- The status of the patient's disability, including an estimated time that the patient can return to work, or any estimated permanent disability. If this changes from the doctor's report of first injury, it should be brought to the attention of the insurance carrier so that it may adjust funding to cover the new situation.
- A treatment plan including a description of the planned course, scope, frequency, and duration of treatment and an estimated date of completion.

specified form, and some states use the same form for both subsequent and final reports. The Physician's Final Report should indicate that the patient has been discharged, the level of the patient's permanent disability, if any, and the balance due on the patient's account (usually provided as a patient's statement showing services, dates of service, charges, and any payments rendered). Once this information is received, the WC carrier will establish the level of permanent disability, if any, medical and other expenses will be paid, and the case will be closed.

Billing for Workers' Compensation Services

When billing WC claims, it is important to follow all guidelines and regulations provided by the state WC agency. Using incorrect forms or not following procedures can cause delays in claims, or difficulty in collecting for procedures performed. Following are general guidelines regarding billing WC cases:

1. As mentioned previously, services rendered in a WC case are the responsibility of the employer, not the injured employee.

2. Some states pay WC cases according to a fee schedule, whereas others may use the amounts based on Medicare's allowed amounts. A fee schedule limits the amount providers can charge for services. Each service is given a different allowed amount based on the difficulty of the procedure, the time involved, the risk to the patient, and other factors. Fee schedules prevent doctors from overcharging for services. The amount paid under a fee schedule is considered payment in full for the services and the biller should write off any amounts not covered.

3. If there are unusual factors that affect the amount the physician has charged, documentation should be sent with the claim to substantiate the increased fees charged. The insurance carrier will then determine if the fees are warranted.

4. If any procedures are listed as By Report (BR) on the fee schedule, a complete report of the procedure, initialed by the doctor, should accompany the claim. This report will allow the insurance carrier to determine the appropriate payment for the procedure. Be sure to attach any lab reports, x-rays, or other data which supports either the excess fees, or the BR procedure.

5. As a biller, always remember to ask if a case is work-related when a patient first visits for treatment of an injury, illness, or condition. This prevents billing the wrong party and having to go through costly adjustments and reimbursements. If the case is work-related, the patient should be instructed to provide the doctor's office with the case number as soon as they obtain it.

6. Because WC cases often go before a jury, every contact with the patient, his employer, his attorney, or anyone else related with the case should be documented and placed in the file. This includes contacts in person, by phone, or through a third party. Be sure to include the date and time of the contact, the full name of the person contacted, who initiated the contact (i.e., patient called, carrier called), and the details of the contact.

7. Be sure to use the proper CPT® and ICD-9-CM codes and to complete all boxes on all forms. Incomplete information is one of the main causes of delay in closing a case.

8. In WC cases, all materials and drugs should be itemized in detail and charged at cost.

9. If a patient is injured in one state and then seeks treatment in a different state, the laws of the state where the claim occurred would cover the injured employee. This situation occurs most often in cities that straddle a state line, or in rural areas where the nearest hospital is in a neighboring state.

   The WC carrier should be contacted before treatment, if possible, as some states have restrictions on treatment. If treatment is approved, be sure to get a written authorization for the patient record. Be sure to ask for all necessary forms for physician's first report of illness, progress reports, physician's final reports, and any other reports needed. Also ask about billing requirements. Some states require billing on a CMS-1500 or other form, some states will accept an itemized patient statement or superbill, and other states require electronic billing.

10. Be sure to file claims for workers' compensation services as soon as possible. Many states have time limits on when you can submit a claim to the insurance carrier (i.e., six months after treatment). If you are past the time limit, some WC carriers will cut the benefit payment and others may refuse to pay it completely.

If you have questions regarding the payment of a particular claim, call the WC insurance carrier and ask to speak with the adjuster in charge of the case. General questions regarding the state WC benefits, rules, and legislation information can be obtained from your state's WC Appeals Board.

Third-Party Liability

It is possible to have third-party liability in a WC case. For example, George works at a restaurant and is taking trash out to the trash bin behind the building. A plumber had been visiting the restaurant. On leaving, he backed up without looking and ran over George's leg.

Because George was clearly injured in the normal performance of his duties, the accident would be covered by WC. The WC insurance carrier would be required to pay all benefits George is entitled to. However, as the accident was clearly the plumber's fault, the WC insurance carrier may encourage George to sue the plumber for damages. Automobile insurance and personal liability insurance may be involved if George wins the case against the plumber; the WC insurance carrier has a right to collect all monies it has paid out for George's benefits.

Practice Pitfalls

1500 form

When billing for services rendered to an injured employee, the provider must complete the appropriate billing forms. Some insurance carriers require a specific billing for submission of workers' compensation claims. However, most workers' compensation charges are billed on the CMS-1500 form. Special requirements on the CMS-1500 for workers' compensation claims are as follows:

* Header—enter the name and address of the workers' compensation insurance company.
* Block 1a—enter the patient's WC claim number if available. If not, enter the employer's policy number.
* Block 4—enter the name of the patient's employer.
* Block 6—enter an X in the "Other" box.
* Block 7—enter the address of the patient's employer.
* Block 8—enter an X in the "Employed" box.
* Block 9–9d—leave empty unless claim has not been declared WC.
* Block 10a—enter an X in the "Yes" box.
* Block 10b—only check "Yes" if the accident happened while the patient was performing work-related activities.
* Blocks 11–11c—leave empty.
* Block 12—leave empty.
* Block 13—leave empty.
* Block 14—enter the date of injury or illness in the MM DD YY format.
* Block 16—enter the dates the patient is unable to work if applicable in the MM DD CCYY format.
* Block 17—enter the SSN or EIN of the employer.

Any fees that exceed the payment made by the workers' compensation insurance company may not be billed to or collected from the patient. Providers must accept the workers' compensation payment as reimbursement in full.

Liens

In permanent disability, a compromise and release will be issued by the insurance carrier for the injuries to the patient. If the physician has been seeing the patient and there are unpaid medical expenses, a lien should be filed for payment of services rendered. A **lien** is a legal document that expresses claim on the property of another for payment of a debt **(see Figure 5–4, form may vary depending on the state)**. A lien is completed and submitted to the attorney representing the injured party to be paid on monetary settlement of the WC claim.

A lien should be sent along with the bill for the initial visit. Whenever additional services are rendered, a copy of the bill should be submitted to the attorney so that all concurrent care will be included in the lien. All services must be for the care of the injury covered under the WC claim. Many states have a special lien form for WC purposes. These forms can be obtained through the local Division of Industrial Accidents. (A sample copy of a lien is shown in **Figure 5–5, form may vary depending**

TO: Attorney _____

_____

_____, Confusion

RE: Medical Reports and Insurance Carrier Lien

FOR_____

    I do hereby authorize the above insurance carrier to furnish you, my attorney, with a full report of any records and resultant payments of myself in regard to the accident in which I was involved.

    I hereby authorize and direct you, my attorney, to pay directly to said insurance carrier such sums as may be due and owed for payment of medical services rendered me or the provider of services both by reason of this accident and by reason of any other bills that are due, and to withhold such sums from any settlement, judgment or verdict as may be necessary to adequately protect said insurance carrier. And I hereby further give a lien on my case to said insurance carrier against any and all proceeds of any settlement, judgment or verdict which may be paid to you, my attorney, or myself as the result of the injuries for which I have been treated or injuries in connection therewith.

    I fully understand that I am directly and fully responsible for reimbursement of any payments for all medical bills submitted for services rendered and that this agreement is made solely for said insurance carrier's additional protection and in consideration of its awaiting payment. And I further understand that such payment is not contingent on any settlement, judgment or verdict by which I may eventually recover said fee.

Dated: _____ Patient's Signature:_____

    The undersigned being attorney of record for the above patient does hereby agree to observe all the terms of the above and agrees to withhold such sums from any settlement, judgment or verdict as may be necessary to adequately protect said insurance carrier named above.

Dated: _____ Attorney's Signature:_____
Mr./Ms. Attorney: Please sign, date, and return one copy to our office at once.

Keep one copy for your records.

■ **Figure 5–4** Sample Lien Letter

on the state.) Complete the lien form and send copies to the WC appeals board, the patient's employer, the patient, and the WC insurance carrier. A copy also should be kept for the files.

If a lien is not filed, all monies recovered at the close of the case officially belong to the patient. It is then the patient's responsibility to cover the medical expenses. If any liens are filed, the patient must first pay the liens and

---

WORKERS' COMPENSATION APPEALS BOARD

STATE OF CONFUSION

CASE NO. _____

NOTICE AND REQUEST FOR ALLOWANCE OF LIEN

_____

LIEN CLAIMANT   ADDRESS
VS.

_____

INJURED WORKER   ADDRESS

_____

EMPLOYER   ADDRESS

_____

INSURANCE CARRIER   ADDRESS

The undersigned hereby requests the Workers' Compensation Appeals Board to determine and allow as a lien the sum of
_____ dollars ($_____) against
any amount now due or which may hereafter become payable as compensation to _____
                                                                              INJURED WORKER
on account of injury sustained by him/her on _____.
                                              DATE

This request and claim for lien is for: (Mark appropriate box)
- ❑   The reasonable expense incurred by or on behalf of said injured worker for medical treatment to cure or relieve from the effects of said injury; or
- ❑   The reasonable medical expense incurred to prove a contested claim; or
- ❑   The reasonable value of living expenses of said injured worker or of his dependents, subsequent to the injury, or
- ❑   The reasonable living expenses of the wife or minor children, or both, of said injured worker, subsequent to the date of injury, where such injured worker has deserted or is neglecting his family; or
- ❑   The reasonable fee for interpreter's services performed on _____.
                                                                  DATE

NOTE: ITEMIZED STATEMENTS MUST BE ATTACHED
The undersigned declares that he delivered or mailed a copy of this lien claim to each of the above-named parties on

_____

ATTORNEY FOR LIEN CLAIMANT   DATE

_____

ADDRESS OF ATTORNEY FOR LIEN CLAIMANT   LIEN CLAIMANT

INJURED WORKER'S CONSENT TO ALLOWANCE OF LIEN

I consent to the requested allowance of a lien against my compensation.

_____

ATTORNEY FOR INJURED WORKER   INJURED WORKER

DEPARTMENT OF INDUSTRIAL RELATIONS
DIVISION OF INDUSTRIAL ACCIDENTS

■ **Figure 5–5** Sample Lien Form

then pay any other resultant expenses. Therefore, if the lawyer files a lien and his fees exhaust most of the money, there will be little or none left for other expenses. If at all possible, patients should be persuaded to pay for medical services before settlement of the claim.

If a lien is filed, the biller should have their copy of the lien letter signed by the patient and the patient's attorney. This makes the attorney responsible for payment of the physician's bills. If the attorney does not remit the necessary funds from the patient's settlement, the attorney must cover the medical expenses.

A lien should have a specified time limit on it; this often is a period of one year. If settlement has not been reached by that time, or there are ongoing charges on the patient's account relating to the WC injury, an amended lien should be filed. The subsequent lien should state the balance of the patient's account, and should have the word AMENDED stamped across the top or below the Appeals Board Case Number.

The biller should place all files with liens in a special section and hold them until the cases have been settled. It is illegal to continually bill or harass the patient when a lien agreement has been signed.

In effect, the lien acknowledges the provider's agreement to wait for reimbursement until the case has been settled. The biller should contact the patient's attorney at least once every quarter for an update on the case and to determine when settlement is expected to occur. The attorney also should be contacted within two weeks after the date settlement is expected to find out the results of the case and ask when payment can be expected.

In some states, the law allows the provider to be paid prior to the attorney or patient collecting any monies from the settlement. Statutes in your state should be checked to protect you. If your state has such a provision, attorneys may not collect their fee and then state that insufficient funds were recovered to cover your total bill. Some states also allow the physician to bill the patient for any funds that were not received from the settlement. Once again, check with the laws of your state to determine if patients can be billed or if any amounts not collected should be written off.

Liens are an inexpensive way of ensuring that the physician will be reimbursed for their services. The cost is much lower than suing the patient and assures that payment will be received when the dispute between the patient and the WC insurance carrier is settled. A lien is a legal document that will be recognized by the court and will provide protection in the event of litigation.

On the Job Now

Directions: Complete a lien letter and a lien form for the following case. Refer to the Patient Data Table and Provider Data Table in Appendix C for additional information. Bobby Bumble states that on 9/11/CCYY, as he walked down the stairs into the reception area to pick up a fax his office had received, he slipped on a banana peel, causing him to injure his back.

Case Number:	54321B
Lien Claimant:	Paul Provider
Injured Worker:	Bobby Bumble
Employer:	Blue Corporation
Insurance Carrier:	Ball Ins. Carriers
Lien Sum:	$31,792.00
Date of Injury:	09/11/CCYY
Attorney for Lien Claimant:	Faren Ekual, Esq.	9354 Doublemint Place, Anytown, USA 12345
Attorney for Injured Worker:	Idee Fendu, Esq.	4345 Justiceville Place, Anytown, USA 12345

Delinquent Claims

If payment is not received within 45 days of billing the WC insurance carrier, the biller should contact the adjuster in charge of the case and ask the reason for the delay. Often, the proper forms have not been received from one party or another. If this is the case, ask which form is missing and who is responsible for sending it. If the form is required by another person (i.e., the employer) contact that person and request that the form be completed as soon as possible so you may receive payment.

If the employer or other party has not completed the necessary item within 30 days of your contacting them, send a letter to the WC Board or Industrial Accidents Commission in your state. The letter should state that you are requesting their help in securing the necessary items from the party. Be sure to include the case number, the name, address, and phone number of the party who should provide the item, the patient's name and address, the date of the injury, and the name and address of the insurance carrier or other person the item should be sent to. Also list the patient's balance due.

Delay of Adjudication

When a patient is released to work, all benefits have been paid, and the case is closed, the claim is said to have been adjudicated. Often adjudication occurs within two to eight weeks after the physician submits the final report, stating that the patient has been discharged and is able to return to work.

If the patient suffers a permanent disability, adjudication can take much longer, especially if the amount of permanent disability is protested and a lawsuit ensues. Additional factors that may delay the close of a case include:

1. Confusion or questions on any of the reports submitted by the employer, injured employee, or physician. This can include conflicting information from one or more parties, or vague or ambiguous terminology (especially by the physician) or illegible items.
2. Omitted information on a report, including incomplete forms, boxes not filled in, or signatures not included.
3. Incorrect billing or questions on the billing provided by the physician.

4. Insufficient progress reports to update the insurance carrier on the status of the patient.

Workers' Compensation Appeals

If you disagree with a decision made on a workers' compensation claim, you may appeal that decision. During an appeal, the facts of the case are reviewed, including any new information that is provided. An appeal usually can only be filed by an injured employee or employer.

For most states, there are two levels of appeal. The first level is a request for review of an adjudicator's claim decision. This appeal is usually forwarded to a hearing officer or an Administrative Law Judge.

The second level review is an appeal from the first level review, to a workers' compensation tribunal or workers' compensation board. This level of review is usually final.

Reversals

Occasionally, an accident that was thought to be WC will turn out not to be. This can happen when a patient hides or omits facts regarding when and how the accident occurred. It also can be found that there is a non-industrial, underlying condition that caused the accident. For example, a patient may have epilepsy and suffer a seizure at work. Any injuries directly received on the job site could be considered WC; however, the treatment of the underlying epileptic condition would not be WC.

In some cases, the injured employee may be found to be negligent in their actions, or willfully not abiding by established workplace rules. In such cases, injuries sustained as the result of negligence of the injured employee may not be considered industrial accidents. For example, if the injured employee is told they must refrain from wearing hoop earrings but they chose to anyway, they may be considered liable if the earrings are caught on machinery and ripped from the ear.

In such cases, the WC board would deny payment on the claim. All claims for treatment should then be sent to the patient's regular insurance carrier with the denial notice from the WC Board. A letter also should be sent to the injured employee notifying them that their claim was denied and that their regular insurance is being billed for the charges.

CHAPTER REVIEW

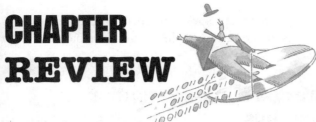

Summary

- WC insurance is a separate medical insurance program that covers work-related injuries, disabilities, and death. A wide range of activities may be covered under WC laws.
- WC provides coverage for nondisability claims, temporary disability claims, permanent disability claims, death benefits, and rehabilitation benefits to injured workers.
- Vocational rehabilitation or training in a different job field is allowed by many states.
- The Doctor's First Report of Injury/Illness is a major factor in the employer's or insurance company's decision to accept or contest the workers' compensation claim. The basic information requested on the form is the date, time, and location of the injury/illness and treatment rendered.
- The Physician's Final Report is usually the last report submitted stating that the patient has been discharged.
- The physician must notify the WC carrier that no further treatment is needed.
- Using incorrect forms or not following procedures can cause a delay in your claim. It is extremely important to follow all guidelines and regulations. The claim is said to be adjudicated when all the benefits have been paid and the patient is released to work.
- Some factors that may delay the close of a case are confusion or questions on any of the reports, omitted information on a report, incorrect billing or questions on the billing, and insufficient progress reports.

Assignments

Complete the Questions for Review.
Complete Exercises 5–1 and 5–2.

Questions for Review

Directions: Answer the following questions without looking back into the material just covered. Write your answer in the space provided.

1. What is workers' compensation? _____

_____

_____

2. What items are likely to cause a delay in adjudication of a case? _____

_____

_____

_____

3. What do you do if a patient states this is a WC injury but he has nothing from the employer to prove it? _____

_____

_____

_____

4. What is a lien? _____

_____

_____

5. Why should you file a lien? _____

_____

6. What signatures should you get on a lien? _____

_____

7. Define Temporary Disability. _____

_____

_____

8. Define Permanent Disability. _____

_____

_____

9. What is a nondisability claim? _____

_____

10. If an employee is injured while at a company-sponsored game, is it considered a WC case? _____

If you are unable to answer any of these questions, refer back to that section in the chapter, and then fill in the answers.

Exercise 5-1

Directions: Complete the crossword puzzle by filling in a word from the keywords that fits each clue.

Across

6. A separate medical and disability reimbursement program that provides 100% coverage for job-related injuries, illnesses, or conditions arising out of and in the course of employment.

Down

1. The doctor must file this report regardless of the type of workers' compensation claim or benefits. This form requests basic information on the date, time, and location of the injury/illness and treatment, the patient's subjective complaints and objective findings, the diagnosis, and the treatment rendered.

2. A benefit provided to retrain an injured employee in a physical ability that will help them to seek future employment.

3. Minor injuries that will not require the patient to be kept from his job.

4. An evaluation that provides medical evidence for the purpose of proving or disproving medical issues in a contested workers' compensation claim.

5. Compensates the family of a deceased employee for the loss of income that the employee would have provided to the family.

7. The report notifying the WC carrier that no further treatment is needed (or that no further treatment will significantly alter the patient's condition) and that the patient has been discharged. The report should indicate that the patient has been discharged, the level of the patient's permanent disability, if any, and the balance due on the patient's account.

Exercise 5-2

Directions: Find and circle the words listed below. Words can appear horizontally, vertically, diagonally, forward, or backward.

1. Lien
2. Medical Service Order
3. Permanent Disability
4. Subjective Findings
5. Temporary Disability
6. Treating Physician

```
X Y Z P Z S W J O R E I K D E P D R Y
J T Q L S Z I M K W F M P W S T R R W
Y L R I X T V H L F I F J Q Z W U Z F
D S G N I D N I F E V I T C E J B U S
V F M J D J D T O U C I P K N C B H X
F T R E A T I N G P H Y S I C I A N X
P S R A V R F L P K G Z F M S Q B T J
M J L X L D M Y Y D K O Q V T X I K G
Y T I L I B A S I D T N E N A M R E P
M E D I C A L S E R V I C E O R D E R
Z O L J G E P E O I W B C P X M J K A
B L C N Y W T P Y N R R D S U W N W L
N A L P T N E M T A E R T Q Z J K P C
T E M P O R A R Y D I S A B I L I T Y
Q N F L T X L M A F K A M Y Y I T R J
N F E S Q A E O U B R G H F T T Z V D
H M R I E S W E E S I S A E A M L X G
T I W G L N N E M K F K K H A V W X A
F H D K G X T K Z S J O O W K H E X Z
```

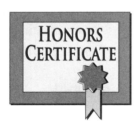

Honors Certification™

The certification challenge for this chapter will be a written test of the information contained in this chapter. Each incorrect answer will result in a deduction of up to 5% from your grade. You must achieve a score of 85% or higher to pass this test. If you fail the test on your first attempt, you may retake the test one additional time. The items included in the second test may be different from those in the first test.

6
Managed
Care

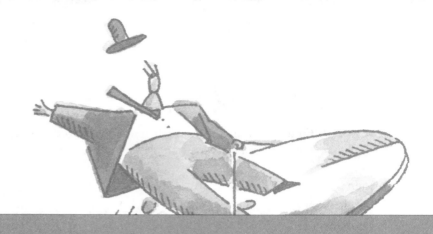

After completion of this chapter
you will be able to:

- List the reasons for rising healthcare costs.
- Describe ways that insurance carriers decrease costs.
- Describe the main types of managed care organizations and their function.
- List the common HMO benefits.
- Describe the various types of Preferred Provider Organizations and their function.
- Explain the purpose of the membership card and eligibility rosters.
- Explain the difference between reporting patient encounters on a CMS-1500 and billing on a CMS-1500.
- Describe how risk for expenses is shared between groups/IPAs and MCPs.
- Explain how providers are reimbursed in a capitation agreement.
- Describe the proper handling of the patient's medical record.

- Properly handle authorizations, referrals, and second opinion referrals using a given scenario.
- List the steps in the second opinion process.
- List the steps to be taken in the case of a member grievance or complaint.
- Properly complete a grievance log.
- State the reasons why a member may be disenrolled and the information that must be documented in a disenrollment.
- Describe the standard provisions for continuing care when a provider terminates their agreement with an MCP.
- Properly generate a payment to an outside provider using a given scenario.
- Properly complete a denial notice.
- Describe stoploss and the procedures for obtaining stoploss reimbursement from the MCP.

Keywords and Concepts
you will learn in this chapter:

- Active Member Roster
- Capitation
- Clean Claim
- Complaints
- Copayment
- Disenrollment
- Eligibility Roster
- Exclusive Provider Organization (EPO)
- Grievances
- Health Maintenance Organizations (HMOs)

- In-Network Providers
- Independent Physician Associations (IPAs)
- Individual Practice Organization (IPO)
- Managed Care
- Management Service Organization (MSO)
- Out-of-Network Providers
- New Member Roster
- Physician Hospital Organization (PHO)

- Preferred Provider Organizations (PPOs)
- Primary Care Provider (PCP)
- Reinsurance
- Self-Insurance
- Social Health Maintenance Organization (S/HMO)
- Stoploss
- Terminated Member Roster
- Utilization Review (UR)
- Withhold

Managed care contracts were created in an attempt to bring healthcare costs under control by having providers share some of the financial risks of health care with the patient and the insurance carrier.

Rising Healthcare Costs

There are numerous reasons for the rising cost of health care in America. Some of the most common include:

1. The higher costs of doing business, including rising rents, employee salaries, and so on.

2. The rising costs of education for medical professionals.

3. Little or no competition among providers. It is not customary for doctors to advertise their prices. Additionally, the American consumer often does little comparison shopping on the basis of cost when trying to find a physician, especially when insurance carriers cover most of the cost of services.

4. Little or no control by traditional plans on the utilization of care. These plans normally paid on claims with little or no restrictions.

5. Greater number of lawsuits, causing ever increasing malpractice insurance premiums. Additionally, many doctors are ordering more tests and trying more treatments in order to protect themselves against possible lawsuits.

6. Higher utilization of medical services. Many people visit the doctor for even the most insignificant reason.

7. The cost of new medical technology. Patients like to see doctors who have the latest technology and equipment. Unfortunately, this equipment costs a tremendous amount of money. Some medical equipment can cost over $500,000.

8. More people are living longer, and those over 65 use more of the medical services than any other age group.

9. Millions of people do not have health insurance. These people utilize services and then are unable to pay, or pay on a delayed timetable. The costs associated with treating the uninsured often are passed on to those patients with insurance.

10. There are more catastrophic illnesses in the world today.

Managed Care

Managed care is a system for organizing the delivery of health services so that the cost of care is reduced and the quality of care is maintained or improved. There are many different types of managed care organizations, including Health Maintenance Organizations, Preferred Provider Organizations, Exclusive Provider Organizations, Physician Hospital Organizations, and Management Service Organizations.

Health Maintenance Organizations

Health Maintenance Organizations (HMOs) are one of the most common managed care trends. Many other managed care models may start with an HMO base and modify it based on the needs of the members. HMOs are organizations or companies that provide both the coverage for care, and the care itself. See **Figure 6–1** for an overview of an HMO. A **Social Health Maintenance Organization (S/HMO)**, also known as a Medicare HMO, is an organization that provides the full range of Medicare benefits offered by standard HMOs plus additional services.

Under an HMO setup, members pay a set amount every month and the HMO agrees to provide all their

---

PATIENTS

- Choose an HMO and contract with that HMO to provide all medical care for a set monthly premium,
- Choose a provider who has contracted with the HMO as their primary care physician, and
- Visit the chosen primary care physician for all medical needs unless an emergency situation exists, and pay a copayment for each medical visit.

HMOS

- Collect premiums from patients,
- Contract with providers to provide certain services,
- Oversee quality of care, and authorize and pay for services not covered by the doctor's capitation plan.

PROVIDERS

- Provide all capitated care for patients,
- Refer patients to specialists when needed,
- If specialist services are not covered by capitation, obtain authorization for referral from HMO, and
- If specialist services are covered by capitation, provide reimbursement (payment) to the specialist from their capitation amount.

GROUPS/IPA

- Contract with providers to join a group so they have greater bargaining power with the HMOs, and
- Contract with the HMOs to provide care for HMO patients in a specified region.

SPECIALISTS

- Treat patients referred by provider and authorized by provider or HMO, and
- Bill provider or HMO for services, and may sign a contract with the provider or HMO to limit charges for services to managed care patients.

■ Figure 6–1 HMO Overview

---

care, or to pay for the covered care they cannot provide. The HMO hires physicians and sets up hospitals (or contracts with existing physicians and hospitals). The member chooses a specific provider for their care (commonly called a **primary care provider** or primary care physician [PCP]).

Health Maintenance Organizations are so named because of their initial belief that healthcare costs could be controlled by providing services that maintained and encouraged the health of its members. By adding benefits such as low-cost physician visits and annual check-ups, the HMOs sought to encourage members to seek medical attention for minor medical problems before they became serious medical emergencies.

There are several different types of HMOs. The most common include those listed here.

Staff Model

This is the original concept of HMO services. A physician or provider is hired to work at the HMO's facility. They are usually paid a salary and may receive additional bonuses. The provider works only for the HMO and does not see outside patients.

Group Model

The HMO contracts with providers or provider groups to render services. These providers agree to only provide care for HMO members, but they do so at their own facilities. In the group practice model care is often provided at a centrally located facility. The HMO may have several facilities in the region they service, or just a few, depending on the size and diversity of the population they serve.

The HMO also will own one or more hospitals that provide the inpatient services which members need. All physicians and other personnel are on staff and paid a salary by the HMO. Any specialists needed to treat the patients are provided by the HMO.

Some HMOs contract with hospitals for a specified number of beds, or for a wing of an existing hospital, rather than build their own facilities. This is because of the increased costs associated with building a new hospital and the decreased utilization of hospitals. Sharing a facility can be a good way to provide an HMO the resources and treatment options needed, while at the same time increasing the revenues of the hospital. HMO personnel normally provide care to HMO patients at these facilities.

Individual Practice Organizations (IPOs)

An **Individual Practice Organization (IPO)** (sometimes called Independent Practice Association or IPA) is a legal entity, comprised of a network of private practice physicians, who have organized to negotiate contracts with insurance companies and HMOs.

There are two arms to this type of organization. The HMO arm acts as an insurer, oversees the program, enrolls members, collects premiums, and handles the claims. The IPOs organize physicians and contract with the HMO for discounted rates on services. The medical group as a whole is paid a capitation amount for each member, and the group oversees the care of the members and attempts to control costs.

The individual physicians (who are members of the medical groups) agree to see patients in their own offices along with their regular fee-for-service clients. The providers were able to easily gather a large number of patients by joining the IPO, and at the same time they retained their autonomy and freedom, unlike the traditional HMO providers who were hired by the HMO and placed on salary.

This type of arrangement allows the HMO to add numerous providers, which allows patients a wider freedom of choice. Because providers are paid a capitation amount according to the number of members they see, there is no additional cost to the HMO for adding numerous additional providers.

Network Model

In this type of arrangement, the HMO contracts with several providers in a given area, allowing some overlap in a geographic region. This allows more of a choice for subscribers and allows an HMO to increase its subscriber base without worrying about unduly overloading a single provider. In the network model, providers see not only the HMO members but also continue to see their regular fee-paying patients as well.

HMO Coverage

Most HMOs offer a higher level of coverage than traditional indemnity plans. For example, not only do HMOs cover physician visits and necessary testing but also treatment by a specialist (when the patient is referred by their PCP) is often covered. HMOs also tend to cover prenatal care, emergency care, home health care, skilled nursing care, drug and alcohol abuse treatment, physical therapy, allergy treatment, and inhalation therapy, often to a higher degree than coverage provided by indemnity plans. Most physician visits require a small copayment from the member.

Hospitalization is usually covered in full by most HMO plans. However, many plans require a per-day inpatient copayment, and if a patient is seen in the emergency room there often is a copayment.

Additionally, HMOs often cover preventive services. Preventive coverage provides for services such as an annual physical, cancer screening (pap smears, mammograms, etc.), flu shots, immunizations, and well-baby care. Many HMO plans also cover health education, cessation of smoking classes, nutrition counseling (especially for diabetics and those needing weight control), or exercise classes. Traditional indemnity plans either limit or restrict coverage of such services.

Eye exams for both children and adults are covered by most HMOs; however, additional vision services (glasses, contacts, etc.) may not be covered.

For those plans that cover prescription drugs, there often is a small copayment required from the member for each prescription. Prescriptions are often limited to a 30-day supply, but many HMOs have no limit to the number of prescriptions that may be filled in a month.

Mental health treatments often require a higher copayment than physician visits and are often limited to short-term care. There also are usually limits on the number of visits.

Physical therapy is often covered only for a brief period of time and only if significant improvement is expected for the patient.

Controversial or experimental procedures (i.e., temporomandibular joint (TMJ) surgery, laser surgery, and gastric stapling) often are not covered. Cosmetic procedures are almost never covered.

Those HMOs that are federally qualified must provide the following minimum benefits:

1. Preventive care.
2. All hospital inpatient services with no limits on costs or days.
3. Hospital outpatient diagnosis and treatment services, including rehabilitative services, with some limitations.
4. Skilled nursing home and home healthcare services.
5. Short-term detoxification treatment for drug and alcohol abuse.
6. Medical treatment and referral for substance abuse.

Preferred Provider Organizations

Preferred provider organizations (PPOs) are the second most common managed care alternative. They are, in essence, a hybrid mix of an HMO and traditional plan.

In a PPO, the insurance carrier contracts with providers to provide services at a contracted rate. These providers are called **in-network providers**. These providers agree to provide services at a reduced amount in exchange for the referrals from the carrier. Additionally, the carrier agrees to reimburse providers in their network at a higher percentage than providers outside their network.

In a PPO, the insurance carrier will contract with a group of hospitals or physicians to provide services at a set fee for each service. Some services may be covered by a capitation amount. Those fees that are not covered by the capitation amount will be billed on a discounted basis to the carrier.

Many services will be covered by the insurance carrier in full. Other services will have a standard coinsurance percentage (e.g., 80%).

Patients may choose to go to an in-network provider or they may go to a provider who has not contracted with the insurance company (**out-of-network providers**). However, if a patient chooses to visit an out-of-network provider the benefits may be reduced.

Additionally, when a patient visits an in-network provider, the provider is usually contractually obligated to handle the claims submission paperwork for the patient.

Exclusive Provider Organization

In an **Exclusive Provider Organization (EPO)**, the patient must select a PCP and can use only those physicians who are part of the network or who are referred by the PCP. These types of organization usually do not provide coverage for care performed outside of the EPO network or facilities. EPO providers are paid as services are rendered.

Physician Hospital Organization

A **Physician Hospital Organization (PHO)** is an organization of physicians and hospitals that band together for the purpose of obtaining contracts from payer organizations. The PHO bargains as an entity for preferred provider status with various payers. The organization also refers clients to each other.

Management Service Organization

A **Management Service Organization (MSO)** is a separate corporation set up to provide management services to a medical group for a fee. Individual physicians and providers contract with the MSO for services. An MSO may be owned by a single hospital, several hospitals, or investors.

On the Job Now

Directions: List the four types of Preferred Provider Organizations and describe the structure of each.

1. _____

   _____

2. _____

   _____

3. _____

   _____

4. _____

   _____

Self-Insurance

Many employers are turning to a concept called **self-insurance**. Instead of paying monthly premiums to an insurance carrier, they place the money in an escrow account. When an employee receives medical attention, they submit the claim to their employer and are reimbursed according to the terms of the employer's contract.

This idea works well for employers with large numbers of employees, but not as well for those with few employees. For example, a company with only 10 employees that pays $1,000 a month in healthcare premiums would have $12,000 in their account for use each year. One employee with a catastrophic illness could wipe out this account with only a few weeks of treatment.

However, if the employer has 1,000 employees, with premiums of $100,000 a month, the account would accumulate a total of $1,200,000 during the year, which is more than enough to handle most cases.

These companies, in essence, create their own little insurance company. They must hire employees to oversee the collection of premiums from employees (if any), the accounting of the department, the processing of claims, and all other aspects an insurance company covers, perhaps with the exception of a marketing department. These additional employees generate additional costs.

To help manage these costs, some companies hire Administrative Services Only (ASO) companies or Third Party Administrators (TPAs) to handle the processing of claims. The employee sends any claims directly to the ASO, and may not even know that the plan is self-funded by their employer. This often happens in the cases of large insurance carriers that have an ASO arm, such as Blue Cross/Blue Shield. The ASO handles the paperwork, processes the claims, and pays benefits out of the escrow account.

Companies who select to be self-insured run the risk that their employees may utilize more care than the premiums they would have paid. They could then lose money. However, by tightening controls or altering benefits, they can keep costs under control.

One reason this strategy works is that employees tend to be healthier, as a whole, than the general population. There are no elderly, and most of the people are well enough to show up to work on a regular basis.

Many self-insurance plans purchase **reinsurance**, also known as stoploss insurance. Reinsurance is an insurance policy that protects the company against catastrophic medical costs levied against their plan, either by a single employee or by all employees as a whole. This protects the employer in cases of a company disaster (i.e., plant collapsing and injuring numerous workers, fire, chemical poisoning, etc.), a non-work-related disaster (i.e., earthquake, flood, tornado, with numerous injuries to employees and their families), a generally unhealthy year, or when the payment amount exceeds a certain dollar threshold.

Billing Managed Care Plans

Providers who treat patients covered by managed care plans (MCPs) create the same bills they would for any other insured patient. The main difference is in preapprovals and in the patient's choice of providers.

Billing MCPs

MCPs, however, have specific rules and regulations that must be followed regarding the keeping of patient charts, determining member eligibility, and all other pertinent data. These rules will be set forth in a Policies and Procedures manual, which will be given to each provider/group/IPO on the signing of a contract with the MCP. It is important that all office staff understand the rules and regulations contained within this manual.

Disobeying any of the rules could result in substantial loss of revenue to the provider or in termination of their contract with the MCP.

The Membership Card

On enrollment, each MCP member is issued a membership card. This card shows the member's name and will contain a record number or other means of identifying the patient. Often there will be a magnetic strip on the back of the card that will have additional information encoded on it.

The membership card also may list a plan number or type that will indicate the benefits covered for this individual. The reverse of the card may show contact numbers for authorization of emergency treatment.

If an MCP member transfers from one medical group to another, or changes their benefits, the MCP may issue a new membership card.

Practice
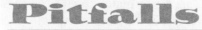

Whenever a member seeks treatment, the provider should check the identification card to verify eligibility and to ensure that the correct patient chart has been pulled. If necessary, the provider may request an additional piece of identification to ensure that the person using the card is actually the member to whom it was assigned.

Eligibility Rosters

Because the membership card is retained by the patient and remains unchanged from month to month, many MCPs may have an **eligibility roster** to assist the provider in determining who is eligible for treatment. These rosters list those patients who have chosen the provider as their PCP. There often will be several different rosters.

The **active member roster** lists those whose coverage has continued into the next month. This usually means that the insured or their employer has paid the monthly premium to continue coverage for another month.

The **new member roster** shows those patients who have signed up for MCP coverage and have chosen the provider as their PCP. In addition to members who have just begun coverage, the new member roster shows those existing patients who have recently chosen this provider as their PCP.

The **terminated member roster** shows those members whose coverage has been terminated or who have chosen to terminate this provider as their PCP. For those whose eligibility has terminated, this list is most accurate for those whose coverage is handled by their employer. In such a case, the employer will notify the MCP that the employee is no longer with the company and that their benefits are being terminated.

There may be those patients who do not show up on any of the rosters. This may be because they have not formally terminated their coverage; however, they did not pay their monthly premium prior to the time the rosters were created. If a patient is seeking treatment and their name does not show up on any of the rosters, contact the MCP to verify that they are still eligible for coverage before providing services. If they are still eligible for coverage, see the following guidelines under SUPPLEMENTAL CAPITATION to ensure that the provider receives the capitation amount for these patients.

The roster also may contain information in addition to the patient's name. This may include identifying information such as Social Security number, date of birth, gender, insurance information such as covered benefits, the employer group number, the plan effective date, and other data.

Member rosters are the primary means of identifying eligibility for a patient. The medical group should verify the member's eligibility every time they seek treatment. If the provider of service provides services without verifying eligibility, the provider is at financial risk for the services it provides, and may not receive reimbursement from the MCP.

Practice
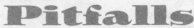
Pitfalls

Be sure to verify the following before the provider renders services: that the member is eligible for service for the month and that they have chosen this provider as their PCP, the amount of their copayment, and the correct group or plan number they are covered under.

Copayment Amounts

MCPs have very few deductibles that must be satisfied each year. The primary form of patient contribution by the member is in the form of a **copayment**. A copayment is a fixed amount a member must pay for a covered service.

The eligibility roster, or the group designation chart, will identify the services covered by the capitation amount. It also will identify the copayment amount that should be collected from the patient for each visit. This copayment is per provider visit. Therefore, if a patient sees one provider in a medical group and is referred to a different provider within that group, the group should collect the copayment twice, once for each visit with each provider. If this money is not collected at the time of the visit, the provider must absorb the loss of this amount.

Copayment amounts may be different for different services. For example, the member may have a $25 copayment for outpatient visits, and a $50 copayment for inpatient visits. For this reason it is important to check the contract for each of the services performed.

For purposes of copayments, services are often broken into the following five categories:

- **Outpatient services**, including physician office visits, outpatient lab and radiology, outpatient surgery, durable medical equipment, home health services, and so on.
- **Inpatient services**, including facility charges, drugs, anesthesia, inpatient laboratory and radiology, emergency services, and so on.
- **Pharmacy and prescription services**.
- **Vision care services**.
- **Dental care services**.

Some contracts may not cover some of these services (i.e., vision and dental care), and some contracts may not cover items that are listed under a specific type of service (i.e., durable medical equipment).

Occasionally, there may be two designated copayment amounts because of the different types of services performed in a single visit. In such a case, only one copayment should be collected from the member. Most provider groups/IPAs will collect the higher of the two amounts.

On the Job Now

Directions: List the five categories of copayments.

1. _____
   _____

2. _____
   _____

3. _____
   _____

4. _____
   _____

5. _____
   _____

Patient Encounter Forms

Some MCPs require that all patient encounters (i.e., visits) be reported to the MCP. This reporting is often done using an encounter form. The MCP may specify the use of a designated form for reporting encounters, or they may use the CMS-1500.

Groups/IPAs

Medical groups are groups of physicians who are signed under or work for the same company. **Independent Physician Associations (IPAs)** are groups of providers who have banded together for the sole purpose of signing a contract with an MCP.

Most MCPs require the group or IPA to have a certain number of physicians in varying specialties. For example, they must often have a general practitioner or internist, a pediatrician, an obstetrician/gynecologist, or a cardiologist. This allows the group to treat all

Practice Pitfalls

Some MCPs have their providers or group/IPAs report patient encounters on a CMS-1500. If there are services that a provider renders that are not covered by the capitation amount, the amount for these charges should be placed in block 24F. If the charges are covered by a capitation amount, and there is no charge for the service, $0 would be listed in block 24F. The total charges and the balance due would be indicated as charged if not covered under the capitation amount, or as $0 if there are no total charges or balance due.

Some MCPs may have providers or group/IPAs submit charges that are the MCP's responsibility on a separate claim form from those that are covered under capitation. Thus, two claim forms for the same provider, patient, and dates of service may be necessary.

aspects of the patient's care and to provide appropriate services to all members who choose that group/IPA as their PCP.

MCP to Group/IPA Risk

MCPs often use existing providers to deliver care to their patients by signing the providers to contracts. They introduce a mechanism for financial risk-sharing by providing cost incentives to providers in order to contain their expenditures (i.e., the provider is paid a set amount, regardless of the services they provide to the patient).

In many MCP situations, the risk for patient services is shared between the group/IPA and the MCP. The contract between the MCP and the group/IPA will outline who is responsible for what services and any conditions or limitations that apply to those services.

Risk determinations are usually considered to be:

- **No risk**—the MCP collects and keeps the monthly capitation amount, and merely pays providers on a fee-for-service basis for the treatment rendered to members. This is similar to a regular insurance carrier setup, except that the member pays only the copay amount, no deductibles or copayment percentage. This arrangement is almost never seen.
- **Partial risk**—the MCP is responsible for most services; however, the capitation covers basic services.
- **Shared risk**—the MCP and the group/IPA share the responsibility for services. A contract will designate which services or treatments are covered by the MCP and which are covered by the provider.
- **Full risk**—the group/IPA is responsible for most, if not all of the services. The MCP is just in the business of selling policies and writing contracts with groups/IPAs.

Most MCP contracts with providers are on a shared-risk basis. The MCP will provide a list to the group/IPA of all possible services (often indicated by CPT® codes and descriptions), and an indication of who is responsible for those services (**see Figure 6–2**). A letter code will often designate who is responsible for payment for that service (i.e., G = Group/IPA responsibility, H = MCP/HMO responsibility, etc.).

This document also will list any services that are denied and the appropriate copayment amount for many of these services. It is important to note that, if

Practice **Pitfalls**

If an MCP offers numerous different types of policies (i.e., group coverage, individual coverage, Medicare HMO coverage, etc.), then each of these plans may be listed on the same sheet. It is important for the biller to be sure they are looking at the correct procedure code and the correct plan to determine who is financially responsible for a service.

the plan is a S/HMO, any services that normally are covered by Medicare should be covered services under the S/HMO contract (regardless of whether the group, MCP, or the HMO has financial responsibility). Therefore, if Medicare determines that they will begin covering a specific type of treatment, then the S/HMO also must begin covering that type of treatment.

Group/IPA to Physician Risk

In addition to the MCP transferring all or part of the risk to the group/IPA, the group/IPA may transfer some or all of their risk to an individual capitated provider as well. The levels of risk transferred to the capitated provider include:

- **No risk**—the group/IPA keeps the entire capitation payment and providers are paid on a fee-for-service basis. There are usually no withholds or bonuses as part of the provider's contract. However, there will often be a fee schedule incorporated as part of the contract agreement, so the amount that the provider receives for services will be determined by the fee schedule.
- **No referral risk transferred**—all or part of the payment to the provider involves risk, but that the risk is not tied to referrals. Only the capitation amount, bonuses, and withholds are at risk (i.e., the provider may perform more services than the capitation, withholds, and bonuses cover). Under this arrangement, referral means any service not provided for by the provider. Essentially, it is expected that the capitation, withholds, and bonuses are the only payments for any and all care that the provider renders to the member. The provider is not responsible for paying for referrals, and the amount of money paid to the provider is not affected by the decision of the provider to make referrals to other providers.

Covered Services	MEDICARE		COMMERCIAL						
	Standard	Medi-Medi	AMG	Rocky	CAT	MIPC	CAIT	SBA	RICE
Abortion - Elective (CPT 59840 - 59841) Note: Refer to Super Panel contracts for financial responsibility for specific procedures	G/P^1	G/P^2	G/P^2	G/P^1	G/P^2	$G/P^{2,3}$	G/P^4	G/P^4	G/P^4
Abortion - Therapeutic (CPT 59812 - 59857) If the life of the mother could be endangered if the fetus is carried to term, or in cases of fetal genetic defect.	-	G	G	G	G	G	G	G	G
Acupuncture	-	-	-	-	-	-	-	-	G
Acute Care • Facility Component • Hospital Based Physicians, including clinical and anatomical pathologist (CPT 80002 - 83999), radiologist (CPT 70010 - 76499), anesthesiologist (CPT 00100 - 01999, 99100 - 99140)	P P	P P	P P	P P	P P	P P	P P	P P	P P
• Professional Component, including consultations and follow up care visits (CPT 99217 - 99239, 99251 - 99275)	G	G	G	G	G	G	G	G	G
• Closed panel physicians under contract with a hospital for test reading (e.g. EKG)[5]	P	P	P	P	P	P	P	P	P
• Special services and reports, miscellaneous (CPT 99000 - 99000, 99175 - 99199)	G	G	G	G	G	G	G	G	G

[1]Not covered except in cases of rape or incest, or when the life of the mother would be endangered if the fetus were brought to term.
[2]Covered for the first thirteen (13) weeks of pregnancy only.
[3]Copay for HIPC is the same as for in-patient hospitalization.
[4]Covered through the second trimester (24 weeks) of pregnancy only.
[5]Plan to confirm closed panel status.

Legend: G = Medical Group Responsibility; P = Plan/HMO Responsibility; G/P = Shared Responsibility;   -- = Not Covered

This chart shows a sampling of CPT codes and the party that bears responsibility for covering costs for each procedure under numerous different plans. It is important to check the correct column for the plan being processed to determine if services are covered or not.

■ **Figure 6–2** Distribution of Responsibility

- **Referral risk is transferred, but is not substantial**—part of the payment to the provider is dependent on the decisions the provider makes to refer patients to other providers. However, that part of the payment is not substantial (i.e., is under 25%). Therefore, if this type of provider makes too many patient referrals to other providers, up to 25% of his or her capitation amount may be withheld.

- **Substantial risk for referrals is transferred, but stoploss protection is in place**—if more than 25% of total payments to the provider are at risk for referrals, the medical group/IPA must have aggregate or per-patient stoploss protection in place. Stoploss protection means that if the costs to the provider exceed a specified amount, the provider will be reimbursed by the group/IPA for at least 90% of expenditures over that amount.

In general, the higher the risk that is transferred to the provider, the higher the capitation amount. If less risk is transferred to the provider, the group/IPA keeps a higher percentage of the capitation amount to cover its expenses.

Capitation Payments

Capitation is the practice of paying a provider a set amount per month to provide treatment to MCP members and for providing other administrative duties. When a contract is signed between an MCP and a provider, an agreement is made regarding a capitated fee. This fee often is dependent on the type of plan under which the patient is covered. Varying factors such as the gender and age of the patient and their overall health also may be considered. The provider and MCP will also agree which services are covered by the capitation amount.

Often, capitation amounts pay for all the basic treatment the patient needs during the month. If the patient does not see the physician that month, the physician keeps the fee. If the patient becomes ill and requires treatment, the physician is expected to provide the necessary services without additional compensation by the MCP. Usually, the amount saved and the extra amount spent balance out.

The capitation amount for each provider is determined by those who are included on either the active or new member roster. The PCP usually receives capitation payments for the previous month. The amount of

the capitation payment will vary according to the coverages or plans that have been selected. Additional amounts may be provided for patients who have entered a hospice or skilled nursing care facility, as well as those who have been diagnosed with specific diseases (i.e., HIV or ESRD) (see the Additional Capitation Section).

The MCP may retain a portion of the monthly capitation amount to protect the HMO from inadequate patient care or financial management by the PCP. This amount is called a **withhold**. They also may withhold a portion to ensure the quality of care given to patients and promptness of payments to outside providers. This amount is outlined in the contract signed by the group and the MCP.

Practice Pitfalls

The 123 MCP withholds 3% of the capitation amount to cover financial insolvency and unpaid claims by the group/IPA. If all obligations have been met, this amount will be returned when the group terminates its contract with the MCP. Additionally, the 123 MCP will withhold 5% of the capitation for its Medical Management Incentive Program. This program stipulates that the 5% will be reimbursed to the group/IPA if the following guidelines are met:

- 25% of the withheld amount will be reimbursed if the provider/group/IPA has submitted less than their budgeted amount of hospital expenses which are covered by the MCP.

- 10% of the amount will be reimbursed for customer satisfaction. The MCP will randomly survey patients to determine their satisfaction with the provider and the services rendered. If the provider is above the average in customer satisfaction, he or she will receive this amount.

- 10% of the withheld amount will be reimbursed for low disenrollment. If the provider/group maintains less than 2% disenrollment (those terminating MCP coverage or transferring to another provider), then they will receive this amount.

- 40% of the withheld amount will be reimbursed for quality of care. This will be determined by a review of medical records by the MCP. If the Medical Review Panel agrees with the treatment given at least 80% of the time, the provider will receive this amount.

- 15% of the withheld amount will be reimbursed for protocol compliance. This is calculated as follows:
  - 5% for compliance with all facility requirements as determined by an audit of the facility.
  - 5% for timeliness of claim payments.
  - 5% for timeliness in submission of all contractually required statements to the MCP.

If the provider meets all the stipulations outlined, they will keep the 5% quality care amount.

You can see how the things you do as a biller may affect the amount the provider receives in his or her monthly capitation check. If you are rude to a patient and a complaint is made, or if a member chooses to transfer to another provider, it could cost the group/IPA. If you do not process claim payments promptly, submit statements to the MCP on time, or let the providers in the group know that they are near the limit on their hospital costs, there will be additional amounts withheld. It is important that the biller understand all factors that can cause withholding from the provider's capitation amounts, and do their best to see that the goals are met for compliance with MCP guidelines.

Supplemental Capitation

On occasion, an eligible member will not appear on the eligibility rosters. The biller should keep a list of all eligible patients seen by the provider (**see Figure 6–3**). If at any time a patient does not show up on an eligibility roster, the biller should contact the MCP to determine the reason.

There may be a legitimate reason (i.e., the patient has transferred to another PCP, but you have not yet received the transfer paperwork), or the patient may have been inadvertently left off the list. If you discover a patient who should have been on the roster and was not, contact the MCP to determine the correct procedure for having the patient's name placed on the roster. Also, ask what paperwork is required to receive the capitation amount for this patient.

Additionally, there will be many patients who sign up for MCP coverage but who do not immediately choose a PCP. These people may not choose a PCP until they feel the need for treatment. At that time they will choose a provider and will be added to that provider's new member roster.

The billing office should contact the new members as soon as possible to determine how long they have been a member and what precipitated their decision to choose this provider as their PCP. If they have been an MCP member for a while but simply had not requested a specific provider, the MCP has been keeping the capitation amounts for that patient and not assigning them to a specific provider. The contract between the provider and the MCP, or the MCP and the member, may stipulate that the MCP will assign a PCP to any enrollee who does not choose one within a specified time. If this is not being done, the physician/group should be notified that they may want to contact the MCP regarding the matter. They may be due additional patients (and capitation amounts) because of new members, who should be assigned to a PCP.

Additional Capitation Amounts

Many MCPs will pay an amount in addition to the regular capitation amount for those patients who have been diagnosed with certain illnesses or whose illness or condition has required them to enter a hospice or skilled nursing facility.

It is the responsibility of the provider to inform the MCP of changes in the patient's status in order to receive the additional reimbursement. The biller should consult the MCP's Policy and Procedure Manual to determine which conditions allow for additional reimbursement and which form to file to obtain this reimbursement. The biller should then make a list of those conditions which qualify for additional reimbursement and the time limits and other conditions for applying for the reimbursement.

As with supplemental capitation, there are usually specific forms and deadlines which must be met in order for a provider to receive the additional capitation. For example, if the deadline for submitting the paperwork is not met, the MCP may refuse to add the additional capitation amount until the following month and the provider may forfeit the additional capitation for the current and preceding months.

Billing for Services

Although the monthly capitation amount covers most services, some services will be reimbursed on a fee-for-service basis. This means that the provider will bill the MCP for these services when they are performed. Most agreements between a provider and an MCP will have a list of those services that are covered by the capitation amount, or those that are considered to be on a fee-for-service basis. Fee-for-service procedures are

Provider Medical Group			
Supplemental Capitation Request			

TO: _____ FROM:_____
     Provider Network Manager   Medical Group Name and Number

Date Submitted: _____ For Eligibility Month/Year:_____

Member Name	Plan Type	Member Number	DRG/Diagnosis

■ **Figure 6–3** Supplemental Capitation Request Form

usually billed on a CMS-1500 form the same as non-MCP services, or they may be electronically billed if required.

The medical biller should familiarize themselves with those services that are covered and those that are billed before treating a patient. They also should collect the copayment amount from the patient before treatment is rendered by the provider.

Appointment Scheduling

The MCP will usually dictate the maximum amount of time a patient must wait for an appointment (i.e., the appointment must be scheduled within four weeks of the patient's request for an appointment). Different time frames may be given for routine appointments than for urgent care appointments.

Many MCPs require that there be a certain number of appointments set aside for emergencies. This allows a patient to be seen within 24 hours if an emergency situation arises. All decisions as to whether a patient should be seen immediately are the responsibility of the provider. At no time should a medical biller attempt to determine the emergent nature of the patient's condition. All triage and assessment, including over the phone, should be performed only by a licensed medical provider.

It is important that these time frames be met. Failure to do so could result in sanctions against the provider. Numerous sanctions could result in the provider losing their contract with the MCP.

If the provider is unable to meet the patient's request for an appointment within the allotted time, the provider should refer the patient to another appropriate provider who can see the patient within the allotted time. The charges for this appointment will be the responsibility of the provider.

If you are scheduling elective surgery, whether inpatient or outpatient, you should avoid the ending and the beginning of the month so that eligibility may be cleared. Additionally, many MCPs will insist that the surgical procedure be performed on the first day of admission. Any necessary preadmit testing should be done on an outpatient basis the day before surgery. If this is not possible, the documentation to substantiate the need for an overnight stay before surgery should be attached to the Treatment Authorization Request (TAR).

Missed Appointments

Each time a patient misses an appointment, the provider must review the patient's chart and determine the appropriate follow-up activity. This decision should be documented in the patient chart and initialed by the provider. The following are appropriate follow-up activities:

- No follow-up needed. Wait for patient to call for a new appointment.
- Send a letter to the patient advising them that they should call to reschedule an appointment.
- Telephone the patient to reschedule the appointment.

If the appropriate follow-up was a letter, the letter should contain the member's name, the date and time of the missed appointment, the reason for the appointment, the provider's name and address, and a phone number which the patient can call to reschedule their appointment.

If the appropriate follow-up is a phone call to reschedule the appointment, record any phone calls or attempts to contact the member in the patient record. This should include the date and time of the call, name and title of the person making the call, and the outcome of the call (i.e., new appointment scheduled, left message, no answer, etc.).

If the physician notes that the patient should be seen as soon as possible, the biller should attempt to contact the member the same day as the missed appointment. The member should then be scheduled for the first available emergency appointment.

If there is no telephone number, or if there has been no contact after three attempts, a letter should be sent to the member requesting that they call the office to reschedule their appointment. A copy of this letter should be placed in the patient chart.

If any correspondence to the patient is returned by the postal service as undeliverable, it should be date stamped and filed in the patient's chart. The doctor should be informed, and a notation of his or her decision of follow-up placed in the patient's chart.

Authorizations, Referrals, and Second Opinions

It is important that the medical biller familiarize themselves with the agreement between the MCP and the provider. Often the MCP will require a second surgical opinion (SSO) or preauthorization for treatment. If the patient is to be admitted to the hospital, precertification may be required. These items will often have timeliness limits on when they are to be performed. For example, precertification must often take place at least five days before a scheduled inpatient admission and emergency treatments require notification to the MCP within 48 hours of admission.

With precertification and preauthorization, the MCP will evaluate the proposed treatment and inform the provider and patient as to whether or not they will cover the services. If the MCP decides that the services are not necessary, they will deny payment. The provider and patient must then decide whether they will abandon the treatment, seek authorization for an alternate treatment, or if they will go ahead with the treatment with the understanding that the patient is completely responsible for the charges.

Preauthorization

It is important to obtain preauthorization for services that are the responsibility of the MCP. If these services are performed without preauthorization, the group/IPA may be responsible for payment of services. Each MCP may have their own specific Treatment Authorization Request (TAR) form.

Often a TAR approval will be valid for a limited time, usually 30 days. If services are not performed within that time, you will need to complete an additional TAR and obtain another preauthorization. In the case of ongoing treatments (i.e., chemotherapy, dialysis), you often will need to obtain monthly authorizations of services covered by the MCP.

If you have not received the authorization back from the MCP within 10 to 15 days, you should contact the MCP. If they never received the TAR, you may need to reschedule the patient and resubmit a new TAR. For this reason, it is best to choose a date which is several weeks in the future. However, you also should attempt to avoid the beginning and ending of the month because the patient's eligibility may change and the MCP will insist that all routine follow-up care or hospital stays be included in the one authorization.

TARs often are three- or four-part forms. If they are not, be sure to make a copy of the TAR for your records before sending it in to the MCP. If you feel additional documentation is necessary to substantiate the need for services, this should be included with the TAR, and firmly attached to it.

If it is not possible to reschedule the patient's surgery as a result of the nature of the treatment, many MCPs have an emergency request procedure that allows faxing of the TAR and overnight approval. If the patient cannot wait for this approval, they should be instructed to go to the emergency room and the hospital will call the MCP and request approval for an emergency admit.

If you list a specific date of surgery on the TAR, surgery must be performed on that date. TARs may not be valid for any dates other than the date listed. In these cases, the group/IPA or provider may be responsible for payment of services, not the MCP.

The MCP also will indicate the number of days allowed for the patient to remain in the hospital (if it is an inpatient admission). If it becomes necessary for the patient to remain in the hospital for a longer period (i.e., as a result of complications), then the group/IPA should submit a request to the MCP as soon as possible with the documentation to substantiate the need for additional inpatient days.

Utilization Review

Utilization review (UR) is a process whereby insurance carriers review the treatment of a patient and determine whether or not the costs will be covered. Many insurance carriers began creating utilization review departments in an effort to control costs and avoid unnecessary procedures. Although this process was started with traditional insurance carriers, managed care carriers have taken the concept a step further, creating complete UR departments and reviewing every outside procedure that may require additional costs and every referral to a specialist.

Many providers dislike the utilization review process. They feel the UR committee cannot always make an effective decision based on the data provided in the medical report. They dislike being second-guessed by a committee that is not familiar with the patient and their problems. Many providers have found a need to hire an additional office person just to review medical information over the phone with the insurance companies in order to get their procedures approved.

However, insurance carriers insist that the process has prevented numerous unnecessary surgeries and helped providers to consider alternate forms of treatment that may be as much or more beneficial to the patient.

Additionally, UR committees are becoming more selective in the items and providers they choose to review. There are some procedures that are nearly always allowed, for example, a cystourethroscopy, whereas more questionable procedures, such as MRIs on the knees, are being reviewed. Additionally, some insurers are tracking the records of providers. Those that are known for ordering tests or procedures that are nearly always necessary are less closely watched than those who have a history of ordering questionable procedures.

Specialist Referrals

If a member requests to see a specialist, the provider must discuss the request with the member. If the request is denied, the procedures for denial of services must be followed, including sending a denial letter to the member. If the provider agrees with the member's request, or recommends the member to see a specialist, an appropriate referral form should be completed and approved. The decision to refer or not to refer a member is a medical decision that should be made by the provider.

The group/IPA must provide a written notice of its decision to the member. If the request is approved, the notice must advise the member of the name, address, and phone number of the consultant and either state an appointment time, or inform the member of the way to schedule an appointment.

The group/IPA is required to have contracts with its specialists. They must maintain contracts with a sufficient number of specialists so that members are not inconvenienced by excessive appointment waiting times. The provider's office also should keep a Specialist Referral Log of all patients referred to a specialist. This log should include:

- The name of the member or patient.
- The request date.
- The appointment date.
- The referring physician.
- The consulting physician or specialist.
- The problem or reason for the referral.
- The date the report was received from the specialist.
- Any comments.

This log can help the practice keep track of patients who have been seen by a specialist and whether or not the results of that referral have been received from the specialist.

Denial of Services to Members

If a member requests a specific treatment and the provider/group/IPA determines that the treatment or service is not medically necessary, would be detrimental to the patient, or would provide no medical benefit to the patient, they may deny the service (i.e., refuse to perform the treatment). The provider should discuss with the patient why they feel these services would not be beneficial. If the patient wishes to pursue the request, they can ask for a second opinion, or ask the provider to reconsider the treatment.

Second Opinions

Many MCPs have a second opinion policy designed to resolve differences of opinion regarding proposed treatment among providers, members, consultants, or the MCP. Second opinions are often provided in the following instances:

- At the request of the member before a surgical or other invasive procedure.
- If the provider's opinion is contrary to the member's expressed expectations, even after the physician has counseled the member.
- If the opinion of the provider differs substantially from the recommended treatment plan of the specialist on the case.
- At the request of the MCP.

There are several steps to the second opinion process.

1. A request is made by the provider, member, consultant, or MCP for a second opinion. This request may be either verbal or in writing.
2. The patient's chart is documented with the request.
3. An internal review is performed. This is a second opinion performed by another physician affiliated with the same group/IPA as the provider.
4. If the member is still dissatisfied, or if the two opinions differ substantially, an external review may be performed. This is an opinion provided by a physician who is not a member of the group/IPA to which the member belongs. If the member is still dissatisfied, they should contact the MCP to request the external review. The MCP reviews the records and, if they deem it necessary to have an external review, they will inform the provider and the member. The MCP may send the member to a physician of their choosing.
5. All records are forwarded to the MCP's Chief Medical Officer, who makes a determination of the proper course of treatment. The provider will then be informed of the decision and it is their responsibility to carry out the proposed treatment plan. This may mean treating the patient themselves, or referring the member to a specialist for treatment.

Financial responsibility for second opinions is usually shared among the group/IPA and the MCP as follows:

1. The provider/group/IPA is responsible for the internal review.
2. The MCP is responsible for the external review unless the provider/group/IPA failed to document the internal review, did not properly complete a TAR and obtain authorization before sending the member for an external review, or if the opinion of the external review physician differs substantially from the provider/group/IPA decision.

All activities regarding the second opinion process must be thoroughly documented in the patient's record. Any time that the MCP must bear financial responsibility for any services, including the external review, a TAR must be completed and the treatment preauthorized.

Because of substantial delays in receiving authorizations or referrals, and member complaints, some MCPs are now allowing members to refer themselves for a second opinion. However, they are limited to obtaining a second opinion from another provider who is affiliated with the same MCP, and the number of times they may refer themselves for a second opinion is limited (i.e., once every six months).

Denials of Service after a Second Opinion

Once the member has exhausted the second opinion process, or chooses not to proceed with the process (i.e., accepts the decision of the internal review), the provider/group/IPA must send a denial letter to the member. A copy of this letter also must be sent to the MCP along with any supporting documentation.

This letter must state the patient's name, the date services were requested, the services that were requested, and the reason for the denial of services.

The MCP often will keep a log of these denials. If they feel a provider/group/IPA is denying too many treatments, they may ask for a review of the record to monitor the quality of care given to the patients.

Member Appeals of Denied Services

Members may appeal any decision that involves the denial of services that they believe should have been performed or covered. This includes the right to appeal decisions both before and after the service has been performed. It also applies to the proposed termination of treatment that the patient is currently receiving (i.e., termination of a hospital stay or continued plan of treatment).

To file an appeal, the member must contact the MCP, usually in writing, and include the following items:

- Patient name.
- Member name (if different from patient).
- Member identification number.
- Member address.
- Phone number.
- Name of provider/group/IPA.
- Name of provider.
- Date service was rendered if previously done.
- Complete description of the problem or why they feel services should not have been denied.
- Member signature.

If the member delivers this appeal to the provider/group/IPA, they should be told to mail it to the MCP, or the provider/group/IPA may be required to accept the appeal and mail it to the MCP themselves.

The MCP will review the appeal and all appropriate supporting evidence. They also will look up the denial and supporting evidence that was filed by the provider/group/IPA. This is why it is so important that the group/IPA file their notices of denial in a timely manner with all necessary supporting documentation.

Within a specified time limit (usually 30 days), the MCP will make a decision regarding the denial of services. If they determine that the services should have been covered or performed, they will instruct the provider/group/IPA to do so. If they uphold the decision of the provider/group/IPA that the services were correctly denied, they will inform the member by letter. A copy of this letter also will be forwarded to the provider/group/IPA and should be placed in the patient's record.

For services that have not yet been rendered, some MCPs have an expedited appeal process in which the MCP is required to make a decision within a few days. This expedited appeal process is required to be available to Medicare members but also may be available to other members.

Member Grievances and Complaints

Grievances are written complaints made by a member regarding quality of services, access to care, interpersonal communication, or any other aspect of their care or relationship with their provider. **Complaints** are verbal expressions regarding the above dissatisfactions. Members may file a grievance or complaint with the provider, the group/IPA, or the MCP.

If the member files the grievance or complaint with the provider or the group/IPA, the following steps should be taken:

1. The provider or group/IPA should attempt to resolve the issue through patient counseling, whether in person or over the phone.

2. If the provider or group/IPA is unable to resolve the grievance or complaint, or it is outside his or her scope of responsibility (i.e., the member is dissatisfied with their MCP contract), the provider must refer the grievance to the MCP. There is usually a time limit associated with this procedure. Often the provider must refer the grievance within one working day of receiving it

if they are unable to resolve it. For this reason, it is imperative that all members of the provider/group/IPA and their staff take complaints from member very seriously.

3. If the grievance or complaint has been resolved at the provider level, the provider/group/IPA must send a letter confirming the resolution of the issue to the member. A copy of this correspondence and any supporting documentation also must be mailed to the MCP.

4. If the provider is unable to resolve the complaint within a specified time limit (i.e., 30 days), they must give the member the opportunity to file a written complaint with the MCP.

5. If the grievance or complaint concerns any aspect of medical care, it must be reviewed by the provider/group/IPA medical director.

Grievance Logs

Often, provider/group/IPAs are required to keep a log of all grievances in addition to documenting all grievances in the patient chart. Some MCPs require that a copy of this log be forwarded to them at set intervals (i.e., every 30 days). If a copy of the log is required but no grievances or complaints have been received, the provider/group/IPA must submit a log with the words "NO GRIEVANCES" printed on it.

The following items are often required on a grievance log:

1. Member name.
2. Member identification number.
3. Date of grievance or complaint.
4. Type of grievance or what the grievance was about.
5. Date of resolution letter or date referred to MCP.

If numerous grievances or complaints are received, the MCP may withhold a portion of the monthly capitation amount, or may terminate their relationship with the provider/group/IPA.

Transfers

A member may transfer from one provider to another at any time. Often, the MCP will require the patient to complete a request for transfer. There will then be a waiting period while the MCP verifies that the member is eligible for coverage and has chosen a provider who is contracted under the member's plan. The transfer will then become effective at the beginning of the next

month. Because capitation amounts are paid month to month, this eliminates the need to split a capitation amount between two or more providers.

Usually, if one member of a family chooses to transfer to another medical group as a provider, then all members of the family must transfer to the same medical group. However, each family member may see a different provider within that medical group. This often is the reason that a medical group will be required to have providers of different specialties within their group (i.e., general practitioner, pediatrician, cardiologist, etc.).

Any member requesting a transfer must complete a transfer request form. This form also must be completed if a patient chooses to transfer from one provider to another within the same medical group. On receipt of the transfer form, the medical group must forward a copy of the patient's medical records to the MCP. The MCP will then forward them to the new provider. If there is no chart available (i.e., the patient has never visited the provider), then the original provider must inform the MCP that there is no chart on this patient.

If the provider feels a need to have a copy of the patient chart, a copy should be made prior to sending the chart to the MCP. This copy should be notated that the patient has been transferred to another facility and the date, and then the entire file should be placed in an "inactive" file. If the biller for a medical group receives a notice that a patient is transferring into their medical group, it is their responsibility to be sure that they have received a copy of the patient's medical record before treating that patient.

Disenrollment

When a patient transfers their care from a provider, they are considered to have "**disenrolled**" from that provider. A patient may disenroll from a provider at any time by requesting a transfer to another provider. A patient also may disenroll from the MCP program by stopping the payment of their premiums or by seeking other insurance coverage. Additionally, the MCP must have the required number of physicians within the designated area to ensure that each patient can receive proper care without excessive travel or undue hardship (i.e., waiting incessantly for appointments).

Because an MCP is responsible for all care given to a patient, there is often no secondary insurance coverage under an MCP. Many MCPs will include a provision in their contract with the patient that states that if the patient enrolls in another MCP or obtains other insurance coverage, their policy with the MCP will be immediately terminated.

MCP Initiated Disenrollment

The MCP may disenroll a member for various reasons. These reasons must have been previously stated in the contract with the member, and verified by documentation by the provider or the MCP.

The reasons for disenrollment can include but are not limited to:

1. The member disregards the enrollment agreement by habitually seeking covered services, other than emergency care, from a provider who is not a contracted provider.

2. The patient/physician relationship has broken down. This can be evidenced by a pattern of broken appointments and refusal to follow physician advice or orders. The MCP may require that the member be referred for psychiatric evaluation prior to initiating this type of disenrollment to ensure that the patient can be held mentally competent and legally responsible for their actions.

3. Physical or verbal abuse of the provider or his or her staff. This often must be documented and a police report filed. The MCP also may require these members to be sent for psychiatric evaluation before initiating disenrollment.

4. The member moves out of the service area covered by the MCP.

5. Failure to pay the required monthly premium.

Each pattern of missed appointments, abusive behavior, or failure to follow medical advice must be carefully documented by the provider and made a part of the patient's record.

Once a provider has documented a habitual problem, they may request disenrollment of the patient. This is often accomplished by filing a request for disenrollment form. These forms vary from one MCP to another but usually contain only basic patient information. The request must then be substantiated with documentation. This documentation should include the following:

1. Documentation in the patient record or progress notes showing dates of visits or missed appointments, or a listing of these. There should be a sufficient pattern shown to document the "habitual" nature of the offense.

2. Documentation in the patient record or progress notes or in a grievance log showing the date, time and subject of any counseling the member received from the provider/group/physician's staff in an effort to prevent or repair the breakdown in the relationship.

3. Explanation of why the problem cannot be resolved.

4. If appropriate, a discussion of why a change to another provider is not appropriate or has not been done.

5. Copies of any correspondence sent to the member in an effort to resolve the situation, or to assist the member in understanding the plan procedures (i.e., when to use the emergency room, need for prior authorization, importance of keeping medical appointments, etc.).

6. Evidence that the member has demonstrated a total lack of cooperation with the plan, has continued to misuse services, or has been physically or verbally abusive after receipt of the correspondence or other written attempts to correct the problem. In many cases, a police report will meet this requirement.

7. Evidence that the noncompliant or abusive member has been referred to a psychiatrist, or evidence showing the reason why this action was not appropriate.

The provider will be required to continue treating the patient until they are officially notified by the MCP that the member has been disenrolled.

Continuing Care

There are times when a provider or group chooses to terminate their contractual obligation with the MCP. If a physician terminates their contract with the MCP or with the group, the remaining members of that group continue to be responsible for the treatment for that patient. Members are assigned to a group, as well as to a physician within that group, and that relationship will continue regardless of whether one provider removes himself from the group or not.

However, if an entire group/IPA terminates their contract with the MCP, there may be a need for continuation of coverage for some members who were being treated by the terminating group. Continuation of coverage exists when a specified treatment was begun by the terminating group/IPA, and must be continued by the newly assigned provider or group/IPA. For continuing care coverage to exist, the following rules often apply:

- The patient must be involved in a specific treatment plan that has been previously authorized by the medical director of the terminating group/IPA.

- The treatment has a clearly identifiable termination (ongoing treatments for a condition that has no cure [i.e., diabetes] would not be reimbursable under continuing care rules).
- Medical care was terminated as a result of the group/IPA situation rather than through any fault of the member.
- If the patient is pregnant, specific rules may apply regarding the length of the gestation and time left to the termination of treatment.

In such cases, the newly assigned group may be allowed additional compensation for the continuing care treatment that is provided to these patients. For example, the provider may be reimbursed by the MCP for each treatment that he provides in relation to the continuing care at the normally contracted rate. The regular capitation amount will apply for all treatments that are provided for a reason other than the continuing care.

Specific rules must be followed to obtain the proper reimbursement, and the Policies and Procedures manual should be checked before rendering services. For example, in order to qualify for an additional reimbursement under continuing care rules, the provider may need to seek preauthorization for all treatments.

It is often the responsibility of the group/IPA that receives the member to identify the need for continuing care coverage. These people should be identified as quickly as possible so that proper rules and reimbursement can be applied.

Miscellaneous Services

Certain rules can apply to select types of services under an MCP agreement. These services can include outpatient surgery, emergency room services, durable medical equipment, and prescriptions.

Outpatient Surgery

Some MCPs will provide a list of surgeries that must be performed in an outpatient setting. This is most often done in a shared risk contract when the group/IPA is financially responsible for outpatient services and the MCP is responsible for inpatient services.

It is important to know which surgeries must be performed on an outpatient basis. If these guidelines are not followed, the group/IPA may be financially responsible for all inpatient costs in relation to the surgery.

Practice
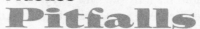
Pitfalls

The biller should be aware of this list and keep it handy. If he or she receives a TAR for services that should be performed on an outpatient basis, but the provider is requesting inpatient authorization, inform the provider immediately. If the provider feels the surgery should be done inpatient because of complications or other circumstances, the documentation for these circumstances should accompany the TAR.

Emergency Room Services

If the provider/group/IPA is considered financially responsible for emergency room services, then they are responsible for managing the member's utilization of ER services and for paying for the cost of these services. The provider/group/IPA must provide written information to its members on how to access these services. The provider/group/IPA must have procedures for the authorization of these services. Payment may not be denied based on lack of notification or lack of authorization for these services.

Practice
Pitfalls

If a biller receives a call requesting authorization for emergency services, it is important that he or she transfer the call to the appropriate person immediately, or get any necessary information so that the provider may return the call as quickly as possible. The biller should not authorize or deny services. The authorization or denial of services should be done only by a licensed medical professional.

Durable Medical Equipment

All durable medical equipment (DME) must be ordered and prescribed by the physician for the patient's use. If the financial responsibility for durable medical equipment lies with the provider/group/IPA, it is imperative that authorization be obtained as soon as possible. Requests and prescriptions for durable medical equipment must include a specified time period. Often MCPs only will authorize the rental of DME for a month at a time. Thus, the authorization must be requested each and every month for patients with chronic conditions (i.e., a glucometer for a diabetic). Also, each request for DME must be on a separate prescription or authorization request form. Thus, it is possible for one patient to have several outstanding DME authorizations (i.e., for oxygen, bed, wheelchair). Each specific DME request will be assessed based on member eligibility and medical necessity. Therefore, it may be necessary to include a copy of the documentation with each DME request.

Prescription Coverage
When an MCP offers prescription coverage to a member, there often are limitations:

1. The member must purchase the drugs from an MCP contracted facility. If they obtain prescriptions from a noncontracted pharmacy, the member will bear the cost of the pharmacy services. There may be exceptions to this rule for emergency situations, or situations in which the patient is outside the service area, or the prescription is not available from a contracted pharmacy.
2. They may limit drugs and medications to a 30-day supply.
3. They will only cover prescription drugs. Over-the-counter medications are not covered.
4. They may only include oral and topical drugs. Injectable drugs often are not covered under the pharmacy benefit. They may, however, be covered under the medical benefit. This is especially true for injectable medications that the patient needs for survival (i.e., insulin for a diabetic).
5. They also may insist that the generic equivalent of a drug be prescribed if it is available. If there is no generic equivalent, the MCP will often cover the brand name at the standard copayment amount. However, if there is a generic equivalent, the MCP may only cover the cost of the generic equivalent. Thus, the member will be charged the standard copay, plus the difference between the generic and the brand name medication.

Some generic drugs are not the same as their brand name counterparts. They may have a similar, but different, active ingredient, or they may be in a different dosage amount from the brand name drug. In such a case they are not considered to be therapeutically equivalent. For these drugs, the MCP may require the physician to prescribe the generic drug, or they may allow the full benefit for the brand name drug.

Sanctions
If a provider/group/IPA fails to meet the quality standards, reporting requirements or any other provisions

of its contract with the MCP, the MCP may impose sanctions on the provider/group/IPA or the individual provider. These sanctions usually include the withholding of specified amounts or not allowing any new members to be enrolled to that provider/group/IPA.

It is not uncommon for sanctions to escalate for additional offenses. Therefore, an MCP may impose a $1,000 (or 5% of capitation) sanction for the first offense, $3,000 (or 10% of capitation) for the second offense and $10,000 (or 15% of capitation) for the third offense. If there are additional offenses, the provider/group/IPA or the individual provider may be terminated.

Because of these sanctions, it is important that all reports, forms, or claim payments be properly completed in a timely manner and all rules be expressly followed.

Claim Payments
If a provider is deemed to be responsible for payment of services, then the provider/group/IPA must either provide these services, or pay for the providing of these services. Often groups/IPAs will attempt to sign a wide variety of providers to their group/IPA so that they do not need to refer patients to outside providers. This often means that they will enter into a contractual agreement with a specific provider (i.e., a chiropractor) in their area to provide services for their patients at a specified rate. This specified rate may be on a fee-for-service basis or on a capitation basis.

Clean Claims
Claims from providers outside the group/IPA must be paid from group/IPA funds if the group/IPA is contractually obligated to cover or provide these services. There usually are time limits on how long a provider may take to pay a clean claim.

A claim is considered "clean" if all information to process the claim is within the plan or group/IPA. A **clean claim** is defined as one that can be paid as soon as it is received because it is complete in all aspects, including patient information, coverage information, coding, itemization, dates of services, and billed amounts.

If a claim is submitted without a piece of information that is included in the group/IPA patient chart, omission of this information alone will not make it an unclean claim. For example, if preauthorization was required, the leaving off of an authorization number alone should not make the claim unclean. The group/IPA should have this information available in the patient chart.

Additionally, the need for medical review of a claim to determine appropriateness of services does not make it an unclean claim.

When a claim is unclean (it does not have the necessary information to be processed), the group/IPA must send a written notice to the provider advising the provider of the information needed to process the claim. Many providers have a standard form letter for this purpose.

If you do not receive a response within 30 days, send a denial notice stating that the services were denied. A copy of a denial notice is shown in **Figure 6–4**.

Date:

Member Name
Address
City, State Zip

File # _____

Dear:

We have received your request for the specific service or referral described below.

Service/Referral Requested: _____
_____

This Service/Referral request is being denied for the reason(s) shown below:
_____   Services are not a covered benefit with your plan.
_____   You have exhausted the benefit for this particular service.
_____   Service/Referral request denied because _____
_____
_____
_____

If you believe this determination is not correct, you have the right to request a reconsideration. You must file the request in writing within 60 days of the date of this notice. File the appeal with: Your HMO, Attn: Member Services, Address, City, State, Zip.

In addition to the complaint process described above, you may also contact the Department of Corporations (DOC). The DOC is responsible for regulating health care service plans in this state. The DOC has a toll-free number (1-800-XXX-XXXX) to receive complaints regarding health plans. If you have a grievance against the health plan, you should contact the plan and use the plan's grievance process. If you need the DOC's help with a complaint involving an emergency grievance or with a grievance that has not been satisfactorily resolved by the plan, you may call the DOC's toll free number.

Please include your name and date of birth on all correspondence. If you have any questions about this notice, please call YOUR HMO at 1-800-XXX-XXXX.

Sincerely,

Name of Medical Group/IPA

cc: Member Services
     Quality Assessment
     Primary Care Provider

■ **Figure 6–4** Denial Notice

Group/IPA Payment Responsibility

When a claim is received from a provider outside the group, or is paid on a fee-for-service basis, the following steps need to be taken:

1. Date stamp the claim and any supporting documents. This will help to prove the timeliness of your claim payments. There are state and federal laws governing how soon you should pay a claim (usually within 30 days). Additionally, the MCP may require that the claim be paid within a specified time period or the provider may forfeit a portion of his capitation amount (see Capitation Payments).

2. Notify the provider in writing if the claim is incomplete, improperly completed, or if additional reports or documentation need to be attached. A copy of this notification should be attached to the claim.

3. Complete eligibility verifications and any internal review (i.e., were treatments authorized or allowed, or did the member choose to see the provider on their own?).

4. Prepare a proper remittance advice or denial notice in the case of denied claims.

5. Determine the proper payment amount.

6. Prepare and mail a check. For timeliness guidelines, a claim is usually considered paid when the check is placed in the mail.

Additionally, the provider/group/IPA is required to provide a check voucher or remittance advice to any fee-for-service provider showing the patient information, service rendered, date of service, amount billed, disposition of copayment (if any), amount group/IPA is paying, and a reason code for any denied services or amounts.

If the provider is paid on a capitated basis, the group/IPA must provide a count of members listed by plan, a payment amount for each plan, and copies of the member rosters. In essence, the same type of document that the group/IPA receives from the MCP when they are paid their monthly capitation amounts must be provided.

Determining the Proper Payment Amount

If there is no contract in place between the provider and the provider/group/IPA before services are rendered, the group/IPA has no legal basis for discounting payment to a provider. They must pay the full amount of the bill, minus any copayment amounts that should have been collected from the patient.

Legally, if a member has met their contractual obligations (i.e., seeking preauthorization or emergency authorization for treatment), they have no responsibility for payment for services other than the copayment amount stipulated in their contract. Therefore, the provider/group/IPA must pay a provider's billed amount, minus any copay. A statement should accompany payment to the provider stating that the copayment is the only amount which may be collected from the patient.

If there is a contracted amount for services, the terms in the contract should be adhered to. Usually, a fee schedule will accompany contracted terms. This fee schedule may be different for each provider with whom the provider/group/IPA contracts. The proper contract should be pulled and the correct allowed amount determined. The member's copayment amount should then be subtracted from this amount, and the remainder paid to the provider. A notice should accompany the check voucher or remittance advice stating that this is the contracted amount for this service and no amounts other than the copayment may be collected from the member.

It is the responsibility of the provider/group/IPA to ensure that neither the member nor the MCP incurs any financial responsibility for claims that are contractually deemed to be the responsibility of the provider/group/IPA.

For services rendered to seniors who are covered by Medicare HMOs, the fee schedule may indicate that fees are limited to the Medicare Fee Schedule. Under this arrangement, Medicare participating providers are limited to the allowed amount as determined by the most recent Medicare Fee Schedule. Nonparticipating providers would be paid the non participating fee amount. The non-participating fee equals 95% of the participating fee amount. The maximum amount a nonparticipating physician or supplier will receive is the Medicare limiting charge, which is equal to 115% of the allowable charges.

In either case, if the fee is being limited by contractual agreement with the provider, a copy of the contract and the accompanying fee schedule should be attached to the claim when it is filed.

Claim Files

Claims are usually filed in a separate claim file, along with all documentation submitted by the provider, and a copy of the explanation of benefits (fee-for-service providers) or member rosters and capitation amounts (capitated providers).

Additionally, a copy of the claim or some documentation showing the services rendered should be placed in the patient chart. If any of the documentation supporting the claim payment is pertinent to further treatment of the patient, this information should also be copied and filed in the patient chart. At no time should any information regarding capitation payments be placed in the patient chart. This information is a part of the contract between the provider and the group/IPA and should be considered privileged information.

Denial of a Claim or Service

If a claim or service is denied, a denial letter must be included with a remittance advice indicating the reason for the denial. The denial notice also must include a statement that the provider has the right to appeal the denial within 60 days, and the address of where to file an appeal.

If the claim is for emergency services, the member or provider is requested to notify the MCP within 48 hours of the initiation of care. However, some MCPs may limit the ability of a provider/group/IPA to deny claims based on the lack of notification within this 48-hour period.

If it is believed that these services were not medically necessary, or were not true emergency services, then the claim must be sent through a medical review process. The medical review should use the presenting diagnosis rather than the discharge diagnosis as the basis for their decision making, and must consider the member's understanding of the medical circumstances that led to the emergency service.

If this medical review determines that the services were not medically necessary or were not true emergency services, then a specific denial letter is required for these claims. This denial letter must meet federal requirements. The MCP often will provide a copy of an appropriate denial letter in their Policies and Procedures Manual. In such a case, this letter should be used verbatim, and the wording left unaltered.

All denial notices must contain an explicit reason, in layman's terms, of why the service(s) are being denied. If the MCP provides a list of denial reasons, then the appropriate denial reason should be written on the denial letter. You may not use a code unless you indicate the meaning of that code in the denial letter. Additionally, all denial letters must meet the following criteria:

1. The decision to deny must be correct and based on approved medical practices.
2. The denial reason must be clear to the member and must use CMS-approved denial reasons.
3. The denial letter must include mandated appeals language and the correct health plan address.
4. The denial letter must be sent to the appropriate parties (the provider, the member, or both).
5. The denial notice must be issued within required time frames.

There are additional guidelines that mandate which items must be included and what size the type used must

be. The MCP should furnish all providers with copies of appropriate denial letters, and these should be used by the provider.

If the member is not covered by the provider/group/IPA, then certain steps must be taken before the claim can be denied. First, call the MCP to determine if the member was covered at the time services were rendered, and who the assigned provider was at that time. If the member was not covered at all, then the claim may be denied for that reason. If the member was not eligible under the provider/group/IPA, but was a covered member under the MCP, then the claim must be forwarded to the MCP.

Additionally, any claims that have been denied by the provider/group/IPA must be sent to the MCP with a copy of any contact or denial letters to the member or provider. Many MCPs also require the use of a denied claim log that includes the following information:

- Current month and year.
- Group name.
- Contact person.
- Phone number.
- Member name.
- File/member number.
- Provider name.
- Whether the provider was contracted or noncontracted.
- Date of service.
- Reason for the denial.
- Date the claim was received.
- Date the notice was sent to the member.
- Date the notice was sent to the provider.

A copy of this log should be forwarded to the MCP on a regular basis. If there are no denials for the month, a copy of the log should still be forwarded to the MCP with the words "NO DENIALS" on the first line of the log.

Appeals

Any member or provider has the right to appeal a denied claim. All denial letters, by law, must include a statement saying that the receiver has the right to appeal the decision and whom to contact to begin the appeal process.

If a member or provider appeals a denied claim, the MCP will review the claim and make a determination of whether to uphold or reverse the denial. If the MCP determines that the services should have been covered, it will inform the provider/group/IPA of its decision and will instruct the provider/group/IPA to pay the claim.

The payment should be generated immediately and a copy of the proof of payment should be sent to the MCP. If the MCP does not receive proof of payment in a timely fashion, it has the right to pay the claim and deduct the payment from the provider/group/IPA's capitation amount. The MCP may have a fund set up under the provider's name in which it has withheld a portion of the provider/group/IPA's monthly capitation amount (i.e., 3%). If so, the claim will be paid from this fund.

If the MCP processes the claim and makes payment to the provider, it not only goes against the provider's record but also the MCP has the right to charge an administrative fee for processing the claim. This fee can be usually ranged from $100–$250.

Medical billers should be aware of the appeals process and should routinely appeal all claims in which services performed by their provider were denied. If possible, additional information substantiating the need for the services or the urgent nature of the services should be included with the appeal.

MCP Responsibilities

If the provider/group/IPA determines that the MCP is responsible for payment of a claim, they must forward the claim to the MCP. The following steps should be completed:

1. Determine which services, if any, are the responsibility of the provider/group/IPA and process these claims according to the guidelines given in this chapter.
2. Indicate on the remittance advice or write a letter stating which services are the responsibility of the MCP, and indicate that the claim is being forwarded to the MCP for payment.
3. There is usually a transmittal form which must be sent with any claims. A copy of this form is shown in **Figure 6–5**.

Provider Network Services

CLAIMS TRANSMITTAL FORM

Date: _____

To: Claims Services

From: _____, Administrator for _____

The attached claims are the responsibility of [the HMO].

Authorization Number _____

____ Inpatient Hospital (IP) Charges

____ Outpatient Surgery (OPS) Facility Charges

____ Anesthesia for approved IP or OPS

____ Radiology for approved IP, OPS or SNF

____ Pathology for approved IP, OPS or SNF

____ Emergency services which resulted in admission to Inpatient status

____ Ambulance

____ Durable Medical Equipment

____ Dialysis Facility Charges

____ Radiation Therapy

____ Member not on roster for date of service. Include relevant roster page(s).

NOTE: Use a separate form for each type of Plan expense. Multiple providers may be grouped if the authorization number is the same.

[The HMO] will not send denial notices for services which are the responsibility of the Group/IPA.

Refer to the Medical Services Agreement for questions of coverage and financial responsibility.

■ Figure 6–5 Transmittal Form

Reinsurance/Stoploss

Stoploss is an attempt to limit payments by an insured person, or a provider/group/IPA in the case of a catastrophic illness or injury to a member.

Many MCP contracts have a stoploss or reinsurance clause included in them. This clause may state that the provider/group/IPA will be financially responsible for the first set amount (i.e., $7,000) in expenses for each member in a contract year. After those expenses have been paid, the MCP will reimburse the provider/group/IPA for verified expenses which exceed the set amount.

If the provider's contract has a stoploss clause, it is important that the medical biller be aware of the set amount. They will need to file a claim with the MCP for any services which exceed that set amount. The biller also should be familiar with that portion of the provider's contract with the MCP, as there are often limits put on the billing. For example, the MCP may require that claims be submitted within a specified time period, or that preauthorization be obtained before the services are rendered. Some contracts also may stipulate that the year runs from July 1 to June 30. If the biller is unfamiliar with the terms required to achieve stoploss reimbursement, the provider could stand to lose a substantial sum of money.

Often the MCPs will require that a claim for reimbursement be submitted on specific forms. An example of this form is shown in **Figure 6–6**.

Incorrect Denials

If a provider/group/IPA arranges, refers, or renders services or equipment that are not covered under a plan, the provider/group/IPA must inform the member ahead of time that the services or equipment are not covered by the plan and that the member is liable for coverage. The provider/group/IPA should have a form for the member to sign stating that they understand that such services are not a covered expense. If the member is not informed of the noncoverage and financial liability in advance, the member cannot be held liable for the cost of the services or equipment.

If the MCP has a Medicare HMO plan, they must agree to cover at least the minimum of services that are covered under Medicare. Therefore, it is important that providers and their billers understand what items are covered under Medicare so that these items are not denied.

Many MCPs have a limit on the number of visits or units that a member may utilize during a year (i.e., 20 chiropractic visits). When the member has exhausted their benefits under such an arrangement, it is important to notify the member that they have reached their limit and any additional treatments will not be covered by the plan. Failure to do so could cause the provider/group/IPA to be liable for the services.

It is important that billers note in a patient's file if they are covered under an MCP plan. If a member receives services that should have been preauthorized, and the provider is a contracted member with a plan, the provider forfeits their fee for those services.

Figure 6–6 Excess Risk (Stoploss) Form

Practice Pitfalls

Example: Sarah James is seen by Dr. Dorman. She indicates that she is covered by Medicare when she is actually covered by a Medicare HMO. Dr. Dorman is contracted with the Medicare HMO to which Ms. James belongs. Thinking that Ms. James is covered by Medicare, he renders services that need preauthorization by the HMO. Because the provider did not inform Ms. James in advance that the services were not preauthorized or were not covered by the HMO, the services will be denied. Because he is a contracted provider with the HMO, Dr. Dorman is not allowed to bill the patient for these services. Therefore, the provider forfeits his fee.

To prevent this from happening, it is important to verify insurance coverage before the first visit, and also to ask each patient if their insurance coverage has changed since their last visit on any subsequent visits.

CHAPTER REVIEW

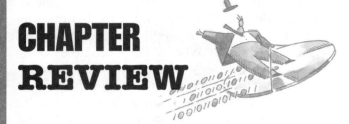

Summary

- Managed care contracts were created in an attempt to bring healthcare costs under control by having providers share some of the financial risks of healthcare with the patient and the insurance carrier.

- There are numerous types of managed care organizations, including HMOs, PPOs, EPOs, PHOs, and MSOs.

- HMOs are one of the most common managed care trends. HMOs pay providers a set capitation amount each month for the patients on their eligibility roster, and in return the provider is expected to cover many of the services that member needs. A written contract will dictate those services that the provider will cover and those that the HMO will cover.

- There are numerous forms that the provider must complete to keep the MCP informed of services rendered and the daily operations of the practice.

Assignments

Complete the Questions for Review.
Complete Exercise 6–1 through 6–3.

Questions for Review

Directions: Answer the following questions without looking back into the material just covered. Write your answers in the space provided.

1. What is a PPO? _____

_____

_____

2. What should a biller do if a patient requests treatment and they are not included on the provider's eligibility roster?

_____

_____

3. What is a TAR and what is its purpose? _____

_____

_____

4. What is an HMO? _____

_____

_____

5. What is stopless? _____

_____

If you are unable to answer any of these questions, refer back to that section in the chapter, and then fill in the answers.

Exercise **6-1**

Directions: Find and circle the words listed below. Words can appear horizontally, vertically, diagonally, forward, or backward.

1. Active Member Roster
2. Clean Claim
3. Copayment
4. Eligibility Roster
5. In-Network Providers
6. New Member Roster
7. Self-Insurance
8. Withhold

```
S I V K G T H E T C B E G I C A B R R I C G V P X J S E U U
R R X F E T W Q L Z E L S U C W E C E R L D N Y H Y E M J I
X N E Q U T N E M Y A P O C G T S T T L I J F B X Y L Z S F
F W A D N W A I V A A D S Q S J R Q S M F H Q G Z X F Y A A
A H H K I N P P F E U S E O X I L K O F M Y F X F J I C B R
O H N O C V F M P I D B R Z E Z B B R I U V D Y L W N N T Q
S A I L R G O N N G I Y G Z M H M A R H G P X Z E E S G Z N
N L A Z W I S R K C T N E W M E M B E R R O S T E R U P I R
M I Y S H K A K P I W X B T J W D E B U E A J W H Y R D H Z
M B F Y L O K O L K J U Y L P T E O M Y U K B Y M E A N N Y
K D E G H L T I C Z R X U U X M J K E A G Y K N S V N A T Z
O O F K V K B F L E K O E P S W U Y M E F C P B G S C L K V
T L F F N I U S H P O O W T N L J I E C Y J U L T O E S F B
Z S V R G B Y E Z N S M F T K O P C V H K D U T W H Q G G T
G X B I G Q A Q E D O X R A E K I Z I N U S H M G M U V D J
Z A L C V X R K C R R O Q O C N K U T A W P W F K H H Q K N
D E T T H J D F O U R V L H A L N X C H B H V L A L N E P Q
J R H E G T A X P J P M K D N P I I A P Z C H K V D L J U A
W D M B K S D H K M N H H S L N I F U X S V Y T R R O N L I
Z H K X B E E R M J H P H N N O X N T C R B T T C U Q U Y U
N X N F U Q E C W E P Z U S P S H B B H M B D V U W Z Z P T
R G E E U O C P A B X F T Y L J F H X O Z N T W Y F B G A L
D Q B Y C Q V R E B N Z A X Q E G Y T R R B C U V M G F G E
Q X W P X T L T C R N B Z V D O N I L I F X K V O M T R S F
L F H B I Q B Y J P P I W L X B E M K W W A P J J K Q T C E
Z Y Z H O V W L B V Q P X M M B O X D N I N U F P X K O E J
I V J A A B E O Y C Z O O U D K C Z E H L J E B A C X J U X
N W R M D E L H T M N L I V L Y H D I A Z F P B W C Y I G O
U H B B C G U S F V W L I V C F R W T E M T N W O H A J H M
G L Z Y M C D M I K D B A J K W A K L S X Q H T J V H N I Z
```

Exercise 6-2

Directions: Complete the crossword puzzle by filling in a word from the keywords that fits each clue.

Across

6. An attempt by insurers to control healthcare costs using a number of different methods.

7. A monthly payment made to a provider in exchange for providing the healthcare needs of a member.

8. An attempt to limit payments by an insured person or a group/IPA in the case of a catastrophic illness or injury to a member.

9. Verbal expressions of dissatisfaction with a provider or services.

Down

1. When a patient transfers their care from a provider.

2. An insurance policy that protects the company against catastrophic medical costs levied against their plan, either by a single employee or by all employees as a whole.

3. Providers that do not agree to provide services at a reduced amount in exchange for the referrals from an insurance carrier within a PPO.

4. A process whereby insurance carriers review the treatment of a patient and determine whether or not the costs will be covered.

5. Written complaints made by a member regarding dissatisfaction with a provider or services.

Exercise 6-3

Directions: Match the following terms with the proper definition by writing the letter of the correct definition in the space next to the term.

1. _____ Individual Practice Organization

2. _____ Health Maintenance Organizations

3. _____ Exclusive Provider Organization

4. _____ Social Health Maintenance Organization

5. _____ Terminated Member Roster

6. _____ Management Service Organization

7. _____ Primary Care Provider

8. _____ Physician Hospital Organization

9. _____ Preferred Provider Organization

a. An organization that provides the full range of Medicare benefits offered by standard HMOs plus additional services.

b. A plan where the insurance carrier contracts with providers to join their network and to provide services at a contracted rate. These providers agree to provide services at a reduced amount in exchange for the referrals from the carrier, and the carrier agrees to reimburse network providers at a higher percentage than providers outside the network.

c. The provider a patient has chosen for their primary medical care.

d. A separate corporation set up to provide management services to a medical group for a fee.

e. A plan in which the patient must select a Primary Care Provider and can use only physicians who are part of the network or who are referred by the PCP.

f. An organization of physicians and hospitals that band together for the purpose of obtaining contracts from payer organizations.

g. Lists those members whose coverage has been terminated or who have chosen to terminate this provider as their PCP.

h. A legal entity, comprised of a network of private practice physicians, who have organized to negotiate contracts with insurance companies and HMOs.

i. Organizations or companies that provide both the coverage for care, and the care itself. Members pay a set amount every month and the HMO agrees to provide all their care, or to pay for the covered care they cannot provide.

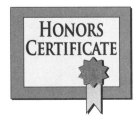

Honors Certification™

The certification challenge for this chapter will be a written test of the information contained in this chapter. Each incorrect answer will result in a deduction of up to 5% from your grade. You must achieve a score of 85% or higher to pass this test. If you fail the test on your first attempt, you may retake the test one additional time. The items included in the second test may be different from those in the first test.

CHAPTER 7   MEDICAL PRACTICE ACCOUNTING

7
Medical Practice
Accounting

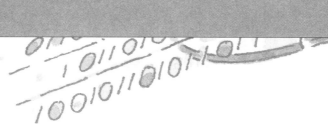

After completion of this chapter
you will be able to:

- Explain and use the ledger card and patient statements.
- Properly post payments to the patient account.
- Properly create a payment plan.
- Properly handle a collections call.

- Explain and use the daily journal.
- Properly balance petty cash using a petty cash count slip and petty cash receipts.
- List the main reports a medical office may use and their purposes.

Keywords and Concepts
you will learn in this chapter:

- Accounting Control Summary
- Accounts Receivable
- Accounts Payable
- Adjustments
- Balance Billing
- Bankruptcy
- Cumulative Trial Balance
- Daily Journal
- Day Sheet

- Defendant
- Deposit Slip
- Deposit Ticket
- Dunning Notice
- Explanation of Benefits (EOB)
- Insurance Tracer
- Patient Aging Report
- Patient Ledger Card
- Patient Receipt

- Patient Statement
- Pended
- Petty Cash Count Slip
- Petty Cash Fund
- Petty Cash Receipt
- Post
- Skip
- Statement of Account
- Statute of Limitations

Patient Accounting

Billing is not the only function of the medical biller. Once a bill has been sent out, it is the biller's responsibility to collect on that bill and to make sure that the patient's account is properly credited.

Often the biller begins by submitting a claim to the patient's insurance carrier. When payment is received from the carrier it is credited against the patient's account. The patient, or a secondary insurance carrier if there is one, is then billed for any remaining amount left unpaid on the claim.

If payment is not received from the insurance carrier in a timely manner, an insurance tracer is sent on the claim. If payment is not received from the patient in a timely manner, the medical biller is responsible for handling collections on the account. If necessary, the account may be sent to small claims court in an effort to collect.

Accounts Payable/Receivable

The main function and purpose of any bookkeeping system is to provide a way to keep an accurate account of money being received and paid out. Most accounting systems are set up on a principle of accounts payable and accounts receivable. In simple terms, money being received is considered **accounts receivable** and money paid out is referred to as **accounts payable**. In any business, the objective is to have more money coming in (accounts receivable) than there is going out (accounts payable).

Because the medical office provides a service and also functions as a business, one of the responsibilities of the medical biller includes the continued updating of financial records.

In the medical office, the biller often is responsible for collecting payments for services from patients. This amounts to most if not all of the accounts receivable that a medical practice may have. Therefore, it is important for the medical biller to ensure that all accounts are paid in a timely manner.

Because of this, billers must keep highly accurate records of patients and the services they receive, bill for those services promptly, record payments, do balance billing in a timely manner, and institute collections procedures when necessary.

Often, the practice will have a second person (if not the doctor themselves) who is responsible for handling all accounts payable. However, it is important that the medical biller be aware of any major purchases that the practice may make, and also have a general idea how much the office expenses are each month. If the medical biller is aware that the practice has approximately $10,000 in expenses each month, they will know what they need to collect to cover those expenses.

Several bookkeeping systems may be used in the medical office to keep track of incoming and outgoing finances.

There are two main ways of keeping patient accounts: by computer and manually. Most computerized billing systems also allow you to handle patient accounting. Thus, they not only generate the claim, but also they record all charges and payments into the system.

If you use a computerized system, the accounting system is automatically set up when you enter patient information into a record. When a claim is created, it is automatically posted to the patient's account. To **post** means to list items such as payments or charges in a log.

When payments are received the information is recorded on a payment screen, and the amount paid is automatically deducted from the patient's account.

The pegboard system is one of the most frequently used manual systems because it is the simplest to use. Ledger cards, charge slips, and daily journal sheets all are used in the pegboard system. This system uses NCR (no carbon required) material on its forms to allow information written on one form to be recorded on all the rest.

Patient Ledger Card/Statement of Account

The patient's account information is often kept on a Patient Ledger Card, also known as a **Statement of Account (see Figure 7–1)**. The **patient ledger card** is used to indicate a chronologic record of all services rendered to a patient and record all payments and adjustments made on their account.

Each service, payment, or adjustment should have its own line or column on a ledger card. Any services provided are added to the remaining balance (if there is one), and any payments received are subtracted from the remaining balance. **Adjustments** are changes that can either increase or decrease the remaining balance on an account.

Items should be entered in chronological order. Thus, the charges for services performed would be entered before any payments for those services. The remaining balance shown on the last line of the

Paul Provider, M.D.
5858 Peppermint Place
Anytown, USA 12345
(765) 555-6768

Ledger Card/Statement of Account

RESPONSIBLE PARTY: _____

ADDRESS: _____

TELEPHONE #: _____

PATIENT NAME: _____PATIENT ACCOUNT #: _____

SPECIAL NOTES: _____

Date	Description of Service	Charge	Payments	Adjustments	Remaining Balance

■ **Figure 7–1** Patient Ledger Card/Statement of Account

ledger card is the amount that is still owed on the patient's account.

To post items to a ledger card, complete the items as listed below.

- **Responsible Party:** Enter the name of the person ultimately responsible for payment of this bill. This is often the patient, or the parent or guardian of a minor patient.

- **Address:** Enter the address of the person ultimately responsible for payment of this bill.

- **Telephone #:** Enter the telephone number of the person ultimately responsible for payment of this bill.

- **Patient Name:** Enter the name of the patient. Each patient should have their own separate ledger card. Never place more than one patient's account information on a card.

- **Account Number:** Enter the patient's account number.

- **Special Notes:** This is where you may enter any special circumstances regarding this patient and their account.

- **Date:** Enter the date of the transaction. This is the date services were rendered in the case of most charges, or the date a payment was received for services.

- **Description of Service:** Enter a description of the reason this account is being changed. If you are recording charges, indicate the services that were performed. If you are recording a payment, indicate that it is a payment, and who is making the payment (i.e., Green Insurance Carrier Payment, check #1234). If you are recording an adjustment, indicate the reason for the adjustment (i.e., adjustment to Medicare-allowed amount).

- **Charge:** Indicate the charge for any services that were performed. If you are recording a payment, leave this space blank.

- **Payments:** Enter the amount of the payment. If there is no payment, leave this space blank.

- **Adjustments:** Enter the amount of the adjustment. If there is no adjustment, leave this space blank.

- **Remaining Balance:** Add the amount of any charges to the previous amount in this field. Subtract the amount of any payments from the previous amount in this column. Adjustments can be either increases or decreases to the patient's account.

It is important to always keep the patient's ledger card updated. Any changes to the patient's account should be promptly noted. This can prevent numerous problems with the patient's account, including interest charges or late charges being assessed.

Insurance Payments

The insurance carrier is often the first entity to make a payment on a claim. Once the insurance carrier has processed the claim, they will send an Explanation of Benefits with the check (if applicable) to the party designated as the payee. If benefits are assigned, this would be the provider. If benefits are not assigned, this would be the patient. If the patient is designated as the payee, the provider will not receive any contact from the insurance carrier. It is the biller's responsibility to collect the full amount due for services from the patient.

Understanding an EOB

When benefits are assigned to the provider, the insurance carrier will create an **Explanation of Benefits (EOB)** for the claim and send payment directly to the provider. This EOB will list the patient, the date of the service, and the service performed. It also will list the amount that was allowed for the procedure, the percentage covered by insurance, and the amount that the insurance carrier will pay.

If benefits are not assigned to the provider, the EOB will be sent to the patient, along with the payment amount. The full amount should be collected from the patient, regardless of what was paid by the insurance carrier (unless Medicare or Medicaid is involved).

It is important to check the EOB carefully against the patient's account. Be sure that the codes that were paid were the ones that were billed. Errors can often occur in the inputting of codes, thus causing improper calculation of the benefits.

There are many different EOB styles and formats. EOBs may list one patient or they may list several on the same page. If several are listed together, be sure that you are crediting the payment to the proper patient. Some providers will choose to list each procedure separately on their records and record the amount received for each service. Others will combine all the services provided on the same date and apply the payment to that total.

```
                        Rover Insurers, Inc.
                         5931 Rolling Road
                         Ronson, CO 81369


December 15, CCYY
Claim For: Abby Addison
Claim Number: 478-78-4
Group Policy Number:  41935
Member's ID Number:  001-00-RED

Dear Ms. Addison:

We received a claim for you. The following details the benefits which were paid on this claim. Please save this
form for your tax records. If you have any questions, please contact the customer service office.
```

DATE OF SERVICE	PROCEDURE	BILLED AMOUNT	ALLOWED AMOUNT	% OF PAYMENT	PAYMENT AMOUNT	DENIED AMOUNT	REASON CODE
11/06/CCYY	HOSP CONSULT	$200.00	$140.00	90%	$ 36.00**	$ 60.00	55
11/07-08/CCYY	HOSP VISIT	$150.00	$100.00	90%	$ 90.00	$ 50.00	55
11/09/CCYY	HOSP D/C	$100.00	$ 75.00	90%	$ 67.50	$ 25.00	55
TOTAL		$450.00	$315.00		$193.50	$135.00	

```
55   Denied amount exceeds the amount covered under your plan.
**   $100 applied to deductible.
```

■ **Figure 7–2** Sample EOB

If the EOB combines payments for several dates of service, be sure that you separate the amount of the payments according to the proper dates. Some EOBs do not contain information that is detailed enough to do this. In such a case, add together the amounts billed on the claim and apply the total amount against this.

See the sample EOB in **Figure 7–2**. On this EOB, Abby Addison received a hospital consultation, two hospital visits, and a hospital discharge. All charges were allowed (though not at the billed amount), and were paid at 90%. However, the patient had not yet met $100 of her deductible, so this amount was taken from the $126 that otherwise would have been paid on the first line item.

On this claim, the billed amount was $450. Because the insurance only paid $193.50, the patient (or any additional insurance if the patient is covered by more than one policy) should be balance billed for the remaining $256.50.

On the Job Now

Directions: Using the Explanation of Benefits in **Figure 7–2**, please answer the following questions.

1. Indicate the name of the patient. _____

2. Indicate the total amount billed on the claim. _____

3. Indicate the total amount allowed on the claim. _____

4. Indicate the total claim payment. _____

5. Indicate the total amount denied. _____

6. Indicate the reason for the denied amount. _____

7. How much was applied to the deductible? _____

8. Indicate the EOB date. _____

9. Indicate the name of the insurance company. _____

10. What was the percentage at which the allowed amount was covered? _____

Patient Payments

When a patient visits the provider they may wish to make a payment for the amount owed on their account, or the estimated amount owing after insurance benefits are paid. A receipt should be given to the patient at the time the patient makes payment. A **patient receipt (see Figure 7–3)** is a written acknowledgment that a specific sum of money has been received. A patient walk out receipt outlines the total activity pertaining to the patient's visit that day. This type of receipt is usually generated from a computerized medical billing system.

Posting Payments

When payment on the claim is received, you will need to post the payment to the patient's account. This can be done on a computerized system or with a manual system.

Be sure to record all the pertinent information regarding a payment. This should include not only the name of the person or entity making the payment, but also the type of payment (i.e., cash, check, money order), and the number of the check or money order.

Post each of the appropriate amounts from the EOB onto the patient's account. In the case of a Medicare or Medicaid Remittance Advice, be sure to write off any amounts that were not allowed. Next, determine the amount that is still owed on the claim.

Balance Billing

If there are any remaining amounts owed, you will need to balance bill. **Balance billing** is sending an additional bill to another party for payment of any remaining amounts on a claim. If the patient has more than one insurance carrier, a second copy of the claim should be sent to the secondary carrier to coordinate benefits between the two carriers. Be sure to attach a copy of the primary carrier's EOB so that the secondary payer may see how much was paid by the primary payer. Do not alter any of the information on the form. You should send an exact copy of the form to the secondary insurance carrier. Many CMS-1500 forms have several carbon copies for this purpose.

If there is no second insurance carrier, the patient should be balance billed for any remaining amounts. Patients are usually billed using a patient statement. Most insurance carriers will send a copy of the EOB to the patient at the same time they send one to the provider. However, some providers prefer to include a copy of the EOB to allow the patient to view how the payment was credited to the account.

Patient Statements

A **patient statement** is an individual summary (either by patient or by family) that lists all the services,

■ Figure 7–3 Patient Receipt

charges, payments, adjustments, and balances due that occurred during the month. This statement is sent to the patient every month. It acts as both a statement of his or her account and as a bill.

Often these statements contain a **dunning notice**, which is a statement or sentence reminding the recipient to make a payment on their account. There are certain days that are more appropriate for sending out patient statements. These dates are usually between the 8th and the 12th of the month and between the 20th and the 27th of the month. Sending out patient statements on these dates receives a higher response, because most people receive their paychecks on the 15th and the 30th or 31st of the month.

Follow-Ups

A claim may be denied or **pended** (held for further information) by the insurance carrier if there are omissions or errors on the form. The most common reasons why claims are denied include missing or incomplete diagnoses, diagnoses not corresponding with services rendered, incorrect dates, charges not itemized, incorrect patient insurance information, incorrect procedure codes, and documentation not submitted to substantiate services rendered.

If the claim was denied or pended for these or any other reasons, complete or correct the information and resubmit the claim.

If the payment was denied on all or part of a claim and you feel the denial is incorrect, write to the insurance carrier and ask for a review or appeal of the claim. Every insurance carrier has an appeals process and will give you the required directions and information or forms to use.

Make sure that you have a good system set up to remind you when to follow up on a claim. If you have not heard from the carrier six weeks after you have filed a claim, it is definitely time to follow up.

When a Claim Is Rejected

An insurance carrier may reject all or part of a claim. Before billing the patient for the remaining balance, be sure you determine why the claim was rejected. Many claims are rejected because of minor errors that can be fixed easily, including:

1. The patient is not listed as covered under the mentioned policy. Many insurance carriers (and their computer systems) track patients according to policy numbers, group numbers, or Social Security numbers. If any of these numbers is incorrect, the claim may be rejected because the patient and the policy numbers do not match up.

2. Office visits are rejected because they fall within the follow-up days for a surgical procedure. If the office visit was for a reason (diagnosis) other than as a follow-up to the surgery, be sure this is clearly indicated on the claim. Box 24e of the CMS-1500 should reference the additional diagnosis. Modifier-24 also can be used to indicate unrelated E/M services by the physician during a postoperative period. Some providers (including Medicare) may require additional documentation proving that the visit was unrelated to the surgical procedure.

3. The claim (or some services) is rejected as not being medically necessary. If procedures seem unrelated to the listed diagnoses, those procedures may be rejected. Be sure that each procedure has an appropriate diagnosis listed for it. If you need additional room for more diagnoses, list procedures on two separate CMS-1500s, according to their related diagnoses.

4. Item 12, release of information, was not completed. After ensuring that the signature is on file, type the words "Signature on File" in the box. Some insurance carriers require that the patient's name or the name of the person who signed the release appear in this field, and will reject claims with "Signature on File."

5. The patient was not covered at the time the treatment was begun. If special conditions exist that negate the preexisting provisions, be sure to attach this information. These special conditions can be the meeting of certain requirements such as the patient being treatment free for a specified period of time, or the patient's medical insurance transferred when the patient moved from one job to another.

6. The claim is rejected because the facility or doctor is incorrect for the type of procedure being performed. For example, if ear surgery is being performed by an obstetrician, it would probably be rejected. Be sure that the procedure codes listed are correct for those procedures that were performed.

7. The claim is rejected because the patient's gender or age is incorrect for the type of procedure being performed. For example, a male is not treated for gynecological procedures. If the gender is listed incorrectly on the patient's form, the claim could be resubmitted.

Carriers are required to provide the reason why the claim or procedure was denied. If you do not understand the wording of why the claim was denied, contact the person (or department) listed on the EOB to inquire.

If the error is a minor one, fix the error and resubmit the claim. If more explanation is needed (i.e., an operative report to justify services performed), include the additional information and resubmit the claim.

If everything on the claim is correct and you disagree with the claims examiner's judgment on the claim, contact the claims examiner and discuss the situation. If you cannot come to an agreement on the claim, ask what the appeals process is for such a situation. All companies have an appeal or claim review process.

Insurance Tracer

If you have not received payment from an insurance carrier within six weeks of sending in the claim, you should submit an insurance tracer. An **insurance tracer** is a form or letter sent to the insurance carrier to inquire about the disposition of a previously submitted claim. Be sure to include the patient's name, their Social Security number or insurance number, their policy name and number, and the patient's address. You also should include the date of services, the diagnosis, and information regarding their employer.

Many medical offices have a form letter for this purpose (**see Figure 7–4**). Payments from insurance carriers should normally be received within four to six weeks. When the payment is received, the amount of payment should be compared with the actual claim originally sent. The payment should then be posted to the patient's account.

Collections

The patient is always financially responsible for payment of services rendered, regardless of whether or not he is covered by insurance. The following are two exceptions: (1) if the patient is a minor, in which case the financial responsibility lies with the parent(s) or legal guardian; or (2) if the patient was injured on the job and the services rendered are related to this injury.

On the Job Now

Directions: Use the following information to complete an insurance tracer form for each patient. For additional information refer to the patient chart or to the Patient Data Table and Provider Data Table in Appendix C.

	Patient	Date Billed	Date of Service	Date of Illness	Diagnosis	Amount Billed
1.	Abby Addison	02/01/CCYY	01/16/CCYY	01/16/CCYY	401.9	$210.00
2.	Bobby Bumble	02/01/CCYY	01/16/CCYY	05/04/CCPY	250.0	$103.00
3.	Cathy Crenshaw	02/01/CCYY	01/16/CCYY	01/16/CCYY	491.9	$160.00
4.	Daisy Doolittle	02/08/CCYY	01/16/CCYY	01/16/CCYY	243	$120.00
5.	Edward Edmunds	02/08/CCYY	01/16/CCYY	05/07/CCYY	414.00	$165.00

Paul Provider, M.D.
5858 Peppermint Place
Anytown, USA 12345
(765) 555-6768

INSURANCE TRACER

Date: _____

Dear Insurance Carrier:

We sent a claim to you over six weeks ago and have not heard back from you.
Patient:
Insured:
Address:
SSN/Birth Date:
Group Number:
Claim Amount:
Date Billed:
Date of Services:
Date of Illness or Injury:
Diagnosis:
Employer:
Address:

Please supply the following information on the above named claim within ten days. Payment on this claim is overdue and we would like to avoid involving the patient and the state insurance commissioner in a reimbursement complaint.

Claim pending because:_____

Payment in progress. Check will be mailed on:_____

Payment previously made. Date: _____

To whom:_____

Check #: _____ Payment Amount: _____

Claim denied. Reason: _____

Patient notified: Yes   No

Remarks: _____

Thank you for your assistance.

Completed by: _____

■ **Figure 7–4** Insurance Tracer

In the case of (2), the company's workers' compensation carrier would be responsible for payment.

After the claim is paid by the insurance carrier and the payment is posted to the patient's account, any remaining balance is billed to the patient. If no payment has been received within 30 days, a follow-up reminder should be sent.

If payment is not received within 15 days of the second notice, send a courteous collection notice reminding the patient that payment is now seriously delinquent, followed by a courtesy call 10 days later. Keep accurate records of when each contact was made and the outcome of that contact. Also record the date you should follow up if you have not received payment.

The longer an account ages, the less likely you will be to recover the money due. This can be as much as 40% or more if the bill is overdue by six months or more.

Often, providers are wary of becoming "bill collectors" because the image is not consistent with that of a healer. However, if revenues are not collected in a timely manner, it can be difficult for the provider to meet the cost of their overhead and other obligations.

Therefore, a balance must be achieved that allows for the collection of revenues without tarnishing the provider's image. The best way to achieve this is to set reasonable credit limits and to stress to patients that they are responsible for payment of the bill. Create a credit agreement, and then ask each patient to sign and date it. Also make sure that the patient understands that by signing the credit agreement, she agrees to abide by its terms.

Do not make your credit policy too stringent. You do not want to lose patients because they cannot afford your terms. If you need to put a little pressure on clients without alienating them, try using a third party (i.e., your accountant).

When collections are being made by telephone, there also are laws to be followed under the Fair Debt Collection Practices Act. Harassing, frightening, or abusive calls are a violation of this act, along with calling during odd hours, or calling friends or neighbors.

A **statute of limitations** is the maximum time that a debt can be collected from the time it was incurred or became due. The statute of limitations varies from state to state, so check with your state legislature.

When all other methods of collection are exhausted, a collection agency may be retained to collect delinquent accounts. Most collection agencies charge a percentage of the account once the debt is collected. Therefore, usually only large amounts are sent to a collection agency.

Many companies use a standard collection letter (**see Figure 7–5**).

If the standard collection notice does not gain a response within 30 days, a delinquent notice should be sent (**see Figure 7–6**).

Collections Procedures

The medical biller often needs to work as a bill collector in order to obtain reimbursement for amounts not covered by insurance or other sources. Usually, these amounts need to be collected from the patient. Occasionally, as a result of an error on a previous claim payment, it may become necessary for a medical biller to recover monies that were paid in error. For these reasons, we will cover the basic laws and regulations regarding collections.

Although the specific laws and regulations vary from state to state, you should become familiar with several general guidelines. These include:

1. You are never allowed to make frightening or abusive calls. This includes making any threats to the person, calling names, or making derogatory statements. Racial or ethnic statements should never be made.

Paul Provider, M.D.
5858 Peppermint Place
Anytown, USA 12345
(765) 555-6768

Dear Sir/Madam:

We are currently showing a past due amount on your account. According to our records your payment of $____ was due on/by _____. As of this date, payment has not been received.

Please remit payment as soon as possible. If you have recently sent payment, please disregard this notice.

Sincerely,

Collections Representative

■ **Figure 7–5** Collection Letter

Paul Provider, M.D.
5858 Peppermint Place
Anytown, USA 12345
(765) 555-6768

Dear Sir/Madam:

Your account is seriously delinquent. According to our records we have not yet received your payment of $_____. This payment was due by _____ and reflects services which were rendered on _____.

If payment is not received by _____ we may be forced to send your bill to collections. Doing so may damage your credit rating.

If you are unable to pay the full amount, please contact our office immediately to set up a payment plan.

Sincerely,

Collections Representative

■ **Figure 7–6** Deliquent Notice

2. It is illegal to call people at odd times of the day. In most states, this means any time between 8 P.M. and 8 A.M. In some states, it is also illegal to contact people at their place of employment.

3. It is illegal to request collection through another party, including friends or neighbors. This means that you are not allowed to leave a message with anyone other than the debtor concerning details of the collection attempt. This includes, but is not limited to, the amount you are trying to collect, any payment amounts or details that may have been worked out, and the nature of the bill. If you call the debtor and reach a family member or roommate, you are allowed to leave a message giving your name, company, and phone number, and a request that the person you are trying to contact return your call.

4. You are not allowed to harass the person from whom you are trying to collect. The legal definition of harassment varies from state to state; however, it is illegal to do things such as call and speak to the debtor several times a day or even several times a week. For this reason, it is important that you remind them of the debt and then ask when you can expect to receive payment. If they are unable to pay in full and if your company allows payment plans, try to work out a payment plan for the amount owed. Make detailed notes of the conversation in the patient file. You

should not contact the person again until after the date payment is expected.

Payment Plans

If the patient cannot pay the entire bill when contacted and your company allows it, payment arrangements should be made. If a payment plan was worked out—whether over the phone or in person—it is advisable to write down the terms of the agreement and have it signed by both parties (the debtor and a representative of the company to which the money is owed).

If the payment requires more than four installments, the federal Truth in Lending Act will apply. Regulation Z of the Truth in Lending Act requires that a written disclosure be made. When the installment plan is being discussed, the following important points should be covered:

* The amount of the debt.
* The amount of the down payment.
* The estimated date of final payment.
* The amount of each installment.
* The date each payment is due (**see Figure 7–7**).

A statute of limitations is the maximum time a debt can be collected from the time it was incurred or became due. Remember that the statute of limitations varies from state to state, so check with your state legislature. You should always be aware of the statute of

Paul Provider, M.D.
5858 Peppermint Place
Anytown, USA 12345
(765) 555-6768

Date:
Doctor:
Patient's Name:
Patient's Address:

Cash price (total fee):
Less cash down payment:
Unpaid balance of cash price:
Amount financed:
FINANCE CHARGE:
ANNUAL PERCENTAGE RATE:
Total of payments:
Deferred payment price:

Patient hereby agrees to pay to (provider's name) at the address shown above, the total payments shown above in _____ monthly installments of $____, first installment being payable _____ 20 ____, and all such installments on the same day of each consecutive month until paid in full.

Signature _____ Date _____

■ **Figure 7–7** Payment Plan Letter

limitations within your state, as the entire debt must be paid off before this time or the physician will forfeit any amounts remaining unpaid.

Truth in Lending Form

Many doctors have a preprinted form for payment plans. This ensures that they comply with all requirements of the Truth in Lending Act. The following form meets all requirements of this act if it is printed on the provider's letterhead. Please note that the words "FINANCE CHARGE" and "ANNUAL PERCENTAGE RATE" must appear in capital letters.

Payment Schedule Form

A Payment Schedule Form is designed to track the payment history of a patient making payments through an installment plan. Some providers prefer to use a payment schedule that may be placed on half of an 8.5 × 11 inch sheet of paper (with the Truth in Lending Form contained on the right-hand side of the paper), or with a payment schedule attached to or printed on the back of the Truth in Lending document.

A payment schedule lists the due date of each installment, the paid amount of the installment, the date

the payment was received, and any follow-up notes (usually notes of a phone call if the payment was not received on time). Some practices will use the follow-up area to include the check number of the payment. This helps to track the payment if there are any questions.

Using a form such as this allows the biller to easily see how many payments have been received and if the patient is behind or ahead in their payments. It also helps to determine if a patient has missed a payment. Occasionally, a payment will be missed, and the patient will then pay subsequent payments on the due date. The patient may believe they are up-to-date on their payments when in fact they are a month behind. By using a Payment Schedule Form this information can be quickly accessed.

Tracing a Skip

A **skip** is defined as a person who has received services without payment and has moved and left no forwarding address. Skips are usually identified by mail being returned to the medical office by the post office and postmarked "return to sender" or "address unknown." In attempting to trace a skip, use the information on the patient information sheet. The person shown in the "person to contact in case of emergency" space should be contacted. Another source is the local Department of Motor Vehicles. If the patient owns a car, it must be registered. The motor vehicle department may be able to provide information regarding the patient's whereabouts. Under no circumstances should information regarding the patient's medical condition be given to the third party.

Tracing a skip is a very tedious and challenging task, and it requires tact as well as patience. If the methods mentioned here prove to be futile, the account may be written off or turned over to a collection agency.

Bankruptcy

Bankruptcy laws allow protection for a debtor. By filing for **bankruptcy**, a debtor announces that he no longer has the ability to pay his creditors and requests relief for his debts from the bankruptcy court. A provider who is owed money by a patient is considered to be a creditor for that patient.

If the patient includes the outstanding provider's fees as part of a bankruptcy filing, the fees owed may be discharged by the court. This means that the debtor does not have to pay the debt.

A claim should be filed on all bankruptcy proceedings, regardless of whether one is requested or not. This protects the provider in case he or she does not receive notice that a claim is required. If a claim is not filed within a specified period of time (usually 90 days) the credi-

tor relinquishes his claim on the debtor. The proper claim forms can be obtained from the bankruptcy court, or standard forms are available in many stationery stores.

As soon as an office is informed that a patient has filed bankruptcy, you are no longer allowed to attempt collection on that account. This often includes not only the patient, but also accounts for all members of the patient's family. If the account was turned over to a collection agency, immediately notify the collection agency that the patient has filed bankruptcy. Many doctors will write off the patient's debt when they are notified of the bankruptcy filing. This prevents statements from continuing to be sent out.

A letter should be sent by certified mail to the patient if the provider wishes to discontinue treatment for the patient. Even if the patient refuses to sign and return the letter, the provider is allowed to discontinue treatment of the patient 30 days after receipt of the letter and not be charged with patient abandonment. See **Figure 7–8** for a sample discontinuance of treatment as a result of a bankruptcy filing letter.

Small Claims Court

At times, a patient who is able to pay his account will refuse to pay. In such cases, it may be necessary to take the patient to small claims court and ask for a judgment against the person.

Paul Provider, M.D.
5858 Peppermint Place
Anytown, USA 12345
(765) 555-6768

Dear _____:

We are sorry to hear about your recent financial difficulties. Unfortunately, due to your situation, Dr. --- will no longer be able to treat you and your family. We will continue treatment for the next 30 days to allow you to find a new physician; however, during this period payment must be made in cash prior to services rendered. We will be happy to inform you of an estimate of the cost of services prior to an appointment to allow you to bring in the required funds.

When you have chosen a new physician, and upon your written request, we will be happy to provide copies of any medical reports or information on your treatment to the new physician.

Please sign and date one copy of this letter to acknowledge understanding, and return it to our offices in the enclosed envelope. Thank you very much.

Sincerely,

Paul Provider, M.D.

■ **Figure 7–8** Letter for Discontinuance of Treatment as a Result of Bankruptcy Filing

Attorneys are not allowed in small claims court, so each party represents themselves. Each side tells their side of the story and the judge renders a decision. There is a maximum limit of $5,000 per case in most areas. Your claim should ask for all money which the defendant owes you, plus any collection costs, court costs, and any other costs incurred in attempting to collect the debt.

Before filing a claim, you must show that you attempted to recover the money and that your efforts have not been successful. This means that you should bill the patient at least three times, and send collection letters demanding payment. If the patient makes no attempt to pay the bill, contact the Municipal Courthouse in your area and request a plaintiff claim form.

Complete the plaintiff claim form and send it to the court with any required filing fees. The **defendant** (the person you are suing), will be notified of the lawsuit and you will be given a court date.

On the scheduled date, show up in court and bring any and all available documentation to support your case. You should include copies of the pertinent portion of the medical record showing the services performed, the billing for those services, and any letters or copies of statements that show collection attempts.

The judge will take all the evidence into consideration and render a verdict. Often the verdict will come several weeks after the court date. If the decision is in your favor, the defendant will be ordered to pay you the money. If not, you are unable to collect the money requested.

Many states have a provision for the defendant to pay "through the court." In such a case, the court collects the money and reimburses you. There is usually a charge for this service, often based on the amount of money being collected. However, this charge can be much less than trying to collect from a defendant who still refuses to pay, even though the court has ruled against him.

If you choose this option, be sure to discuss it with the clerk of the court before trial.

Practice Accounting

As a medical biller, you are often responsible for keeping a petty cash drawer to use when collecting payments from patients as well as for reconciling the amount in petty cash. At the end of each day, you will prepare a deposit slip indicating all payments received that day. You should recount the petty cash to ensure that the same amount remains at the end of the day as

there was at the beginning. Also be sure that the money in petty cash is sufficient for making change for customers.

When a patient makes a payment, place the check or cash into the petty cash drawer. If change is needed, remove the proper change from the petty cash drawer.

Petty Cash

Most offices have a **petty cash fund** to start the business day. This fund is used to make change for patients who are making cash payments and for purchasing miscellaneous small office supplies. Keeping track of this fund on a daily basis is essential.

Petty Cash Count Slips

Most offices use a **petty cash count slip (see Figure 7–9)** to keep track of the amount of money kept in petty cash. The petty cash count slip has space to write the date and time at the top. The remainder of the slip shows various denominations of currency and coins.

To use the petty cash count slip, count the number of each denomination you have. Put the number of

```
┌─────────────────────────────────┐
│        PETTY CASH COUNT          │
│                                  │
│  DATE _____  │
│  TIME _____  │
│           QUANTITY      AMOUNT   │
│  CURRENCY                        │
│    $100   _____    _____  │
│    $50    _____    _____  │
│    $20    _____    _____  │
│    $10    _____    _____  │
│    $5     _____    _____  │
│    $1     _____    _____  │
│  TOTAL                _____  │
│  COINS                           │
│    $1     _____    _____  │
│    Half $ _____    _____  │
│  Quarters _____    _____  │
│    Dimes  _____    _____  │
│   Nickels _____    _____  │
│   Pennies _____    _____  │
│   TOTAL               _____  │
│  RECEIPTS TOTAL + _____  │
│                                  │
│  GRAND TOTAL          _____  │
└─────────────────────────────────┘
```

■ **Figure 7–9** Petty Cash Count Slip

items on the first line. Then multiply the denomination by the number of items. This is the amount of money you have for that denomination.

Once you have counted all the money in the drawer, total the amount on the petty cash count slip. Most offices also will require the person making the count to sign the slip with their name or initials.

This count is often performed at the beginning of the day, before any money is taken from or added to petty cash, and at the close of the day.

The morning's petty cash count slip is usually kept in the petty cash box for the day.

When closing at the end of the day, all monies added to the petty cash drawer should be taken out. These will be deposited in the bank. The remaining amount is counted using a second petty cash count slip. Although the denominations of the currency or coin may change a bit, the total amount in petty cash should be the same at the end of the day as it was at the beginning, unless money was removed to purchase supplies or other items.

Petty Cash Receipts

At times, the money in petty cash will be needed to pay for small office supplies or other items for the office (i.e., a cake to celebrate an employee's birthday).

There are usually only a few people who are allowed to take money from petty cash. Each time cash is removed, the medical biller should get the permission of a supervisor. This is usually documented using a **petty cash receipt (see Figure 7–10)**.

Each person who takes money from petty cash should sign a petty cash receipt showing the date the money was taken, the amount, and what it is to be used for.

Petty cash receipts should be kept in the petty cash box until a purchase receipt and change are obtained. This allows all reimbursements and outgoing monies to be monitored and approved by a supervisor.

After purchases are made, the receipt and any change should be returned to the petty cash drawer. Be sure that the amount of the receipt and the change equal the amount that was originally taken from petty cash. Indicate on the petty cash receipt the amount of change returned. Then staple the purchase receipt to the petty cash receipt.

At times, someone may purchase an office supply with their own money and need to be reimbursed with petty cash funds. A petty cash receipt also should be completed for these types of purchases. The exact amount should be returned to the person, and the purchase receipt stapled to the petty cash receipt.

Petty cash receipts should be kept in the petty cash drawer. When reconciling funds at the end of the day, petty cash vouchers should be counted as cash. This will help you to determine if your amounts have balanced.

All petty cash receipts should be consecutively numbered and treated as amounts paid out.

The Day Sheet/Daily Journal

At the end of the day, the day sheet, also known as the **daily journal**, will need to be balanced. The **day sheet** is used as a balance sheet. This form indicates the patient's name, the individual fee charged for the day, any payments made, and the current balance (**see Figure 7–11**). All receipts for the day and any insurance or other payments should equal the cash/check total collected on the daily journal.

The beginning line on the daily journal should be the petty cash total for the day. All entries should be made on the journal for insurance payments, cash payments, or any other miscellaneous payments or adjustments. To balance, make a total of the cash receipts for the day, any petty cash disbursements, and the petty cash on hand. A receipt should be made for all payments made in the office or by mail. Total all insurance payments received. Combine the receipts total and the

Figure 7–10 Petty Cash Receipt

Paul Provider, M.D.
5858 Peppermint Place
Anytown, USA 12345
(765) 555-6768

Day Sheet/Daily Journal

Date	Name	Description of Service	Charge	Payments	Adjustments	Remaining Balance

■ **Figure 7–11** Day Sheet/Daily Journal

insurance payments total. Total the payments column on the daily journal. This total is equal to the combined insurance payments, cash receipts, and petty cash totals.

If the daily journal does not balance, go back through the charge slips and ledger cards for the day. By comparing the amounts written, you should be able to find your error.

Deposit Slips

All checks should be stamped on the back with a bank deposit stamp and entered on a deposit slip (**see Figure 7–12**). A **deposit slip (also referred to as deposit ticket)** is an overview and balance of monies being deposited.

Be sure to fill out the correct deposit slip. Several companies have more than one bank account. The deposit slip has space for coin, cash, and check deposits. Add up the amount of money you have in coins and enter it in the first box. Next, add up the amount of cash you have and list it in the second box.

Checks are listed individually. Fill in the bank number of the check. This is a four- to six-digit number with a hyphen in the middle (i.e., 66-123). This number refers to the bank and the branch of the bank that the check is drawn on. Next to this number and below the previous amounts, list the amount of the check. If you run out of space for all of your checks, there is usually additional space on the back of the deposit slip.

When all amounts have been entered, total them and put the amount at the bottom. This will give you the total amount of your deposit.

Office Reports

There are numerous reports designed to help the medical office run smoothly and to keep track of the cash flow. These include the daily journal, patient statements, the accounting control summary, cumulative trial balance, and patient aging report.

Accounting Control Summary

The **accounting control summary** is a weekly or monthly report form that shows each day's charges, payments, and adjustments for the period indicated. The medical biller uses this form to double-check the figures against his or her records. This ensures that all information that is to be input reaches the computer properly and has been entered correctly. It also lists items that were not entered.

Items may not be entered or "held in suspense" for a variety of reasons, including wrong account numbers, incorrect spellings, missing code numbers, and no master record for the family.

Cumulative Trial Balance

The **cumulative trial balance** lists each patient alphabetically and shows any charges, payments, or adjustments to the patient's account. This allows the medical office to keep track of all accounts and the amounts that are owed and have been paid.

Patient Aging Report

A **patient aging report (see Figure 7–13)** allows the medical biller to categorize a patient account's outstanding balance by the length of time the charges have been due.

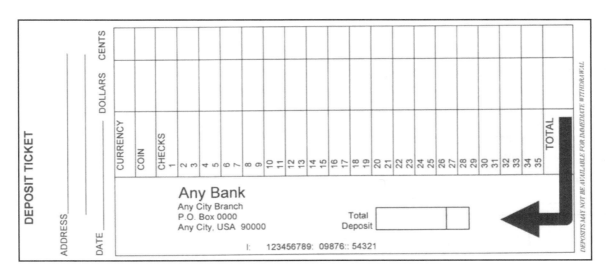

■ **Figure 7–12** Deposit Slip/Deposit Ticket

PAUL PROVIDER
5858 Peppermint Place
Anytown, USA 12345
(765) 555-6768

Patient Aging Report

Patient	Current	31 – 60 Days	61 – 90 Days	91+ Days	Total

■ **Figure 7–13** Patient Aging Report

CHAPTER REVIEW

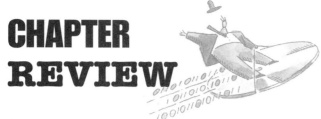

Summary

- Keeping accurate patient accounts is one of the most important jobs of a medical biller. Patients must not only be billed for the services they receive, but insurance carriers must be billed, payments must be posted to accounts and the patient must be balance billed for any remaining amounts on the claim.

- If payment is not received from an insurance carrier in a timely manner, an insurance tracer must be completed.

- Collections also are an important aspect of the job. Some patients will refuse to pay their bill and collection attempts must be made. At times, this involves tracing a skipped patient or filing a claim in small claims court. If the patient files bankruptcy, all collections on the account must stop and the patient must be properly informed if the provider refuses to continue to treat the patient.

- It is important to keep a daily journal of the office transactions, an accounting control summary, a cumulative trial balance, and patient aging reports. It is the medical biller's responsibility to reconcile petty cash and prepare a deposit slip of the day's receipts.

Assignments

Complete the Questions for Review.
Complete Exercises 7–1 through 7–4.

Questions for Review

Directions: Answer the following questions without looking back into the material just covered. Write your answers in the space provided.

1. What information is listed on a patient statement? _____

   _____

   _____

2. Under the Truth in Lending Act, what items must be included in a payment plan? _____

   _____

   _____

3. What is the purpose of the ledger card? _____

   _____

4. If you are attempting to collect on a bill, is it legal to call the person names or to make derogatory comments regarding them, their sex, race, or ethnic background? _____

5. What information are you allowed to give if you call a debtor and speak with a roommate or other family member? _____

_____

6. What is the purpose of the petty cash count slip and how do you use it? _____

_____

_____

7. What is the purpose of the daily journal? _____

_____

8. What is included on a daily journal? _____

_____

_____

9. What is the purpose of the petty cash receipt? _____

_____

10. What are some of the most common accounting reports used in a medical office and what is their purpose?

_____

_____

_____

If you are unable to answer any of these questions, refer back to that section in the chapter, and then fill in the answers.

Exercise 7-1

Directions: Find and circle the words listed below. Words can appear horizontally, vertically, diagonally, forward, or backward.

1. Accounting Control Summary
2. Adjustments
3. Cumulative Trial Balance
4. Defendant
5. Explanation of Benefits

6. Patient Aging Report
7. Pended
8. Post
9. Statute of Limitations

```
Y T P Z N B W G Y Y V T U I E B J X Q I V E E J X I F R Y N
D R V A D I W N P K F Y S C T B B F L X S C U G V S B X R S
M P A Z T X S S Q L V G N O M B W W A T T N W W L P P L T X
E I N M P I H L V Y M K P W P I K A I H G A J J Z I B Z K K
V P Y R M L E V L B B W S G S Q S F V R X L O P N X C K A C
Q S P D T U C N T D O I B G H G E E J U O A E D Q W A H E I
P C F Z R E S M T W D M S D U N N V H Z Z B J A V L G Z L I
Q Z O H E F I L R A M G K E E X O J B F V L C I D J X C P Q
F S M J G H P I O L G M X B D H P W N K P A H N X Y D L W A
X H K Q V K K Q W R K I F F B M H W J U U I G Z F B W Y B P
K C L H G F N W E P T O N O Q U W Y Z Q D R C Z M G A U U M
E X U Q O P P Z Q J N N K G K X X A C L B T S W T F B N B X
J R O P C O C R D O Q K O D R B L R T K C E Z E E Y X G T X
H P O J M L V E I N N F H C X E I E J B U V E L S K Y M W Q
L S K J J Y F T X M G S P Z G N P W N C U I O G S Q C O E K
M J D M U E A E U M D K K Z U N H O X N G T T X O F V X A B
E Q T B N N Q Z R T N S Q M Q V I C R D A A Y L K N Y E Y W
E X B D A B H R L S Z V K X Q R Z T D T C L S S T E B I G V
Z Y A L D A A I A Q T L S R P J W R N E G U V M G T H E Y P
B N P F D K D A Y Q S N U E E H L Q H U M M O M A S P A U Y
T X D E D N E P Z E T A V R J B J D Z R O U K N D O T X H A
E S T A T U T E O F L I M I T A T I O N S C K Y J G T I C H
L H R R D U N F R H Z D D H B U S Z X B X V C M U H Q T O M
Y K Y Q X O V L N X N D D E O Q B I R Z I Z K A S V V K S P
P F B I K A K H O P X O A V J T T T L L H R P J T K U V C M
A A Z P W H D F S Y D Z K W H V C M V H Y N W Z M V H V Q K
B E A H U F H R F F P Z W X X B P Z D E G E H X E T D H J C
C R W A H P Q L B H S T U R K R J Z P A X A R D N N M O A O
K U M Y E F P U J R J J I A S D P M S H V Z A H T S D L R N
A F L M Q V E T L S X M W Y V Z Q C P O T L N C S I M L I Z
```

Exercise 7-2

Directions: Complete the crossword puzzle by filling in a word from the keywords that fits each clue.

Across

4. An overview and balance of monies being deposited.
7. Money being received by a business.

Down

1. This is used to keep track of the amount of money kept in petty cash.
2. The act whereby a debtor announces they no longer have the ability to pay creditors and asks for relief from the federal courts.
3. A fund that is used for providing change to patients who are making cash payments, and for buying miscellaneous small office supplies.
4. A daily balance sheet that shows the patient's name, the individual fee charged for the day, any payments made, and the current balance.
5. A card used to indicate a chronologic record of all services rendered to a patient.
6. A person who has received services without payment and has moved and left no forwarding address.

Exercise 7-3

Directions: Match the following terms with the proper definition by writing the letter of the correct definition in the space next to the term.

1. _____ Accounts Payable

2. _____ Statement of Account

3. _____ Balance Billing

4. _____ Petty Cash Receipt

5. _____ Daily Journal
6. _____ Patient Statement

7. _____ Dunning Notice

8. _____ Insurance Tracer

a. A daily balance sheet that shows the patient's name, the individual fee charged for the day, any payments made, and the current balance.

b. A form or letter sent to the insurance carrier to inquire about the disposition of a previously submitted claim.

c. A statement or sentence reminding the recipient to make a payment on their account.

d. An individual summary (either by patient or by family) that lists all the services, charges, payments, adjustments, and balance due that occurred during the month.

e. Money paid out, usually for goods or services.

f. Sending an additional bill to another party for payment of any remaining amounts on a claim.

g. A form that is used whenever money is removed from the petty cash fund indicating how much money was removed and who received it.

h. A card used to indicate a chronologic record of all services rendered to a patient.

Exercise 7-4

Directions: Based on the following scenarios and using Dr. Paul Provider's information complete an encounter form and patient receipt. Then post the payment to the patient ledger card. Next, balance the day sheet/daily journal. Finally, create a bank deposit slip for the payments made. Refer to the Patient Data Table and Provider Data Table in Appendix C for additional information.

1. The following services were billed for: Abby Addison   Date of Service: 01/16/CCYY
   Diagnosis: Hypertension
   99205–Comprehensive High Complexity Exam ($160)
   8100–Urinalysis ($30)
   36415–Venipuncture ($20)
   Patient made a cash payment of $60 on this visit.

2. The following services were billed for: Bobby Bumble   Date of Service: 01/16/CCYY
   Diagnosis: Diabetes
   99211–Minimal Exam ($35)
   81000–Urinalysis ($30)
   82948–Glucose Fingerstick ($18)
   36415–Venipuncture ($20)
   Patient made a payment by check of $75 on this visit.

3. The following services were billed for: Cathy Crenshaw   Date of Service: 01/16/CCYY

    Diagnosis: Chronic Bronchitis

    99204–Comprehensive Moderate Complexity Exam ($140)

    36415–Venipuncture ($20)

Patient made a payment by check of $110 on this visit.

4. The following services were billed for: Daisy Doolittle   Date of Service: 01/16/CCYY

    Diagnosis: Congenital Hypothyroidism

    99203–Detailed Low Complexity Exam ($100)

    36415–Venipuncture ($20)

Patient made a cash payment of $15 on this visit.

5. The following services were billed for: Edward Edmunds   Date of Service: 01/16/CCYY

    Diagnosis: Coronary Artery Disease

    99214–Detailed Moderate Complexity Exam ($60)

    93000–EKG ($55)

    81000–Urinalysis ($30)

    36415–Venipuncture ($20)

Patient did not make a payment.

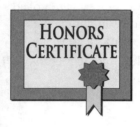

Honors Certification™

The certification challenge for this chapter will be a written test of the information contained in this chapter. Each incorrect answer will result in a deduction of up to 5% from your grade. You must achieve a score of 85% or higher to pass this test. If you fail the test on your first attempt, you may retake the test one additional time. The items included in the second test may be different from those in the first test.

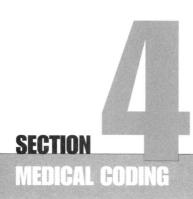

SECTION 4
MEDICAL CODING

8
Reference
Books

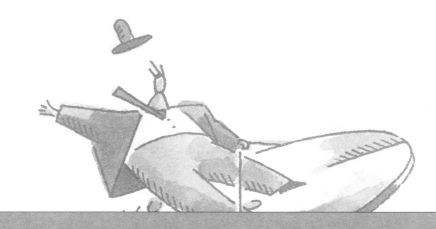

After completion of this chapter
you will be able to:

- Recognize the *Merck Manual, PDR*, Medical Dictionary, *CPT*® and *ICD-9-CM*, and explain their use.
- Determine if a pharmaceutical is a prescription or a nonprescription drug.
- List the sections of the *Physicians' Desk Reference* and the information each section contains.

- Properly use the *Physicians' Desk Reference*.
- Explain the purpose and use of the Health Care Procedure Coding System (HCPCS).
- Describe the two levels used in HCPCS coding.
- Properly code procedures or items using HCPCS.

Keywords and Concepts
you will learn in this chapter:

- Air Ambulance
- Base Call Charge
- Chemotherapy Drugs
- Controlled Drugs
- Durable Medical Equipment (DME)
- Enteral Therapy
- Generic Drugs
- Health Care Procedure Coding System (HCPCS)
- Immunosuppressive Drugs

- International Classification of Diseases—9th Revision Clinical Modification (ICD-9-CM)
- Legend
- Legend Drugs
- Medically Oriented Equipment
- Medical Dictionary
- Medications
- Nonlegend Drugs
- Orthotics

- Over-the-Counter Drugs (OTC)
- Parenteral Therapy
- Pharmaceuticals
- Physician's Current Procedure Terminology (CPT®)
- Physicians' Desk Reference (PDR)
- Proprietary Drugs
- Prosthetic Devices
- Reference Book

A **reference book** is a source of information to which a reader is referred. In health claims billing, coding, and examining, there are a number of books that are used as reference books. These include the *International Classification of Diseases—9th Revision (ICD-9-CM), Physician's Current Procedure Terminology (CPT®), Relative Value Study (RVS), Health Care Procedure Coding System (HCPCS), Physicians' Desk Reference (PDR)*, the medical dictionary, and the *Merck Manual*. We will discuss each of these books briefly in this chapter. The ICD-9-CM and CPT® have their own chapter to discuss their use in further detail.

ICD-9-CM

The *International Classification of Diseases—9th Revision Clinical Modification* (**ICD-9-CM**) is an indexing of diseases and conditions. The ICD-9-CM serves a dual purpose for health benefits personnel: first, it enables the medical biller and the claims examiner to convert English language descriptions of an illness, injury, or other condition into a numerical code, and, second, it allows for the classification of diseases for statistical purposes. Symptoms, diseases, injuries, and routine services are identified with either a three-, four-, or five-digit code, which may be entirely numerical or a combination of alphanumeric.

The ICD-9-CM consists of three volumes:

* Volume I—A tabular listing of diseases.
* Volume II—An alphabetical listing of diseases by English language description.
* Volume III—A numerical and alphabetical listing of surgical or nonsurgical procedures that may be performed by a physician.

The order of use and the degree of use of these volumes vary. The ICD-9-CM and its use will be discussed in detail in Chapter 9.

CPT®

The *Physician's Current Procedure Terminology* (**CPT®**) is a systematic listing for coding the procedures or services performed by a physician. Within this text, the word "physician" is used generically to apply to any provider of services other than a hospital or other facility. Each procedure is identified with a five-digit numerical code. The purpose of the CPT® is to provide a uniform method of accurately describing medical, surgical, and diagnostic services, which facilitates an effective means of communication among physicians, patients, and claim administrators.

The CPT® has six major sections:

1. Evaluation and Management—99201–99499.
2. Medicine—90001–99199.
3. Surgery—10000–69999.
4. Anesthesia—00100–01999.
5. Radiology/Nuclear Medicine—70000–79999.
6. Pathology & Laboratory Tests—80000–89999.

The CPT® and its use will be discussed in detail in Chapter 10.

Medical Dictionary

Medical dictionaries list medical terms and their definitions, synonyms, illustrations, and supplemental information. Numerous medical dictionaries are available. As a rule, this manual should be used mainly for verifying a diagnosis or affected body area, or checking definitions and the spelling of terms. As with most dictionaries, entries are arranged alphabetically.

When using the medical dictionary, it is important that you first read through the foreword and any instructions or general guidelines contained in the front of the book. Because each publisher uses different symbols and information, you must read these instructions to understand the symbols and terms and their meanings. In addition to basic definitions, many medical dictionaries include other information regarding the word or term.

When using the medical dictionary it is imperative that the medical biller read through the entire entry. If terms are used in the definition that the medical biller does not understand, the unknown word also should be looked up, either in the medical dictionary (if it is a medical term) or in a standard dictionary (if it is not).

There are numerous diseases, conditions, or terms that are very similar to each other in spelling or pronunciation but vastly different in meaning. It is important to use the proper term and its proper spelling when billing and coding a claim.

Merck Manual

The *Merck Manual* is used to assist in identifying the symptomatology, prognosis, treatment protocols, etiology, and other miscellaneous information regarding diagnoses.

The *Merck Manual* has two main sections, a listing of diseases and an index. The index is arranged alphabetically by disease. To find a particular disease simply locate the disease and its corresponding page number in the index. The information provided includes the diagnosis, symptoms, prognosis, and treatment.

On the Job Now

Directions: Determine the correct reference book needed to answer the following questions, then use that reference to find the answer. Do not be concerned if you do not understand all the words in the description or answer.

1. What is a synonym (word with the same meaning) for the common cold? _____

_____

2. How long is a person contagious with the common cold? _____

_____

3. Name two symptoms or signs. _____

_____

_____

4. What causes the common cold? _____

_____

5. What is the incubation period for this disease? _____

Physicians' Desk Reference

Medications are drugs (often called **pharmaceuticals**) used to treat diseases, symptoms, or discomforts (i.e., pain medications). The *Physicians' Desk Reference* **(PDR)** is a medical reference book that provides comprehensive information about the particular use of a drug, how the drug works in the body, possible side effects, warnings against use for the elderly, pregnant, and for people with other health complications. The PDR is published annually with supplements published as necessary during the year. Two types of drugs are listed in the PDR, legend and nonlegend. **Legend drugs** are drugs requiring a prescription. The pharmaceutical manufacturer's warning "Caution: Federal law prohibits dispensing without a prescription," called the "legend," appears on the label. Legend drugs are indicated with the symbol Rx. **Nonlegend drugs** are drugs not requiring a prescription. Nonlegend drugs also are known as **over-the-counter drugs (OTC)**. There also are drugs that are closely monitored or controlled, and consequently are called controlled drugs. **Controlled drugs** are drugs that are tightly controlled by federal mandates because of their addictive, experimental, toxic, or other highly volatile properties.

The PDR is divided into six sections:

1. Manufacturers' Index.
2. Product Name Index.
3. Product Category Index.
4. Product Identification Section.
5. Product Information Section.
6. Diagnostic Product Information.

Manufacturer's Index (white)—arranged alphabetically by manufacturer, then by drug name. The name and address of the manufacturer are included. This section includes prescription and nonprescription drugs.

Product Name Index (pink)—arranged alphabetically by drug name. Prescription and nonprescription drugs are included. This section is usually used first to locate the manufacturer's name and the page number for further information.

Product Category Index (blue)—arranged alphabetically by drug action category, that is, according to the most common use of the drug. If the drug is an antidepressant, it is listed under the antidepressant category; if it is an antacid, it is listed under the antacid category.

Product Identification Section (gray)—arranged alphabetically by manufacturer; then by brand name. This section contains the actual size and full-color reproductions. Only the reproductions submitted by the manufacturer are included.

Product Information Section (white)—arranged alphabetically by manufacturer, then by brand name. Most pharmaceuticals are described by indications and usage, dosage, administration, description, clinical pharmacology, supply warnings, contraindications, adverse reactions, overdosage precautions, and other miscellaneous information.

Diagnostic Product Information (green)—arranged alphabetically by manufacturer, then by product. This section provides a description of diagnostic products only.

Generic versus Brand Name Drugs

A pharmaceutical manufacturer bears the cost of all research, development, and testing of a new drug. When a pharmaceutical company develops a drug, they can file for and may receive patent protection for that particular drug. **Proprietary drugs** are drugs that are patented or controlled by a manufacturer. The manufacturer copyrights the trade or brand name. This allows the pharmaceutical company the right to manufacture the drug exclusively under a brand name for a period of time. After the patent has expired, any company may manufacture the drug. Other companies that begin manufacturing the drug after the time period expires do not have the research and development costs. Therefore, they can produce an equivalent drug for a lot less money. The drugs produced by other manufacturers are generic drugs. **Generic drugs** are nonproprietary drugs not protected by trademark, and usually are descriptive of the drug's chemical structure.

When making a generic drug, the manufacturer must provide appropriate safety data to the Food and Drug Administration (FDA). This data includes sufficient proof that the generic product has the identical active ingredient(s) and is as effective as the brand name drug in all aspects. When the generic drug meets these requirements, it is considered "therapeutically equivalent."

Most manufacturers of generic drugs also make brand name drugs. In fact, 70% to 80% of all generic drugs are made by the same manufacturers that make the brand name drugs. The profit made on the generic drugs helps to offset some of the research and development costs of other brand name drugs.

Prescription Plans

Prescription medications are usually covered under benefit plans in one of two ways: (1) under a separate, free standing plan for outpatient, prescription medicines only; or (2) under Major Medical as any other eligible expense, subject to all applicable deductibles, copayments, limitations, and exclusions.

Separate prescription service plans establish networks of participating pharmacies and then assume responsibility for the claims processing. Such plans usually include some if not all of the following components:

1. The claimant is not required to pay for his or her prescription with a large cash outlay. Instead, a small specified copayment amount, chosen by the group, is paid by the claimant for each prescription (copayments usually range from $8 to $30).

2. The pharmacy accepts an identification card as evidence that payment will be made by the plan; it then bills the plan for the unpaid balance.

3. A claim form is not required from the cardholder. The pharmacy bills the payer directly.

4. The member is required to go to a participating pharmacy to fill prescriptions. Otherwise, the claimant will be responsible for full payment of the medication, or a reduced percentage may be paid.

5. Each prescription filled will provide a supply for a specified number of days—30-, 60-, or a 90-day maximum.

Prescription service plans typically exclude the following types of expenses:

1. Devices or medical/surgical supplies of any type such as bandages, gauze, and so on. Hypodermic needles and syringes may be covered for diabetics.

2. Drugs dispensed while the member is confined in a facility, including those given on the day of discharge.

3. Immunization agents, biological sera, blood, plasma, or other blood agents.

4. Investigational or experimental drugs.

5. Health foods, food supplements, vitamins, and appetite suppressants.

As with most other plan provisions, the covered and excluded charges vary from plan to plan. Therefore, the benefits should be verified.

On the Job Now

Directions: Look up the following medications in the PDR. Indicate in the space provided whether or not the drug is prescription by writing in the status symbol. Also, indicate the trade name if the generic name is given; indicate the generic name if the trade name is given. The manufacturer's name is indicated in parentheses.

	Name	Symbol
1. Fluorouracil Cream (Roche)		
2. Proventil (Schering)		
3. Spectazole (Ortho-McNeil)		
4. Fenfluramine Hydrochloride (Robins)		
5. Valium Injectable (Roche)		
6. Klonpin (Roche)		
7. Psyllium Husk Fiber (Proctor & Gamble)		
8. Metaproterenol Sulfate (Boehringer Ingelheim)		
9. Pentazocine Hydrochloride and Acetominophen (Winthrop)		
10. Flonase (Glaxo-Smith-Kline)		
11. Dilantin Injection Parenteral (Parke-Davis)		
12. Sotradecol Injection (Elkins-Sinn)		
13. Aldomet Tablets (Merck)		
14. Mandol (Lilly)		
15. Viagra (Pfizer)		

HCPCS

The *Health Care Procedure Coding System* (HCPCS) is a listing of codes and descriptive terminology used for reporting the provision of supplies, materials, injections, and certain services and procedures. These codes were most often used for billing Medicare services. HCPCS is now mandatory for all transactions involving health care to comply with HIPAA. The HCPCS system has two levels of coding:

- Level I—uses the current CPT® codes for most procedures.
- Level II—uses the HCPCS codes listed in the HCPCS manual.

Before January 2004, there was a Level III that used codes that were specific to the local Medicare carrier. Level III codes were eliminated by CMS to conform to the HIPAA laws.

To properly code using the HCPCS system, check Level II codes first. If no code exists for the service or item you are billing, you should use the appropriate CPT® code.

Historical Information

The Healthcare Common Procedure Coding System (HCPCS) was established to provide a standardized system to code items and services provided in the delivery of medical care. This system was established in 1978 and is necessary to ensure that insurance claims processed by Medicare, Medicaid, and other health insurance programs are processed in a consistent manner. HCPCS is based on the American Medical Association (AMA) Current Procedure Terminology (CPT®) with additional codes and modifiers developed by HCFA. HCPCS is made up of two coding levels:

- Level 1: The first level contains only the CPT® codes and modifiers. Maintenance of these codes is the responsibility of the AMA, and updates are done on a yearly basis. There are over 7,000 CPT® codes; however, the CPT® is limited in its selections for materials, supplies and injection codes. For example, the code 99070 is used for all supplies.
- Level 2: The second level includes the HCFA designated codes. These are nonphysician services such as Durable Medical Equipment, Prostheses and Orthoses. A few physicians' services that were not found in the CPT® codes

were assigned HCFA codes, such as J codes for injections. HCFA codes are alphanumeric beginning with A0000 and continuing through V9999. There are over 2,400 HCPCS codes which are updated yearly.

Although the acronym HCPCS is technically used to denote both levels of the coding system, it is commonly used to denote just the Level 2, which differs from the more commonly used CPT® codes.

Because there are numerous changes to the CPT® and HCPCS codes every year, it is imperative that the biller use the most current edition of the CPT® and HCPCS manual.

Coding Using the HCPCS Manual

Procedure coding is a way for providers to report to an insurance carrier the exact service(s) performed for their patients. While the CPT® covers many provider services, it is not all-encompassing. Medicare carriers required more detailed information on certain types of services. These often included medical equipment, supplies, and the injection of drugs. The CPT® only provides five codes for injectable drugs:

90782—Subcutaneous or intramuscular injection

90783—Intra-arterial injection

90784—Intravenous injection

90788—Intramuscular injection of antibiotic

90799—Unlisted injection

These codes do not indicate the type of drug being injected or its use (i.e., pain management, alleviation of symptoms, etc.).

With the advent of the HCPCS J codes, the biller can now enter a code to indicate which drug is being given to the patient.

Most versions of the HCPCS manual contain an index. This index lists most of the procedures or items that are included in the manual. However, not all items may be included. For example, some HCPCS indexes do not list all the drugs included in the J code section. But most of the drugs are listed in alphabetical order, making it easy to locate the correct code.

To locate a HCPCS code for an item or service, use the index. The index will provide you with the specific HCPCS code for that item or service. If there is more than one applicable code, the index will list all codes or may list a range of codes (i.e., L3810–L3860). However, just looking in the index is not enough. After identifying the code, locate the code in the lettered section and read the information provided. There may be additional information regarding the code, or there may be references to other codes that may be more appropriate.

As with the CPT® and ICD-9-CM, the HCPCS manual uses semicolons. Thus, if a code is indented, the full description of that code includes everything in the unindented code directly above it, up to the semicolon. For example, use your HCPCS manual to locate code L3805. The correct description for this code would be: Wrist-hand-finger-orthoses (WHFO); long opponens, no attachment, custom fabricated.

On the Job Now

Directions: Determine the correct HCPCS codes for the following procedures/items.

1. Injection of thiamine HCl, 100 mg.

2. Injection of azithromycin, 500 mg.

3. Injection of testosterone suspension, up to 50 mg.

4. Injection of lorazepam (Ativan), 2mg.

5. Injection of iron dextran 50 mg.

1. _____

2. _____

3. _____

4. _____

5. _____

Sections of the HCPCS Manual

The HCPCS manual is categorized into numerous sections (**see Table 8–1**). Each section begins with a letter, and within that section each code begins with the same letter.

Transportation Services

These codes are used to report transportation services, including ambulance and air ambulance services. Ambulance expenses are expenses that are incurred to transfer an injured or sick person to a medical facility. These expenses are not considered professional or hospital services.

Transportation Services	A0000–A0999	**Chemotherapy Drugs**	J9000–J9999
Medical and Surgical Supplies	A4000–A7509	**Temporary Codes for DMERCS**	K0000–K9999
Miscellaneous and Experimental	A9000–A9999	**Orthotic Procedures**	L0000–L4999
		Prosthetic Procedures	L5000–L9999
Enteral and Parenteral Therapy	B0000–B9999	**Medical Services**	M0000–M9999
Temporary Hospital Outpatient PPS	C0000–C9999	**Pathology and Laboratory**	P0000–P9999
Dental Procedures	D0000–D9999	**Temporary Codes**	Q0000–Q9999
Durable Medical Equipment	E0000–E9999	**Diagnostic Radiology Services**	R0000–R9999
Temporary Procedures and Professional Services	G0000–G9999	**Private Payer Codes**	S0000–S9999
		State Medicaid Agency Codes	T0000–T9999
Rehabilitative Services	H0000–H9999	**Vision Services**	V0000–V2999
Drugs Administered Other than Oral Method	J0000–J8999	**Hearing Services**	V5000–V5999

Table 8–1 **Categorization of HCPCS Manual**

An ambulance expense is covered under the following conditions:

1. The ambulance must be medically necessary and not for the patient's convenience.
2. Transportation is provided by a professional ambulance/paramedic service.
3. Transportation is to the nearest facility capable of treating the patient.
4. Transportation is provided from one facility to another when the necessary treatment cannot be obtained from the first hospital.
5. Transportation to home from a facility is provided if the patient is unable to travel in an upright position. Exceptions such as this vary by plan, so refer to the plan provisions before processing.
6. Charges for ambulance services are covered when either emergency room or inpatient hospital charges also are billed. An exception would be in the case of an insured who is dead on arrival at the hospital.
7. Transportation to a facility if the claimant is dead on arrival, even though no treatment or charges are incurred at the facility.

Expenses commonly billed by an ambulance service include:

- **Base call charge.** This is the amount automatically charged for the ambulance to respond to a call even if the patient is not subsequently transported.
- **Oxygen** and oxygen supplies.
- **Mileage.**
- **Linens.**
- **Emergency response charge.** This is an extra expense in addition to the base charge, which may be added if the patient's condition is severe enough that resuscitation efforts or other types of stabilization measures are required.
- **Paramedic response charge.** If paramedics rather than emergency medical technicians (EMTs) are used, an extra expense may be added.

Air Ambulance

An **air ambulance** is a helicopter or other flight vehicle used to transport a severely injured or ill person to a hospital. Air medical transport may be covered if:

1. The facility in the area where the patient is injured cannot manage the patient's condition and it is medically necessary to transfer the patient by air to another facility more equipped to treat the patient.
2. Ground transport time would be prolonged and, thus, compromise the patient's medical status.

Coverage is limited to the regular air ambulance charge for transportation to the nearest facility that can handle the case.

On the Job Now

Directions: Determine the correct HCPCS codes for the following procedures/items.

1. Ambulance service, basic life support emergency transport.   1. _____

2. Ambulance service, advanced life support emergency transport.   2. _____

3. BLS routine disposable supplies.   3. _____

4. Ambulance oxygen and oxygen supplies, life-sustaining situation.   4. _____

5. Advanced life support, level 2.   5. _____

Medical and Surgical Supplies

Perishable medical and surgical supplies may be covered under the plan if the items can be used only by the patient and are medically necessary in the treatment of the illness or injury. Medical and surgical supplies include:

1. Disposable, nondurable supplies and accessories required to operate medical equipment or prosthetic devices.
2. Necessary drugs and biological items put directly into equipment (such as nonprescription nutrients).

3. Initial and replacement accessories essential for operating medical equipment.
4. Supplies furnished and charged by a hospital, surgical center, or physician as part of active therapy, such as elastic bandage, cast, and cervical collar.

Examples of medical supply items include diabetes testing strips, catheters, syringes, ostomy pouches, and so on. Do not include items or supplies that could be used by the patient or a member of the patient's family for purposes other than medical care.

On the Job Now

Directions: Determine the correct HCPCS codes for the following procedures/items.

1. Ostomy pouch, drainable; for use on barrier with locking flange (two-piece system).
2. Tracheostomy care kit for new tracheostomy.
3. Paraffin, per pound.
4. Surgical trays.
5. Vabra aspirator.

1. _____
2. _____
3. _____
4. _____
5. _____

Miscellaneous and Experimental

This section is used to code services that are considered to be experimental or investigational in nature. These services often are not covered by insurance carriers.

Patients who receive these services should be informed ahead of time that the services may not be covered. They can then make an informed decision regarding their care.

If patients are involved in an investigational study (i.e., to study the effectiveness of a drug or procedure), their costs may be covered by the entity that is monitoring the study.

Enteral and Parenteral Therapy

Enteral therapy involves the administration of nutritional products directly into the intestines. A tube is inserted through the nasal passage into the stomach. This is used for patients who are unable to chew or swallow.

Parenteral therapy involves administering substances to a patient via a tube inserted into a vein. (i.e., medications or nutritional supplements). Nutrition may be given to patients whose digestive system cannot tolerate food.

This section of the HCPCS manual includes codes for both the equipment used to deliver the therapy, and the nutritional solutions themselves. When coding for these services, be sure to include all codes that apply to the given situation.

Temporary Hospital Outpatient PPS

The codes in this section are used to bill for services that are covered under the Outpatient Prospective Payment System. This system uses the Ambulatory Payment Classifications (APCs) to bill for outpatient hospital services. This payment classification system will be discussed in detail in the chapter on Hospital Billing Procedures.

Dental

The codes included in this section are comparable with those included in the Current Dental Terminology (CDT) book released by the American Dental Association (ADA). Although most dental procedures are not covered by Medicare, there are times when a procedure may be covered. The reasons include:

- Accident.
- Dental treatment required as a result of a medical procedure.
- Restorative treatment.

Dental Procedures

Some procedures performed on the mouth or teeth are covered under dental plans, but others may be covered under Major Medical plans. This holds true even though the services were performed by a dentist or an oral surgeon rather than an MD. These can include the following services:

1. Accidental injury to the teeth (see the section on dental accidents).
2. Surgery to remove impacted, unerupted, or supernumerary teeth. Major Medical benefits are generally paid in the case of tissue-impacted, partly bone-impacted, or totally bone-impacted teeth.
3. Jawbone surgery.
4. Tumors or cysts within the oral cavity.
5. Nasal, auricular, orbital, or ocular prosthesis.
6. Obturators or repair of the cleft palate.
7. Complex, subperiosteal, or endosseous implants.
8. Lab charges such as urinalysis, hemoglobin, hematocrit, and complete blood count.
9. Repair of fractures of the mandible, maxilla, or facial bones.

Dental Accidents

Many carriers cover accidental injury to permanent natural teeth under medical benefits. For the injury to qualify as an accident, you should be able to place the exact date, time, and place at which the accident occurred. However, damage as a result of chewing or biting is generally not considered accidental.

Under the provisions of most contracts, the teeth must be permanent natural teeth that were in place before the accident. Often dentures, partials, or "nonnatural" teeth are excluded. In this case, if there was damage to the pontic and the adjoining abutment teeth, the abutment teeth would be covered but the pontic would not. However, if the teeth were evulsed (knocked out) as the result of an accident, fixed or removable prosthetics may be covered as "required to alleviate the damage." Likewise, deciduous teeth are often not covered as they are not permanent teeth.

Some plans may restrict payment to "sound" natural teeth. The term "sound" natural teeth defines teeth that are in good condition, without substantial restoration, fractures, cracks, extensive decay, or damage as a result of periodontal disease. The "good condition" clause applies to the crown of the tooth and also to the root structure and the supporting structures of the tooth.

Durable Medical Equipment

Durable medical equipment (DME) is an item that can be used for an extended period of time without significant deterioration (i.e., it can stand repeated use). Therefore, an item that can be rented and returned for reuse would meet the requirement for durability. Medical supplies of a disposable nature, such as incontinent pads and surgical stockings, would not qualify as durable.

Medically oriented equipment is primarily and customarily used for medical purposes (i.e., it is designed to fulfill a medical need). Therefore, it is generally not useful in the absence of an illness or injury. For example, an air conditioner may be used in the case of a heart patient to lower room temperature and reduce fluid loss. However, because the primary and customary use is nonmedical in nature, an air conditioner cannot be considered medical equipment. If the item could be used in a regular manner in the absence of a diagnosis, it is probably nonmedical in nature.

DME Billing Procedures

Most plans allow for the purchase or temporary rental of equipment and supplies when prescribed by a physician. However, certain requirements must be satisfied.

Basically, three tests must be applied to items billed as DME in determining whether or not the items may be covered under a plan:

1. Does the item satisfy the definition of DME?
2. Is the item reasonable and necessary for the treatment of an illness or injury or for improvement of the functioning of a malformed body part?
3. Is the item prescribed for use in the patient's home?

Only when all three conditions are met will the item be covered by the plan.

An item may meet the definition of DME and yet not be covered by the plan. Two things to be considered are:

1. **Reasonableness.** This evaluates the soundness and practicality of the DME approach to therapy, including factors such as:
   a. Is the need for the unit based on failures of other less costly approaches?
   b. Have more conservative means been attempted?
   c. What benefits will be derived from the unit?
   d. Do the benefits justify the expense?
2. **Necessity.** Equipment is necessary when it is expected to make a meaningful contribution to the treatment of the patient's illness or injury or to the improvement of the functioning of a malformed body part.

Many plans cover the use of oxygen under DME benefits. Even though the oxygen itself is not durable, the canister in which the oxygen is contained and transported is durable, and it therefore falls under the category of DME. Charges for delivery of the DME and oxygen are usually covered.

Rental versus Purchasing Determinations

If the rental fee is greater than the purchase price, rental is allowed up to but not exceeding the purchase price. Purchase of the item is not required. However, the member should be notified that an expense that is higher than the purchase price may not be allowed.

For DME to be purchased or rented temporarily, the equipment must be prescribed for use in the home. Therefore, any facility that meets at least the minimum requirements of the definition of a hospital or skilled nursing facility is usually excluded from consideration.

A patient's home can be considered, but is not limited to:

- His or her own home, apartment, or dwelling.
- A relative's home.
- A home for the elderly.
- A nursing home.

Repairs, Replacement, and Delivery

Repairs are covered when necessary to make the equipment functional. If the expense for repairs exceeds the estimated cost of purchasing or renting new equipment for the remaining period of medical need, payment is limited to the lower amount.

Replacements are usually covered in cases of irreparable damage or wear or when the patient's physical condition has changed. Replacements as a result of wear or changes in the patient's physical condition must be supported by a current physician's order. Replacements as a result of loss may or may not be covered, depending on the circumstances. Usually, replacement is not covered when disrepair or loss results from a patient's carelessness.

DME Billing Requirements

All claims for DME should be documented with the following information:

1. A description of the equipment prescribed by the physician. If the item is a commonly used item, a detailed description may not be necessary. However, with new equipment, it is important to try to obtain a marketing or manufacturer's brochure that indicates how the item is constructed and how it functions.
2. A statement of the medical necessity of the equipment. This should be in the form of a prescription showing the imprinted name, address, and telephone number of the prescribing physician. The related diagnosis should also be indicated.
3. An indication as to whether the item is to be rented or purchased, and the rental or purchase price.
4. The estimated length of time that the equipment will be needed. This information will aid in the analysis of whether a rental or a purchase is more economical.
5. An indication as to where the equipment will be used and for how long.

Procedures and Professional Services

The codes listed in this section are often temporary codes set up to identify professional services for which no corresponding CPT® code exists. These often are

On the Job Now

Directions: Determine the correct HCPCS codes for the following procedures/items.

1. Over-bed table.   1. _____

2. Walker, folding, wheeled, adjustable or fixed height.   2. _____

3. Raised toiled seat.   3. _____

4. Hospital bed, fixed height, with any type side rails with mattress.   4. _____

5. Dry pressure mattress.   5. _____

services that are covered by Medicare but may or may not be covered by other insurance carriers. For example, flu shots for the elderly or those in need are covered by Medicare. However, most traditional insurance carriers consider these shots to be preventive medicine. If the plan does not cover preventive medicine, flu shots may not be covered.

Many of these codes are deleted when a corresponding CPT® code is created. Thus, it is important to use the HCPCS manual for the current year when coding these services.

Rehabilitative Services

The codes in this section identify rehabilitative services, such as alcohol or drug abuse treatment. These services are often covered under the mental/nervous portion of a health plan.

Many insurance carriers are recognizing the role that drug and alcohol abuse plays in affecting the health of the patient. For that reason, many carriers will reimburse for rehabilitative services. Additionally, many companies will cover the costs for these services if they feel it will help them to retain a good employee.

Many of these codes are specific to a certain type of facility. It is important to determine the type of facility providing the treatment before using the codes in this section.

Drugs Administered by Other than Oral Method

This is one of the most frequently used sections when coding administration of medications. J codes indicate the type of drug being administered to a patient.

When coding drug usage, it is important to note the dosage amount contained in the code description. This amount is often a standard dosage amount, or portion of a dosage amount. Check the amount actually administered to the patient. It is important to note the method by which the drug was administered. This section of the HCPCS manual includes all drugs that are administered other than orally. That can include an injection, inhalation, suppository, insulin pump, and so on. Each method of administration can have a different code. In order to code properly, you must take into account the drug used, the amount given, and the administration method.

Although the drugs in this section are somewhat alphabetical, there are many drugs that will appear out of order. They may be in order of their brand name, as that is the name that was applied to the drug when it first came out (and when the HCPCS code was first assigned).

Immunosuppressive Drugs

Immunosuppressive drugs included in this category are for the suppression of the immune system. These drugs may be administered orally.

Patients who have received a transplanted organ need to keep their immune system suppressed or their bodies may reject the new organ. There also may be additional reasons for administering immunosuppressive drugs.

Chemotherapy Drugs

Chemotherapy drugs are those drugs administered to help fight cancer and other serious diseases. The guidelines regarding checking dosage, brand versus generic names, and so on, apply to this section the same as they applied to the section for drugs administered other than orally.

Temporary Codes for DMERCs

This section contains codes that were temporarily assigned for use by Durable Medical Equipment Regional Carriers (DMERCs). All Medicare DME claims should be submitted to one of four regional carriers. The proper regional carrier for the claim is dependent on the residence of the beneficiary, not the point where the DME item was purchased. For a list of the DMERCs and the areas they serve, you can go to the Medicare Web site at <http://www.medicare.gov>. Because DME claims are sent to and processed by different carriers than are regular services, it is important not to mix DME and services on the same claim.

These codes often will further define a piece of durable medical equipment that was ordered for a patient. For example, this section will list several additional types of wheelchairs and wheelchair attachments. The codes in this section are often deleted when no longer needed. This can be a result of an additional code being created in the regular DME codes (E Codes), or from the equipment no longer being considered valid treatment for a given condition or situation. These codes should only be used when you are instructed to do so by the DMERC in your area. Otherwise, the closest regular DME codes should be used.

Because these codes are temporary, there are numerous changes to this listing every year. For that reason, it is important to always use a current HCPCS manual when coding in this section.

Orthotic Procedures

Orthotics are devices used to correct a deformity or disability. They also are used to correct misalignment of the joints, especially the joints used for walking. Orthotics can be as small as a lift placed inside the shoe, or as large as a brace to correct curvature of the spine.

When billing for an orthotic device, you will need to include a copy of the prescription with the complete diagnosis. Some carriers may even require pictures to be taken to document the need for the device. Other carriers may request literature from the manufacturer of the device explaining how the device is used and the benefits to the patient.

Before billing for these items, it is best to contact the insurance carrier and ask what their guidelines are. They can inform you of any documentation you will

need to submit with the claim. Submitting the documentation at the same time as you submit the claim can prevent a delay in processing.

Prosthetic Procedures

Prosthetic devices are designed to replace a missing body part or to restore some function to a paralyzed body part.

Prosthetic devices include the making and application of an artificial part medically necessary to replace a lost or impaired body part or function, such as an artificial arm or leg.

Prosthetics are intended to replace body parts that are permanently damaged. Many carriers will accept the provider's decision that the body part needs to be replaced. If the judgment of the attending physician is that the condition is of long or indefinite duration, the test of permanence is met.

Covered expenses associated with prosthetics include:

- Shipping and handling as part of the purchase price.
- Temporary postoperative prostheses.
- Replacement charges when replacement is a result of a change in the patient's physical condition. (Children often need replacement prostheses every six to 12 months, depending on their growth rate and other factors.) Replacement is not covered for wear and tear.

Medical Services

This section contains very few codes. The reason this section is so small is that most procedures that would be listed here are already listed in the CPT®. Thus, the CPT® would be the main coding manual for these medical services. Often, the codes that are included in this section are considered new or experimental.

The modifiers included in this section will often designate the type of provider involved. This can include psychologists, clinical social workers, and so on.

Pathology/Laboratory

The codes in this section are for pathology and laboratory tests. Many of these codes are not listed in the CPT®.

Some of the codes in this section are for the testing of blood or blood parts (i.e., plasma, platelets), to ensure that it is free of disease before being transfused into a patient. There also are codes for the separation of blood into the various specific components that a patient might need.

A few of the tests in this section (i.e., pap smears), can be split into the technical component (the person or facility taking the test or drawing the blood), and the professional component (the person interpreting the test results). If the provider performs the test, but does not interpret the results, it is important to use the modifier –TC.

Temporary Codes

This section is used for creating temporary codes. This list will contain codes that are current, as well as codes that have been superceded by a permanent HCPCS code. Some codes will be superceded by a CPT® code that has been added to the CPT®.

This section includes many different types of procedures and services. Many of these codes pertain to new drugs that have been added to the market. As with the other temporary code sections, the items in this section will be changed frequently, so it is important to use the current HCPCS manual when coding.

Diagnostic Radiology Services

This short section is for recording transportation of x-ray or EKG equipment to a nursing home or other facility. In situations in which there is more than one patient to be seen, or where the patient is too fragile to be moved, it is easier to transport the equipment to the patient.

Vision Services

The codes in this section are used to report services performed on or pertaining to the eyes. These can include eyeglasses, contacts, prosthetic eyes, lenses, or other items pertaining to the care and use of the eyes or eyeglasses.

The codes in this section can be very specific regarding the type of lenses used in the glasses and other

factors. Because of this, special training may be needed to code these services properly. Any devices ordered in this section must have a prescription written by an authorized provider. A copy of this prescription should be submitted with the claim.

Hearing Services

The codes in this section are used for reporting services in regards to hearing. This includes hearing testing, as well as devices used to assist those who are hearing impaired (i.e., hearing aids). Other assistive living devices (i.e., telephone amplifier, television caption decoder) are also included in this section. There also are codes for speech-language services such as speech screening.

Any devices ordered in this section must have a prescription written by an authorized provider. A copy of this prescription should be submitted with the claim.

Modifiers

Each section of the HCPCS manual has modifiers that are unique to that section. It is important that medical billers check the modifiers for each section before billing a claim. Without the proper modifiers, claim payment may be delayed or denied. This is especially true in the case of Medicare claims. Not including the appropriate modifier also can cause incorrect reimbursement.

Modifiers in the HCPCS manual are usually two-digit letter codes. In some cases, two separate one-digit letter codes will be combined to make up a single two-digit letter code. For example, in the transportation services section, the first letter indicates from where the patient was picked up and the second letter indicates to where the patient was delivered.

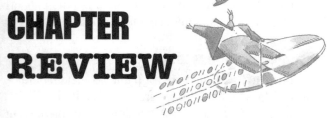

CHAPTER REVIEW

Summary

- The ICD-9-CM is used to code diagnoses and conditions.
- The CPT® is used to code procedures and services rendered by providers.

- The PDR assists in determining whether a drug is prescription or nonprescription, and lists some of the properties (i.e., manufacturer, chemical makeup, side effects, appearance) of a specific drug.
- Medical dictionaries list medical terms and their meanings.
- The *Merck Manual* can assist in determining whether a service or procedure is appropriate for a given diagnosis or condition.

- There are two levels of HCPCS coding:

  Level 1: Contains only the CPT® codes and modifiers.

  Level 2: Includes the codes found in sections A through V of the HCPCS manual.

Assignments

Complete the Questions for Review.
Complete Exercises 8–1 through 8–8.

Questions for Review

Directions: Answer the following questions without looking back into the material just covered. Write your answers in the space provided.

1. Which manuals are used for coding diagnoses? _____

_____

2. The full name of the PDR is _____

3. If you needed to verify a diagnosis, affected body area, or spelling of terms and definitions, you would probably refer to the _____

4. What are medications? _____

_____

5. Explain the difference between a legend and a nonlegend drug. _____

_____

6. Name the six sections of the PDR.

   1. _____

   2. _____

   3. _____

   4. _____

   5. _____

   6. _____

7. (True or False?) Controlled drugs can be purchased over the counter. _____

8. What is the HCPCS book used for? _____

_____

9. What are the two coding levels of HCPCS?

1. _____

_____

2. _____

_____

10. What are the three tests that are applied to DME items to determine if they will be covered under a plan?

1. _____

_____

2. _____

_____

3. _____

_____

If you are unable to answer any of these questions, refer back to that section in the chapter, and then fill in the answers.

Exercise 8-1

Directions: Determine the correct reference book needed to answer the following questions, and then use that reference to find the answer. Do not be concerned if you do not understand all the words in the description or answer.

1. What do the initials AIDS and HIV stand for? _____

_____

2. Which of the following is the correct diagnosis code for AIDS? 079.53, V01.7, 042, or 795.71? _____

3. Describe the disease from question 2. _____

_____

_____

4. How is the disease transmitted among adults? _____

_____

_____

5. How is the disease transmitted to infants? _____

_____

6. What is the description of the code 43842 and is it an appropriate treatment for an AIDS patient? _____

_____

_____

7. What are the descriptions of the codes 86701, 86702, and 86703, and are any of them an appropriate procedure for a suspected AIDS patient? _____

_____

_____

_____

8. If the patient is a Medicare patient and receives an injection of Interferon, would you use the code J9213 or 90772, and why? _____

_____

_____

9. What precautions should medical personnel take when treating someone with AIDS? _____

_____

_____

_____

10. What book would tell you if a specific drug was considered effective against the given condition? _____

_____

Exercise 8-2

Directions: Determine the correct reference book needed to answer the following questions, and then use that reference to find the answer. Do not be concerned if you do not understand all the words in the description or answer.

1. What is the English-language description for the diagnosis code 696.1? _____

_____

2. Describe the disease from question 1. _____

_____

_____

3. What are erythematous papules? _____

_____

4. What is the cause of the disease in question 1? _____

_____

5. Name two symptoms or signs of this disease. _____

_____

_____

6. Name two possible treatments for this disease. _____

_____

_____

7. What is the English-language description for the procedure code 97028? _____

_____

8. Is procedure code 97028 a valid treatment for diagnosis code 696.1? _____

_____

9. Should a patient with this disease expose themselves to sunlight? _____

_____

10. Does smoking affect this condition? If so, in what way? _____

_____

Exercise **8-3**

Directions: Write at least one diagnosis that the indicated medication is normally used to treat.

1. Atromid

2. Inderal LA

3. Quibron

4. Ortho-Novum

5. Pro-Banthine Tablets

6. Sus-Phrine Injection

7. Tofranil Tablets

8. Lanoxin Injection

9. Diethylstilbestrol

10. Parafon Forte

Exercise **8-4**

Directions: Determine the correct HCPCS codes for the following procedures/items.

1. Moisture exchanger, disposable, for use with invasive mechanical ventilation.   1. _____

2. Detailed and extensive oral evaluation—problem focused.   2. _____

3. Application of desensitizing medicaments.   3. _____

4. Injection of calcium gluconate, per 10 ml.   4. _____

5. Air pressure mat.   5. _____

6. Cellular therapy.   6. _____

7. Stomach tube-levine type.   7. _____

8. Sitz bath chair.   8. _____

9. Jaw motion rehabilitation system.   9. _____

10. Dialysis equipment, unspecified.   10. _____

11. Replace quadrilateral socket brim; molded to patient model.   11. _____

12. Cardiokymography.   12. _____

13. Lenticular, nonaspheric, per lens, bifocal.   13. _____

14. Speech screening.   14. _____

15. Assessment for hearing aid.   15. _____

16. Oral thermometer, reusable.   16. _____

17. Collagen skin test kit.   17. _____

18. Injection, tetracycline, 200 mg.   18. _____

19. Ambulatory surgical boot.   19. _____

20. Prosthetic implant.   20. _____

21. Potassium hydroxide (Koh) preparation.   21. _____

22. Transportation of portable EKG to nursing home.   22. _____

23. Infusion of normal saline solution, 250cc.   23. _____

24. Botulinum toxin type A, 2 units.   24. _____

25. Orthodontic treatment (non-contract fee).   25. _____

26. House call.   26. _____

27. Rollabout chair, 6 inch casters.   27. _____

28. Dialysis blood leak detector.   28. _____

29. Splint.   29. _____

30. Mens' orthopedic oxford shoes.   30. _____

Exercise 8-5

Directions: Determine the correct HCPCS codes for the following procedures/items.

1. Synthetic vascular graft material implant.   1. _____

2. Artificial larynx, BV type.   2. _____

3. Thoracic low profile extension, lateral.   3. _____

4. Azithromycin dihydrate capsules, 1 gm.   4. _____

5. Infusion chemo treatment.   5. _____

6. Triam A injection, 10mg. 6. _____

7. Sterile syringe, 30cc. 7. _____

8. Amalgam, 2 surfaces, primary. 8. _____

9. Tigan Injection, 100 mg. 9. _____

10. Raised toilet seat. 10. _____

11. Apnea monitor, with recording feature. 11. _____

12. Dexasone LA injection. 12. _____

13. Assessment for hearing aid. 13. _____

14. Epoetin alpha injection, 1500 units, (non ESRD). 14. _____

15. Hot water bottle. 15. _____

16. Bed board. 16. _____

17. Cervical collar molded to patient. 17. _____

18. Celestone soluspan, 3 mg. 18. _____

19. Nonelastic binder for extremity. 19. _____

20. Canal preparation and fitting. 20. _____

21. Pediatric speech aid. 21. _____

22. Fresh, frozen plasma. 22. _____

23. Preparation of vaginal wet mount. 23. _____

24. Gas impermeable contact lens. 24. _____

25. Reverse osmosis water purifier. 25. _____

26. Reimplantation of tooth. 26. _____

27. Tylenol, nonprescription. 27. _____

28. Duoval PA. 28. _____

29. Hemodialysis machine. 29. _____

30. Insulin injection, 100 units. 30. _____

Exercise **8-6**

Directions: Find and circle the words listed below. Words can appear horizontally, vertically, diagonally, forward, or backward.

1. Chemotherapy Drugs
2. Enteral Therapy
3. Generic Drug
4. Medications
5. Orthotics
6. Pharmaceuticals
7. Physicians' Desk Reference
8. Proprietary Drug
9. Prosthetic Devices

```
Y S U X N C J F S J K A X C O U D I N C T X P Q N N T Y L P
L M E H Y B U Z B H S S S S G V I J C A B H R X T S K D C L
Z F P C A G O L F C H X G Q U G A N Z I Y W N J F I H S F M
Q R X A I N W Y G Y E G R S P L H D D S I L O L M W P Y U S
V B J K T V T H A Z X I O T W E E O I S Y X K I E W M D B C
N W J D A Y E Z D S Y X R G C K R C E T D O L H D U X W E V
U F H N D F K D C R Y G L L G R I I R M L L I X I L D M W H
P K H R T F I I C N Y N D U K A T V J L N E Q C C O D L S T
X P B N M M D R B I O G R A N Y Q M J D P A U Z A A E F G V
K E A A O R P Z R S T D U S G U R D Y P A R E H T O M E H C
U M P D W W U Y X W Y E D V X X K U O R D P O N I J Y N X Q
E X U C Q F Z K F R K E H V T Z U I S J S H S G O X E X R A
A E L B X Q G R A J S O U T D X M N L U S B F X N J M Z M C
D T N F F M N T Q K Z G G B S V D Y A X Y E T Z S H K O P E
V X Y Q D A E T R C O T T E T O Q Q C B Z P Y V Y K R W G K
W C Z F Y I U E L M L N T L N Z R P I R M Z T W E T X L I F
F T B M R L F H D J N B D P I E C P T P W Z D T H R W T Q I
O S R P R E Q L T Y N V T N A Z R T U N N F C O S P K I N R
X A O L R C E V P J H W N S G M H I E R S C T U L W H I W V
E R N E N T E R A L T H E R A P Y Y C X E I F W I U A S H U
P T N W C N F Q Q S L U B G W R S G A D C C Q L Q L F X Q H
G C L T H O U V X O O M I M M T M I M S R G Y L S J Y Y J K
E G D L J A W I Q S V U P F F Z C M R N H U U U Q W U B E P
U Q A P C V G P E P D R I K J I P G A W R C G H M C J F A X
A I R I W P N W A C M U G Q E V X Q H N G S F A D Z S W X D
F U Z I M Q Y N C P R M X L Z M L G P G V F Y O W K U Y E O
H T B D D R E K R M Q M K P Y Y U G U H L O L W H J X B K P
A O M R Z G F L Y U N A C Z B C V E P B M X F F L G P U L Y
P Z N A S V U D W A L T N W W T U M C H B G G V U M R M J K
X P O L F P W N C C M V E C A V M R D J S U R F W J U R I O
```

Exercise **8-7**

Directions: Complete the crossword puzzle by filling in a word from the keywords that fits each clue.

Across

7. Drugs requiring a prescription. The "legend" always appears on the label.
8. A label inscribed as follows: "Caution: Federal (United States) law prohibits dispensing without a prescription."

Down

1. Therapy that involves administering substances to a patient via a tube inserted into a vein (i.e., medications or nutritional supplements).
2. A helicopter or other flight vehicle used to transport severely injured or ill persons to a hospital.
3. Drugs not requiring a prescription.
4. Drugs that are tightly controlled by federal mandates because of their addictive, experimental, toxic, or other highly volatile properties.
5. Lists medical terms and their definitions, synonyms, illustrations, and supplemental information.
6. The amount automatically charged for an ambulance to respond to a call even if the patient is not subsequently transported.

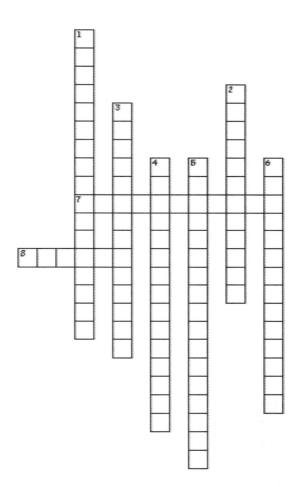

Exercise 8-8

Directions: Match the following terms with the proper definition by writing the letter of the correct definition in the space next to the term.

1. _____ Reference Book

2. _____ Durable Medical Equipment

3. _____ Physician's Current Procedure Terminology

4. _____ Immunosuppressive Drugs

5. _____ International Classification of Diseases-9th Revision Clinical Modification

6. _____ Medically Oriented Equipment

7. _____ Health Care Procedure Coding System

8. _____ Over-the-Counter Drug

a. An index used for billing injections, medication, supplies, and durable medical equipment.

b. Equipment that is primarily and customarily used for medical purposes.

c. A drug that may be purchased without a prescription. Also known as a nonlegend drug.

d. An indexing of diseases and conditions.

e. Source of information to which a reader is referred.

f. Drugs for the suppression of the immune system.

g. A systematic listing for coding the procedures or services performed by a physician or provider.

h. An item that can be used for an extended period of time without significant deterioration (i.e., it can stand repeated use.

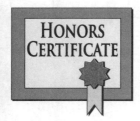

Honors Certification™

The certification challenge for this chapter will be a written test of the information contained in this chapter. Each incorrect answer will result in a deduction of up to 5% from your grade. You must achieve a score of 85% or higher to pass this test. If you fail the test on your first attempt, you may retake the test one additional time. The items included in the second test may be different from those in the first test.

9

International Classification
of Disease (ICD-9-CM) Coding

After completion of this chapter
you will be able to:

- Discuss the history of the ICD-9-CM and why it was created.

- Describe the contents of each volume of the ICD-9-CM.

- Describe how each volume of the ICD-9-CM is arranged.

- State the guidelines concerning ICD-9-CM coding.

- Describe the main terms and how they are used.

- Identify and describe the common signs and symbols used in the ICD-9-CM.

- List the important factors to be aware of when using ICD-9-CM codes for billing.

- Describe how to handle downgrading of codes and concurrent care situations.

- Convert the English-language description of an illness or injury into a numeric ICD-9-CM code.

Keywords and Concepts
you will learn in this chapter:

- Benign
- Cancer in Situ
- Concurrent Care
- Eponyms

- ICD-9-CM
- Main Term
- Malignant
- Malignant Primary

- Malignant Secondary
- Neoplasm
- Subclassifications
- V Code

ICD-9-CM refers to the *International Classification of Diseases—9th Revision Clinical Modification*. This is a coding system devised to provide standardization of the coding of diseases, conditions, impairments, and symptoms by the medical and insurance industry.

History of the ICD-9-CM

The **ICD-9-CM** is a statistical coding of medical diagnoses and procedures that has been around (under different titles) since the early 1900s. It is based on the World Health Organization's (WHO's) International Classification of Diseases (ICD).

WHO originally created the ICD as a means of compiling data on morbidity and allowing hospitals and clinics to restore and retrieve diagnostic data.

In 1956, the American Hospital Association and the American Association of Medical Record Librarians (later known as the American Medical Record Association) undertook a study of the efficacies of coding systems for diagnostic indexing. Their study concluded that the ICD provided a good framework for hospital indexing.

In 1977, the National Center for Health Statistics convened a steering committee to provide advice and counsel on revisions that should be made to the ICD-9-CM. This created the ICD-9-CM, which is a clinical modification of WHO's ICD-9-CM.

Each year the ICD-9-CM is updated. On release of the revised information by the U.S. Department of Health and Human Services, numerous publishing companies print their own version of the information contained in the ICD-9-CM. These versions all contain the same basic information. However, various options are added in an effort to make their book more preferred. These options can include color coding, tabs, numerous symbols, and various instructions and aids.

The decision of which publisher's version of the ICD-9-CM to use is simply a matter of individual or company choice.

Contents of the ICD-9-CM

The ICD-9-CM is comprised of three volumes.

Volume I—The tabular or numerical listings of diagnoses are structured numerically according to body system. Volume I is used when:
- An ICD-9-CM code is provided, but there is no language description of the diagnosis, or

- A language diagnosis is included, but an ICD-9-CM code is not indicated and the terms used by the provider cannot be found in Volume II. If you can identify the body system, you may be able to locate an appropriate ICD-9-CM code.

A number in parentheses after a code is the page number in Volume II that can be checked to verify the code. Table 9–1 shows the organization of Volume I.

Volume II—The alphabetic listings of diagnoses. This section is most commonly used first. It is divided into four sections:
- An alphabetical index of diseases and injuries.
- A table of drugs and chemicals.
- An alphabetical index of external causes of injuries and poisonings (accidents) (E codes).
- A listing of factors affecting the health status of an individual (V codes).

Volume III—A numeric listing of surgical procedure codes. Volume III contains both a tabular listing and index. The tabular listing has procedures arranged according to body sections. The body sections are arranged as follows:

1. Operations on the Nervous System.
2. Operations on the Endocrine System.
3. Operations on the Eye.
4. Operations on the Ear.
5. Operations on the Nose, Mouth and Pharynx.
6. Operations on the Respiratory System.
7. Operations on the Cardiovascular System.
8. Operations on the Hemic and Lymphatic System.
9. Operations on the Digestive System.
10. Operations on the Urinary System.
11. Operations on the Male Genital Organs.
12. Operations on the Female Genital Organs.
13. Obstetrical Procedures.
14. Operations on the Musculoskeletal System.
15. Operations on the Integumentary System.
16. Miscellaneous Diagnostic and Therapeutic Procedures.

The index has procedures listed in alphabetical order. The medical biller should confirm their choice of code by looking in the tabular listing and checking all referrals, exclusions, and notes included.

How to Use the ICD-9-CM

The ICD-9-CM is structured to move from a general diagnosis to a more specific diagnosis by adding on digits. It uses three-, four-, or five-digit codes. Three-

Number	Body System/Classification
00–13	Infective and Parasitic Diseases
14–23	Neoplasms
24–27	Endocrine, Nutritional, Metabolic Diseases
28	Diseases of the Blood and Blood-Forming Organs
29–31	Mental/Nervous Disorders
32–38	Diseases of the Nervous System and Sense Organs
39–45	Diseases of the Circulatory System
46–51	Diseases of the Respiratory System
52–57	Diseases of the Digestive System
58–62	Diseases of the Genito-Urinary System
63–67	Complications of Pregnancy, Childbirth and the Puerperium
68–70	Diseases of the Skin and Subcutaneous Tissue
71–73	Diseases of the Musculoskeletal System and Connective Tissue
74–75	Congenital Anomalies
76–77	Certain Causes of Perinatal Morbidity and Mortality
78–79	Symptoms, Signs and Ill-Defined Conditions
80–86	Fractures, Dislocations, Sprains and Internal Injuries
87–90	Lacerations
91–99	Other Accidents, Poisoning and Violence (nature of the injury)
V0–Y24	Miscellaneous Informative Codings (a particular diagnosis is not indicated)

Table 9–1 **Organization of Volume I**

digit codes are the most general. By adding additional digits, a more precise diagnosis is identified.

The requirements of various processing systems or clients vary. Most require very precise coding, and the use of five digits would be required.

When performing ICD-9-CM coding, the medical biller should always code to the highest number of digits possible; the highest degree of specificity. This includes four- and five-digit subclassifications wherever they occur. **Subclassifications** are secondary classifications under a main classification.

General Guidelines

Some basic guidelines should be kept in mind when coding and using the ICD-9-CM. The following are general guidelines to keep in mind when trying to locate the proper ICD-9-CM code:

1. Read through the introduction of the ICD-9-CM to ensure understanding of any color coding, symbols, abbreviations, and terms that the book uses.

2. Always use both the Index Listing (Volume II) and the Numeric Listing (Volume I). Volume II alone will not give you any exclusions, referrals, or instructions for the codes, including the need for four- or five-digit subclassifications.

3. Always code the principal diagnosis. The principal diagnosis is the condition that is established as being chiefly responsible for requiring the patient to seek medical care.

   a. Do not code symptoms or the suspected condition if a final diagnosis is indicated. Symptoms and suspected conditions are usually accompanied by terms such as "probable," "suspected," "questionable," or "Rule out (R/O)."

   b. It is understood that some conditions will not be fully diagnosed until test results have provided further understanding of the condition; in such cases, code conditions to the highest degree of certainty for the encounter. For example, many codes contain a fourth or fifth digit, which is for "unspecified" conditions or types. Often this will be indicated by the abbreviation NOS for "Not Otherwise Specified." These codes are acceptable if this is the highest level of certainty documented by the physician at this encounter.

4. Code diagnosis to the highest number of digits possible. For example, do not use only three digits to describe a condition when four- and five-digit subclassifications exist for that category.

5. Code only the diagnosis determined by the physician and any complications. Do not list any codes for previous conditions that were previously treated and that no longer exist.

6. The main diagnosis, condition, or reason for the encounter should be listed first. All other conditions that coexist at the time of treatment and that affect the treatment are to be coded following the main reason. If several conditions equally resulted in the encounter, the doctor or medical biller is free to list whichever they choose first.

7. When a patient is seen for ancillary diagnostic services only, the appropriate V code should be listed first, and the diagnosis or condition that is the underlying reason for the tests should be listed second. If a second code is not listed, delays in claim processing or denial of benefits may result.

   For example, if a chest x-ray is taken (coded V72.5) and no second code is listed, the claim may be denied if there are no benefits for routine chest x-rays.

8. When a patient is seen for ancillary therapeutic services only, the appropriate V code should be listed first, and the diagnosis or condition that is the underlying reason for the services should be listed second.

9. Diagnosis codes for chronic diseases or conditions may be coded as often as needed when the patient has repeated encounters for the chronic disease or condition.

10. Diagnoses that relate to earlier episodes of care or are chronic and have no bearing on the current treatment are to be excluded.

11. When billing for surgical procedures, use the correct code to indicate the diagnosis or reason for the surgery. If a postoperative diagnosis is different from the preoperative diagnosis, and the postoperative diagnosis is known at the time the claim is submitted, you should code the postoperative diagnosis.

12. Adjectives (acute, chronic, and the like) may appear as subterms. For example, the diagnosis of Acute Pelvic Inflammatory Disease may be located in the following manner:

   a. Look up the condition—disease,

   b. Under disease, refer to the subheading (site) of pelvis, pelvic,

   c. Locate the specific condition—inflammatory (female) (PID), and

   d. Finally, locate manifestation, acute—614.3.

13. Cross-reference to synonyms, closely related terms, and code categories beginning with "See" and "See also," for example, "Pelvic-peritonitis (See also peritonitis, pelvic, female)."

14. Carefully read any and all notes under the main term. These can include exclusions, referrals, and examples of diagnoses or conditions.

15. Carefully note any modifiers associated with the main term. Compare these with any qualifying terms used in the diagnosis statement.

16. Watch for subterms listed under a main term. Subterms become more specific the further down they go.

These guidelines should be memorized and used whenever you are attempting to locate an ICD-9-CM code. They will ensure a higher degree of accuracy and a higher rate of correct benefit payment on claims.

Main Terms

The Alphabetic Index is arranged by condition, disease, or syndrome. These identifying names are called the Main Terms and are the keys by which this volume is structured. The **Main Terms** usually identify disease conditions rather than locations. The Main Terms may be listed as proper medical terms or ill-defined terms or as eponyms. **Eponyms** are illnesses or conditions named after a person (i.e., Gerhardt's Disease). Certain conditions may be listed under more than one term.

Practice
Pitfalls

Carefully read through the beginning sections of your ICD-9-CM manual. This will give you a lot of additional information on properly using the manual. This is one of your best sources for learning how to use the ICD-9-CM.

For example, in the following cases, the Main Terms are underlined.

Streptococcal <u>tonsillitis</u>—This can be located in two ways:

- Under tonsillitis (subheading streptococcal)
- Under infection (subheading streptococcal, site—sore throat)

Streptococcal is not a condition; it is the type of organism involved in an infection.

Some other examples include the following:

- <u>Dislocated</u> shoulder.
- Pulmonary <u>edema</u>.
- Pelvic <u>abscess.</u>
- <u>Prolapsed</u> uterus.
- <u>Fractured</u> radius.
- Sick sinus <u>syndrome.</u>
- Chronic <u>hepatitis.</u>
- External <u>hemorrhoids</u>.

On the Job NOW

Directions: Identify the Main Term and write it in the space provided.

Acute Bronchitis _____

Heart Palpitations _____

Rectal Leukoplakia _____

Pernicious Anemia _____

Bacterial Meningitis _____

Ulcerative Colitis _____

Rosacea Acne _____

Recurrent Urethritis _____

Diabetes Mellitus _____

Internal Hemorrhoids _____

Exceptions

In some instances, the ICD-9-CM is organized differently so that the Main Terms do not identify disease conditions. These exceptions include:

1. Obstetric conditions, which are found under "Delivery," "Pregnancy," or "Puerperal." (Puerperal refers to the period immediately following delivery.)
2. Complications of medical and surgical conditions, which are located under "Complications."

However, they can also be found under the condition. For example, "evisceration" of an operative wound can be found under evisceration and complication. It is recommended that you look under the condition.

3. Late effects of diseases and injuries, which are under the Main Term "late effects."
4. In some situations, a claim or bill may provide a "diagnosis" that is not a sickness or injury per se. For example, exposure to, history of, problem with, or vaccination are not diagnoses but may be considered appropriate Main Terms.

Practice
Pitfalls

The medical biller is limited to the available number of spaces on the billing form. List only the main conditions up to the number of spaces provided.

Once you have identified the code in the indexed listing (Volume II), cross-reference your selection with the Tabular listing in Volume I. This will ensure that you have selected the proper code. It also will allow you to code to the highest degree of specificity.

Be sure to research any exclusions, referrals ("See Also"), and examples to ensure that your code is correct. Also be sure to refer to the three- and four-digit classification headings. These headings often have further information or list the fourth and fifth digits that apply to all following codes in that classification.

For example, let's use the dislocated shoulder mentioned previously. The index lists the three-digit classification for a dislocated shoulder as 831. However, a four-digit classification will tell whether the injury is open or closed, and a five-digit classification will pinpoint the diagnosis as to the more precise location of the injury. Also, note that a chronic or recurrent shoulder dislocation has an entirely different three-digit classification of 718.

Now turn to classification 831 in the tabular listing. You will see that the five-digit subclassifications are listed directly below the three-digit classification heading. This is followed by the three-digit classifications and the four-digit classifications.

The reason for this order can be better understood when you look at the codes 800–804. Each of these codes is for a fracture of the skull. The five-digit codes that immediately follow the classification heading can be used with any of the three- or four-digit classifications that begin with the numbers 800, 801, 803, or 804. The classifications for 804 appear several pages later. This is why it is important to always look back to the four- and three-digit classification headings when coding.

Appropriate sites or modifiers are listed in alphabetical sequence under the Main Terms with further subterm listings as required. For example, the diagnosis of Open Tibia/Fibula Fracture may be located as follows:

See Fracture heading

Locate tibia as a subheading

Site—with fibula

Description—open = 823.92

Neoplasms

A **neoplasm** is a growth (tumor) that results from abnormal cell activity. Selecting an ICD-9-CM code for a neoplasm involves identifying the following factors:

- The pathologic status of the growth—benign or malignant.
- The site of the growth—breast, lung, bladder.
- The cell type (i.e., oat cell).

This information is not always provided on medical reports, claims, or bills. Therefore, as with any other diagnosis, the code selected will be based on the available information. The more information provided, the more specific the code.

For coding growths or tumors, you need to become familiar with the ICD-9-CM Neoplasm Table (NT) located in Volume II. This table is organized alphabetically by site (location). Because the site is not always known, there is an entry for "unknown site or unspecified."

On the right side of the Neoplasm Table are six columns from which to select an ICD-9-CM code based on the given diagnosis. The terms used in these columns are defined as follows:

Malignant primary—Primary means that the site of the tumor is the point of origin of the neoplasm. **Malignant** means that the cancer or growth is growing. Malignant growths will spread throughout the body until they kill the patient.

Malignant secondary—Secondary means that the site of the tumor in question is not where the disease originated. It has spread to this location from the primary site.

Malignant CA in situ—In situ means that the malignant growth is still localized in one area and has not spread.

Benign—Localized growth that does not spread (metastasize) and is not usually terminal.

Uncertain Behavior—Usually a particular type of growth is either always malignant or always benign. There are, however, some growths that may be either. In cases in which the information does not establish which type of manifestation is present and the growth could be either, this coding may be used. As a rule, this column should be used only when the neoplasm's behavior is stated to be uncertain by a pathologist or physician or is listed as such in the Alphabetic Index.

Unspecified—A growth is unspecified when it is not identified as benign or malignant and the type of growth is always one or the other.

The first step in coding growths is to determine whether the growth is benign or malignant. If the status is indicated, go directly to the table under either the malignant or benign column, according to the site of the growth. Choose the malignant column based on the specifics of the diagnosis—primary, secondary, or in situ.

For example:

Diagnosis: Benign Breast Tumor

ACTION: **1.** Find "breast" alphabetically.
       2. Look at the benign column.
       3. The code is 217.

Diagnosis: CA in Situ—Uterus

ACTION: **1.** Find "uterus" alphabetically.
       2. Look under Malignant-CA in situ.
       3. The code is 233.2.

Diagnosis: Brain Tumor

ACTION: **1.** Find "brain" alphabetically.
       2. Look under Unspecified.
       3. The code is 239.6

If a growth is identified as malignant, but is not further identified as primary, secondary, or CA in situ, assume that it is primary.

The terms CA, cancer, carcinoma, and sarcoma always indicate a malignancy. Other terms, such as fibroma and adenoma, require you to check the alphabetical listing (not the Neoplasm Table) of Volume II to determine whether the condition is benign or malignant. Subsequently, the proper column in the Neoplasm Table can be referenced.

For example:

If the diagnosis is:	Look under the Main Term:
Pelvic Fibroma	Fibroma
Adenoma	Adenoma
Adenosarcoma	Adenosarcoma
Papilloma, eyelid	Papilloma
Osteosarcoma	Osteosarcoma

On the Job Now

Directions: Locate the appropriate ICD-9-CM code and write it in the space provided.

1. Benign Breast Tumor   _____

2. CA in Situ, Uterus   _____

3. Lung Tumor   _____

4. Secondary CA, Pancreas   _____

5. Primary CA, Pylorus   _____

6. Cancer in Situ, Trachea   _____

7. Malignant Tumor Duodenum   _____

8. Cancer, Rectum   _____

9. Sarcoma, Skin   _____

10. Brain Tumor   _____

In most cases, looking under the appropriate Main Term will direct you to the correct column in the Neoplasm Table. In some circumstances, however, you will be given a valid ICD-9-CM code by the provider and you will not need to reference the Neoplasm Table at all.

As you can see, the reference under the Main Term identifies whether the neoplasm is benign or malignant. In the case of adenosarcoma, a valid ICD-9-CM code (189.0) is given and the Neoplasm Table did not have to be checked. Remember that M codes are disregarded. Also note that the "See Also" reference, which is usually optional, must be followed in the case of neoplasms. Over time, you may learn which neoplasms are benign or malignant and may be able to go directly to the Neoplasm Table.

Lesions

Although lesions are similar to neoplasms, they are treated differently by the ICD-9-CM. Lesions should be handled as indicated in the following statements:

If the diagnosis simply states "lesion," look under the Main Term "lesion" alphabetically in Volume II.

If the diagnosis is "benign lesion," look under the Main Term "lesion."

If the diagnosis is "malignant lesion," look under one of the malignant columns in the Neoplasm Table in Volume II.

Sprains/Strains

Sprains and strains are coded according to the site of injury. Strains of the musculoskeletal system are included under the Main Term, Sprain. There is a separate Main Term reference for strains that are not related to the musculoskeletal system (such as eyestrain). If the location of a musculoskeletal strain or sprain is unknown, use code 848.9 (musculoskeletal system). Normally, 848.9 is used as a temporary code while additional information is requested from the provider.

Dislocations

As with strains and sprains, dislocations are coded according to the site of injury. Code 839.8 should be used if the exact injury site is unknown. See previous paragraph.

A closed dislocation includes simple, complete, partial, uncomplicated, and unspecified (type). Open dislocations include infected, compound, and dislocation with a foreign body.

"Chronic," "habitual," "old," or "recurrent" dislocations may be coded as "dislocation, recurrent, and pathologic."

Fractures

As with strains, sprains, and dislocations, fractures are coded according to the site of injury.

Closed fractures include the following descriptions, with or without delayed healing: comminuted, linear, depressed, march, elevated, simple, fissured, slipped epiphysis, greenstick, spiral, impacted, and unspecified.

Open fractures include compound, infected, missile, puncture with or without a foreign body, with or without delayed healing.

Assume that the fracture is closed unless there is wording that indicates otherwise.

When multiple fractures are involved, it is easier to look under the names of the bones involved than to look under "Fracture, multiple."

V Codes

The **V code** listing is a supplementary listing of factors that affect the health status of the patient. Often there are reasons for an encounter that relate to a disease or condition but do not constitute a diagnosis. There are three main types of occurrences:

1. When a person who is not ill has an encounter with a healthcare provider for a specific purpose that is not in and of itself a disease or condition. These encounters can include a visit from a person who is getting a vaccination or a check-up, who is acting as an organ or tissue donor to another person, or who wants to discuss a problem that is not considered a disease or condition (i.e., fertility problems, genetic counseling).

2. When a patient with a chronic or recurring condition visits a healthcare provider for service associated with treatment of that condition. This can include a cast change, dialysis for renal disease, monitoring of pacemaker, and other similar situations.

3. When a situation arises that influences the person's health, but is not a disease or condition. Such situations include exposure to potential health hazards (i.e., tuberculosis, polio), animal bites that require rabies vaccination, and the fact that a person's physiology or family history suggests a factor that should be borne in mind when treatment is received (i.e., carrier of suspected infectious diseases, history of cancer or other diseases, allergies to medicines).

When performing diagnosis coding in circumstances 2 and 3 above, the V code should be used as a supplementary code (not the primary diagnosis code). The diagnosis or condition that underlies the reason for the treatment (circumstance 2) or that caused the patient to seek medical attention (circumstance 3) should be coded as the primary diagnosis. V codes are arranged according to the following headings:

V01–V09 Persons with potential health hazards related to communicable diseases

V10–V19 Persons with potential health hazards related to personal and family history

V20–V29 Persons encountering health services in circumstances related to reproduction and development

V30–V39 Liveborn infants according to type of birth

V40–V49 Persons with a condition influencing their health status

V50–V59 Persons encountering health services for specific procedures and aftercare

V60–V68 Persons encountering health services in other circumstances

V70–V82 Persons without reported diagnosis encountered during examination and investigation of individuals and populations

As a medical biller, you should examine the V codes and familiarize yourself with the situations they define.

E Codes

The E code listing is a supplementary classification of external causes of injury and poisoning. E codes are used to indicate the cause of the injury, not the injury itself. Therefore, an E code should always be an additional code, not a primary diagnosis code. For example, a patient was a pedestrian struck by a car and suffered a fractured femur. The diagnosis would be fractured femur (code 821.00), and the cause would be pedestrian struck by automobile (E814.7).

To correctly code E codes, consult the index located in section 3 of Volume II (behind the table of drugs and chemicals). This index is used the same way the index to diseases and conditions is used. First, locate the cause in the index, then turn to the tabular listing to confirm your choice and to ensure correct four- and five-digit subclassifications.

The beginning of the E code section contains definitions of the terms involved in describing causes. The medical biller should familiarize him or herself with these definitions because they are vital to proper coding. When coding transport accidents, the following headings are used:

* Railway (E800–E807)
* Motor Vehicle (E810–E825)
* Other road vehicles (E826–E829)
* Water Transport (E830–E838)
* Air and Space (E840–E845)

If you are coding an accident that involves more than one type of vehicle, the order listed here should be followed. For example, let's code an accident between a car and a streetcar. Since a streetcar is considered a railway vehicle, the car would take precedence. Therefore, you would look under the motor vehicle section to find motor vehicle accident involving collision with train (E810). The four-digit subclassification would then be added to this number to describe the activity of the patient at the time of the accident (see motor vehicle accident section heading).

If you are coding machinery accidents (nontransport vehicles), you should use category E919.x. This allows for a broad description of the type of machinery and activity that made up the cause of the injury. If you wish to provide a more detailed description, the Internal Labor Office has created a Classification of Industrial Accidents According to Agency. However, this classification should be used in addition to the appropriate E code, not in place of it. Some versions of the ICD-9-CM reproduce this classification listing.

Practice
Pitfalls

The diagnosis coded must support the services rendered. On the claim form, the diagnosis that relates to each procedure performed is placed next to the procedure code. Therefore, each procedure performed should have a diagnosis that substantiates the need for that procedure.

Signs and Symbols Used in the ICD-9-CM

Most coding books have different signs and symbols to alert you to specific situations with codes. However, different versions of the coding books may have different signs and symbols, or none at all.

Listed below are some of the common signs and symbols used in the ICD-9-CM.

- • This code is new to this edition of the ICD-9-CM. It has just been added to the list of ICD-9-CM codes.
- m This code has been changed from last year's edition of the ICD-9-CM.
- fl A fourth digit is required to properly use this code.

   A fifth digit is required to properly use this code.

Many ICD-9-CMs also have signs or symbols for nonspecific codes or unspecified codes. These codes should only be used as a last resort when no other code is appropriate.

Some ICD-9-CMs also will use colors to signify the fourth- or fifth-digit requirement. For example, a pink box may appear behind the code number.

It is important to understand the meanings of these signs and symbols as they are used in your version of the ICD-9-CM. Without understanding them, your chances of improperly coding a claim can increase greatly.

The details of the signs and symbols used in your version of the ICD-9-CM should appear in the beginning of the book. You should read this section carefully before beginning coding.

Concurrent Care

Often, reimbursement problems occur when two doctors are seeing a patient at the same time for two unrelated medical conditions. This is known as **concurrent care**. Claims were frequently denied as duplication of services when the patient was seen by two physicians on the same day, when no duplication actually occurred.

Before 1992, there was a CPT® modifier (−75) that notated concurrent care. This modifier has since been dropped. Now there are two ways to ensure that there is a possibility of payment from the payer:

1. Submit two separate claim forms, one for each physician, which list two completely separate

diagnoses and the related services that were provided.

2. If the separate providers were members of the same medical group and payment is to be made to the medical group, then all services should be submitted on the same claim form. However, two separate diagnoses should be listed, and the procedures performed for each should be substantiated by the referencing of the separate diagnoses next to the procedure.

ICD-10-CM

Each year the ICD-9-CM is updated, incorporating new diagnoses and revising or eliminating old ones. However, since these are limited revisions, the book continues to be called the ICD-9-CM. The version is indicated by the year.

Each time there is a major revision of the ICD, it is assigned a new version number. The ICD-9-CM is for the ninth such revision.

Recently, the American Medical Association developed the ICD-10-CM. This is a major revision of the International Classification of Diseases. Texts have been developed regarding the use of this new coding book; however, the actual book itself is still going through the numerous revision and approval processes necessary before it can be adopted. Because the actual revision itself is not complete, any current manuals give instructions on what they presume the new version will eventually look like. Additionally, although the contents of the ICD-10-CM will change, the new volume is expected to be used much like the ICD-9-CM. Therefore if you can comfortably use the ICD-9-CM, the transition to the ICD-10-CM should not prove too difficult.

For these reasons, and because numerous changes are expected before the introduction of the ICD-10-CM, we have chosen not to include a detailed description of the book here. However, medical billers and health claims examiners should be aware that this text is coming, and, when it is adopted, should be used in place of the current ICD-9-CM.

CHAPTER REVIEW

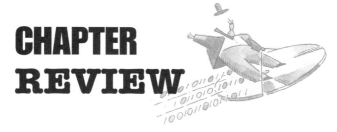

Summary

- The ICD-9-CM is the primary book used when coding diagnoses on health claims. It is made up of three volumes. Volume I is the tabular listing of diagnoses and conditions. Volume II is the indexed or alphabetic listing of diagnoses and conditions. Volume III is the tabular and alphabetic listing of procedures.

- To accurately code a diagnosis, locate the Main Term for the condition under the indexed listing in Volume II. The numeric code located should be checked against the information provided in Volume I, and all referrals, exclusions, and additional digit subclassifications should be consulted to ensure that the right code has been chosen.

- When coding procedures in Volume III, first consult the index, then cross-reference the code with the information provided in the tabular listing.

- Diagnoses that do not substantiate services rendered, match the proper location of services, or otherwise conflict with additional information on the claim form will result in delays and denials of benefit payments.

Assignments

Complete the Questions for Review.
Complete Exercises 9–1 through 9–10.
Correct the exercises on completion. If you are billing correctly less than 90% of the time, more practice is needed.

Questions for Review

Directions: Answer the following questions without looking back into the material just covered. Write your answers in the space provided.

1. Volume _____ is the tabular listing of diagnoses.

2. If only a language description of the condition is provided, Volume _____ should be used to locate the numerical listing.

3. Main Terms are used to identify the _____

4. (True or False?) Benign lesions are listed in the Neoplasm Table. _____

5. (True or False?) Always assume fractures are "open" unless otherwise indicated. _____

6. (True or False?) The more digits in the code, the more general the diagnosis. _____

7. (True or False?) Obstetrical related conditions are handled differently than other Main Terms. _____

8. (True or False?) "Rule Out" is a definitive diagnosis. _____

9. Volume II is used in some instances to determine whether a neoplasm is_____ or
   _____.

10. The ICD-9-CM is comprised of _____ volumes.

If you are unable to answer any of these questions, refer back to that section in the chapter, and then fill in the answers.

Exercise 9-1

Directions: Based on the condition, look up the appropriate ICD-9-CM code and write it in the space provided. Also underline the Main Term.

Condition	Code
1. Tuberculous Pleurisy	1. _____
2. Nontoxic Nodular Goiter	2. _____
3. Pernicious Anemia	3. _____
4. Bacterial Meningitis	4. _____
5. Tricuspid Valve Disease	5. _____
6. Upper Respiratory Infection (acute)	6. _____
7. Bronchitis	7. _____
8. Acute Bronchitis	8. _____
9. Diabetes Mellitus Without Mention of Complication	9. _____
10. Normal Delivery	10. _____
11. Metacarpus Osteoarthrosis	11. _____
12. Other Dyspnea and Respiratory Abnormality	12. _____
13. Exposure to Hepatitis	13. _____
14. Gallbladder Disease	14. _____
15. Acne	15. _____
16. Murine (Endemic) Typhus	16. _____
17. Ulcerative Colitis	17. _____
18. Malignant Neoplasm of Orbit	18. _____
19. Urticaria Pigmentosa	19. _____
20. Malignant Neoplasm of Cerebrum	20. _____
21. Degenerative Skin Disorders	21. _____
22. Rosacea Acne	22. _____
23. Artificial Insemination	23. _____

24. DTP Inoculation   24. _____

25. Generalized Hyperhidrosis   25. _____

26. Swimmer's Ear (acute)   26. _____

27. Heart Palpitations   27. _____

28. Paramacular Lesion of the Retina   28. _____

29. Rectal Leukoplakia   29. _____

30. Plasma Cell Leukemia Not in Remission   30. _____

Exercise 9-2

Directions: Based on the diagnosis description, look up the appropriate ICD-9-CM code and write it in the crossword puzzle space provided.

Crossword Game #1

Across
1. Atrophic skin spots
2. Open wound of pharynx
3. Relapsing fever
4. Malignant neoplasm of parotid gland

Down
1. Hallucinations
2. Foot and mouth disease
3. Malignant neoplasm of nasopharynx lateral wall
4. Headache due to lumbar puncture

Crossword Game #2

Across
1. Acute appendicitis with peritoneal abscess
2. Blister on heel
3. Femoral artery aneurysm
4. Big spleen syndrome

Down
1. Urethral calculus
2. Chronic coronary insufficiency
3. Mumps
4. Fish Tapeworm Infection

Exercise 9-3

Directions: Based on the condition, look up the appropriate ICD-9-CM code and write it in the space provided. Also underline the Main Term.

Condition	Code
1. Proximal Fibular Open Dislocation	1. _____
2. Gangrene of the Tunica Vaginalis	2. _____
3. Obstructed Gangrenous Hernia	3. _____
4. Hypercholesterolemia	4. _____
5. Other Ovarian Dysfunction	5. _____
6. Sudden Infant Death Syndrome (SIDS)	6. _____
7. Glomerulohyalinosis Diabetic Syndrome	7. _____
8. Gonococcal Salpingo-oophoritis (chronic)	8. _____
9. Bladder Neck Stricture	9. _____
10. Popliteal Thrombophlebitis	10. _____
11. Ulcerative Colitis	11. _____
12. Superior Mesenteric Artery Syndrome	12. _____
13. Renal Artery Thrombosis	13. _____
14. Recurrent Urethritis	14. _____
15. Enuresis	15. _____
16. Diabetes Mellitus	16. _____
17. Endogenous Obesity	17. _____
18. Essential Hypertension	18. _____
19. Inguinal Hernia	19. _____
20. Tendon Sheath Ganglion	20. _____
21. Borderline Glaucoma	21. _____
22. Glioblastoma of the Forearm	22. _____
23. Ulcerative Gastroenteritis	23. _____

24. Hallux Valgus

24. _____

25. Heart Disease

25. _____

26. Heat Prostration

26. _____

27. Epidural Hematoma of the Brain

27. _____

28. Internal Hemorrhoids

28. _____

29. Familial Hypercholesterolemia

29. _____

30. Endocrine Imbalance

30. _____

Exercise **9-4**

Directions: Starting with the marked line, look up the ICD-9-CM codes and enter one digit on each line. Use the last number of the previous code as the first number of the following code (for example, ICD-9-CM codes 001.3, 384.5, and 500.23 would be written 0 0 1 3 8 4 5 0 0 2 3).

Never-ending Circle

Game #1

1. Complicated open wound of ear
2. Deprivation of water
3. Stuttering
4. Chicken pox
5. Overdose of appetite suppressants
6. Blackwater fever
7. Patella fracture
8. Quartan malaria
9. Hemophilia C
10. Other nonthrombocytopenic purpuras

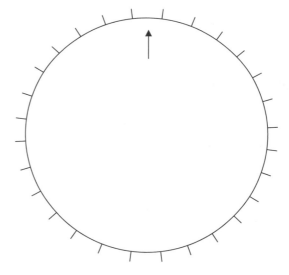

Never-ending Circle

Game #2

1. Abscess on the chin
2. Tuberculosis of the eye
3. Culture shock
4. Insect bit on the lip
5. Hemorrhoids without complication
6. Vaginal Infertility
7. Acute bronchitis
8. Tetanus
9. Diaphoresis
10. Eye penetrated with FB

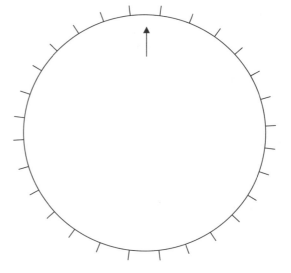

Exercise 9-5

Directions: Based on the condition, look up the appropriate ICD-9-CM code and write it in the space provided. Also underline the Main Term.

Condition	Code
1. Hypothyroidism	1. _____
2. Fetal Alcohol Intoxication	2. _____
3. Diabetic Iritis	3. _____
4. Loss of Appetite	4. _____
5. Embryonal Liposarcoma	5. _____
6. Atrophic Spots of Skin	6. _____
7. Necrosis of the Liver	7. _____
8. Ameloblastic Sarcoma	8. _____
9. Septicemia Salmonella	9. _____
10. Squamous Cell Carcinoma of the Skin, In Situ	10. _____
11. Open Cuboid Infected Fracture	11. _____
12. Recurrent Elbow Dislocation	12. _____
13. Weight Gain Failure	13. _____
14. Anemia in End Stage Renal Disease	14. _____
15. Thyroid Disease	15. _____
16. Degenerative Nephritis	16. _____
17. Neurofibromatosis	17. _____
18. Cardiovascular Observation	18. _____
19. Tibial Osteosarcoma	19. _____
20. Stirrup Otosclerosis	20. _____
21. Ruptured Spleen	21. _____
22. Skin Sepsis	22. _____
23. Anaphylactic Shock	23. _____
24. Diaphysitis	24. _____

25. Carotid Artery Stenosis

25. _____

26. Post Status Asthmaticus

26. _____

27. Capsulitis of the Knee

27. _____

28. Glue Ear Syndrome

28. _____

29. Epilepsy

29. _____

30. Trichinosis

30. _____

Exercise 9-6

Directions: Based on the diagnosis description, look up the appropriate ICD-9-CM code and write it in the crossword puzzle space provided.

Crossword Game #1

Across

1. Cheek Abscess
2. Arteriosclerotic vascular
3. Sebaceous cyst, breast
4. Secondary malignant neoplasm of the skin of the breast

Down

1. Maternal obesity syndrome
2. Elbow strain
3. Malignant lymphoma
4. Chronic gonorrhea

Crossword Game #2

Across

1. Accident involving two cars colliding, driver injured
2. Temporal bone fracture, open
3. Generalized osteoarthrosis, lower back
4. Dysgammaglobulinemia
5. Salmonella osteomyelitis

Down

1. Failure of sterile precautions during a surgical operation
2. Sphenoid bone fracture, open with subdural and extradural hemorrhage
3. Histoplasmosis pericarditis
4. Diabetes mellitus without complication
5. Small round virus

Exercise 9-7

Directions: Based on the condition, look up the appropriate ICD-9-CM code and write it in the space provided. Also underline the Main Term.

Condition	Code
1. Abnormal Movements	1. _____
2. Hurthle Cell Benign	2. _____
3. Pregnant with Twins	3. _____
4. Twisted Umbilical Cord (During Delivery)	4. _____
5. Metastasis to the Pancreas	5. _____
6. Semilunar Cartilage Cyst	6. _____
7. Endometrioid Cystadenocarcinoma of Middle Lobe of Lung	7. _____
8. Premature Heart Contractions	8. _____
9. Severe Sunburn of the Back	9. _____
10. Chemical Burn of Gums	10. _____
11. Struck by a Falling Object	11. _____
12. Deaf Mute	12. _____
13. Cruveilhier's Disease	13. _____
14. Cholecystic Chlamydial Disease	14. _____
15. Alzheimer's Disease	15. _____
16. Fractured Mandible, Open	16. _____
17. Fractured Larynx	17. _____
18. Fractured Femur, Subtrochanteric	18. _____
19. Fractured Tibia and Fibula	19. _____
20. Compound Fx, Trochanter	20. _____
21. Fx Skull with Concussion	21. _____
22. Fx Ribs (Six), Open	22. _____
23. Sprained Ankle	23. _____
24. Strain, Knee	24. _____

25. Sprain, Elbow   25. _____

26. Sprained Foot   26. _____

27. Eye Strain   27. _____

28. Dislocated Joint (Infected), Open   28. _____

29. Dislocated Jaw, Recurrent   29. _____

30. Dislocated Collar Bone, Open   30. _____

Exercise 9-8

Directions: Based on the condition, look up the appropriate ICD-9-CM code and write it in the space provided. Also underline the Main Term.

Condition	**Code**
1. Giant Cell Carcinoma	1. _____
2. Dermatofibroma Protuberans	2. _____
3. Leydig Cell Tumor (male)	3. _____
4. Glomangioma	4. _____
5. Intramuscular Lipoma	5. _____
6. Sebaceous Cyst	6. _____
7. Leukemia	7. _____
8. Oat Cell Lung Carcinoma	8. _____
9. Papillary Hydradenoma	9. _____
10. Mucoid Adenoma of the Auricle	10. _____
11. Juxtaglomerular Tumor	11. _____
12. Malignant Insulinoma	12. _____
13. Basophil Adenoma of the Nose	13. _____
14. Malignant Renal Intraductal Papilloma	14. _____
15. Abdominal Fibromatosis	15. _____
16. Aldosteronoma	16. _____
17. Epithelial Neoblastoma	17. _____
18. Nabothian Gland Neoplasm (secondary)	18. _____
19. Myxochondrasarcoma	19. _____

20. Plasmacytoma, Esophagus

20. _____

21. Bowen's Disease

21. _____

22. Papillary Intraductal Carcinoma, Salivary Duct

22. _____

23. Carcinomatous Cyst of the Breast

23. _____

24. Ciliary Epithelium Diktyoma

24. _____

25. Wrist Disgerminoma

25. _____

26. Ependymoblastoma, Spinal Cord

26. _____

27. Femur Osteofibroma

27. _____

28. Jadassohn's Blue Nevus

28. _____

29. Hutchinson's Melanotic Freckle

29. _____

30. Myxofibroma, Connective Tissue

30. _____

Exercise 9-9

Directions: Find and circle the words listed below. Words can appear horizontally, vertically, diagonally, forward, or backward.

1. Cancer in Situ
2. Main Term
3. Malignant
4. Malignant Primary
5. Neoplasm

```
T S R H F W P N C Z G T X Z E N C C X H A X D E E
K Z S S Q U X I G Y T C L B M W I G T S D Y L T F
P C B U Y R A M I R P T N A N G I L A M R A M C X
O O C S T Y F W H A A U Z Y L C P R W K V J S O A
N N J X A I V G B L V K H X M V F R U G I P M G G
F T B Z R L S C X K G A J J J C H K G Q G X U V K
S R O L F T Y N Q S C R M E X W H A Z Z C F F Z D
N E O P L A S M I J W N G J H I X J S F C L Q F Y
M H G E D L O F I R J X F N D O N Y D Z F J V I A
N U N P S W K R Q X E E X K I E S Y D S I M J K H
P K O B X Y W W T T I C X R F O R E P E R T A M I
M I L X H L Z G Y U E C N D E H E U S M I O E C T
T K D U K D X V Q A A G A A X Q D R G P T G A B U
F Q Y E L H L R B I Z M N D C W Z A F I N R V H U
U L W D V K B O L S P P R N B A S J Q C A G P T P
H Y H K Y C V M Y X Q G C S U F Y Z Q I N E Y B E
E K Q Z V S R A Z L E G U S M X F K T P G A Q J U
K C P S B E Y W V J I T C X A C Y Z H G I D T Y P
F I Y O T V J U O P H Y R F L V Z L L U L J Y O W
C X E N R B I L P O I B H D U I O A I R A H D H V
R L I I D U F W G K U D R W Q E E N I J M W B H Y
Y A L Z K V I M F V D T M C K C I A L S I T J U Z
M N B W Q D S O N R R K D O D A S W M L D S U W Y
G M K V J E J Z F C N B P I W G U R J O N L F M H
W H S T I N G Q H B V S Z G I A X E T L A D F I Q
```

Exercise **9-10**

Directions: Complete the crossword puzzle by filling in a word from the keywords that fits each clue.

Across

5. Secondary classifications under a main classification.

Down

1. Means that the site where the growth is growing is not where the disease originated. It has spread to this location from the primary site.

2. Illnesses or conditions named after a person.

3. Localized growth that does not spread (metastasize) and is not usually terminal.

4. A statistical coding of medical diagnoses and procedures.

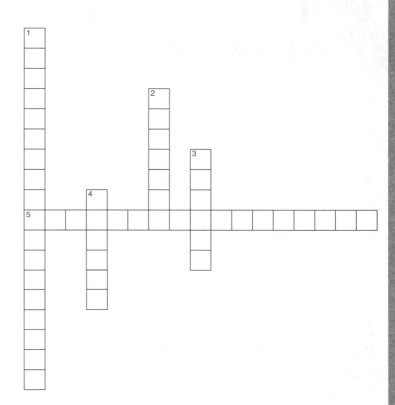

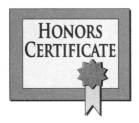

Honors Certification™

The certification challenge for this chapter will be a written test of the information contained in this chapter. Each incorrect answer will result in a deduction of up to 5% from your grade. You must achieve a score of 85% or higher to pass this test. If you fail the test on your first attempt, you may retake the test one additional time. The items included in the second test may be different from those in the first test.

10
Current Procedural
Terminology (CPT®) Coding

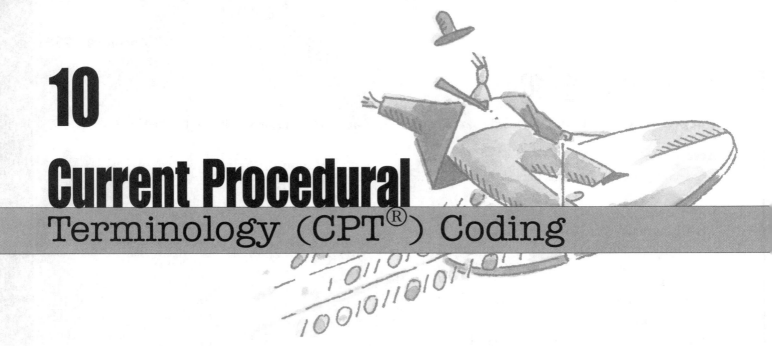

After completion of this chapter
you will be able to:

- Name the six sections of the CPT® and RVS manuals.

- Use the CPT® to properly code procedures and services.

Keywords and Concepts
you will learn in this chapter:

- Bilateral Procedures
- Biofeedback
- Block Procedures
- Consultation
- CT Scans (Computed Tomography)
- Current Procedural Terminology (CPT®)
- Custodial Care
- Diagnostic X-Rays
- Dialysis
- Emergency

- Evaluation and Management Codes
- Follow-Up Days
- Home Services
- Hospital Inpatient Services
- Laboratory Examinations
- Modifiers
- Multiple Procedures
- Nuclear Medicine
- Occupational Therapy
- Office Visits
- Physical Medicine

- Physical Therapy
- Preventive Medicine
- Psychiatric Services
- Qualifying Circumstances
- Radiation Oncology Services
- Relative Value Study (RVS)
- Second Opinion
- Skilled Nursing Facility (SNF)
- Speech Therapy
- Therapeutic Injections
- Ultrasonography
- Unlisted Codes

The **Current Procedural Terminology (CPT®)** is the coding reference manual most commonly used by medical billing personnel. The CPT® provides a listing of descriptive terms and identifying codes for reporting medical services and procedures performed by providers. It uses a five-digit code to identify procedures and services, which not only simplifies reporting but also allows for compilation of data. The purpose of the CPT® is to provide a uniform system that will accurately describe medical, surgical, and diagnostic services.

The CPT® was originally created by the American Medical Association in 1966. Since that time, it has undergone extensive revisions. Revisions are made every year with additional updates as needed. Because of the extensive changes that sometimes appear, it is important to use the correct version of the CPT®. Using an outdated CPT® may result in using codes that have been changed or deleted, and may cause a delay or denial of a claim payment.

The **Relative Value Study (RVS)** is a listing of procedures and their appropriate codes, along with a unit value that has been assigned to the procedure. Often the names CPT® and RVS are used interchangeably. However, the CPT®, not the RVS, should be used when coding procedures. When billing claims, it is important for the biller to understand the difference between the two books and to use the appropriate book when billing claims.

The CPT® and RVS reference books have six major sections **(see Table 10–1).**

The RVS uses the same codes for anesthesia as for surgery; however, the use of a modifier denotes that services are for anesthesia rather than surgery.

Using the CPT®

To properly code using the CPT®, choose the numerical code associated with the English-language descrip-

Evaluation and Management		99201—99499
Anesthesia:	CPT®	00100—01999
	RVS	10021—69990
		99100—99140
Surgery		10021—69990
Radiology/Nuclear Medicine		70010—79999
Pathology and Laboratory Tests		80048—89356
Medicine		90281—99199
		and 99500—99602

Table 10–1 **Sections of the CPT®/RVS**

tion of the procedure performed. Sometimes the procedure will be phrased in different terminology (i.e., testectomy is found under orchiectomy even though both are legitimate medical terms). Therefore, it is important to check all related codes and alternate terminology for a procedure. It also may be necessary to consult a medical dictionary for alternate terminology for a specified procedure.

Each section of the CPT® has specific instructions relating to that section before the code listing. It is important that you read each of these instructions in order to properly code the procedures contained in that section.

Semicolons in the CPT®

Some descriptions in the CPT® are subprocedures of other descriptions. These subheading descriptions will be indented under the main procedure. To properly understand an indented procedure, read the description of the main procedure (the one not indented) up to the semicolon. Next, add the remaining description found in the indented wording.

For example, codes 21208 and 21209 read as follows:

21208   Osteoplasty, facial bones; augmentation
21209   reduction

Therefore, the correct description for 21209 is Osteoplasty, facial bones; reduction. It is important to carefully read the full description of all related procedures before choosing the one which best describes the procedure performed. A slight change in the main description can significantly alter the meaning of the indented procedure.

Signs and Symbols Used in the CPT®

Most coding manuals have different signs and symbols to alert you to specific situations with codes. However, different versions of the coding manuals may have different signs and symbols, or none indicated at all.

Listed below are some of the common signs and symbols used in the CPT®.

- • This code is new to this edition of the CPT®. It has just been added to the list of CPT® codes.

- ▲ This code has been changed from last year's edition of the CPT®.

- ( ) This code was deleted. It appears in last year's CPT®, but is not valid for this year. Do not use this code.

- + Add on code. This code must be used with an additional code. This procedure is performed in addition to or in conjunction with another procedure.

- φ This code is exempt from the use of modifier -51 (modifier -51 indicates multiple surgery).

Many CPT® manuals also contain signs or symbols for nonspecific codes or unspecified codes often indicated by color blocks. These codes should only be used as a last resort when no other code is appropriate.

The details of the signs and symbols used in your version of the CPT® should appear in the beginning of the book. You should read this section carefully before coding.

Using the CPT® Index

The CPT® index lists all main procedures, often with a choice of several codes. Again, some procedures are indented, indicating that the unindented procedure listed directly above them is part of the description.

Listings in the CPT® are arranged by the procedure done, then by the site of the procedure. For example, the heading "Amputation" then lists numerous portions of the body that can be amputated and their related codes. Some portions of the body also have a heading.

Modifiers

Modifiers are two-digit codes that can be added to CPT® codes to denote unusual circumstances. These modifiers more fully describe the procedure that was

performed. In addition, modifiers alter the valuation of the procedure by increasing or decreasing the allowed amount.

For example: Modifier −80 denotes the work of an assistant surgeon. Because the assistant surgeon is merely assisting and is not responsible for the primary care of the patient, he is paid substantially less.

Some commonly used modifiers include:

-21 Prolonged evaluation and management services

-22 Unusual procedural services

-24 Unrelated evaluation and management service by the same physician during a postoperative period

-26 Professional component

-32 Mandated service

-47 Anesthesia by surgeon

-50 Bilateral procedure

-51 Multiple procedures

-52 Reduced services

-57 Decision for surgery

-62 Two surgeons

-80 Assistant surgeon

Unlisted Codes

Listed at the end of each CPT® section and subsection are "**unlisted codes**." These are the codes that end in "99." Procedures that are unusual or new and, therefore, do not have a designated code to describe them are coded by the appropriate unlisted code (based on body section or type of service). These codes are to be used only when no other appropriate code is available.

The following coding sections deal specifically with using the CPT® manual. Only those sections that need additional explanation are included. Because the CPT® is the main reference manual used by medical billing personnel, it is vitally important that its usage be thoroughly understood. You also should go through the general guidelines listed in the CPT® to assist in coding each section.

Evaluation and Management Codes

Evaluation and management codes designate procedures used to evaluate the patient's condition and to assist the patient in managing that condition (**see Table 10–2**).

Office or Other Outpatient Services	**99201–99215**
Hospital Observation Services	**99217–99220**
Hospital Inpatient Services	**99221–99239**
Consultations	**99241–99255**
Emergency Department Services	**99281–99288**
Pediatric Critical Care Patient Transport	**99289–99290**
Critical Care Services	**99291–99292**
Inpatient Neonatal and Pediatric Critical Care Services	**99293–99296**
Continuing Intensive Care Services	**99298–99300**
Nursing Facility Services	**99304–99318**
Domiciliary, Rest Home, or Custodial Care Services	**99324–99328**
Domiciliary Rest Home, or Home Care Plan Oversight	**99339–99340**
Home Services	**99341–99350**
Prolonged Services	**99354–99360**
Case Management Services	**99361–99373**
Care Plan Oversite Services	**99374–99380**
Preventive Medicine Services	**99381–99429**
Newborn Care Services	**99431–99440**
Special Evaluation and Management Services	**99450–99456**
Other Evaluation and Management Services	**99499**

Table 10–2 **Evaluation and Management Codes Subsections**

The key components in determining the proper code are history, examination, and medical decision making. Additional components that are considered include counseling, coordination of care, nature of presenting problems, and time. For further instructions regarding proper coding, see the general guidelines contained in the CPT® manual.

Office or Other Outpatient Services 99201–99215

Office visits are the evaluation and management of a patient's condition in a physician's office, clinic, or outpatient department of a hospital.

Specialized care such as chiropractic, physical therapy, and psychiatric counseling is located in other coding sections. Specialized care is coded based on the type of treatment provided, not the location of service. The place of the treatment could be anywhere, although it is usually in an office.

If care is provided outside of normal office hours, codes 99050 through 99054 are used in addition to the regular office visit code. This allows the provider to obtain extra compensation for the inconvenience of care provided outside the usual business hours.

Hospital Inpatient Services 99221–99239

Hospital inpatient services are the evaluation and management of a patient provided in a hospital setting. These services are sometimes referred to as medical while hospitalized (MWH).

Coding for these services is based on whether the patient is a new or established patient, the time, and the complexity of the case.

Consultations 99241–99255

Usually a **consultation** is provided at the request of another physician. The specialist may request diagnostic services and may make therapeutic recommendations to the referring physician. However, the specialist does not usually take over the day-to-day treatment or management of the patient. In fact, for the service to qualify as a consultation, the physician cannot be responsible for the regular management of the patient.

If the physician subsequently assumes responsibility for the routine care of the patient, the services should be coded as visits and not consultations. If the consultant is seeing the patient in addition to the regular attending physician, 99231–99233 should be used.

Second Surgical Opinion Consultations (SSOs) (99271–99275) are also a part of this group. A **second opinion** is designed as a benefit to the patient by confirming the need for a surgery.

Many plans provide a special benefit called an SSO benefit, which usually provides 100% payment for services provided by a second, independent specialist whom the patient consults before scheduling the surgery.

Normally, for an SSO benefit to be payable, the following requirements must be satisfied:

1. The second or third opinion physician must be totally uninvolved with the original recommending physician. Therefore, he cannot be part of the same medical group and will often be picked by the administrator, medical management firm, or payer.
2. The consultation must be completed before scheduling the surgery.
3. The second-opinion provider cannot perform the recommended surgery.

Emergency Department Services 99281–99288

When a patient goes to the outpatient or emergency department of a hospital, there usually is a physician in attendance who provides professional care at the facility. The physician's charges may appear on the hospital bill or may be billed separately.

Many hospitals have two types of outpatient departments: (1) the emergency room (ER) and (2) outpatient medical clinics.

If the patient wants to have his regular physician in attendance and the physician is called in from outside the hospital to provide services, code 99056 should be used.

If the patient visits the outpatient clinic of a facility, regular office visit coding should be used because a clinic is conceptually the same as an office.

Pediatric Critical Care Patient Transport 99289–99290

These codes are used to bill for direct face-to-face care by a physician during the transfer of a pediatric patient from one facility to another. The patient must be critically ill or injured and must be 24 months old or younger. These services are coded according to the amount of time spent in transport care, not the specific services required during the time of that care.

Nursing Facility Services 99304–99318

A **skilled nursing facility (SNF)** is primarily engaged in providing skilled nursing care and related services for residents who require medical or nursing care; or rehabilitation services for the rehabilitation of injured, disabled, or sick persons.

An individual is often admitted to a Skilled Nursing Facility (commonly referred to as an SNF) from an acute care facility. This may occur because the acuteness of the patient's condition has been stabilized and only time and continued noncritical treatments are required.

Domiciliary, Rest Home, or Custodial Care Services 99324–99328

Custodial care is primarily for the purpose of meeting the personal daily needs of the patient and could be provided by personnel without medical care skills or training. For example, custodial care includes assistance with walking, bathing, dressing, eating, and other activities. Skilled nursing personnel are not required for this nonmedical type of care, which is commonly referred to as "assisting with the activities of daily living" of the patient.

Home Services 99341–99350

As the name implies, **home services** are visits performed by a provider in the patient's home. The coding of these services is based on the same factors as office visits. In the absence of a proper description, use code 99351.

Preventive Medicine Services 99381–99429

Preventive medicine is, as the name implies, routine, well care provided when there is not an active illness or disease. If there is any credible diagnosis indicated, do not code as preventive. (Some of the services may still be considered preventive and may not be covered, for example, immunizations.)

Modifiers

All evaluation and management services are billed by use of the five-digit CPT® code and the code may be detailed by adding a modifier to it. Some of the modifiers that may be used with evaluation and management codes are:

-21—Prolonged evaluation and management services.

-24—Unrelated evaluation and management service by the same physician during a postoperative period.

-25—Significant, separately identifiable evaluation and management service by the same physician on the same day of the procedure or other service.

-32—Mandated service.

-52—Reduced services.

-57—Decision for surgery.

Anesthesia

The CPT® code range for anesthesia is 00100–01999 (**see Table 10–3**). The RVS code range for anesthesia is 10021–69990 (same as surgery).

Anesthesia unit values are listed in the RVS for procedures that require anesthesia administered by an

On the Job Now

Directions: Based on the service description, look up the appropriate evaluation and management CPT® code and write it in the space provided.

Description   **Code**

1. Office visit, evaluation of established patient medical decision low complexity, expanded problem focused history.   1. _____

2. Rest home visit, evaluation of new patient, medical decision making moderate complexity, expanded problem focused history and exam.   2. _____

3. Initial hospital visit, new or established patient, detailed or comprehensive history and exam, straightforward medical decision.   3. _____

4. Subsequent, hospital care, medical decision of moderate complexity, expanded problem focused history.   4. _____

5. Admission to SNF, established patient, medical decision of low complexity. Detailed history, comprehensive exam.   5. _____

6. Limited follow-up care in a convalescent facility, straightforward medical decision, problem focused history and exam.   6. _____

7. Emergency department care, minimal care, straightforward medical decision, problem focused history and exam.   7. _____

8. Initial inpatient consultation, new patient, medical decision of moderate complexity, comprehensive history and exam.   8. _____

9. Complex comprehensive initial consultation, office, medical decision of high complexity.   9. _____

10. Follow-up minimal consultation, office, straightforward medical decision making, problem focused history and exam.   10. _____

Practice

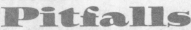

The following are billing tips on using the CPT®.

1. As long as you document the time you spent and the reason why, you can bill for the higher level E&M codes (and receive the higher reimbursement).
2. Make sure the diagnosis code you submit is consistent with the level of the visit you are billing for.
3. If the code you are submitting is a high-level code or is unusual, include documentation to support the services when the claim is submitted.

Head	00100–00222
Neck	00300–00352
Thorax	00400–00474
Intrathoracic	00500–00580
Spine and Spinal Cord	00600–00670
Upper Abdomen	00700–00797
Lower Abdomen	00800–00882
Perineum	00902–00952
Pelvis (Except Hip)	01112–01190
Upper Leg (Except Knee)	01200–01274
Knee and Popliteal Area	01320–01444
Lower Leg	01462–01522
Upper Arm and Elbow	01710–01782
Forearm, Wrist, and Hand	01810–01860
Radiological Procedures	01905–01933
Burn Excisions or Debridement	01951–01953
Obstetric	01958–01969
Other Procedures	01990–01999

Table 10–3 Anesthesia Codes Subsections

anesthesiologist. Remember that local anesthesia (anesthesia that only numbs a local area) is never allowed separately. Therefore, anesthesia benefits are those that are allowed on procedures that require more than local anesthesia. These units (for all schedules) are used under the following conditions:

- The anesthesia is personally administered by a licensed provider.
- The provider remains in constant attendance during the procedure for the sole purpose of rendering the anesthesia service.

Anesthesia Base Units

Anesthesia base units are designed to allow for the preparation for anesthesia, the administration of the anesthetic, and the administration of fluids and blood incident to the anesthesia or surgery. The surgical unit values include surgery, local infiltration, digital block, or topical anesthesia.

Anesthesia Time Units

The length of time that a patient is under anesthesia determines the amount of money that will be allowed for the procedure. Anesthesia time begins when the anesthesiologist starts to prepare the patient for the induction of anesthesia in the operating room area (or its equivalent). The time ends when the anesthesiologist is no longer in constant attendance, usually when the patient is ready for postoperative supervision. This time should always be indicated on the claim form when billing for anesthesia services.

Actual anesthesia time should be reported in minutes. Convert hours into minutes and enter the total minutes in block 24G.

Modifiers

All anesthesia services are billed by use of the anesthesia five-digit CPT® code plus the addition of a physical status modifier. The use of other optional modifiers may be appropriate.

Physical status modifiers are represented by the initial P followed by a single digit from 1 through 6, as follows:

P1—A normal healthy patient.

P2—A patient with mild systemic disease.

P3—A patient with severe systemic disease.

P4—A patient with severe systemic disease that is a constant threat to life.

P5—A moribund patient who is not expected to survive without the operation.

P6—A declared brain-dead patient whose organs are being removed for donor purposes.

On the Job Now

Directions: Starting with the marked line, look up the codes and enter one digit on each line. Use the last number of the previous code as the first number of the following code (for example, codes 00133, 38405, and 50023 would be written 0 0 1 3 3 8 4 5 0 0 2 3).

Never-ending Circle

1. Insertion of tissue expander(s) for other than breast, including subsequent expansion

2. Anesthesia for all procedures on esophagus, thyroid, larynx, trachea, and lymphatic system of neck; not otherwise specified, age one year or older

3. Anesthesia for intracranial procedures; not otherwise specified procedures in sitting position

4. Molecular diagnostics; molecular isolation or extraction interpretation and report

5. Percutaneous skeletal fixation of humeral epicondylar fracture, medial or lateral, with manipulation

6. Repair of dural/cerebrospinal fluid leak, not requiring laminectomy

7. Radiologic examination, ribs, bilateral; three views including posteroanterior chest, minimum of four views

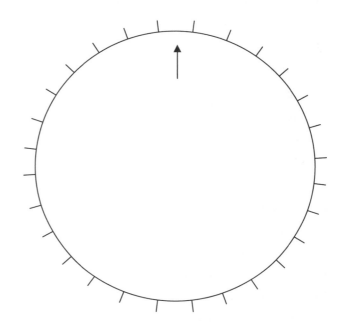

Under certain circumstances, it may be necessary to use other modifiers for anesthesia services as follows:

-**22**—Unusual services.

-**23**—Anesthesia.

-**32**—Mandated services.

-**51**—Multiple procedures.

Qualifying Circumstances

Many anesthesia services are provided under particularly difficult circumstances because of factors such as extraordinary condition of the patient, notable operative conditions, or unusual risk factors. This section includes a list of important **qualifying circumstances** that significantly impact on the character of the anesthetic service provided. These procedures would not be reported alone but would be reported as additional procedure numbers qualifying an anesthesia procedure or service. More than one code may be selected.

99100—Anesthesia for patient of extreme age, under one year or over 70 years.

99116—Anesthesia complicated by utilization of total body hypothermia.

99135—Anesthesia complicated by utilization of controlled hypotension.

99140—Anesthesia complicated by emergency conditions.

Emergency conditions need to be specified. An **emergency** is defined as existing when delay in treatment of the patient would lead to a significant increase in the threat to life or body part.

On the Job Now

Directions: Based on the service description, look up the appropriate anesthesia CPT® code and write it in the space provided.

Description	Code
1. Routine obstetric care w/antepartum care, vaginal	1. _____
2. Excision of tonsil tags	2. _____
3. Anoscopy	3. _____
4. Arthroscopy, ankle surgical removal of FB	4. _____
5. Laryngoscopy	5. _____
6. Proctoscopy	6. _____
7. Bronchoscopy	7. _____
8. Ophthalmoscopy	8. _____
9. Femoral artery ligation	9. _____
10. Orchiopexy, unilateral or bilateral	10. _____
11. Biopsy of liver	11. _____
12. Catheterization, urethra; simple	12. _____
13. Treatment of spontaneous abortion	13. _____
14. Adrenalectomy	14. _____
15. Urethroplasty; first stage	15. _____
16. Laminectomy	16. _____
17. Sigmoidoscopy	17. _____
18. Renal biopsy, percutaneous	18. _____
19. Liver transplant (recipient)	19. _____
20. Myringotomy	20. _____
21. Thoracoplasty	21. _____
22. Repair blood vessel, direct; neck	22. _____
23. Pneumocentesis	23. _____
24. Circumcision, using clamp; newborn	24. _____
25. Salpingo-oophorectomy; complete	25. _____
26. Bronchoplasty, graft repair	26. _____
27. Tracheoplasty, cervical	27. _____
28. Treatment of closed metacarpal fracture; single	28. _____
29. Cryotherapy	29. _____
30. Treatment of closed distal tibial fracture	30. _____

Surgery

The surgery section of the CPT® book is arranged according to body systems (i.e., integumentary, respiratory) **(see Table 10–4)**. Within each body system, surgeries are arranged according to their anatomic position from the head downward toward the feet.

The RVS lists unit values for surgical procedures, which include the surgery, local anesthesia, and the normal, uncomplicated follow-up care associated with the procedure for the time period indicated in the column titled "Follow-up Days."

Integumentary System	10040–19499
Musculoskeletal System	20000–29999
Respiratory System	30000–32999
Cardiovascular System	33010–37799
Hemic and Lymphatic Systems	38100–38999
Mediastinum and Diaphragm	39000–39599
Digestive System	40490–49999
Urinary System	50010–53899
Male Genital System	54000–55899
Intersex Surgery	55970–55980
Female Genital Surgery	56405–58999
Maternity Care and Delivery	59000–59899
Endocrine System	60000–60699
Nervous System	61000–64999
Eye and Ocular Adnexa	65091–68899
Auditory System	69000–69979
Operating Microscope	69990
Cardiac Catheterizations	93501–93581

Table 10–4 Surgery Codes Subsections

Modifiers

Surgical procedures are billed by use of the five-digit CPT® code and the code may be detailed by adding a modifier to it. Some of the modifiers that may be used with surgical CPT® codes are as follows:

-22—Unusual Procedural Services.

-26—Professional Component.

-32—Mandated Services.

-47—Anesthesia by Surgeon.

-50—Bilateral Procedure.

-51—Multiple Procedures.

-52—Reduced Services.

-54—Surgical Care Only.

-62—Two Surgeons.

-66—Surgical Team.

-76—Repeat Procedure by Same Physician.

-77—Repeat Procedure by Another Physician.

-80—Assistant Surgeon.

-81—Minimum Assistant Surgeon.

-90—Reference (Outside) Laboratory.

-99—Multiple Modifiers.

Multiple or Bilateral Procedures

Multiple procedures are more than one surgical procedure performed during the same operative session. The first procedure to be listed when reporting multiple surgical procedures is the procedure with the highest fee. All additional surgical procedures should be listed in descending fee order followed by modifier -51. The provider's full fee should be listed for each procedure billed.

Block procedures are multiple surgical procedures performed during the same operative session, in the same operative area, usually in the integumentary system. The objective of these codes is to handle multiple repetitions of the same service. A block procedure consists of a primary code and subsequent modifying codes.

For example:

11100—Biopsy of skin, subcutaneous tissue or mucous membrane; single lesion.

11101—Each separate additional lesion.

11200—Removal of skin tags, up to 15 lesions.

11201—Each additional 10 lesions.

Procedure	Billed Amt	Allowed
Tonsillectomy (42821)	$600	$600
Eustachian Tube Inflation (69400)	300	200

Bilateral procedures are surgeries that involve a pair of similar body parts (i.e., breasts, eyes). There are two main types of operative sessions for multiple or bilateral procedures.

Same Time, Different Operative Field, Incision, or Orifice

When more than one surgery is performed during the same operative session but through a different orifice (opening) or incision or in a different operative field, code each procedure separately with the

On the Job Now

Directions: Based on the service description, look up the appropriate CPT® code and write it in the crossword puzzle space provided.

Across

1. Ventriculucisternostomy, third ventricle; stereotactic, neuroendoscopic method
2. Thoracentesis with insertion of tube with or without water seal
3. Laminotomy with decompression of nerve root(s), including partial facetectomy, foraminotomy and/or excision of herniated intervertebral disk; one interspace, cervical, one interspace, lumbar
4. Treatment of superficial wound dehiscence; simple closure
5. Conization of cavix, with or without fulguration, with or without dilation and curettage, with or without repair; cold knife or laser, loop electrode excision

Down

1. Stereotactic biopsy, aspiration, or excision of lesion, spinal cord
2. Open treatment and reduction of vertebral fracture, posterior approach, one segment, thoracic
3. Incision of soft tissue abscess; superficial, deep or complicated
4. Anesthesia for all procedures on esophagus, thyroid, larynx, trachea and lymphatic system of neck; not otherwise specified, age 1 year or older needle biopsy of thyroid
5. Simple repair of superficial wounds of scalp, neck, axillae, external genitalia, trunk and/or extremities 2.6 cm to 7.5 cm

primary procedure listed on the insurance claim form first. Bilateral procedures follow the same rules as multiple procedures performed through different incisions.

Same Time, Same Operative Field, Incision or Orifice

Sometimes, when multiple procedures are performed during the same operative session through the same incision, orifice, or operative field, the additional procedures are considered to be incidental.

An incidental procedure is one that does not add significant time or complexity to the operative session. In this case, the allowable amount would be that of the primary procedure only. No additional amount would be allowed for the extra procedures. However, if the additional procedures are not incidental, then the rules for handling multiple procedures explained earlier would be applied.

Following the rules previously indicated, the payer would allow 100% of the primary procedure plus 50% of the secondary procedure. Therefore, in this example, the allowable amount would be 100% of $600 + 50% of $200 for a Total Allowance of $700.

Practice Pitfalls

It is important to understand which procedure is the primary procedure and which is the secondary procedure.

For example, let's look at the same procedures as those just reviewed, billed as follows:

Procedure	Billed Amt	Allowed
Tonsillectomy (42821)	$300	$600
Eustachian Tube		
Inflation (69400)	$600	$100
Total	$900	$700

The primary procedure is the tonsillectomy, and the inflation is the secondary procedure. Therefore, using the multiple surgery rules but following the doctor's billing, the allowed amount would be:

100% of $600 up to the actual charge	$300
50% of $200 or the actual charge, whichever is less	+100
Total Allowance would be	$400

As you can see, incorrect billing would substantially reduce the claim payment amount.

Assistant Surgery

As mentioned briefly in the modifiers section, some surgical procedures require an assistant surgeon. When billing for assistant surgeon services, modifier -80 or -81 should be added to the appropriate CPT® code.

Unbundling

Unbunding happens when a provider bills separately for procedures that are a part of the primary procedure. For example, a hysterectomy can be performed with or without the removal of the ovaries or the fallopian tubes. Therefore, a provider billing for a hysterectomy and separately billing for removal of the ovaries is unbundling.

Follow-Up Days

Follow-up days are days immediately following a surgical procedure for which a provider must monitor a patient's condition in regard to that particular procedure. Surgical procedures include the surgery, local anesthesia, and the normal, uncomplicated follow-up care associated with the procedure.

Practice Pitfalls

1. Two codes are reported, but one of the codes includes both services and should have been the only code reported. Claim is billed as follows.

   a. 11750 Excision of nail and nail matrix, partial or complete for permanent removal.

   b. 11752 Excision of nail and nail matrix, partial or complete for permanent removal; with amputation of tuft of distal phalanx.

   Since the excision of nail and nail matrix is part of 11752, only 11752 should be reported. Payment for 11752 includes payment for both the excision and the amputation.

2. Two or more CPT® codes for distinct services are reported, but there is a single code that combines the two. Claim is billed as follows:

   a. 43453 Dilation of esophagus, over guide wire or string.

   b. 43200 Esophagoscopy, rigid or flexible fiberoptic; diagnostic procedure.

   A dilation of the esophagus via an esophagoscope could be reported correctly with a single code or incorrectly with two codes. The correct billing for the services above is:

   43226 Esophagoscopy, rigid or flexible fiberoptic; with insertion of guide wire followed by dilation over guide wire.

Complications or other circumstances requiring additional or unusual services concurrent with the procedure or procedures, or during the listed period of normal follow-up care, may warrant additional charges on a fee-for-service basis. All visits occurring within the listed follow-up days should be combined with the surgical charge. There are several categories for follow-up care:

Follow-up care for diagnostic procedures (i.e., endoscopy, injection procedures for radiology) includes only care that is related to recovery from the diagnostic procedure itself. Care of the underlying condition for which the diagnostic procedure was performed or other accompanying conditions is not included and may be charged separately in accordance with the services rendered.

Follow-up care for therapeutic procedures generally includes all normal postoperative care.

On the Job Now

Directions: Starting with the marked line, look up the codes and enter one digit on each line. Use the last number of the previous code as the first number of the following code (for example, codes 00133, 38405, and 50023 would be written 0 0 1 3 3 8 4 5 0 0 2 3).

Never-ending Circle

1. Chemosurgery for second stage, fixed or fresh tissue, up to five specimens

2. Cystourethroscopy, with steroid injection into stricture

3. Rhinoplasty for nasal deformity secondary to congenital cleft lip or palate, including columellar lengthening; tip, septum, osteotomies

4. Radical resection for tumor, radial head or neck

5. Closed treatment of carpal scaphoid fracture; without manipulation

6. Open treatment of rib fracture without fixation, each

7. Renal endoscopy through established nephrostomy or pyelostomy, with or without irritation, instillation, or ureteropyelography, exclusive of radiologic service; with removal of foreign body or calculus

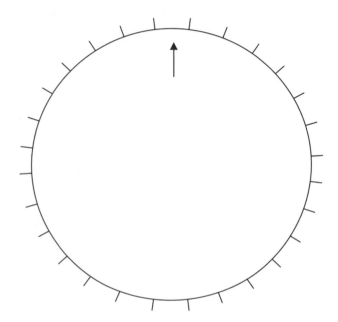

Complications, exacerbations, recurrence, or the presence of other diseases or injuries requiring additional services concurrent with the surgical procedure(s) or during the indicated period of normal follow-up care may warrant additional charges coded and allowable separately.

When additional surgical procedure(s) are carried out within the listed period of follow-up care for a previous surgery, the follow-up periods will run concurrently through their normal termination.

Maternity Expenses

The services normally provided in maternity cases include all routine, antepartum care (prior to delivery), delivery, and all routine, postpartum care (after delivery). The maternity procedure codes are based on this premise unless the specific code indicates otherwise. Antepartum care (prenatal) includes:

- Initial and subsequent history.

- Physician's exams, usually one per month for the first eight months, then weekly during the ninth month.

- Weight, blood pressure, urinalysis (monthly or weekly).

- Fetal heart tones.

- Maternity counseling on food requirements, vitamins, and related items.

Delivery includes:

- Vaginal delivery (with or without episiotomy, forceps, or breech delivery).

- Cesarean delivery.

Postpartum care (after delivery) includes:

- Postdelivery hospital visits.

- Postdelivery office visits (usually one or two routine check-ups) during the first six weeks following delivery.

Cosmetic Surgery

Although some procedures are cosmetic in nature and are performed solely to improve the appearance, they may also be performed for functional reasons. For instance, a blepharoplasty is the removal of excessive skin and fat from the eyelids. Certainly, removal of excessive skin and fat improves the person's appearance. However, most plans cover blepharoplasty when the skin overhang is so extensive that it interferes with the patient's vision. Therefore, the fact that a cosmetic procedure is performed does not necessarily mean that it is considered solely cosmetic.

When the restorative or cosmetic nature of the procedure is not obvious, billers should include documentation to verify the need for services. This documentation often includes:

- Hospital admission history and physical.
- Operative report.
- Pathology report.
- Pre- and postoperative photographs.
- A narrative report from a referring physician, if available.

On the Job Now

Directions: Based on the surgery service description, look up the appropriate surgical CPT® code and write it in the space provided.

Description	Code
1. Excision of mediastinal cyst	1. _____
2. Pyelotomy; with exploration	2. _____
3. Repair, laceration of palate; up to 2 cm.	3. _____
4. Resection of external cardiac tumor	4. _____
5. Wedging of clubfoot cast	5. _____
6. Puncture aspiration of cyst of breast	6. _____
7. Removal of foreign body; intraocular, anterior chamber	7. _____
8. Mastoidectomy; complete	8. _____
9. Open treatment of ankle dislocation	9. _____
10. Nipple/areola reconstruction	10. _____
11. Hysterotomy, abdominal	11. _____
12. Cholecystectomy	12. _____
13. Amniocentesis, any method	13. _____
14. Spinal puncture, lumbar, diagnostic	14. _____
15. Acne surgery, removal of comedones	15. _____
16. Routine obstetric care w/antepartum care, vaginal	16. _____
17. Excision of tonsil tags	17. _____
18. Direct repair of aneurysm, carotid—assistant	18. _____
19. Arthroscopy, ankle surgical removal of FB	19. _____
20. Excision of lesion of pancreas—assistant	20. _____

Diagnostic Radiology	**70010–76499**
Diagnostic Ultrasound	**76506–76999**
Radiation Oncology	**77261–77799**
Nuclear Medicine	**78000–79999**

Table 10–5 **Radiology and X-Ray Codes Subsections**

Radiology/X-ray

The radiology section of the CPT® is arranged according to the anatomic position, and the body part, starting at the head and moving downward toward the feet **(see Table 10–5)**. Knowledge of anatomy will make it much easier to locate to which area of this section to refer. This section is divided into four subsections.

Diagnostic x-rays are all uses of radiant energy in medical diagnosis and therapeutic procedures.

CT scans (computed tomography) are 365-degree pictures of specific body areas. This scan provides a three-dimensional picture of the area and is used to help identify tumors and cancers located in an organ. CT scans are much more definitive than x-rays.

Ultrasonography is a radiological technique in which deep structures of the body are visualized by recording the reflections of ultrasonic waves directed into the tissue.

Radiation oncology services are the use of radiation to treat a condition. This treatment is used in conjunction with chemotherapy to treat malignant cancers. Normally, radiation therapy is composed of multiple treatments and does not include a "picture" of the body part. It is done for treatment purposes only, not for diagnostic reasons.

Nuclear medicine combines use of radioactive elements and x-rays to image an organ or body part. Certain radioactive elements collect in different organs. Therefore, to see whether an organ is working effectively or to determine whether it is enlarged, a radioactive element is injected into the patient, and pictures are taken of the organ at specified intervals to determine how, where, and how much of the element collects in a specific organ.

On the Job Now

Directions: Based on the service description, look up the appropriate radiology CPT® code and write it in the space provided.

Description	Code
1. Platelet survival study	1. _____
2. Intermediate radiology therapeutic treatment planning	2. _____
3. CT, lumbar spine w/o contrast	3. _____
4. A/P abdominal x-ray, single view	4. _____
5. Intravenous kub, pyelography	5. _____
6. B-scan retroperitoneal echography, limited	6. _____
7. Infusion of radioelement solution	7. _____
8. Salivary gland function study	8. _____

9. X-ray knee, A/P and lateral

10. Cephalogram, orthodontic (professional component)

11. X-ray hand; minimum of three views

12. Duodenography, hypotonic

13. Pelvimetry, with or without placental localization

14. X-ray forearm, a/p and lateral (professional component)

9. _____

10. _____

11. _____

12. _____

13. _____

14. _____

Pathology/Laboratory

Laboratory examinations are the analyzing of body substances to determine their chemical or tissue make-up. Body fluids or tissues are collected and then either run through analyzing machines or viewed under a microscope to identify any abnormal substances or tissues. CPT® codes for this section are arranged by the type of testing or service (**see Table 10–6**).

CPT® codes 80048–80076 refer to various types of panel tests. Panel tests are composed of multiple tests that are combined and run from one specimen. The number of tests determines which code to use. Unbundling is also common in this section. When a charge slip is received from the provider listing numerous lab tests, the biller should check to ensure that the tests are not all part of a single panel test.

Organ or Disease Oriented Panels	80048–80076
Drug Testing	80100–80103
Therapeutic Drug Assays	80150–80299
Evocative/Suppression Testing	80400–80440
Consultations (Clinical Pathology)	80500–80502
Urinalysis	81000–81099
Chemistry	82000–84999
Hematology and Coagulation	85002–85999
Immunology	86000–86849
Transfusion Medicine	86850–86999
Microbiology	87001–87999
Anatomic Pathology	88000–88099
Cytopathology	88104–88199
Cytogenetic Studies	88230–88299
Surgical Pathology	88300–88399
Transcutaneous Procedures	88400
Other Procedures	89049–89240
Reproductive Medicine Procedures	89250–89356

Table 10–6 **Pathology/Laboratory Codes Subsections**

On the Job Now

Directions: Please indicate the bundled CPT® code and the charge for the services listed below.

Bill from Provider	CPT® Code	Charge
Calcium	82310	$ 25
Carbon Dioxide	82374	$ 25
Chloride	82435	$ 25
Creatinine	82565	$ 15
Glucose	82947	$ 10
Potassium	84132	$ 15
Sodium	84295	$ 15
Urea Nitrogen	84520	$ 30

CPT® Code _____ **Charge** _____

Practice Pitfalls

There are many laboratory tests that are commonly ordered by most providers. Following is a list of some of these services with general coding and billing guidelines.

1. Urinalysis—If unspecified, use code 81000.
2. Glucose—If unspecified, use 82947.
3. Pregnancy testing—Unspecified, use 84702.
4. TB Test (86580)—Often, this test is covered only if the diagnosis is for a respiratory condition (i.e., URI, rhinitis).
5. Pap smears (88142)—Usually, a covered expense if the patient is being treated for a gynecologic condition, that is vaginitis, pelvic pain, dysmenorrhea.
6. Handling/collection charges—Normally coded 99000–99002. This charge is usually billed when the specimen is obtained in the office but sent to an outside laboratory for analysis.

Component Charges

Whenever a lab or x-ray test is performed, there are two distinct services that are actually completed.

The first service is the taking of the specimen or x-ray. This charge should include the expense for the personnel performing the test and the cost of the necessary equipment. This is called the Technical Component (TC).

The second service is for the interpretation or reading of the results of the test. This is called the Professional Component (PC) and is denoted by adding modifier -26 to the CPT® code.

Medicine

This area of the CPT® includes nonsurgical and medical care services (**see Table 10–7**). Nonsurgical services include optometry care, chiropractic care, acupuncture treatment, physical therapy, and hospital care.

Immunizations 90471–90749

Immunizations are considered to be preventive treatment. Therefore, an active illness or disease is usually not present.

On the Job Now

Directions: Based on the service description, look up the appropriate laboratory CPT® code and write it in the space provided.

Description	Code
1. Wet mount for ova and parasites	1. _____
2. Huhner test and semen analysis	2. _____
3. Comprehensive metabolic panel	3. _____
4. Serum cholesterol, total	4. _____
5. Blood ethchlorvynol	5. _____
6. Feces screening for lipids, qualitative	6. _____
7. Ascorbic acid (vitamin C), blood	7. _____
8. Desipramine, assay	8. _____
9. Digoxin, RIA (reduced services)	9. _____
10. Histamine test	10. _____
11. Galactose test (reference laboratory)	11. _____

Immune Globulins	90281–90399	Endocrinology	95250–95251
Immunization Administration for Vaccines/Toxoids	90465–90474	Neurology and Neuromuscular Procedures	95805–96004
Vaccines/Toxoids	90476–90749	Central Nervous System Assessments/Tests	96101–96120
Hydration, Therapeutic, Prophylactic, and Diagnostic Injections and Infusions	90760–90779	Health and Behavior Assessment /Intervention	96150–96155
Psychiatry	90801–90899	Chemotherapy Administration	96401–96549
Biofeedback	90901–90911	Photodynamic Therapy	96567–96571
Dialysis	90918–90999	Special Dermatological Procedures	96900–96999
Gastroenterology	91000–91299		
Ophthalmology	92002–92499	Physical Medicine and Rehabilitation	97001–97799
Special Otorhinolaryngologic Services	92502–92700	Medical Nutrition Therapy	97802–97804
Cardiovascular	92950–93799	Acupuncture	97810–97814
Non-Invasive Vascular Diagnostic Studies	93875–93990	Osteopathic Manipulative Treatment	98925–98929
Pulmonary	94010–94799	Chiropractic Manipulative Treatment	98940–98943
Allergy and Clinical Immunology	95004–95199	Special Services, Procedures and Reports	99000–99091

Table 10–7 Medicine Codes Subsections

Therapeutic Injections 90760-90779

These codes are used for **therapeutic injections** that are injections required in the treatment of an illness or disease. They are not routine or preventive injections.

Types of therapeutic injections include:

* Subcutaneous—just below the outermost level of skin.
* Intradermal—just below the second level of skin, the dermis.
* Intramuscular—into a muscle.
* Intra-arterial—into an artery.
* Intravenous—into a vein.

Allergy injections should be coded 95115–95134, unless otherwise directed. Most antibiotics are injected intramuscularly.

Psychiatry 90801-90899

Psychiatric services and treatments include treatment for psychotic and neurotic disorders, organic brain dysfunction, alcoholism, and chemical dependency.

The language description generally indicates psychotherapy, individual therapy, or group therapy. The ICD-9-CM coding is usually in the range of 290.00 to 319.00. The providers of service are usually an M.D. (often a psychiatrist) or a clinical psychologist.

Most benefit plans require a referral by an M.D. if one of the following providers is indicated: MFCC (Marriage, Family, and Child Counselor), LCSW (Licensed Clinical Social Worker), or MSW (Master of Social Work).

Psychiatric care may be reported without time dimensions, using CPT® codes 90841 or 90845, or with time dimensions, using CPT® codes 90843 or 90844, based upon practices customary in the local area. Modifiers -50 or -22 may be used to report reduced or unusual service time.

Biofeedback 90901-90911

Biofeedback is training a person to consciously control automatic, internal body functions. For instance, through conscious control, some body rhythms that control the constriction of blood vessels and beating of the heart can be increased or decreased. This type of treatment can be used for a variety of illnesses or symptoms. A common use is for the control of intractable pain.

Dialysis 90918-90999

Dialysis is a maintenance procedure used for end-stage renal disease when the kidneys cease functioning. The fees for dialysis are usually billed on a monthly basis. When coding, the actual dates of service should be indicated, or a monthly from/through date should be used. Normally, the insurance carrier provides coverage only for the first 30 months of treatment. After that time, Medicare becomes the primary payer (refer to the Medicare section for additional information). If the dialysis is performed in an acute facility, the patient may be billed separately for the facility fees and the physician fees. Remember, the CPT® codes are only to be used on physician services.

Ophthalmology 92002-92499

Optometry or ohthalmology care is provided by either an optometrist or an ophthalmologist (M.D.). Most health plans do not cover routine vision care services related to the refraction and subsequent prescription of glasses or contact lenses.

Otorhinolaryngologic Services 92502-92700 (Ear, Nose, and Throat)

Otorhinolaryngologic services are for the care and treatment of the nerves of the hearing organs. Some of the services entail regular hearing tests.

Cardiovascular 92950-93799

The cardiovascular section is very large, and it is heavily used by the medical biller. Following are some of the more commonly billed services:

* EKG 93000.
* EKG Interpretation and Report Only 93010.
* Cardiovascular Stress Test 93015.
* 24-Hour EKG Monitoring 93224.

Physical Therapy 97010-97799

Physical therapy is the science of physical or corrective rehabilitation or treatment of abnormal conditions of the musculoskeletal system through the use of heat, light, water, electricity, sound, massage, and active, passive, or restrictive exercise.

This therapy often follows surgery or an injury to a joint or muscle. When either of these events occurs, the muscles attaching to the affected joint become weak or atrophied. Consequently, to restore full movement, concentrated therapy to the affected area may be required. Physical therapy treatments may include functional activities, mobility training, manipulation, physical modalities, assessment, instruction, and specialized testing or therapeutic exercises.

Although physical therapy is usually performed by a Registered Physical Therapist (RPT), it is not uncommon for chiropractors (DC), podiatrists (DPM) and osteopaths (DO) to bill for these services as well.

Occupational therapy is a type of physical therapy. The objective of this treatment is to either restore normal movement, or, in the case of paralysis, to teach the patient alternative ways of dealing with his or her handicap to meet the demands of everyday living. Occupational therapy is normally billed by an Occupational Therapist (OT), a hospital, or a rehabilitative facility.

Speech therapy is for the purpose of improving speech and verbal communication skills. It is usually performed by a speech therapist.

Physical Medicine 97010-98943

Physical medicine is the manipulation and physical therapy associated with the nonsurgical care and treatment of the patient. The most common form of physical medicine is chiropractic manipulation of the spine. Theoretically, any joint can be involved; the most common is the spinal area.

The chiropractor's scope of practice is limited in most states. For example, in some states chiropractors are not allowed to draw blood or prescribe prescription medicines. The limitations vary by state.

Many chiropractors use an accident diagnosis, 84x.xx series, for billing purposes. If an accident or injury has occurred this should be substantiated with a date, place, and the circumstances of the accident or injury indicated. Otherwise, the coding should be changed to reflect a noninjury skeletal condition (72x.xx).

Specialist Services

The remaining part of this section of the CPT® is composed of services that are usually billed only by specialists within a given field. It is important to take the time to look through this section and to become aware of what services are listed. A brief explanation of some of these sections is provided below.

Gastroenterology 91000-91299

Gastroenterology procedures are those services related to the digestive system, esophagus, stomach, and intestines.

Pulmonary 94010-94799

Pulmonary services include treatment and testing of the respiratory system, in relation to lung function.

Allergy and Clinical Immunology 95004-95199

This section includes allergy testing and desensitization (allergy shots).

Neurology 95805-96004

Neurology includes nerve and muscle testing. These services may be considered lab or medical.

Chemotherapy Administration 96401-96549

Chemotherapy includes administration of chemotherapy agents, usually for treatment of cancer. These codes do not include the cost of the chemical.

Special Dermatological Procedures 96900-96999

Dermatological Procedures are procedures to treat the skin.

Case Management Services 99361-99373

Case management services are services that initiate and coordinate the healthcare treatment team. These services are only required in very complex cases involving multiple body systems that are covered by several providers.

Special Services, Procedures, and Reports 99000-99091

This section includes miscellaneous services not covered elsewhere. It also includes critical care services that are usually considered to be hospital or emergency care.

Some sections of the CPT® Medicine section may be considered diagnostic testing (DXL), medical, or surgical (this varies from payer to payer).

On the Job Now

Directions: Based on the service description, look up the appropriate medicine CPT® code and write it in the space provided.

Description	Code
1. Diathermy with paraffin bath	1. _____
2. Tar and ultraviolet bath, dermatology	2. _____
3. Manipulation for physical therapy by physician, one area	3. _____
4. Electrocardiogram, complete	4. _____
5. Provocative testing, for allergies	5. _____
6. Heart electroconversion	6. _____
7. Gonioscopy	7. _____
8. Psychoanalysis	8. _____
9. Biofeedback training for high blood pressure	9. _____
10. IV therapy for anaphylactic shock, one hour	10. _____
11. Informational book of diabetes care	11. _____
12. Specimen handling fee	12. _____
13. Newborn resuscitation	13. _____
14. Subsequent detailed hospital visit	14. _____
15. Group psychotherapy by a physician	15. _____
16. Emergency department care at hospital, problem focused, tetanus toxoid injection	16. _____
17. Supplies, office	17. _____
18. 25 Minute conference with interdisciplinary health team regarding case management	18. _____
19. Rapid desensitization, 45 min. Allergy immunotherapy	19. _____
20. Cardiopulmonary resuscitation	20. _____
21. Follow-up consultation for complications of diabetes/inpatient, expanded problem moderate complexity	21. _____
22. Injection of penicillin	22. _____
23. Problem focused initial emergency room exam for severe congestion	23. _____
24. Comprehensive exam for new patient with severe arthritis, office, moderate complexity	24. _____
25. Contact lens prescription	25. _____

CHAPTER REVIEW

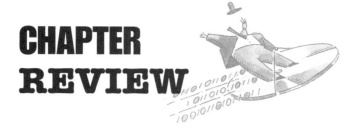

Summary

- The CPT® is used for coding procedures and services rendered by a provider. It provides a uniform means of reporting and allows for computer compilation of data.
- The CPT® reference book has six major sections. The correct code is located according to the section that pertains to the service or procedure performed.
- Modifiers are two-digit codes that can be added to CPT® codes to denote unusual circumstances. These modifiers more fully describe the procedure that was performed. In addition, modifiers alter the valuation of the procedure by increasing or decreasing the allowed amount.
- CPT® coding is one of the most vital functions that a medical biller performs. Without proper CPT® coding, claims may be denied, delayed, or returned for correction.

Assignments

Complete the Questions for Review.
Complete Exercises 10–1 through 10–11.

Questions for Review

Directions: Answer the following questions without looking back into the material just covered. Write your answers in the space provided.

1. What are Evaluation and Management codes? _____

_____

2. What is Physical Medicine? _____

_____

3. In what order is the CPT® surgical section arranged? _____

_____

4. When is modifier -80 used? _____

_____

5. (True or False?) Modifier -50 is used when billing for preoperative care only. _____

If you are unable to answer any of these questions, refer back to that section in the chapter, and then fill in the answers.

Exercise **10-1**

Directions: Based on the service description, look up the appropriate CPT® code and write it in the space provided.

Description	Code
1. Pulmonary stress testing	1. _____
2. 45-minute individual psychotherapy	2. _____
3. Color vision exam	3. _____
4. Extended f/up visit, critical care, one hour	4. _____
5. Prosthetic training, 35 minutes	5. _____
6. Peritoneal dialysis for May, age 35	6. _____
7. Psychological testing, five hours	7. _____
8. Infusion of calcium, 1.5 hours	8. _____
9. Gonioscopy	9. _____
10. Tetanus injection for cut due to rusty can	10. _____
11. Intermediate ophthalmological exam and evaluation for continued care	11. _____
12. Pediatric pneumogram	12. _____
13. Typhoid vaccination	13. _____
14. Initial comprehensive consultation, office, moderate complexity	14. _____
15. ER problem focused exam straightforward	15. _____
16. Initial hospital visit, normal newborn	16. _____
17. Allergy injection	17. _____
18. Allergen serum, one vial, single antigen	18. _____
19. Hearing aid exam	19. _____
20. Initial problem focused consultation, office	20. _____
21. Pulmonary stress, testing	21. _____
22. Psychiatric diagnostic interview examination	22. _____

23. Discharge from hospital

23. _____

24. Detailed office visit; subsequent initial hospital comprehensive admission and history, low complexity

24. _____

25. Minimal office visit, established patient

25. _____

Exercise 10-2

Directions: Based on the service description, look up the appropriate CPT® code and write it in the crossword puzzle space provided.

Across

1. Full thickness graft, free, including direct closure of donor site, trunk; 20 sq cm or less
2. Ureterotomy with exploration or drainage
3. Established office visit, expanded, low complexity
4. Dilation of urethral stricture by passage of sound or urethral dilator; male; initial
5. Anesthesia for procedures on external, middle, and inner ear including biopsy; not otherwise specified

Down

1. Excision, trochanteric pressure ulcer, with primary suture
2. Closure of ureterovisceral fistula
3. Radical resection, proximal or middle phalanx of finger with autograft
4. Anesthesia for procedures on plastic repair of cleft lip
5. Anesthesia for all procedures on the integumentary system, muscles and nerves of head, neck, and posterior trunk, not otherwise specified

Exercise 10-3

Directions: Based on the service description, look up the appropriate CPT® code and write it in the space provided.

Description	Code
1. Urinalysis	1. _____
2. Complete chest x-ray	2. _____
3. ECG, complete	3. _____
4. CBC with differential	4. _____
5. MRI of left hip joint	5. _____
6. Lipid panel	6. _____
7. Erythropoietin bioassay	7. _____
8. CT scan of the abdomen with contrast	8. _____
9. Cardiovascular stress test with exercise, interpretation only	9. _____
10. Cholecystography with contrast	10. _____
11. Streptokinase, antibody	11. _____
12. HIV antigen	12. _____
13. Ultrasound for gestational age, limited	13. _____
14. Doppler EKG, complete	14. _____
15. Facial nerve function study	15. _____
16. Ova and parasites, concentration and identification	16. _____
17. Blood potassium	17. _____
18. Estradiol, ria (placental)	18. _____
19. General toxicology screen	19. _____
20. Cyanocobalamin bioassay (Vitamin B-12)	20. _____
21. Lithium levels, interpretation and report only	21. _____
22. Serum albumin	22. _____
23. Needle biopsy ultrasonic guidance, complete	23. _____

24. Unilateral renal venography, complete   24. _____

25. MRI w/contrast, brain   25. _____

Exercise **10-4**

Directions: Based on the service description, look up the appropriate CPT® code and write it in the space provided.

Description   **Code**

1. Radiologic exam, hand: two views   1. _____

2. Bone age studies   2. _____

3. Xeroradiography   3. _____

4. Mammography; unilateral   4. _____

5. Echography, spinal canal and contents   5. _____

6. Tuberculosis, intradermal   6. _____

7. Theophylline, assay   7. _____

8. Urinalysis, chemical, qualitative   8. _____

9. Obstetric panel   9. _____

10. Iron binding capacity, serum; chemical   10. _____

11. Radiologic examination, abdomen single view   11. _____

12. Radiologic exam, hip; unilateral   12. _____

13. Glucose tolerance test, three specimens   13. _____

14. FSH   14. _____

15. Hepatitis panel   15. _____

16. Entire spine, myelography, super. & inter.   16. _____

17. Cervicocerebral angiography, w/catheter including vessel origin   17. _____

18. Basic dosimetry, radiation therapy   18. _____

19. Laryngography w/contrast super & inter   19. _____

20. Protozoa antibody tube, guide   20. _____

21. Gases, blood PO2 by manometry 21. _____

22. Heparin assay 22. _____

23. Hepatitis Be antigen (hbeag) 23. _____

24. Necropsy (autopsy); forensic examination 24. _____

25. Russell viper venom time, diluted 25. _____

26. Ureterectomy, with bladder cuff (separate procedure) 26. _____

27. Radical abdominal hysterectomy—assistant 27. _____

28. Tenotomy, subcutaneous, toe, single 28. _____

29. Synovectomy, Foot 29. _____

30. Pericardiocentesis; initial 30. _____

Exercise 10-5

Directions: Based on the service description, look up the appropriate CPT® code and write it in the space provided.

Description	**Code**
1. Excision or curettage of bone cyst or benign tumor, talus or calcaneus	1. _____
2. Removal of permanent pacemaker	2. _____
3. Renal biopsy, percutaneous by trocar	3. _____
4. Partial hymenectomy or revision of hymenal ring	4. _____
5. Myringotomy	5. _____
6. Thoracoplasty	6. _____
7. Repair blood vessel, direct; neck	7. _____
8. Colostomy or skin level cecostomy	8. _____
9. Circumcision, using clamp; newborn	9. _____
10. Salpingo-oophorectomy; complete	10. _____
11. Bronchoplasty, graft repair—assistant	11. _____
12. Tracheoplasty, cervical	12. _____
13. Closed treatment of metacarpal fracture; single w/o manipulation	13. _____

14. Cryotherapy

14. _____

15. Open treatment of distal tibial fracture of fibula only

15. _____

16. Vaginal hysterectomy

16. _____

17. Total ankle replacement

17. _____

18. Tympanotomy

18. _____

19. Angioplasty; coronary balloon

19. _____

20. Lithotripsy, extracorporeal shock wave with water bath

20. _____

21. Radial orchiectomy, inguinal

21. _____

22. Repair of cleft plate

22. _____

23. Vulvectomy

23. _____

24. Venous thrombectomy, direct or catheter

24. _____

25. Complete amputation of penis

25. _____

Exercise **10-6**

Directions: Based on the service description, look up the appropriate CPT® and ICD-9-CM code and write it in the space provided.

Description	ICD-9-CM code	CPT® code
1. Glaucoma provocative test	1. _____	_____
2. Diabetic minimal check-up, established	2. _____	_____
3. Hearing loss comprehensive testing	3. _____	_____
4. Allergen immunotherapy injection for grass	4. _____	_____
5. Physical therapy for skeletal pain, 45 minutes	5. _____	_____
6. Follow-up newborn care, in the hospital	6. _____	_____
7. Problem focused follow-up visit to Shady Oaks Rest Home, advanced senility	7. _____	_____
8. Emergency high complexity admit to Hoag Memorial Hospital, pulmonary edema	8. _____	_____
9. Manipulation with hot packs and traction and ultrasound, physical therapy for low back pain	9. _____	_____
10. Therapeutic phlebotomy for URI	10. _____	_____

Exercise 10-7

Directions: Starting with the marked line, look up the codes and enter one digit on each line. Use the last number of the previous code as the first number of the following code (for example, codes 00133, 38405, and 50023 would be written 0 0 1 3 3 8 4 5 0 0 2 3).

Never-ending Circle

1. Detailed office visit, moderate complexity
2. Exploration, repair, and presacral drainage for rectal injury; with colostomy
3. Telangiectasia injection leg
4. Folic acid; serum RBC
5. Thyroid uptake; single determination
6. Anesthesia for vaginal procedures; vaginal hysterectomy
7. Excision of frenum, labial or buccal

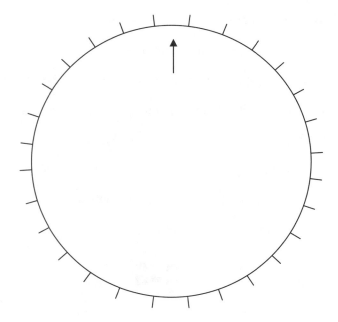

Exercise 10-8

Directions: Find and circle the words listed below. Words can appear horizontally, vertically, diagonally, forward, or backward.

1. Bilateral Procedures
2. Block Procedures
3. Computed Tomography
4. Current Procedural Terminology
5. Follow-Up Days
6. Modifiers
7. Multiple Procedures
8. Psychiatric Services
9. Radiation Oncology Services
10. Ultrasonography

```
G C G D G J Y B Q X I V P O Y F Z C Q P S G J T U M Q N B V
K A Z X E U Q J S S K P N H X I O R R U E F B T V J B U I X
U C A R Q O T D D R B S P E R Z K Z Y E R U C A I M A W L O
X Q N L A S A E G N K A D I L J K M N V U Y F P J D P S A Z
J Z N X W D X W S C R S F M S G S W Y Q D M S C C T L L T M
Q C V I G C I T H G N C K W S C Z J R Y E Y M Y W W N W E H
L L C R B T I A O C Y R R S I G J T Z E C E V R M D K Q R Z
S X O A G U B N T F T N Q R E Y I R E H O H M V E I Q B A O
Y E U Z A B O M X I C H T V R V K B I Q R H L F T N B K L E
P K R D Z S J U O F O H U I C L K A U H P I Q R G F B K P H
R I C U A X P I I D I N F D E F T O K O K O F N I L I Z R N
E I T R D H A R J T I D O E P R H W D J C D C I Q D Y O O X
R T T B Q E Z K R H R F O N I R E O N N O Z M A B D W S C Y
W L W I F B C O N E V P I C C V Q W P T L E J T K Y D N E B
U I X O F J V O D Q V L S E O O Z D P Z B L D X I P E I D S
C U R R E N T P R O C E D U R A L T E R M I N O L O G Y U V
Q W V P J U T D X P R V Z P G S W O S A N T G Y L J X A R G
U Y B A F V C U L V E W A I F T D A G I U C C K B H V N E X
C I N W T I D L I F O L L O W U P D A Y S B L R N Z L U S Y
Q Z Q B K M D C Z D O S P V O I Q K C G S K Y C O W O R V H
V J N B I S E F F K A W Q I A R N F B L W E L R C R B C J T
G K B W S S B K H H Z T B T T N L F U H Y K R D K G U J Y N
Z J N X K Q O V Y G C G U Q N L K I F E O U K V H H L Y G V
T K Z R H V S N C A W H F M I T U Q D W X G C T I C G O Y Y
T F A Y L P V W V A B Y N L H S V M X F Q M V W P C X Y R W
I I C G M L C I L A H J R L X A I Z S K Y C C S B S E M T M
H I R O Q T K T F W U L R H M A Q T M F Q B P S N K U S Y W
Q P D S E G S P T S U A U D C O T K A C X C U L F Q H U N P
Y H P A R G O M O T D E T U P M O C V H E L A Q O K J G A N
S J G D C U P N U K W S S K B T W K X Y I A B P H S W X F O
```

Exercise 10-9

Directions: Find and circle the words listed below. Words can appear horizontally, vertically, diagonally, forward, or backward.

1. Diagnostic X-Rays
2. Laboratory Examinations
3. Physical Therapy
4. Relative Value Study
5. Skilled Nursing Facility

```
L I Y M B F F E A I A M C E F Y V Q F P P S
Z A N D W J W H O P T L Y B P O N N G Q K Y
U M B H U Y S P T M M G F A C Z V I I I Y A
H C Q O H T Y N V T M B R W X N X S L C W R
G Q Z S R P S M D I R E P Y S L Q L R Y K X
W A F Z L A P E R J H J X X O G E J O O N C
Y B Z Z M Q T S U T M X V B V D B Z W Z J I
A B O H Q O N O L L G K D B N X S T Z I H T
Z Y U H Y F Q A R W A E V U I O Y L B B T S
B B N E R U C R T Y D V R A M J M Z A Q F O
I M V E X I N U M U E S E V E O V Z C W F N
O S H H S I K J X A I X X V J Q Z Y S K J G
X U O Y J Y S T X N E V A O I K D V A V T A
S N H B C Q Y M G Y C C Y M K T H B T K H I
C P S M L A J F P Z A W X U I N A T K G M D
X W J A Z A A D C R D U V N Y N K L C Q D H
J H V L J C A T U H T G H W Y L A U E O P O
P F U P I Q S L H X C C E W R I Z T J R R A
G T X L D J D Y U M Z E E C W M J O I U Y Q
C G I U U U X U C D L T V N Q D A I R O G H
T T S E R U D E C O R P T R O P E R Y B N R
Y L G O Q Q R M L A N D C E Q H O H A C I S
```

Exercise **10-10**

Directions: Complete the crossword puzzle by filling in a word from the keywords that fits each clue.

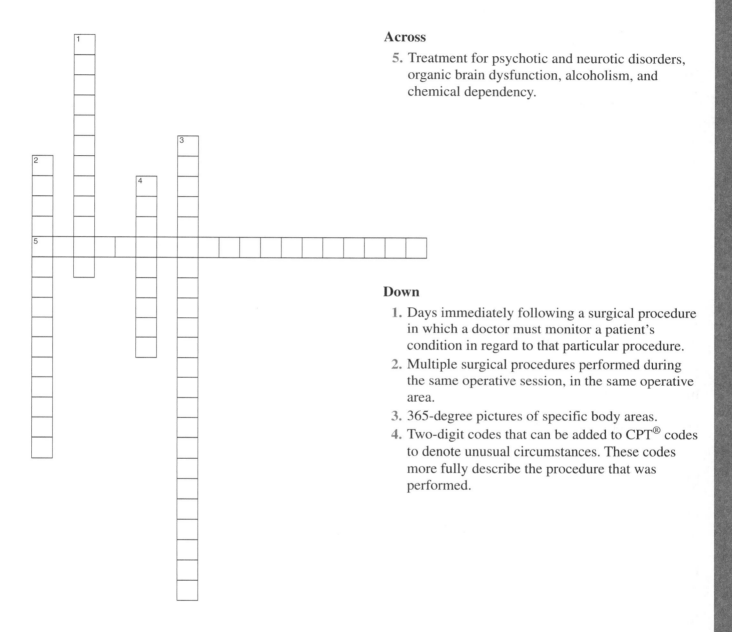

Across

5. Treatment for psychotic and neurotic disorders, organic brain dysfunction, alcoholism, and chemical dependency.

Down

1. Days immediately following a surgical procedure in which a doctor must monitor a patient's condition in regard to that particular procedure.
2. Multiple surgical procedures performed during the same operative session, in the same operative area.
3. 365-degree pictures of specific body areas.
4. Two-digit codes that can be added to CPT® codes to denote unusual circumstances. These codes more fully describe the procedure that was performed.

Exercise 10-11

Directions: Match the following terms with the proper definition by writing the letter of the correct definition in the space next to the term.

1. _____ Biofeedback

2. _____ Custodial Care

3. _____ Dialysis

4. _____ Emergency

5. _____ Evaluation and Management Codes

6. _____ Home Services

7. _____ Hospital Inpatient Services

8. _____ Nuclear Medicine

9. _____ Occupational Therapy

10. _____ Office Visits

11. _____ Physical Medicine

12. _____ Preventive Medicine

13. _____ Second Opinion

14. _____ Speech Therapy

15. _____ Therapeutic Injections

16. _____ Unlisted Codes

a. Combines use of radioactive elements and x-rays to image an organ or body part.

b. Routine, well care provided when there is not an active illness or disease.

c. The manipulation and physical therapy associated with the nonsurgical care and treatment of the patient.

d. Therapy for the purpose of improving speech and verbal communication skills.

e. Care that is primarily for the purpose of meeting the personal daily needs of the patient and could be provided by personnel without medical care skills or training.

f. Injections required in the treatment of an illness or disease.

g. The codes that end in "99" and are listed at the end of each CPT(r) section and subsection.

h. A consultation designed as a benefit to the patient by confirming the need for a surgery.

i. Codes that designate procedures used to evaluate the patient's condition and to assist the patient in managing that condition.

j. Training a person to consciously control automatic, internal body functions.

k. The evaluation and management of a patient's condition in a physician's office, clinic, or outpatient department of a hospital.

l. A maintenance procedure used for endstage renal disease when the kidneys cease functioning.

m. Visits performed by a provider in the patient's home.

n. The evaluation and management of a patient provided in a hospital setting.

o. Defined as existing when delay in treatment of the patient would lead to a significant increase in the threat to life or body part.

p. A type of physical therapy, the objective of which is to either restore normal movement, or, in the case of paralysis, to teach the patient alternative ways of dealing with his or her handicap to meet the demands of everyday living.

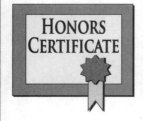

Honors Certification™

The certification challenge for this chapter will be a written test of the information contained in this chapter. Each incorrect answer will result in a deduction of up to 5% from your grade. You must achieve a score of 85% or higher to pass this test. If you fail the test on your first attempt, you may retake the test one additional time. The items included in the second test may be different from those in the first test.

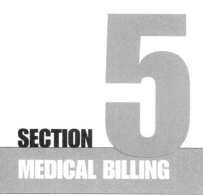

SECTION
MEDICAL BILLING

11

The CMS-1500 Form and
Medical Billing Procedures

After completion of this chapter
you will be able to:

- Properly complete the CMS-1500 claim form.
- Explain the types of services that should be billed on a CMS-1500 form.
- Describe the use of the charge slip and the information it contains.
- List procedures or situations when delayed billing is appropriate.
- Describe items that may affect the billing amount of a service or procedure.
- State the most common billing forms used and their applicability.
- List the guidelines that can facilitate the quickest possible payment of a claim.
- Describe how follow-up days, maternity bundling, unbundling, diagnosis related groups, and ambulatory patient groups can affect the procedures and amounts billed.
- Properly calculate the patient's portion of a bill using a given scenario.
- Describe the purpose of the patient claim form and list the information it contains.

- Discuss how benefits are coordinated with an HMO.
- Explain what a clean claim is and why it is important to submit clean claims.
- Explain the reason for the incomplete data master list and the information entered on it.
- Explain what submission time limits are and how they can affect claim payment.
- Explain electronic claims submission and the benefits of using it.
- List the common billing reports that are used and explain their purpose.
- Explain how to handle denied claims.
- Explain how to handle the resubmission of a claim.
- Explain how to appeal the decision on a claim.
- Explain how to make an adjustment on a claim.
- Discuss the role of the State Insurance Commissioner.

Keywords and Concepts
you will learn in this chapter:

- Acknowledgment Report
- Claim Attachment
- Claim Register
- Clean Claims
- CMS-1500 Claim Form
- Coordination of Benefits (COB)
- Electronic Claims

- Electronic Claim Submission
- Incomplete Data Master List
- Insurance Claims Register
- Optical Character Recognition (OCR)
- Overinsurance
- Patient Claim Form
- Place of Service Code (POS)

- Professional Courtesy
- Prompt Payment Laws
- Self-Funded Plan
- State Insurance Commissioner
- Superbills
- TRICARE

Professional services billing forms usually come in three types: the superbill (also known as a charge slip), the CMS-1500, and patient claim form.

The medical biller will be required to use several types of billing forms, depending on the type of services rendered and to whom the bill is being submitted for payment.

Superbill

Superbills (see Figure 11–1) are billing forms used by many providers of service and suppliers. This form serves as a charging slip to expedite the process of medical insurance reimbursement. The standard form has four copies: one copy for the office, one for insurance filing, one for the patient, and a fourth for the patient's record. As long as a superbill contains the required information, many insurers will accept it for payment; however, Medicare will not.

A charge slip is an invoice and, as such, is subject to the same accountability requirements as other standard billing forms. Superbills and charge slips may be different depending on the provider of service and the form he or she chooses to use. However, the type of information required by payers is generally the same.

CMS-1500 Form

The Centers for Medicare and Medicaid Services (CMS) 1500 is a standardized form approved by both the American Medical Association and CMS for use as a "universal" form for billing professional services **(see Figures 11–2 and 11–3).**

This is the only form acceptable for billing Medicare and Medicaid programs for physician's services or medical supplies (the UB-92 is allowed for use when billing hospital services).

The following listing will assist in explaining the uses of the various blocks on the form. It contains the block number along with the name of the block and a brief description of the information required for proper claim completion. The word "same" refers to a description that is the same as the title of the block.

The various sections of the **CMS-1500** claim form include information categorized as follows: patient, insured, secondary insurance, third-party liability, authorization signature, illness, procedures performed, and provider of services.

Following is a listing and explanation of the date codes used on the CMS-1500 form:

- MM—Month (i.e., October = 10)
- DD—Day (i.e., October 11 = 11)
- YY—Two-Position Year (i.e., 2006 = 06)
- CCYY—Four-Position Year (i.e., 2006 = 2006)
- MM | DD | YY or MM | DD | CCYY—Indicates that a space must be reported between month, day, and year (i.e., 10 | 01 | 06 or 10 | 01 | 2006). This space is delineated by a dotted vertical line on the CMS-1500 form.
- (MMDDYY) or (MMDDCCYY)—Indicates that no space must be reported between month, day and year (i.e., 030106 or 03012006). The date must be recorded as one continuous number.

Paul Provider, M.D.
5858 Peppermint Place
Anytown, USA 12345
(765) 555-6768

Superbill/Charge Slip

Date of Service: _____ Account Number: _____

Name (Last, First): _____

X	Code	Description	Fee	X	Code	Description	Fee	X	Code	Description	Fee
Initial				**Established**				**Special Procedures**			
	99202	Expanded Exam	60.00		99211	Minimal Exam	35.00				
	99203	Detailed Low Complexity	100.00		99212	Brief Straightforward Exam	40.00				
	99204	Comp Moderate Complexity Exam	140.00		99213	Expanded Low Complexity Exam	45.00				
	99205	Comp High Complexity Exam	160.00		99214	Detailed Moderate Complexity Exam	60.00				
					99215	Comp High Complexity Exam	90.00				
Consultations				**Laboratory**				**Prescriptions**			
	99244	Comprehensive	150.00		36415	Venipuncture	20.00				
					81000	Urinalysis	30.00				
					82948	Glucose Fingerstick	18.00				
					93000	EKG	55.00				

X	Code	Diagnosis	X	Code	Diagnosis	X	Code	Diagnosis
	466	Bronchitis, Acute		401	Hypertension		460	Upper Resp Tract Infection
	428	Congestive Heart Failure		414	Ischemic Heart Disease		599.0	Urinary Tract Infection
	431	CVA		724.2	Low Back Syndrome		616	Vaginitis
	250.0	Diabetes Mellitus		278.0	Obesity		490	Bronchitis
	625.3	Dysmenorrhea		715	Osteoarthritis		244	Acquired Hypothyroidism
	345	Epilepsy		462	Pharyngitis. Acute		**ICD-9-CM**	**Other Diagnosis**
	0009.0	Gastroenteritis		714	Rheumatoid Arthritis			

Remarks/Special Instructions	**New Appointment**	**Statement of Account**	
		Old Balance	
		Today's Fee	
Referring Physician	Recall	Payment	
		New Balance	

CPI® codes, descriptions, and two-digit numeric modifiers are copyrighted 2005 American Medical Association. All Rights Reserved

■ **Figure 11–1** Superbill/Charge Slip

Figure 11–2 Front of the CMS-1500 Claim Form

BECAUSE THIS FORM IS USED BY VARIOUS GOVERNMENT AND PRIVATE HEALTH PROGRAMS, SEE SEPARATE INSTRUCTIONS ISSUED BY APPLICABLE PROGRAMS.

NOTICE: Any person who knowingly files a statement of claim containing any misrepresentation or any false, incomplete or misleading information may be guilty of a criminal act punishable under law and may be subject to civil penalties.

REFERS TO GOVERNMENT PROGRAMS ONLY

MEDICARE AND CHAMPUS PAYMENTS: A patient's signature requests that payment be made and authorizes release of any information necessary to process the claim and certifies that the information provided in Blocks 1 through 12 is true, accurate and complete. In the case of a Medicare claim, the patient's signature authorizes any entity to release to Medicare medical and nonmedical information, including employment status, and whether the person has employer group health insurance, liability, no-fault, worker's compensation or other insurance which is responsible to pay for the services for which the Medicare claim is made. See 42 CFR 411.24(a). If item 9 is completed, the patient's signature authorizes release of the information to the health plan or agency shown. In Medicare assigned or CHAMPUS participation cases, the physician agrees to accept the charge determination of the Medicare carrier or CHAMPUS fiscal intermediary as the full charge, and the patient is responsible only for the deductible, coinsurance and noncovered services. Coinsurance and the deductible are based upon the charge determination of the Medicare carrier or CHAMPUS fiscal intermediary if this is less than the charge submitted. CHAMPUS is not a health insurance program but makes payment for health benefits provided through certain affiliations with the Uniformed Services. Information on the patient's sponsor should be provided in those items captioned in "Insured"; i.e., items 1a, 4, 6, 7, 9, and 11.

BLACK LUNG AND FECA CLAIMS

The provider agrees to accept the amount paid by the Government as payment in full. See Black Lung and FECA instructions regarding required procedure and diagnosis coding systems.

SIGNATURE OF PHYSICIAN OR SUPPLIER (MEDICARE, CHAMPUS, FECA AND BLACK LUNG)

I certify that the services shown on this form were medically indicated and necessary for the health of the patient and were personally furnished by me or were furnished incident to my professional service by my employee under my immediate personal supervision, except as otherwise expressly permitted by Medicare or CHAMPUS regulations.

For services to be considered as "incident" to a physician's professional service, 1) they must be rendered under the physician's immediate personal supervision by his/her employee, 2) they must be an integral, although incidental part of a covered physician's service, 3) they must be of kinds commonly furnished in physician's offices, and 4) the services of nonphysicians must be included on the physician's bills.

For CHAMPUS claims, I further certify that I (or any employee) who rendered services am not an active duty member of the Uniformed Services or a civilian employee of the United States Government or a contract employee of the United States Government, either civilian or military (refer to 5 USC 5536). For Black-Lung claims, I further certify that the services performed were for a Black Lung-related disorder.

No Part B Medicare benefits may be paid unless this form is received as required by existing law and regulations (42 CFR 424.32).

NOTICE: Any one who misrepresents or falsifies essential information to receive payment from Federal funds requested by this form may upon conviction be subject to fine and imprisonment under applicable Federal laws.

NOTICE TO PATIENT ABOUT THE COLLECTION AND USE OF MEDICARE, CHAMPUS, FECA, AND BLACK LUNG INFORMATION
(PRIVACY ACT STATEMENT)

We are authorized by HCFA, CHAMPUS and OWCP to ask you for information needed in the administration of the Medicare, CHAMPUS, FECA, and Black Lung programs. Authority to collect information is in section 205(a), 1862, 1872 and 1874 of the Social Security Act as amended, 42 CFR 411.24(a) and 424.5(a) (6), and 44 USC 3101;41 CFR 101 et seq and 10 USC 1079 and 1086; 5 USC 8101 et seq; and 30 USC 901 et seq; 38 USC 613; E.O. 9397.

The information we obtain to complete claims under these programs is used to identify you and to determine your eligibility. It is also used to decide if the services and supplies you received are covered by these programs and to insure that proper payment is made.

The information may also be given to other providers of services, carriers, intermediaries, medical review boards, health plans, and other organizations or Federal agencies, for the effective administration of Federal provisions that require other third parties payers to pay primary to Federal program, and as otherwise necessary to administer these programs. For example, it may be necessary to disclose information about the benefits you have used to a hospital or doctor. Additional disclosures are made through routine uses for information contained in systems of records.

FOR MEDICARE CLAIMS: See the notice modifying system No. 09-70-0501, titled, 'Carrier Medicare Claims Record,' published in the Federal Register, Vol. 55 No. 177, page 37549, Wed. Sept. 12, 1990, or as updated and republished.

FOR OWCP CLAIMS: Department of Labor, Privacy Act of 1974, "Republication of Notice of Systems of Records," Federal Register Vol. 55 No. 40, Wed Feb. 28, 1990, See ESA-5, ESA-6, ESA-12, ESA-13, ESA-30, or as updated and republished.

FOR CHAMPUS CLAIMS: PRINCIPLE PURPOSE(S): To evaluate eligibility for medical care provided by civilian sources and to issue payment upon establishment of eligibility and determination that the services/supplies received are authorized by law.

ROUTINE USE(S): Information from claims and related documents may be given to the Dept. of Veterans Affairs, the Dept. of Health and Human Services and/or the Dept. of Transportation consistent with their statutory administrative responsibilities under CHAMPUS/CHAMPVA; to the Dept. of Justice for representation of the Secretary of Defense in civil actions; to the Internal Revenue Service, private collection agencies, and consumer reporting agencies in connection with recoupment claims; and to Congressional Offices in response to inquiries made at the request of the person to whom a record pertains. Appropriate disclosures may be made to other federal, state, local, foreign government agencies, private business entities, and individual providers of care, on matters relating to entitlement, claims adjudication, fraud, program abuse, utilization review, quality assurance, peer review, program integrity, third-party liability, coordination of benefits, and civil and criminal litigation related to the operation of CHAMPUS.

DISCLOSURES: Voluntary; however, failure to provide information will result in delay in payment or may result in denial of claim. With the one exception discussed below, there are no penalties under these programs for refusing to supply information. However, failure to furnish information regarding the medical services rendered or the amount charged would prevent payment of claims under these programs. Failure to furnish any other information, such as name or claim number, would delay payment of the claim. Failure to provide medical information under FECA could be deemed an obstruction.

It is mandatory that you tell us if you know that another party is responsible for paying for your treatment. Section 1128B of the Social Security Act and 31 USC 3801-3812 provide penalties for withholding this information.

You should be aware that P.L. 100-503, the "Computer Matching and Privacy Protection Act of 1988", permits the government to verify information by way of computer matches.

MEDICAID PAYMENTS (PROVIDER CERTIFICATION)

I hereby agree to keep such records as are necessary to disclose fully the extent of services provided to individuals under the State's Title XIX plan and to furnish information regarding any payments claimed for providing such services as the State Agency or Dept. of Health and Humans Services may request.

I further agree to accept, as payment in full, the amount paid by the Medicaid program for those claims submitted for payment under that program, with the exception of authorized deductible, coinsurance, co-payment or similar cost-sharing charge.

SIGNATURE OF PHYSICIAN (OR SUPPLIER): I certify that the services listed above were medically indicated and necessary to the health of this patient and were personally furnished by me or my employee under my personal direction.

NOTICE: This is to certify that the foregoing information is true, accurate and complete. I understand that payment and satisfaction of this claim will be from Federal and State funds, and that any false claims, statements, or documents, or concealment of a material fact, may be prosecuted under applicable Federal or State laws.

Public reporting burden for this collection of information is estimated to average 15 minutes per response, including time for reviewing instructions, searching existing date sources, gathering and maintaining data needed, and completing and reviewing the collection of information. Send comments regarding this burden estimate or any other aspect of this collection of information, including suggestions for reducing the burden, to HCFA, Office of Financial Management, P.O. Box 26684, Baltimore, MD 21207; and to the Office of Management and Budget, Paperwork Reduction Project (OMB-0938-0008), Washington, D.C. 20503.

■ **Figure 11–3** Back of the CMS-1500 Claim Form

CMS-1500 Block Explanations

The CMS-1500 form requires specific information entry in the various blocks. Refer to the CMS-1500 Matrix in Appendix D for a detailed explanation of the information required for the various blocks on the form.

The following list will assist in explaining the uses of the various blocks on the CMS-1500 form. It contains the block number along with the name of the block and a brief description of the information required. The word "same" refers to a description that is the same as the title of the block.

Information About the Patient

These blocks contain information about the patient.

1 **Medicare, Medicaid, TRICARE (CHAMPUS), CHAMPVA, FECA Black Lung, or Other.** Check the box of the organization to which you are submitting this claim for payment.

2 **Patient's Name.** Same.

3 **Patient's Birth Date and Sex.** All dates should be recorded as Month/Day/Year. Check the box for the appropriate sex.

5 **Patient's Address and Phone Number.** Same.

6 **Patient's Relationship to Insured.** Same.

8 **Patient's Status.** Check applicable boxes.

Information About the Insured

These blocks contain information on the insured, their insurance, and their employment.

1a **Insured's ID Number.** Social Security number, ID number, or policy number of insured.

4 **Insured's Name.** Subscriber's Name.

7 **Insured's Address and Phone Number.** Same.

11 **Insured's Policy Group or FECA Number.** Subscriber's Group Number. This number refers to primary insured listed in 1a.

11a Insured's Date of Birth. Same.

11b Employer's Name or School Name. Employer or school name of insured party.

11c Insurance Plan Name or Program Name. Name of insurance company or group plan.

11d **Is There Another Health Benefit Plan?** Check appropriate box. If "YES" is checked, then items 9A–9D must be completed.

Information About the Secondary Insurance

These blocks contain information about a secondary insurance policy (if any), which may provide coverage on this patient.

9 **Other Insured's Name.** Other insured whose coverage may be responsible, in whole or in part, for the payment of this claim.

9a **Other Insured's Policy or Group Number.** Same.

9b **Other Insured's Date of Birth and Sex.** Same.

9c **Employer's Name or School Name.** Employer or School Name of other insured party.

9d **Insurance Plan Name or Program Name.** Name of insurance company or group plan for other insured.

Information About Third-Party Liability

These blocks contain information on whether a third party may be liable for payment on this claim.

10a Was Condition Related to: Employment? If "YES" is marked, then there is Worker's Compensation Insurance involved. If "NO" is marked, then Worker's Compensation is not involved. Circle whether employment is current or previous.

10b Was Condition Related to: Auto Accident? If "YES" is marked, then check for an injury date (Item 14) and an injury diagnosis (Item 21). The state the accident occurred in should also be indicated. If "NO" is marked then the claim may not be for an auto accident injury.

10c Was Condition Related to: Other Accident? If "YES" is marked, then check for an injury date (Item 14) and an injury diagnosis (Item 21). If "NO" is marked then the claim may not be for an accident injury.

10d **Reserved for Local Use.** Same.

Authorization Signatures

These blocks should be signed by the insured, or a permanent release of information and assignment of benefits should be kept on file. If there is a permanent release of information or assignment of benefits on file, the words SIGNATURE ON FILE should be placed in these boxes.

12 **Patient's or Authorized Person's Signature.** Patient's release of medical information.

13 **Assignment of Benefits.** This box should be signed by the patient in order to allow the insurer to pay the physician directly.

Information About the Illness

These blocks contain information about the current illness.

14 Date of Illness, Injury, Accident, or Pregnancy. All injury claims (i.e., injury diagnosis) must have an injury or accident date. If the patient's condition is a pregnancy, the date of the last menstrual period should be indicated.

15 If Patient Has Had Same or Similar Illness, Give First Date. Same.

16 Dates Patient Unable to Work in Current Occupation. Same.

17 Name of Referring Physician or Other Source. If this patient was referred to the current physician by another physician, hospital, or clinic, the referring party should be listed here. For claims billed by an assistant surgeon or anesthesiologist, the name and credentials of the attending surgeon should be listed here. For durable medical equipment (DME) claims, list the name of the prescribing physician. Also list the referring physician's UPIN in block 17a.

17a I.D. Number of Referring Physician. Same.

18 Hospitalization Dates Relating to Current Services. Same.

19 Reserved for Local Use. Leave blank.

20 Outside Lab. Was laboratory work performed outside your office? If so, check the "YES" box and indicate the total of the charges.

21 Diagnosis or Nature of Illness or Injury. The diagnosis indicates why the patient visited the provider. Both an ICD-9-CM code and a description should be indicated.

22 Medicaid Resubmission Code. Leave blank.

Information About the Procedures Performed

These blocks contain information about the procedures that were performed.

23 Prior Authorization Number. Authorization number for services that were approved before being rendered. Indicate the precertification or preauthorization number here. For DME claims indicate "Prescription on File," if applicable, and for claims requiring a second surgical opinion indicate "SSO Performed," if applicable.

24a Date of Service. The date service was rendered by the provider. A complete date must be given.

24b Place of Service. This is a numerical code to indicate the location where the service was rendered (see Appendix C for further information).

24c Type of Service. Leave blank.

24d Procedures, Services or Supplies. The five-digit procedure code as found in the CPT®/RVS and HCPCS manuals. These are codes that have been assigned to each procedure that the provider can perform. By selecting the proper code, billers can describe the type of service performed with a few numbers. This eliminates the confusion that used to arise from various abbreviations and descriptions of a procedure. It also allows for easy computer tabulation of the different procedures performed.

24d Modifier Code. The two-digit modifier from the CPT®/RVS further describing the procedure code.

24e Diagnosis Code. This is used in conjunction with Item 21. The number placed in Item 24E (i.e., 1, 2, 3, 4) refers to diagnosis 1, 2, 3, or 4, in Item 21. In other words, the doctor can perform different services for different illnesses or injuries on different dates and submit them all on one claim form.

24f Charges. The charge per line of service.

24g Days or Units. The number of times that a service was performed.

24h EPSDT Family Plan. Leave blank.

24i EMG. If service was rendered in the hospital emergency room, place a Y in this item. This information should match the service code in Item 24B.

24j COB. Are there other insurance policies or plans that may be responsible for payment on this claim? Insert Y for yes, N for no.

24k Reserved for Local Use. Leave blank.

28 Total Charge. The total charge of the claim.

29 Amount Paid. The amount paid by the patient or subscriber.

30 Balance Due. The difference between the total charge and the amount paid by the patient or subscriber (if any).

Information About the Provider of Services

These blocks contain information about the provider of services.

25 Federal Tax I.D. Number. If the provider of service is a physician or an individual, his/her

Social Security or Taxpayer Identification Number should be used. If the provider of service is a facility, an Employer Identification Number should be indicated.

26 **Patient's Account Number.** Same.

27 **Accept Assignment for Government Claims.** Refers only to TRICARE or Medicare. Do not use to assign payment on this claim to the provider. Use Item 13 only for your assignment of payment.

31 **Signature of Physician or Supplier of Service Including Degrees or Credentials.** Must be signed by the provider indicating that the said services have indeed been rendered. Degrees or credentials (i.e., M.D., D.O., etc.) should follow the name.

32 **Name and Address of Facility Where Services Were Rendered.** If this information is the same as Item 33, it may be left blank.

33 **Physician's/Supplier's Billing Name, Address, Zip Code, and Phone #.** The name, address, and phone number of the physician or supplier of service. This is the address that payments will be addressed to if assignment of benefits was made in Item 13.

1500 Health Insurance Claim Form (Version 08/05)

The National Uniform Claim Committee (NUCC) was formed in the mid-1990s to establish a standardized data set for use in the submission of both paper and electronic health insurance claims for physicians, suppliers, and ambulance services. NUCC replaces the Uniform Claim Form Task Force.

Minor changes have been made to the 1500 Health Insurance Claim Form (version 08/05) in order to accommodate the National Provider Identifier (NPI), to comply with HIPAA regulations, and to address the needs of electronic claim submission. The 1500 Health Insurance Claim Form was approved by the NUCC in November 2005 and will replace the CMS-1500 (version 12/90). Finalization of the 1500 Health Insurance Form (version 08/05) is expected to take place in the spring of 2006, so changes to this form are anticipated.

The following is a sample of the new 1500 Health Insurance Claim Form (version 08/05), and is for informational purposes only (**see Figures 11–4 and 11–5**). Refer to Appendix D for additional information regarding the new 1500 Health Insurance Claim Form (version 08/05).

Practice Pitfalls

Guidelines for Completing the CMS-1500

Properly completing the CMS-1500 form is vital to getting the proper reimbursement for the services that were rendered. The following guidelines will help to minimize errors and speed claims processing. (Refer to the CMS-1500 Matrix in Appendix C.)

1. Use all uppercase letters.
2. Do not go outside the box lines. Many forms are scanned by computer and exceeding the box limits can cause errors.
3. Fill in all required blocks as appropriate for the claim submission.
4. Be sure that all diagnoses have related procedures and that all procedures have a related diagnosis.
5. Do not write on the form unless it is for the purpose of signing in block 12, 13, or 31.
6. Do not sign or write in red ink.
7. Do not use a highlighter on the form. Some scanners will pick up the highlighter and turn it into a black mark, thus obliterating the information in that item.
9. Substitute a space for dollar signs, decimal points, modifier dashes, and hyphens in Social Security numbers.
10. Include the hyphen in tax and employer identification numbers in block 25.
11. Do not place more than one service or code on each of the service code lines. If more than six procedures were performed, use an additional form.
12. Include only CPT® and ICD-9-CM codes. Do not use narrative descriptions of services or diagnoses.
13. Do not use punctuation. Do not use special characters such as periods, parentheses, dollar signs, and ditto marks.
14. If it is necessary to add attachments, they should be on paper that is 8.5 by 11 inches.

Observing these guidelines will help ensure that claims are scanned in properly, and decrease the chance of errors and delays.

SAMPLE

1500

HEALTH INSURANCE CLAIM FORM

APPROVED BY NATIONAL UNIFORM CLAIM COMMITTEE 08/05

CARRIER

PICA		PICA

1. MEDICARE   MEDICAID   TRICARE CHAMPUS   CHAMPVA   GROUP HEALTH PLAN   FECA BLK LUNG   OTHER
(Medicare #)   (Medicaid #)   (Sponsor's SSN)   (Member ID#)   (SSN or ID)   (SSN)   (ID)

1a. INSURED'S I.D. NUMBER   (For Program in Item 1)

2. PATIENT'S NAME (Last Name, First Name, Middle Initial)

3. PATIENT'S BIRTH DATE   SEX
MM | DD | YY   M   F

4. INSURED'S NAME (Last Name, First Name, Middle Initial)

5. PATIENT'S ADDRESS (No., Street)

6. PATIENT RELATIONSHIP TO INSURED
Self   Spouse   Child   Other

7. INSURED'S ADDRESS (No., Street)

CITY   STATE

8. PATIENT STATUS
Single   Married   Other
Employed   Full-Time Student   Part-Time Student

CITY   STATE

ZIP CODE   TELEPHONE (Include Area Code)
(   )

ZIP CODE   TELEPHONE (Include Area Code)
(   )

9. OTHER INSURED'S NAME (Last Name, First Name, Middle Initial)

10. IS PATIENT'S CONDITION RELATED TO:

11. INSURED'S POLICY GROUP OR FECA NUMBER

a. OTHER INSURED'S POLICY OR GROUP NUMBER

a. EMPLOYMENT? (Current or Previous)
YES   NO

a. INSURED'S DATE OF BIRTH   SEX
MM | DD | YY   M   F

b. OTHER INSURED'S DATE OF BIRTH   SEX
MM | DD | YY   M   F

b. AUTO ACCIDENT?   PLACE (State)
YES   NO

b. EMPLOYER'S NAME OR SCHOOL NAME

c. EMPLOYER'S NAME OR SCHOOL NAME

c. OTHER ACCIDENT?
YES   NO

c. INSURANCE PLAN NAME OR PROGRAM NAME

d. INSURANCE PLAN NAME OR PROGRAM NAME

10d. RESERVED FOR LOCAL USE

d. IS THERE ANOTHER HEALTH BENEFIT PLAN?
YES   NO   If yes, return to and complete item 9 a-d.

READ BACK OF FORM BEFORE COMPLETING & SIGNING THIS FORM.

12. PATIENT'S OR AUTHORIZED PERSON'S SIGNATURE I authorize the release of any medical or other information necessary to process this claim. I also request payment of government benefits either to myself or to the party who accepts assignment below.

SIGNED_____   DATE_____

13. INSURED'S OR AUTHORIZED PERSON'S SIGNATURE I authorize payment of medical benefits to the undersigned physician or supplier for services described below.

SIGNED_____

PATIENT AND INSURED INFORMATION

14. DATE OF CURRENT: ILLNESS (First symptom) OR INJURY (Accident) OR PREGNANCY(LMP)
MM | DD | YY

15. IF PATIENT HAS HAD SAME OR SIMILAR ILLNESS. GIVE FIRST DATE   MM | DD | YY

16. DATES PATIENT UNABLE TO WORK IN CURRENT OCCUPATION
FROM   MM | DD | YY   TO   MM | DD | YY

17. NAME OF REFERRING PROVIDER OR OTHER SOURCE

17a.
17b. NPI

18. HOSPITALIZATION DATES RELATED TO CURRENT SERVICES
FROM   MM | DD | YY   TO   MM | DD | YY

19. RESERVED FOR LOCAL USE

20. OUTSIDE LAB? $ CHARGES
YES   NO

21. DIAGNOSIS OR NATURE OF ILLNESS OR INJURY (Relate Items 1, 2, 3 or 4 to Item 24E by Line)

1. |___.___   3. |___.___
2. |___.___   4. |___.___

22. MEDICAID RESUBMISSION CODE   ORIGINAL REF. NO.

23. PRIOR AUTHORIZATION NUMBER

24. A. DATE(S) OF SERVICE						B. PLACE OF SERVICE	C. EMG	D. PROCEDURES, SERVICES, OR SUPPLIES (Explain Unusual Circumstances) CPT/HCPCS	MODIFIER	E. DIAGNOSIS POINTER	F. $ CHARGES	G. DAYS OR UNITS	H. EPSDT Family Plan	I. ID. QUAL	J. RENDERING PROVIDER ID. #
From			To												
MM	DD	YY	MM	DD	YY										
1														NPI	
2														NPI	
3														NPI	
4														NPI	
5														NPI	
6														NPI	

25. FEDERAL TAX I.D. NUMBER   SSN EIN

26. PATIENT'S ACCOUNT NO.

27. ACCEPT ASSIGNMENT? (For govt. claims, see back)
YES   NO

28. TOTAL CHARGE $

29. AMOUNT PAID $

30. BALANCE DUE $

31. SIGNATURE OF PHYSICIAN OR SUPPLIER INCLUDING DEGREES OR CREDENTIALS (I certify that the statements on the reverse apply to this bill and are made a part thereof.)

SIGNED_____   DATE_____

32. SERVICE FACILITY LOCATION INFORMATION

a. NPI   b.

33. BILLING PROVIDER INFO & PH #   (   )

a. NPI   b.

PHYSICIAN OR SUPPLIER INFORMATION

NUCC Instruction Manual available at: www.nucc.org   OMB APPROVAL PENDING

■ **Figure 11–4** Sample of Front of 1500 Health Insurance Claim Form

■ Figure 11–5 Sample of Back of 1500 Health Insurance Claim Form

Patient Claim Form

In addition to the billing forms, a medical biller may occasionally receive a **Patient Claim Form (see Figures 11–6 and 11–7)**. This form is provided by self-funded plans. A **self-funded plan** is a company that insures itself and its own workers.

The information contained on this form is self-explanatory. The member should complete the information entitled "To Be Completed by Member" and the provider of services should complete the information entitled "To Be Completed by Physician."

Patient Claim Form

Information must be printed or typewritten. Claim form must be completed and returned to us at the indicated address.

Medicare Patients: Submit this claim to Medicare FIRST! A copy of the Medicare Explanation of Benefits must be submitted with this claim form.

TO BE COMPLETED BY MEMBER

1. Information Pertaining To Member			
Name: Last, First, M.I.	Sex:	Date Of Birth	Member ID #
Home Address: Street City State Zip			Telephone Number
Marital Status	Name Of Spouse	Spouse's Date Of Birth	Member ID #
Is Spouse Employed?	If Yes, Name And Address Of Employer		Employer Phone Number
2. Information Pertaining To Patient			
Patient Name: Last, First, M.I.	Sex	Date Of Birth	Member ID #
Home Address: Street City State Zip			Telephone Number
Is Patient Employed? Full-Time Part Time No	Relationship To Employee?	If Dependent Child Over 19, Name Of School Where Full-time Student:	
3. Information Regarding Current Treatment			
Related To Illness?	Related To Pregnancy?	Related To Work?	Description Of Illness Or Injury
Date Of Accident	Where Happened?	Describe Accident	
4. Information Regarding Insurance			
Are You, Your Spouse or Dependent Children Covered By Any Other Insurance?		Name Of Insured	
If Yes, Name And Address Of Insurance			Insurance Phone Number
Patient's Or Guardian's Signature I certify that the above information is true and correct and I authorize the release of any medical information necessary to process this claim. Signed: Date:			
Assignment of Benefits: I assign payment of benefits to the following provider:			
Address: Street City State Zip			Telephone Number

■ **Figure 11–6** Patient Claim Form Side 1

Billing for Services

After the patient has been seen by the doctor, the doctor will complete a charge slip or fee ticket. The charge slip is a form used by the provider to indicate the services rendered, the diagnosis for the visit, and whether a return visit is required. This form usually has a list of service descriptions along with the corresponding numeric billing codes, and a list of diagnosis and diagnosis codes.

The charge slip is given to the patient after the visit is complete. The patient will in turn give the charge slip to the receptionist for payment to be

TO BE COMPLETED BY PHYSICIAN

Patient's Name: Last, First, M.I.

Home Address: Street	City	State	Zip	Telephone Number

Is Condition Due To Illness?	Injury?	Work Related?	Pregnancy?	If Yes, Date Of Last Menstrual Period

Diagnosis Or Nature Of Illness Or Injuries. Give Description And ICD-9 Code.

_____

_____

Date Of Service	Place Of Service	Description Of Medical Services Or Supplies Provided	CPT® Code	ICD-9-CM Code	Charge

Date Of First Symptoms	Date Of Accident	Date Patient First Seen	Total Charges	
Dates Patient Unable To Work From To:	If Still Disabled, Date Patient Should Return To Work		Amount Paid	
Patient Still Under Care For This Condition?	Date Of Same Or Similar Illness Or Condition		Does Patient Have Other Health Coverage?	

Under Section 6019 Of The Internal Revenue Code, Recipients Of Medical Payments Must Provide Identifying Numbers To Payors Who Must Report Such Payments To The Internal Revenue Service.   Taxpayer ID Number: _____ Social Security Number: _____

Physician's Name: _____   Signature: _____

Street Address	City	State	Zip

INFORMATION REGARDING THIS CLAIM FORM

A Separate Claim Must Be Filed For Each Different Injury Or Illness.

A Claim Must Be Filed Within 90 Days of The Date Of Service Or Claim Benefits May Be Reduced.

If Patient Is Medicare Eligible, Claim Must First Be Submitted To Medicare For Payment. We Cannot Process Claim Without Information Regarding Medicare's Payment.

■ **Figure 11–7** Patient Claim Form Side 2

made and a return visit to be scheduled, if required. At that time, the receptionist should collect any amount that the patient owes. For cash patients (those without insurance or responsibility by a third-party payer), the entire amount often is collected, or a payment plan is set up. For many patients covered by insurance, a small copayment will be required. The receptionist should issue a receipt for any monies collected and list the amount re-

ceived and the form of payment (cash or check) on the charge slip.

The patient also should be given or sent a copy of the billing information. If the charge slip or superbill has carbon copies, one of these may be used as a bill for the patient. For patients covered by insurance, the medical biller will eventually prepare a claim to be sent to the insurance carrier.

On the Job Now

Directions: Based on the following scenarios, complete a Patient Claim Form for the following patients. The provider of services is Paul Provider, M.D. Refer to the Patient Data Table and Provider Data Table in Appendix C for additional information.

1. The following services were billed for: Abby Addison   Date of Service: 01/16/CCYY

    Diagnosis: Hypertension

    99205–Comprehensive High Complexity Exam ($160)

    81000–Urinalysis ($30)

    36415–Venipuncture ($20)

    Patient made a cash payment of $60 on this visit.

2. The following services were billed for: Bobby Bumble   Date of Service: 01/16/CCYY

    Diagnosis: Diabetes

    99211–Minimal Exam ($35)

    81000–Urinalysis ($30)

    82948–Glucose Fingerstick ($18)

    36415–Venipuncture ($20)

    Patient made a payment by check of $75 on this visit.

3. The following services were billed for: Cathy Crenshaw   Date of Service: 01/16/CCYY

    Diagnosis: Chronic Bronchitis

    99204–Comprehensive Moderate Complexity Exam ($140)

    36415–Venipuncture ($20)

    Patient made a payment by check of $110 on this visit.

4. The following services were billed for: Daisy Doolittle   Date of Service: 01/16/CCYY

    Diagnosis: Cogenital Hypothyroidism

    99203– Detailed Low Complexity Exam ($100)

    36415–Venipuncture ($20)

    Patient made a cash payment of $15 on this visit.

5. The following services were billed for: Edward Edmunds   Date of Service: 01/16/CCYY

    Diagnosis: Coronary Artery Disease

    99214–Detailed Moderate Complexity Exam ($60)

    93000–EKG ($55)

    81000–Urinalysis ($30)

    36415–Venipuncture ($20)

    Patient did not make a payment.

Delayed Billing

If a procedure is expected to take an extended period of time (i.e., pregnancy, multiple surgeries), billing for the procedure should be delayed until the entire process is complete. The appropriate CPT® code usually covers all services. For example, in the case of a pregnancy, all prenatal visits for nine months before the delivery are included under CPT® code 59400, as well as the delivery of the baby and the postpartum care. If the provider were to bill before the delivery, several scenarios could cause an error in billing. The patient could be rushed to the hospital in advanced labor and the baby could be delivered by another doctor, or a complication could occur that requires the baby to be taken out by Cesarean section.

It is impossible to determine exactly what procedures a doctor will perform until they are actually done, so billing should be postponed until all related services have been performed. Also, billing for procedures that have not been performed (even if you expect to perform them in the future) is considered fraud.

Incomplete Data Master List

Patient data that is incomplete is a major source of delay in both billing for services and in payment for those services. Without complete patient data, it can be difficult to complete a billing form properly. Additionally, many insurance carriers will refuse to pay a claim that is not completed properly. Problems of incomplete data often occur because of a discrepancy between the forms the patient completes and the information needed for proper patient chart maintenance.

An **Incomplete Data Master List** is a complete listing of patients whose patient chart does not have properly filled out or completed patient forms. A master list for patients with incomplete data can help an office solve this problem quickly and efficiently.

A sample Incomplete Data Master List is shown in **Figure 11–8**. To complete the form, fill in data as detailed for the following fields:

Date: Indicate the date that you first noticed the information was missing.

Patient: Enter the patient's name.

Data Missing: List the data that is missing. Be sure to clearly list all items that are missing. Each piece of missing data should be placed on a separate line.

Why: List the reason why the data is missing. This can alert you to possible problems with your intake forms. For example, if a specific item is consistently overlooked by patients, perhaps it needs to be highlighted.

Disposition: When the information has been obtained, list the date obtained and the means by which the information was obtained.

Comp: Indicate the date the information was input into the computer.

Incomplete Data Master List

Indicate below all the patients whose data is incomplete at the time the patient data is being put in the computer.

Date	Patient/Account	Data Missing	Why	Disposition	Data	Comp
1/1/ccyy	Kent Wright/12345	Birthdate	IL	PC – 1/10/ccyy	BD:03/15/63	1/10/ccyy
		Marital Status	PO	PC – 1/10/ccyy	Married	1/10/ccyy

Why Codes:
PO – Omitted or overlooked by patient
IL – Data was completed but is illegible
NI – Not included on forms

Disposition Codes:
PC – Phone Call
LS – Letter Sent
AP – Asked in person while patient was in office.

■ **Figure 11–8** Incomplete Data Master List

Because of the limited amount of space on the form, standard abbreviations may need to be used. For example, the form shown in Figure 11–8 lists several codes. Any standard abbreviations created by the facility should be listed at the bottom of the form. This will eliminate confusion as to the proper abbreviation or its meaning.

A letter should be sent to all patients on the Incomplete Data Master List at least once a month, requesting needed information. This can be a simple form letter with space at the bottom for inserting the information requested. Include a self-addressed, stamped envelope with the letter.

Whenever you contact the patient to request missing or incomplete information, be sure to indicate that the information is needed to bill their insurance carrier.

An Incomplete Data Master List also can alert you to information that is needed for your computer program. If there are several pieces of data missing, the practice may want to create an additional form for patients to complete that requests this information.

Determining the Proper Billing Amount

Providers may have different charges for the same service. For example, if the patient is covered by Medicare, there are limits to the amount that Medicare will cover and to the amount that may be collected on the overall bill.

Medicare Limitations

Medicare limits the amount that may be charged by providers to patients. This limit may not always show up on the provider's initial bill.

Network Provider Limits

If the provider has signed a PPO contract, there may be limits to the amounts that the provider may charge for services. The provider must limit balance billing to the patient so that the total amount collected for the service does not exceed the contracted amount.

Before calculating any payments, it is important to determine the amount that the patient should be billed and the total amount that may be collected. This prevents overbilling the patient and having to make a refund at a later date.

If the provider has signed a contract that limits payments, there should be a comprehensive listing of the procedures that have limits and the amounts that

may be charged for these procedures. Billers must first look up the appropriate CPT® or HCPCS code for the services that were rendered. This description of service and code is then compared to the amount listed in the PPO contract. If there is a limit to the charge, it will be listed under the appropriate CPT® or HCPCS code.

There are a number of situations that can affect billing for patient services.

Follow-Up Days

When billing for surgical services, the total surgical care is included in the charge for the surgery. Total surgical care includes the initial visit with the patient before surgery, the surgical procedure, and the routine follow-up care. If visits are related to a prior surgical episode, you cannot bill separately for them. For further information on this issue, see the chapter on CPT® Coding.

Maternity Bundling

All maternity procedures are usually bundled together. This includes one visit per month in the months leading up to the delivery, as well as the actual delivery service itself. Additionally, some carriers consider certain tests to be included in the overall maternity care, for example, urinalysis tests and ultrasounds.

Be sure to determine the exact services that are considered part of maternity care. Any procedures that are not routinely part of this care may be billed separately.

Unbundling

Codes for individual lab tests include the taking of a specimen for each test. If a single blood specimen is collected and a number of lab tests run from that single specimen, a panel test code should be chosen to report the procedure. Panel test codes report multiple tests run from a single specimen.

If you are billing for several laboratory tests together, make sure you use the appropriate code and charge for the combined test.

Unbundling is discussed more fully in the chapter on CPT® Coding.

Diagnosis Related Groups

Some diseases or conditions are covered under a Diagnosis Related Group (DRG) billing. DRG billings lump all charges for hospital treatment of a specific diagnosis under one payment. For example, if a hospital treats a patient for one of these conditions, they will be paid a lump sum charge that will cover all treatment. If the hospital's charges are higher than the amount provided in the lump sum payment, they must write off any charges above the payment. They are not allowed to balance bill the patient for this amount. However, if the hospital's charges are less than the lump sum payment, they are still paid the same amount. The hospital may keep the extra money. DRGs are only for hospital treatment.

Ambulatory Patient Groups

An Ambulatory Patient Group is similar to a Diagnosis Related Group, except that it is for outpatient treatment (treatment outside a hospital setting). The same rules apply regarding the lump sum payment.

There are a number of things to keep in mind when dealing with patients. Of course, customer service should always be your first and foremost concern, but at the same time you need to have regard for the medical office. It is important to obtain all necessary information from the patient. Remember that the primary objective of the medical biller is to minimize the amount of time between the physician's service and the complete payment of the bill.

Special Services

Physicians may bill charges other than medical services. Some medical offices charge for completing insurance or claim forms, late charges on past due amounts, charges for missed appointments, and charges for phone calls by or from patients. These services are usually not covered by insurance carriers and are the sole responsibility of the patient.

A **Professional Courtesy** is when a doctor renders medical services to another professional, such as a doctor, pharmacist, or nurse, or to a relative. Billing procedures vary from not charging the patient to a percentage of the physician's usual charges for these services. You should familiarize yourself with the provider's billing procedures before billing for these services.

Claims Submission Process

Once the provider has seen the patient and the proper billing forms have been completed, it is time to prepare a claim and submit it for payment. There are a number of items that need to be considered before submitting claims. These include whether or not the claims are

Practice
Pitfalls

These information tips are useful in helping to streamline the practice's billing process:

1. Be sure to understand the policies of the office regarding the completion of forms and payment of bills. This way you can explain it accurately to the patient.

2. Ask the patient to fill out all the forms required for the patient file. Give the patient sufficient time to fill out the forms and check that all of the forms have been filled out completely before accepting them. Many offices mail the forms to the patient before their visit to ensure completeness.

3. Use the office forms consistently and accurately so that the tracking of information proceeds smoothly, regardless of who enters the information.

4. Look over the completed forms as soon as they are completed and returned by the patient. If there is information that is incomplete or illegible, ask the patient to clarify the information.

5. Secure all the details of the insurance. If the patient or insured has a card, make a copy of it for the patient file. Make sure the information contains the subscriber's name, the policy number, the effective date, the company that holds the policy or the name of the policy, and the insurance carrier's address.

6. Make sure the patient understands the provider's policy regarding any amounts that the insurance carrier does not pay or does not cover.

7. Complete all insurance forms accurately and completely. This will ensure the prompt payment of claims by the insurance carrier. Also, use the forms preferred by the insurance carrier. Use of other forms can result in a delay in the processing of the claim.

8. Give the patient a copy of the bill when she leaves the medical office. This can be a superbill, a copy (not the original) of the CMS-1500, or a listing of the charges incurred during the current visit.

9. If an Assignment of Benefits Form is not on file or if the patient's insurance carrier requires it, have the patient sign the Assignment of Benefits box on the claim form before leaving the office.

10. Make sure the claims and all necessary papers have been signed by the physician, nurse, and anyone else who is required to do so.

considered clean claims, whether the claims are to be submitted on paper or electronically, and whether or not there are any claim submission time limits.

The first step is to prepare all claim files and print out the claims that will be submitted on paper. After the claims are printed, check over each one to make sure that it fits the definition of a clean claim and that it meets all the requirements for optical character recognition (OCR).

Submission Time Limits

Many payers require that claims be submitted within a specified period from the date that the services were rendered. If claims are not submitted within the time limits, payment may be reduced or denied.

The provider's office should have a chart indicating the time limits for submission of claims. Additionally, it is best to set a standard of submitting all claims within 10 days of the date services were rendered. This keeps claims billings within the time limits set by most carriers, and it also ensures that payment for the services is received as soon as possible.

Claim Attachments

A **claim attachment** is any document providing additional medical information to the claims payer that cannot be accommodated within the standard billing form. These attachments assist in claim adjudication. Claim attachments should have the patient's name and policy identification number on them and should be submitted with the claim.

Common attachments include operative reports, pathology reports, treatment plans, medical necessity reports, progress notes, consultation reports, additional ambulance information, procedure reports, medical history, a prescription for DME, and a copy of an EOB. They are sent to the insurance payer with the original claim or in response to a request for information from the payer.

These attachments and documentation provide the claims processor or medical reviewer with information to determine coverage, medical necessity, and which payer is primary. This is needed to determine the benefit due. Some information is also used to check for fraud and abuse.

The Department of Health and Human Services on September 23, 2005, published a proposed rule to establish national standards for electronic claims attachments. The rulemaking is authorized under the HIPAA administrative simplification provisions. The department proposed standards for six types of electronic attachments: ambulance services, emergency department,

rehabilitation services, clinical reports, laboratory results, and medications. Most healthcare providers will have two years after the final rule is passed to meet the claims attachment standards, and small health plans will have three years.

Optical Scanning Guidelines

All information should be typed or machine-printed. Most insurance carriers' claims are processed using **Optical Character Recognition (OCR)** equipment. OCR is an automated scanning process that reads the information on claim forms. With OCR, claims processing is faster and more accurate than it is when processed manually.

Use the CMS-1500 red ink version for claims submissions. The red ink used to print Form CMS-1500 cannot be duplicated by your PC printer. If you attempt to print red ink versions of Form CMS-1500 from your printer, the insurance company will not be able to process the claim.

Electronic Claims Submission

Many claims are routinely submitted electronically to insurance carriers. These types of claims are called **electronic claims**. **Electronic claims submission** is a process whereby insurance claims are submitted via computerized data (either by data diskette or modem) directly from the provider to the insurance company. When claims are submitted electronically, the claim data is entered directly through the phone lines into the insurance carriers' computer system. The Administrative Simplification and Compliance Act (ASCA) requires claims to be submitted to Medicare electronically, with some exceptions.

Claims submitted electronically usually contain fewer errors; because they eliminate the need for data entry personnel to reenter the information, payment is also generated more quickly. In addition, insurance carriers reduce their management and overhead costs by allowing electronic claims submission. Many payers also process electronic claims faster than paper claim submissions.

Generally, electronic claims submission is performed on a weekly basis. Once a week, the medical biller contacts the insurance carrier using the computer and downloads the information.

An acknowledgment report is generated by the insurance carrier and returned to the practice's office. The report confirms that the file was received and provides a list of the claims that were accepted or rejected. The medical biller should review this report carefully. If claims were rejected, an error number and message are included on the audit report to help explain the reason for rejection. The biller can make necessary corrections to the rejected claim(s) and resubmit them.

It is important to have the proper equipment and forms before attempting to submit claims electronically. The format of the claim form must be approved by the carrier, and an agreement also must be in place between the provider and the insurance carrier. This agreement contains the basic understanding on the means of submitting data and the correct procedure coding system. Because electronic claims submission does not allow the opportunity for the physician to sign the claims, a physician's signature on the agreement will be accepted in lieu of a signature on the claim form. It is also imperative to have a patient signature on file for Authorization to Release Information and Assignment of Benefits.

Occasionally, some data transmission problems will arise as a result of systems that are incompatible, static, other problems on the telephone lines, or other software or hardware problems. For this reason, always keep a backup copy of the information transmitted until the claim has been processed. Also, try to submit claims to the insurance carrier early in the morning or late at night. In this way, you may miss the peak times during which your transmission may be interrupted.

Clean Claims

It is important to be sure that the claims you submit to an insurance carrier are "clean claims." **Clean claims** have all the necessary information to process them quickly for benefits.

Before submitting a claim for processing, be sure to check it and make sure that all necessary information is filled in. If a claim is submitted for payment with incomplete information, many insurance carriers, including Medicare, often will reject it.

Coordination of Benefits

Coordination of Benefits (COB) is a process that occurs when two or more group plans provide coverage on the same person. Coordination between the two plans is necessary to allow for payment of 100% of the allowable expenses but no more.

This process was developed in response to the growing problem of overinsurance. **Overinsurance** occurs when a person is covered under two or more policies and is eligible to collect an accumulation of benefits that will actually exceed the amount charged

by the provider. The purpose of COB is to allow coverage and usually payment of 100% of allowable expenses without allowing the covered member(s) to make money over and above the total costs for care.

Before standardized coordination rules were adopted by the benefits industry, a person covered under two policies could collect full benefits from both. Thus, the individual would make a profit by being sick. In response to the diversity of handling procedures used by various carriers and administrators in coordinating coverages, the National Association of Insurance Commissioners (NAIC) developed a standardized model for COB administration, called the Order of Benefit Determination (see Appendix C). The majority of benefit plans follow this model.

COB with Health Maintenance Organizations

A Health Maintenance Organization (HMO) is a type of prepayment plan in which providers agree to charge members for their services in accordance with a fixed

Practice Pitfalls

1. Batch Medicare, Medicaid, HMO, and PPO claims in separate groups before sending them electronically. This way, each of these types of forms will be processed at one time and you will have a separate batch total for each type.

2. Maintain a copy of all paperwork and claims submitted to the insurance carrier. Also compile and keep an insurance claims register with information on the date of submission of the claim to the insurance carrier.

3. Make sure that the forms that the medical office or the computer service generates are compatible with the required submission format for the insurance carrier.

4. If the practice is considering a new form, send a copy to all the insurance carriers you submit claims to and ask for a written approval of the form. Requesting the approval in writing can solve problems later. It may take six weeks or more to receive form approval.

schedule of rates. The HMO insured may pay a specified copayment at the time that the service is rendered or may not be required to pay anything. The patient and the doctor are never involved in having to complete claim forms for submission to a payer. Instead, the HMO is billed directly or the HMO pays a monthly retainer fee to the physician for membership plus other specified fees.

If the required medical services are available through the HMO but the insured does not go to an HMO provider for the treatment, he or she may be held entirely responsible for all of the expenses.

Prepayment plans are included in the definition of the type of policies to which COB provisions apply. However, many HMOs do not have COB provisions, although more are now starting to incorporate this concept because the spiraling costs of medical care are affecting them as well.

An example of an HMO is Kaiser Permanente. Kaiser provides a prepayment policy for hospital and professional medical services at no cost or at a small fee, as long as the member goes to a Kaiser facility. Subsequently, they provide the member with a "reasonable cost statement," which represents what would have been charged to a nonmember. If the HMO does not have a COB provision, they would be considered the primary payer. To coordinate benefits, a request must be made for receipts or statements showing the actual out-of-pocket expense. The secondary plan would pay no more than the amount that would be considered the allowable expense. If the HMO does have a COB provision, the regular OBD determination rules should be applied.

Collecting the Patient Portion

Many medical offices will collect the estimated amount due from the patient at the time services are rendered. This estimated amount is based on the patient's portion of the coinsurance amount and any deductible that has not yet been satisfied. This practice requires that medical billers contact the patient's insurance company before treatment is rendered (usually within 24 hours of the scheduled appointment). The biller should confirm that the patient is covered by the insurance, determine the correct coinsurance amount, any special circumstances that may apply to the treatment, and any deductible that has not yet been met by the patient.

Once this information has been obtained, the biller should determine the estimated amount that is the patient's responsibility.

Practice Pitfalls

Barney Bumpkiss is scheduled for a high-complexity office visit for the treatment of diabetes ($130). The doctor is expected to perform a glucose monitoring of the patient ($30) and a CBC ($30).

On calling the insurance carrier, you determine that Barney is currently covered by insurance that has a $125 deductible. Barney has received prior treatment, satisfying $75 of his deductible. The remaining services are covered at 80% for medical services and 70% for laboratory services.

The patient's estimated amount should be determined as follows:

Charges

Office visit	$130
Glucose monitoring	$30
CBC	$30
Total	$190

Deductible to Be Satisfied

Amount of deductible	$125
Deductible paid	$75
Deductible remaining	$50

Office visit ($130) − deductible remaining ($50) = $80
$80 × 20% (patient's coinsurance) = $16
Lab charges ($60) × 30% (patient's coinsurance) = $18
Total patient portion ($16 + $18) = $34
+ unmet deductible of $50 = $84 Estimated patient payment due.

Be sure to inform the patient that this is an estimated amount, based on your charges. The insurance carrier may allow a smaller amount, which may result in a higher estimated patient payment.

Collecting from Medicare Patients

If the patient is enrolled in the Medicare program, it is important not to overcollect on the patient's portion of the payment. Because Medicare limits the amount that a provider can collect, it is important to determine the appropriate Medicare-allowed amount before calculating the patient's portion of the payment.

Many medical offices will have a list of their most commonly rendered services and the Medicare-allowed

services. It may be necessary to either
...care carrier and ask what the allowed
...o back through past Medicare payments
...for this patient, if this treatment is for an
...on) to determine the allowed amount.

If an office does not have a listing of approved amounts, the Medicare carrier may have a list they can distribute. If not, the biller should consider creating a list and adding in the Medicare-approved amount from each Medicare Notice that it receives.

Additionally, if Medicare determines that the services are not medically necessary, you must refund all monies paid to the patient, even if you are appealing the decision and are waiting for a final determination.

Remember that any amount collected that is more than the Medicare-allowed amount for the procedure will need to be refunded to the patient. This can prevent ill feelings on the part of the patient, especially Medicare patients who are on a fixed income.

On the Job Now

Directions: Using the following scenarios determine the correct amount to be collected from the patient before rendering services.

Yellow Insurance covers 90% of all procedures except anesthesia, which is covered at 80%. They have a $125 annual deductible.

1. Yvonne Yang is scheduled to receive drainage of a cyst in the mouth ($340), an x-ray of the mouth and throat ($85), and an esophagotomy ($624). She has not met any portion of her deductible.

   Amount to be collected: _____

2. Yasmin Yarrow is scheduled to receive a straightforward office visit, new patient ($100). She has met $10 of her deductible.

   Amount to be collected: _____

Brown Insurance covers patients at 80% for medical services. The carrier requires a deductible of $150 annually.

3. Betty Boston is scheduled to have a straightforward office visit ($85) to have a skin lesion examined. She has met all of her deductible.

   Amount to be collected: _____

4. Betsy Bryman is scheduled to receive the removal of a 2.1 cm lesion on her arm ($560). She has met $30.50 of her deductible.

   Amount to be collected: _____

5. Barry Barker is scheduled to receive a moderate complexity office visit ($110) and an x-ray of his arm ($65). He has met $5 of his deductible.

   Amount to be collected: _____

TRICARE

TRICARE is the medical program for military personnel. TRICARE provides a comprehensive program of healthcare benefits for active duty and retired services personnel, their dependents, and the dependents of deceased military personnel. Persons eligible for TRICARE will be enrolled in the Defense Enrollment Eligibility Reporting System (DEERS). This is a computer database used to verify TRICARE eligibility. The valid uniformed services ID card serves as proof of eligibility for TRICARE coverage. The patient is responsible for appropriate copays, cost shares, and deductibles.

TRICARE is secondary to all other insurance or health policies except Medicaid and TRICARE supplemental insurance. However, most military personnel will be treated free of charge or at a minimal fee at veterans' administrative clinics and facilities. Because of this, many medical billers will never have to bill TRICARE.

There are several different healthcare programs under the TRICARE banner.

TRICARE Prime is a managed care option similar to an HMO. All active duty personnel are required to be enrolled in this option. Their spouses and dependents also are encouraged to enroll, although it is not mandatory for them.

- If a network provider is used, the provider must file the claim.
- If a nonnetwork provider is used or if emergent/urgent care outside the patient's region is required, the provider may file claims on the patient's behalf or the provider may require the patient to pay out-of-pocket and file their own paper claim for reimbursement.

TRICARE Extra is a Preferred Provider Organization. Patients who seek treatment from a network provider are covered at 85% of the allowed amount, whereas those who seek treatment from a nonnetwork provider are covered at 80% of the allowed amount.

- When a network provider is used, the providers must file the claim.

TRICARE Standard is the new name for what was formerly called the Civilian Health and Medical Program for the Uniformed Services (CHAMPUS). This option provides coverage on a fee-for-service basis.

- The provider may file claims on behalf of the patient or require the patient to pay out-of-pocket and file their own paper claim for reimbursement.

TRICARE For Life and TRICARE Plus is a Medigap insurance that covers those who are 65 or over and covered by Medicare.

Balance Billing

According to the Department of Defense Appropriations Act of 1993, providers who do not accept assignment can bill TRICARE patients no more than 115% of the TRICARE maximum allowable charge. Billing a patient more than 115% of the TRICARE maximum allowable charge is considered "balance billing" and can result in exclusion from TRICARE and other government healthcare programs.

"Accepting Assignment" on Claims

By "accepting assignment," a doctor agrees to accept the TRICARE maximum allowable charge as payment in full and to write off the difference between the TRICARE maximum allowable charge and the billed charges. Doctors who accept assignment also agree to file claims for the beneficiary.

The difference between TRICARE maximum allowable charge and the amount TRICARE paid is the patient's responsibility. However, when the patient's other health insurance pays more than the TRICARE maximum allowable charge, the billed item is considered paid in full.

TRICARE as Secondary Payer

TRICARE is always the second payer if the patient has other insurance (including Medicare). The only exceptions are Medicaid and TRICARE supplemental policies.

TRICARE-Certified and TRICARE-Contracted Providers

A **TRICARE-certified (authorized)** provider is a facility, doctor, or other healthcare professional who meets the licensing and certification requirements of TRICARE regulations and practices for that area of healthcare.

TRICARE-certified (authorized) providers may or may not agree to "accept assignment"—that is, accept the TRICARE maximum allowable charge as payment in full for services. If providers do not agree, then they are considered certified (authorized), nonparticipating providers. They may elect to accept assignment on a claim-by-claim basis. These also are known as TRICARE-certified (authorized), nonnetwork providers.

Because a provider is TRICARE-certified (authorized) does not mean that the provider is contracted with TRICARE.

A TRICARE-contracted provider is a TRICARE-certified (authorized) provider who has a contract agreement with a TRICARE Prime Contractor. This provider agrees to accept the TRICARE maximum allowable charge as payment in full and submit claim forms for beneficiaries. A TRICARE-contracted provider is also a certified (authorized), participating provider or a network provider.

Participating providers agree to accept TRICARE payment and any cost share as payment in full. Nonparticipating providers do not agree to accept the TRICARE-determined allowable charge as the total charge for services; they can bill you up to 15% more of the TRICARE allowable charge. TRICARE will send reimbursement to you and you, in turn, will pay the provider.

Billing Reports

There are a number of reports that can help you manage claims that have been submitted or are in various stages of the process. By generating or running these reports on a daily basis, you can be sure that all services are being billed and all claims are proceeding properly.

The most common of these reports is listed here. Some computer programs have the capacity to generate these reports. If the program does not have a report that specifically covers the information desired, some programs will allow you to create a custom report. If this is not possible, a manual report can be created.

Following are various reports, information regarding their purpose, and the information generally included in the report.

Transaction Reports

Many medical billing programs allow you to print a transaction report of the claims that were entered or completed on a given day. By printing out this report, you can compare it to the appointment book to ensure that all services that were completed during the day have been billed for.

Practice
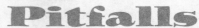

There are many reasons why claims are delayed or denied when they could have been processed if the correct information had been submitted initially. Here are some helpful billing tips to facilitate prompt claim payments.

1. Make sure the Defense Enrollment Eligibility Reporting System (DEERS) information is correct and current. When treating TRICARE patients, be sure to list the name, rank, station, and ID number from the enrollment card on the patient's chart. Also copy the card and place it in the chart.

2. TRICARE claims can be submitted on a CMS-1500. Complete the CMS-1500 and submit it to the fiscal intermediary or submit claims electronically if required.

3. When filing a TRICARE claim, be sure to indicate that someone else may be responsible for payment, such as automobile insurance or possible Workers' Compensation.

4. If there is other health insurance, file the claim with the other health insurance carrier before filing with TRICARE.

5. If the patient is a dual eligible beneficiary (those who are eligible for Medicare and TRICARE benefits), submit claims in the usual manner to Medicare first. Claims will automatically be transmitted from Medicare to TRICARE for secondary claims processing.

6. Keep copies of everything submitted to claims processors.

7. Be sure to send the claim to the correct address to avoid processing delays.

8. Submit claims as soon as possible. Submitting claims quickly will ensure timely reimbursement.

9. Claims must be filed within one year of the date of service to be considered for reimbursement.

Acknowledgment Reports

Acknowledgment reports are generated by an insurance carrier. They indicate the claims that were received electronically. By comparing this report to the information in your daily journal, you can determine if all services that were performed have been billed.

Because claims may be submitted to different insurance carriers, there should be an Acknowledgment Report from each different insurance carrier.

Insurance Claims Register

An **Insurance Claims Register (see Figure 11–9)** lists all claims that have been fully completed and are being submitted to the insurance carrier by the provider's office. This report can be compared to the Acknowledgment Report to ensure that all claims were received by the appropriate carriers.

Claims Register

A **Claims Register** is a database that lists all claims created by a practice. This database can usually be sorted by date, doctor, or patient name.

Prompt Payment Laws

In many states, there is a time limit (often 30 days) by which an insurance carrier must respond to a claim. This response can be payment of the claim, a denial of the claim, or a request for further information.

Payment delays from insurance companies can be a significant problem for a medical practice. Because of this, many states have enacted **prompt payment laws**, also known as fair claims practice regulations. Prompt payment laws dictate how quickly an insurance company must pay a clean claim once it is received. In some states, the law only applies to noncontracted providers.

Tracer Claims/Delinquent Claims

If payment for a claim is not received within 45 days of billing the insurance carrier, the biller should contact the carrier to determine the reason for the delay. Often the proper forms have not been received. If such is the case, ask which form is missing and who is responsible for sending it.

The insurance carrier also may state that they have not received the claim. In such a case, ask if you can fax a copy of the claim to speed up the process. This may be allowed, or some carriers will request that you remail the claim. If the claim was sent electronically, a copy of your electronic claims submission report or the insurance carrier's acknowledgment report may be helpful in locating the missing claim.

If the carrier is still unable to locate the claim, you can resubmit an electronic claim or remail a paper copy.

When speaking with the insurance carrier, try to get an idea of when the claim will be paid. Remember that you should attempt to collect payment on services as soon as possible. The patient record also should be documented to indicate all communications with insurance carriers regarding claim payments.

Denied Claims

When a claim is denied, it is important to determine the reason for the denial. If the claim was denied as a result of incorrect or incomplete information on the part of the provider's office, resubmit the claim using the procedures in the next section of this chapter. It is important to correct and resubmit the claim as soon as possible.

If the claim is denied for other reasons, first identify the reason for the problem and then determine the solution needed to fix the problem. If the insurance carrier says that the patient is not insured by them, ask what information they used to check for coverage. This is often the name of the insured, their ID number, and the policy name or number. If any of these items differ from that in the insurance carrier's records, it can cause the claim to be denied.

Try to determine which piece of information is incorrect. If the information matches what is shown on the forms the patient originally filled out, check the insurance card (you should have made a copy of the insurance card at the time of the patient's first visit). Match the information on the insurance card with that on the claim. If any information is missing or incorrect, correct it in the computer and then resubmit the claim.

If the carrier denies the services as noncovered, request them to identify specifically where in the contract the services are excluded. Be sure to update your files to reflect this information.

PAUL PROVIDER, M.D.
5858 Peppermint Place
Anytown, USA 12345
(765) 555-6768

Insurance Claims Register

Page No. _____

Date Claims Filed	Patient Name	Name of Insurance Policy	Place Claim Sent	Claim Amount	Follow-Up Date	Paid Amount	Remaining Balance

■ **Figure 11–9** Insurance Claims Register

Resubmission of Claims

If the claim was denied because of incorrect or incomplete information on the part of the provider's office, it is important to correct the problem and resubmit the claim as soon as possible.

Some insurance carriers require that you get approval to resubmit a claim before doing so. This is because many insurance carriers' claims processing programs are designed to search for duplicate bills. Thus, the program will log the patient information, the date of services, and the services that were rendered. If a claim is sent in with data that matches these items, the computer will automatically flag the claim as a duplicate claim, and the claim may be denied.

To prevent this from happening, be sure to contact the insurance carrier. Make sure that the information that you are correcting on the claim includes the information that caused it to be rejected. There is no reason to resubmit a claim if the required information is not included in the resubmission.

Also, be sure to ask if an approval number needs to be obtained to resubmit the claim. If so, be sure this approval number is included in the appropriate place on the form. This will prompt the computer or the claims examiner to know that the claim needs to be reprocessed, not just flagged as duplicate.

Adjusted Claims

Sometimes, the insurance carrier will adjust information on your claim. They may bundle together several services, or downcode services they determine were billed inappropriately.

When an adjustment needs to be made to a claim, it is important to perform it as soon as possible.

There are several ways of making adjustments:

Recreate the claim: A new claim can be created that shows only the adjusted information, not the information originally submitted. Because this may cause a discrepancy between what the medical record indicate was done and what the patient was billed for, the medical record will need to be updated. This can be done by adding in the corrected or changed information and indicating that there is an adjustment on the claim. The medical record should indicate exactly what changes were made, and why.

When this type of adjustment is made, you may need to adjust the codes on the original claim and the amounts for the codes. The patient's ledger or statement information or the medical office's accounting records also may need to be revised.

Make an adjustment to the patient account: This second method is more commonly used. Rather than recreate any documents, an adjustment is simply added to the patient's account. This adjustment should list the items being adjusted and the reason for the adjustment.

Because this type of adjustment shows up as an adjustment on the medical office's accounting records, there is no need to rerun any accounting reports for previous periods.

Review and Appeals

If you disagree with the denial or adjustment of a claim, you have the right to appeal the decision. Most insurance carriers have a specific process to be used for appeals. This often includes submitting a copy of the claim along with a letter stating the reason you disagree with their decision.

When writing an appeal letter, it is important to be specific regarding why you feel the claim payment, or lack of payment, is incorrect. Simply stating that you do not feel the insurance carrier paid enough on the claim is not enough. You need to state why the payment is incorrect.

If the claim was downcoded to a lower-valued procedure, double-check your records. If you agree with the downcoding, change it in your records (including the patient's computerized records). If you disagree with the downcoding, submit the claim for appeal. Be sure to attach a copy of the medical records and a letter explaining why you believe that the higher code should be allowed.

Balance Billing Patients for Downcoded or Denied Claims

Before balance billing patients on claims that have been denied or downcoded, you need to assess the situation. You may need to adjust the original bill to reflect the downcoded amount. In some cases, you may need to remove services from the bill if they have been denied by the insurance carrier. This is especially true in the case of Medicare or Medicaid claims.

If a Medicare or Medicaid claim is denied as not medically necessary, you are not allowed to bill the patient for these services unless the patient was informed before services were rendered that Medicare or Medicaid may not cover the services. If the patient was informed, a Medicare Advance Notice must have been completed before the rendering of services. If this notice was not signed before services were rendered, you are not allowed to bill the patient and any denied services must be written off.

If Medicare has downcoded a claim or service, you also must downcode the claim or service on the bill sent to the patient. For example, if you charged the patient for a high-complexity visit and Medicare downcoded the visit to one of moderate complexity, you must downcode the procedure on all billing reports or claims. You are only allowed to collect from the patient the amount that would be due from them for the lower-coded visit.

State Insurance Commissioner

Each state has a **State Insurance Commissioner**. This person is responsible for overseeing the insurance companies and their practices within the state. If a biller has a repeated problem regarding an insurance carrier not properly paying claims in a timely manner, they can file a report with the State Insurance Commissioner.

The State Insurance Commissioner will assign an investigator to the case if they feel that an investigation is warranted. If they find that the insurance carrier is not adhering to state mandates and laws, they can impose sanctions or fines on the insurance carrier.

Because reporting an insurance carrier to the State Insurance Commissioner is a serious situation, you should make all attempts to resolve a situation with the claims examiner or their supervisor first. Then discuss the situation with the provider and allow them to make the determination of whether or not to file a report.

Maximum Reimbursement Guidelines

Following are a few guidelines that will allow you to receive the maximum reimbursement possible on each claim.

1. Be sure that the claim form is filled out completely and accurately.

2. Be sure that each procedure is linked to its appropriate diagnosis and that the diagnosis substantiates the need for the procedure.

3. Check the contract provisions (or contact the insurance carrier to request information regarding contract provisions). Follow all provisions carefully, including precertifying procedures, preauthorization of hospitalizations, need for second surgical opinions, and so on.

4. Be sure that any benefits that are reimbursed at a higher benefit amount are clearly indicated. This can include outpatient surgery being paid at a higher percentage than inpatient surgery; preadmit testing paid at a higher percentage; accident provisions; and so on.

5. If a common accident provision applies, send in the claim for the patient who has previously paid the most toward their deductible first.

6. Make a notation at the top of the filed copy of the claim regarding the benefit level you expect this claim to be paid at and why (i.e., 100% accident benefit). When the claim is paid, double-check the EOB to ensure that the claim was paid at the expected benefit level. If not, contact the insurance carrier for an explanation.

7. Double-check all EOBs to ensure that all procedures were paid or accounted for. In cases of paper claims, it is easy for a single procedure to be omitted.

8. Appeal all decisions that you do not agree with, especially in cases of downcoding or denials because of medical necessity. Be sure to include appropriate information as to why the services should be allowed at the level indicated. Simply adding a modifier is not enough. Provide lab tests, operative reports, or other written data that substantiates your point of view.

CHAPTER REVIEW

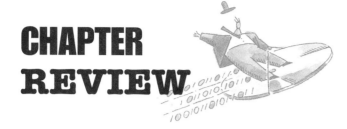

Summary

- The CMS-1500 is the most widely accepted form for billing professional services. It is vital that the correct information be inserted in each item to allow the claim to be processed without delay. Although the completion may seem simple, it takes practice to be able to properly fill out the form in the correct manner.

- Properly handling the billing of claims is the prime responsibility of the medical biller. If the proper general guidelines and procedures are not followed, it can cause a delay in reimbursement for the services.

- If a provider's office has incomplete data on a patient, it is important to obtain that data as quickly as possible. Missing or incorrect data often can cause delays or denials on claim payments. An incomplete data master list can assist in keeping track of incomplete data if the medical biller is unable to obtain the data immediately.

- Two types of billing require special handling: TRICARE and Coordination of Benefits. It is important for the medical biller to understand the basic benefits provided by TRICARE and to know how to coordinate benefits when there is more than one payer who may cover payment for a patient. This will allow the provider to recover the maximum amount possible from the various payers, leaving a smaller balance for the patient to pay or for the physician to write off.

- Electronic claim submission not only cuts down on errors but also dramatically decreases the time needed for payment of the claim and prevents loss of claims through the mail or other courier service.

- It is important for the medical biller to properly submit clean claims. This can be done on paper or via electronic (computer) submission. Regardless of which method you use, it is important to follow the guidelines for that method to ensure that the claim can be processed quickly and easily.

- Many insurance carriers have time limits for submitting claims. Because of this, it is important for the medical biller to submit claims in a timely manner, preferably as soon as services are completed.

- If a claim is downcoded or denied, it is important for the medical biller to assess the situation and decide whether they need to accept the decision and create an adjustment, resubmit the claim with additional information, or file an appeal with the insurance carrier.

Assignments

Complete the Questions for Review.
Complete Exercises 11–1 through 11–4.

Questions for Review

Directions: Answer the following questions without looking back at the material just covered. Write your answers in the space provided.

1. What is the CMS-1500 claim form used for? _____

_____

2. If the provider of service is an individual, what should be placed in the box entitled Federal Tax ID Number?

_____

3. Which box denotes that Workers' Compensation is involved in the claim? _____

4. How would you indicate that the place where services were rendered was an office? _____

_____

5. What are the boxes at the top of the CMS-1500 form, labeled "Medicare, Medicaid, TRICARE, CHAMPVA, Feca Black Lung, and Other," for? _____

_____

6. What does the term "Assignment of Benefits" mean? _____

_____

7. On the CMS-1500, what is Item 24I "EMG" for? _____

_____

8. On the CMS-1500, what does Item 24J "COB" stand for and what does the term mean? _____

_____

9. (True or False?) When a physician or provider of service signs a medical billing form, he/she is legally stating

that the service(s) that they are seeking payment for have actually been performed. _____

10. What does COB stand for? _____

11. What is the purpose of COB? _____

_____

12. List and describe the two ways of making an adjustment.

1. _____

2. _____

If you are unable to answer any of these questions, refer back to that section in the chapter, and then fill in the answers.

Exercise **11-1**

Directions: Complete a superbill/charge slip and a CMS-1500 form for the following scenarios. The provider of services is Paul Provider, M.D. All services are performed at his office. Amounts in parentheses are the amounts the doctor is billing for the procedure. Refer to the Patient Data Table and Provider Data Table in Appendix C for information.

Upon Completion of the CMS-1500, use an Insurance Claims Register (located in Appendix B) and list all claims that have been fully prepared and are ready for submission to the insurance carrier for payment. Enter the date that you created the CMS-1500 in the **Date Claim Filed** column.

1. On 3/4/CCYY Abby Addison comes in to visit the provider. She has a bad case of the flu and receives a problem-focused office visit ($95) and a therapeutic injection (vitamin B-12) ($30).

2. On 3/3/CCYY Bobby Bumble visits the provider for treatment of a superficial abscess on his neck. The provider performs an incision and drainage of the abscess ($95).

3. On 3/4/CCYY Cathy Crenshaw visits the provider for treatment of a cut on her arm. She cut her arm on a broken window at home on 3/4/CCYY. The provider performs a moderate complexity office visit with five stitches ($110) and a tetanus injection ($30). On 3/15/CCYY Cathy comes in to have her stitches removed.

4. On 3/3/CCYY Daisy Doolittle visits the provider for a refill of her contraceptive prescription. The provider performs a problem-focused exam and writes her a new prescription ($95).

5. On 3/3/CCYY Edward Edmunds visits the provider for pain and swelling in his shoulder. The provider does a moderate complexity office visit ($110) and a urinalysis ($30). The final diagnosis is tendonitis. On 3/10/CCYY the provider operates to remove the calcium deposits. The operation was performed inpatient at Provider Medical Center.

Exercise 11-2

Directions: Find and circle the words listed below. Words can appear horizontally, vertically, diagonally, forward, or backward.

1. Claim Register
2. Electronic Claim
3. Overinsurance

4. Professional/Courtesy
5. Prompt Payment Laws
6. Self-Funded Plan

```
N Q C U E F V T H U C E P C C R K M F F F X S P O Z M N V D
I A E R L L V O B C Z C L T H T D U Y V V Y M E V P T E S G E
B Y L I W D E D L M S A J C R W F N G K S H L G O R E J F A
N P B P E K M C P E I V H J P R U E R E Z M F I X E A O S P
O P A Q Y R W Q T M W D L I R F S B C O G E F S X X F X P G
M O R F G R P W R R Y C C M A L P M S L O C U U Y D J G Y E
G P C O U B A E O Q O M N A A A A F P I H E N U R U P C C R
R W F J P G G M C A Z N M N P U L K T G M L D Q B F R Y Z A
B L W K D I P K I X N K I U X I M A D E P W E A I G O L M N
G Y V G S A U C M R M M E C Y H S R C E F X D G J C F V L I
E F O T M P M M W G P O M P C D Q X I B X M P W B G E F R P
E Y E X C E M V Z Y D H K Y I L B M A R S V L A S U S W E R
E R E C N A R U S N I R E V O Y A P V Q C U A F S L S V K X
T R H A C E P A N W O B X K H I C I C J N F N W E F I R H G
A A I I Q Y W E X S V Q V S Z Z N L M P Y J W P K B O S P Z
U B U W A Y T R W S T V H G W J Z I K W K J M F C P N P H E
J F R T U P N G G T C X P B A K F Z J P F H M D H K A L O D
U D W J Y K E N S V F O H K R Z D V A K N X J B U K L T R E
S Z T D O H I B U Y R F D X C I V U R T A S L B E R C N T L
B P R O M P T P A Y M E N T L A W S N H U K J F R W O M T O
C R W I O F Q A V X O R X R N D S O U R P B A I O P U I D J
Z M K I T K G G K C I X Y I N Y F Q E T E R Q O N V R Y N O
U C O I G V E H H A W Q B P W S C C T L L A C P I A T L H W
S R Z G R W H Y Z A C W J T K S Y Y J J J Y K M C T M E D E L
U W E Z B X X M K L Z L J J D N R A O H T M O F Y X S L O S
J W E Z P Q J E O E R Q D R O F D W N W S V B P A T Y X K Y
M E D H A B G U K M J N F L T U H U E L E Y E Z K F G O O F
B Z V A X V L T B L P S F E F Y T C Z A P N Z W A W H M W P
Q A S K J W Z S I R W L G V U S W Z M L Y K I V J V T U B L
C M J V N T Z S N W O O T K O W H P U F T I N C F T C D Z F
```

Exercise 11-3

Directions: Complete the crossword puzzle by filling in a word from the keywords that fits each clue.

Across

6. Claims that have all the necessary information to enable them to be processed quickly.

Down

1. A numerical code to indicate the location where the service was rendered.

2. Reports generated by an insurance carrier. They indicate the claims that were received electronically.

3. These are billing forms used by many providers of service and suppliers. This form serves as a charging slip to expedite the process of medical insurance reimbursement.

4. A form for billing professional services that is provided by self-funded plans.

5. The Department of Defense's healthcare program for members of the uniformed services and their families and survivors, and retired members and their families.

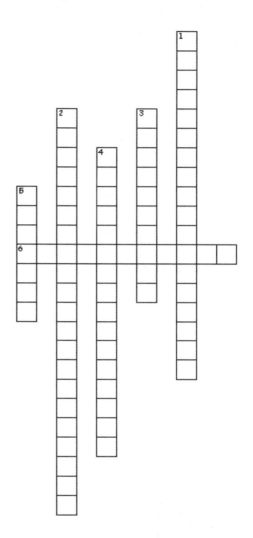

Exercise 11-4

Directions: Match the following terms with the proper definition by writing the letter of the correct definition in the space next to the term.

1. _____ CMS-1500

2. _____ Electronic Claim Submission

3. _____ Incomplete Data Master List

4. _____ Optical Character Recognition

5. _____ Claim Attachment

6. _____ Insurance Claims Register

7. _____ State Insurance Commissioner

a. This person is responsible for overseeing the insurance companies and their practices within the state.

b. Lists all claims that have been fully completed and are being submitted to the insurance carrier by the provider's office.

c. Any document providing additional medical information to the claims payer that cannot be accommodated within the standard billing form.

d. A standardized form for use as a "universal" form for billing professional services.

e. An automated scanning process that reads the information on claim forms.

f. A complete listing of patients whose charts have not been properly filled out or who have not completed patient forms.

g. A process whereby insurance claims are submitted via computerized data (either by data diskette or modem) directly from the provider to the insurance company.

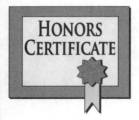

Honors Certification™

The certification challenge for this chapter will be a written test of the information contained in this chapter. Each incorrect answer will result in a deduction of up to 5% from your grade. You must achieve a score of 85% or higher to pass this test. If you fail the test on your first attempt, you may retake the test one additional time. The items included in the second test may be different from those in the first test.

12

The UB-92 Form and
Hospital Billing Procedures

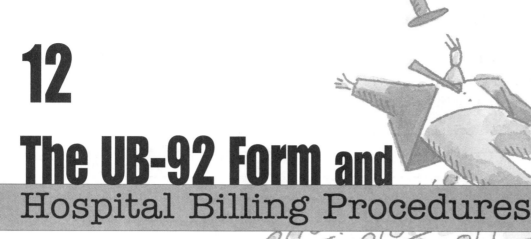

After completion of this chapter
you will be able to:

- Describe the purpose of the UB-92.
- Properly code the type of bill.
- Properly identify condition codes, occurrence codes, and occurrence span codes.
- Properly complete the UB-92 billing form.
- Identify hospital revenue codes.
- Choose the proper form for billing various types of hospital services.
- Describe what personal items are and give examples.
- Describe what APCs are and how they affect payment.

- Explain what DRGs are and how they affect payment on a hospital claim.
- Explain the purpose of a charge master description list and the information contained on it.
- Describe the common methods used for entering hospital charges on a patient's bill.
- Discuss how billing can affect other departments in a hospital.
- Discuss the importance of precertification, preauthorization, and utilization review.
- Describe what an ambulatory surgical center does.

Keywords and Concepts
you will learn in this chapter:

- Admission Kit
- Ambulatory Patient Classifications (APCs)
- Ambulatory Surgical Centers (Surgi-Centers)
- Bar Code

- Chargemaster Description List (CDL)
- Condition Codes
- Interim Billing
- Itemized Bill
- Occurrence Codes
- Occurrence Span Codes

- Personal Items
- Prospective Payment System (PPS)
- Revenue Codes
- Source of Admission Code
- Type of Admission Code
- Uniform Bill-1992 (UB-92)
- Value Codes

The **Uniform Bill-1992 (UB-92)**, also referred to as the CMS-1450, is intended to be used by hospitals or other hospital-type facilities for in-patient and outpatient billing **(see Figures 12–1 and 12–2)**. The data elements and the design of the form were determined by the

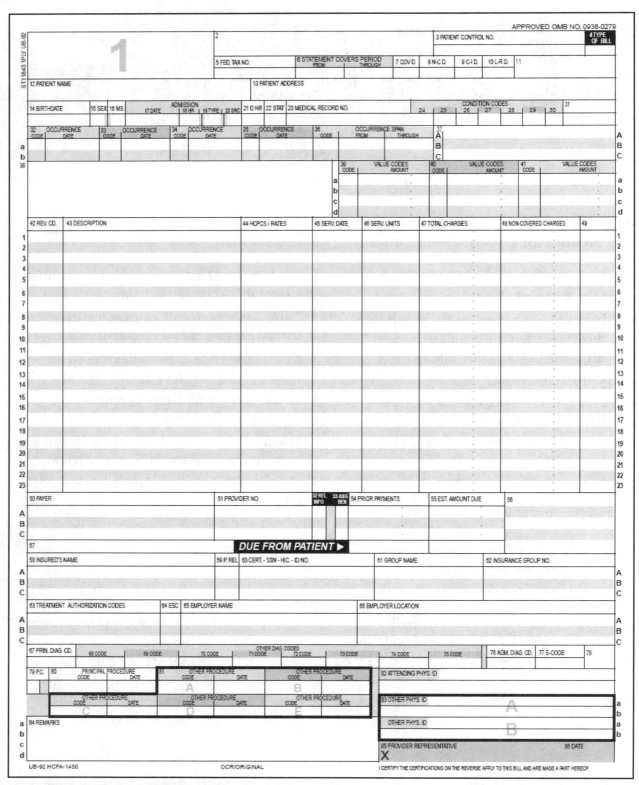

■ Figure 12–1 Sample of Front of UB-92 Billing Form

UNIFORM BILL: NOTICE: ANYONE WHO MISREPRESENTS OR FALSIFIES ESSENTIAL
INFORMATION REQUESTED BY THIS FORM MAY UPON CONVICTION BE
SUBJECT TO FINE AND IMPRISONMENT UNDER FEDERAL AND/OR STATE LAW.

Certifications relevant to the Bill and Information Shown on the Face Hereof: Signatures on the face hereof incorporate the following certifications or verifications where pertinent to this Bill:

1. If third party benefits are indicated as being assigned or in participation status, on the face thereof, appropriate assignments by the insured/beneficiary and signature of patient or parent or legal guardian covering authorization to release information are on file. Determinations as to the release of medical and financial information should be guided by the particular terms of the release forms that were executed by the patient or the patient's legal representative. The hospital agrees to save harmless, indemnify and defend any insurer who makes payment in reliance upon this certification, from and against any claim to the insurance proceeds when in fact no valid assignment of benefits to the hospital was made.

2. If patient occupied a private room or required private nursing for medical necessity, any required certifications are on file.

3. Physician's certifications and re-certifications, if required by contract or Federal regulations, are on file.

4. For Christian Science Sanitoriums, verifications and if necessary re-verifications of the patient's need for sanitorium services are on file.

5. Signature of patient or his/her representative on certifications, authorization to release information, and payment request, as required be Federal law and regulations (42 USC 1935f, 42 CFR 424.36, 10 USC 1071 thru 1086, 32 CFR 199) and, any other applicable contract regulations, is on file.

6. This claim, to the best of my knowledge, is correct and complete and is in conformance with the Civil Rights Act of 1964 as amended. Records adequately disclosing services will be maintained and necessary information will be furnished to such governmental agencies as required by applicable law.

7. For Medicare purposes:

   If the patient has indicated that other health insurance or a state medical assistance agency will pay part of his/her medical expenses and he/she wants information about his/her claim released to them upon their request, necessary authorization is on file. The patient's signature on the provider's request to bill Medicare authorizes any holder of medical and non-medical information, including employment status, and whether the person has employer group health insurance, liability, no-fault, workers' compensation, or other insurance which is responsible to pay for the services for which this Medicare claim is made.

8. For Medicaid purposes:

   This is to certify that the foregoing information is true, accurate, and complete.
   I understand that payment and satisfaction of this claim will be from Federal and State funds, and that any false claims, statements, or documents, or concealment of a material fact, may be prosecuted under applicable Federal or State Laws.

9. For CHAMPUS purposes:

   This is to certify that:

   (a) the information submitted as part of this claim is true, accurate and complete, and, the services shown on this form were medically indicated and necessary for the health of the patient;

   (b) the patient has represented that by a reported residential address outside a military treatment center catchment area he or she does not live within a catchment area of a U.S. military or U.S. Public Health Service medical facility, or if the patient resides within a catchment area of such a facility, a copy of a Non-Availability Statement (DD Form 1251) is on file, or the physician has certified to a medical emergency in any assistance where a copy of a Non-Availability Statement is not on file;

   (c) the patient or the patient's parent or guardian has responded directly to the provider's request to identify all health insurance coverages, and that all such coverages are identified on the face the claim except those that are exclusively supplemental payments to CHAMPUS-determined benefits;

   (d) the amount billed to CHAMPUS has been billed after all such coverages have been billed and paid, excluding Medicaid, and the amount billed to CHAMPUS is that remaining claimed against CHAMPUS benefits;

   (e) the beneficiary's cost share has not been waived by consent or failure to exercise generally accepted billing and collection efforts; and,

   (f) any hospital-based physician under contract, the cost of whose services are allocated in the charges included in this bill, is not an employee or member of the Uniformed Services. For purposes of this certification, an employee of the Uniformed Services is an employee, appointed in civil service (refer to 5 USC 2105), including part-time or intermittent but excluding contract surgeons or other personnel employed by the Uniformed Services through personal service contracts. Similarly, member of the Uniformed Services does not apply to reserve members of the Uniformed Services not on active duty.

   (g) based on the Consolidated Omnibus Budget Reconciliation Act of 1986, all providers participating in Medicare must also participate in CHAMPUS for inpatient hospital services provided pursuant to admissions to hospitals occurring on or after January 1, 1987.

   (h) if CHAMPUS benefits are to be paid in a participating status, I agree to submit this claim to the appropriate CHAMPUS claims processor as a participating provider. I agree to accept the CHAMPUS-determined reasonable charge as the total charge for the medical services or supplies listed on the claim form. I will accept the CHAMPUS-determined reasonable charge even if it is less than the billed amount, and also agree to accept the amount paid by CHAMPUS, combined with the cost-share amount and deductible amount, if any, paid by or on behalf of the patient as full payment for the listed medical services or supplies. I will make no attempt to collect from the patient (or his or her parent or guardian) amounts over the CHAMPUS-determined reasonable charge. CHAMPUS will make any benefits payable directly to me, if I submit this claim as a participating provider.

ESTIMATED CONTRACT BENEFITS

■ **Figure 12–2** Sample of Back of UB-92 Billing Form

National Uniform Billing Committee (NUBC). This form was designed to provide the basic data needed by most payers to adjudicate a large majority of their claims. The objective was to accommodate a wide range of needs while eliminating the need for attachments. The NUBC is also responsible for the design of the UB-92 form and plays a major role in maintaining the integrity of the UB-92 data set.

Field Locator # and Name/Description

The UB-92 form requires specific information entry in the various fields. Refer to the UB-92 Matrix in

Appendix E for an explanation of the information required for the various field locators on the form.

The following list will assist in explaining the uses of the various fields on the UB-92 form. It contains the field locator number along with the name of the item and a brief description of the information required. The word "same" refers to a description that is the same as the title of the item.

Field Locator #:

1 **Provider Name, Address, and Telephone Number.** Name, address, and telephone number of hospital or clinic where services were rendered.

2 **Reserved (untitled).** All unlabeled items are reserved for state or national use. Their use may be assigned by either the state or National Uniform Billing Committee.

3 **Patient Control Number.** Patient's account number.

4 **Type of Bill.** Three-digit code providing information regarding what type of bill is being submitted. (See Appendix C for further information.)

5 **Federal Tax Number.** Provider's Identification Number or Social Security Number.

6 **Statement Covers Period.** The dates of service that this billing statement represents. Dates should match those on the itemized billing statement. For services rendered on the same day, both dates should be the same.

7 **Covered Days.** Number of days that services are covered by primary payer.

8 **Noncovered Days (inpatient only).** Number of days services are not covered by primary payer. For Medicare, the reason for noncoverage should be explained by occurrence codes, PSRO items, or in remarks.

9 **Coinsurance Days.** Number of days for which the patient must pay a portion of the costs of services. For Medicare, the inpatient Medicare days occurring after the 60th and before the 91st day in a single spell of illness.

10 **Lifetime Reserve Days.** Under Medicare, each beneficiary has a lifetime reserve of 60 additional days of inpatient hospital services after using 90 days of inpatient hospital services during a spell of illness.

11 **Reserved for State Assignment.** This field has not been assigned, and use, if any, will be for state identifiers used on a national level.

12 **Patient's Name.** Same.

13 **Patient's Address.** Same.

14 **Birth Date.** Patient's date of birth.

15 **Sex.** Patient's sex.

16 **Marital Status.** Patient's marital status (S = Single, M = Married, X = Legally Separated, D = Divorced, W = Widowed, U = Unknown).

17 **Date of Admission.** Date patient was admitted to hospital.

18 **Hour of Admission.** Hour patient admitted to hospital according to a 24-hour clock (i.e., 10:10 P.M. would be written 22:10). 99 = unknown.

19 **Type of Admission.** Numerical code denoting the priority of this admission (see Appendix C for further information).

20 **Source of Admission.** Numerical code denoting the source of this admission (see Appendix C for further information).

21 **Discharge Hour.** Time patient was discharged from inpatient care. Time should be written according to a 24-hour clock. 99 = unknown. This element is not necessary for outpatient care.

22 **Patient Status.** Numerical code denoting the status of the patient as of the statement–through date. This element is necessary only for inpatient care (see Appendix C for further information).

23 **Medical Record Number.** Number assigned by the provider to the medical record.

24–30 **Condition Codes.** Codes used to identify conditions relating to the claim that may affect payer processing (see Appendix C for further information). No specific date is associated with this code.

31 **Reserved for National Assignment.** This field has not been assigned, and use, if any, will be for national identifiers.

32–35 **Occurrence Codes.** The code and associated date defining a significant event relating to this bill that may affect payer processing.

36 **Occurrence Span.** The code and the related dates that identify an event that relates to the payment of the claim. These codes identify occurrences that happened over a span of time.

37 Internal Control Number. The control number assigned to the original bill by the payer or the payer's intermediary.

38 Responsible Party Name and Address. Name and address of person ultimately responsible for ensuring payment of the bill. This is usually the patient, or the parent or legal guardian if the patient is a minor.

39–41 Value Codes and Amounts. Codes and the related dollar amount that identify data of a monetary nature that is necessary for the processing of this claim.

42 Revenue Code. Revenue code referencing the type of services provided (see the next section of this chapter for further information).

43 Revenue Description. A description of the services provided. Abbreviations may be used. Accommodation (room) descriptions must be entered first on the bill and must be in chronologic order of appearance (i.e., 03/01/89 ICU, 03/02/89 semiprivate room).

44 HCPCS/Rates. The accommodation rate for inpatient bills, or the CPT® or HCPCS code for ancillary or outpatient services. Outpatient Workers' Compensation and Medicaid require HCPCS coding in this space.

45 Service Date. The date the service was provided if this is a series bill where the date of service differs from the from/through date on the bill.

46 Units of Service. Quantitative measure of services, days, miles, pints of blood, units, or treatments (i.e., if a patient was hospitalized for three days, a "3" would be placed here).

47 Total Charges. Total charges for that line of services.

48 Noncovered Charges. The amount per line of service that is not covered by the primary payer.

49 Reserved for National Assignment.

50 Payer Identification. Name of insurer(s) covered by the patient who may be responsible for payment on this bill. Insurers should be listed in order of Primary Payer, Secondary Payer, and Tertiary Payer(s). If required, numbers identifying each payer organization should be listed.

51 Provider Number. The number assigned to the provider by the listed payer.

52 Release Information. A Y (yes) or N (no) designation stating whether or not patient's signature is on file authorizing the release of information. An R also may be entered to show that a hospital has restricted authorization to release information. In such cases, the authorization should be attached. If no Authorization to Release Information is on file, one must be obtained before sending in the claim.

53 Assignment of Benefits. A Y (yes) or N (no) designation stating whether or not patient's signature is on file authorizing the insurer to pay the provider of service directly instead of the patient. If a Y is placed in this item, you must have an assignment of benefits signed by the insured on file in your office. (See the next section of this chapter for further information.)

54 Prior Payments. The amount that has been paid toward this bill before the current billing date. These can include payments by the patient, other payers, and so on.

55 Estimated Amount Due. The amount estimated by the provider to be due from the indicated payer. This is usually the total amount due minus any previous payments.

56 Reserved for State Assignment This field has not been assigned, and use, if any, will be for state identifiers used on a national level.

57 Reserved for National Assignment. This field has not been assigned, and use, if any, will be for national identifiers.

58 Insured's Name. Name of the person listed on the insurance forms (subscriber's name). This may be a spouse or parent of the patient.

59 Patient's Relationship to Insured. Numerical code designation indicating the relationship between the patient and the insured (see Appendix C for further information).

60 Subscriber's Certificate Number. The policy number under which the insured is covered if it is an individual policy. If the insured is covered under a group policy (such as one offered by his/her employer), often the insured's Social Security number is used as the subscriber number.

61 Insured Group Name. The name of the group or company that holds the insured's policy. Often this is the employer of the insured. This information is required by Medicare when Medicare is not the primary payer.

62 Insurance Group Number. The group number denoting the group policy or plan under which the insured is covered.

63 Treatment Authorization Code. A number indicating that the treatment described by this bill has been authorized by the payer.

64 Employment Status Code. A code denoting whether or not the employee is currently employed part or full time, is retired, or is in active military service (see Appendix C for further information).

65 Employer Name. Name of the employer of the insured person.

66 Employer Location. Address of the employer of the insured or responsible party.

67 Principal Diagnosis Code. ICD-9 code for the diagnosis of the patient's condition. The diagnosis shown should reflect the information contained in the patient's medical record for the dates indicated in Item 6 even if the diagnosis is changed at a later date.

68–75 Other Diagnosis Codes. ICD-9, V, and E Codes for any additional diagnosis of the patient's condition.

76 Admitting Diagnosis. The ICD-9 code provided at the time of admission.

77 External Cause of Injury Code (E Code). The ICD-9 Code for an external cause of injury, poisoning or adverse effect.

78 Reserved for State Assignment. This field has not been assigned, and use, if any, will be for state identifiers used on a national level.

79 Procedure Coding Method Used. An indicator code that identifies the coding method used for procedure coding on the claim.

1–3 Reserved for State Assignment
4 CPT®-4
5 HCPCS
6–8 Reserved for National Assignment
9 ICD-9CM

80 Principal Procedure Codes and Date. CPT® code for principal procedure rendered and the date that procedure was rendered. For Medicare, ICD-9 codes must be entered here and on Item 81.

81 Other Procedure Codes and Dates. CPT® code for additional procedures rendered and the dates of those procedures.

82 Attending Physician ID. Name and license number of the physician who is primarily responsible for the patient.

83 Other Physician ID. Name and license number of secondary physician, assistant surgeon, and so on.

84 Remarks. Pertinent data for which there is no other specific place on the form. Often this space is used to record the nature of an accident (i.e., fell and hit head on concrete, 06/09/XX). For Medicaid, required for abortion certification when the attending physician is an employee of the hospital and does not submit a separate bill. Also, multiple visits to the ER on the same day should be recorded.

85 Provider Representative Signature. Signature of provider representative. For hospital billings, it is not necessary for the attending physician to sign, as long as a representative of the hospital signs the form certifying that the information entered is in conformance with the certifications specified on the reverse of the bill. Billers should make sure that the physician's certification is contained in the hospital records.

86 Date Bill Submitted. Date the bill was signed and submitted for payment.

On the Job Now

Directions: Answer the following questions without looking back at the material just covered. Write your answer in the space provided.

1. Where on the UB-92 should the Provider's Identification Number or Social Security Number be placed?

   _____

2. What information should Field Locator 15 include? _____

   _____

3. Where on the UB-92 should you place the Service Date? _____

   _____

4. What information should Field Locator 50 include? _____

   _____

5. Where should you put down pertinent data for which there is no other specific place on the form?

   _____

Uniform Bill (UB-04)

The UB-92 will be replaced by the UB-04. Minor changes have been made to the UB-04 in order to accommodate the National Provider Identifier (NPI), to comply with HIPAA regulations, and to address the needs of electronic claim submission. The UB-04 was approved by the NUBC in February 2005 and will replace the UB-92. There may be additional changes to the UB-04.

The following is a sample of the UB-04 and is for informational purposes only (**see Figures 12–3 and 12–4**). Refer to Appendix E for additional information regarding the UB-04.

Item 42, Hospital Revenue Codes

Hospital **revenue codes** identify a specific accommodation, ancillary service, or billing calculation. Subcategory classifications and standard abbreviations are listed below each major category. The correct subcategory classification should be added to the major category number to create a three-digit number. The use of a fourth digit has been approved by the NUBC for possible future needs. These four-digit numbers are thus far unassigned and therefore are not in use.

For a list of current hospital Revenue Codes, see Appendix C.

SAMPLE

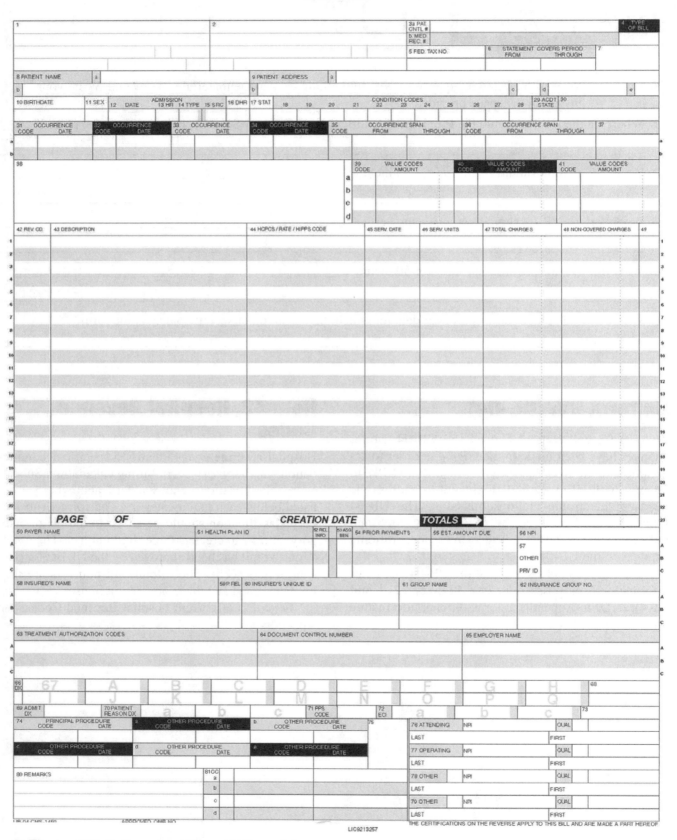

■ **Figure 12–3** Sample of Front of UB-04 Billing Form

■ Figure 12–4 Sample of Back of UB-04 Billing Form

On the Job Now

Directions: List the Revenue Codes for the following services.

Description	Revenue Code
1. Room and Board—Private (Medical or General). Routine service charges for single-bed rooms.	
• General Classification (R&B/PVT)	110
• Medical/Surgical/Gyn (MED-SER-GYN/PVT)	111
2. Medical/Surgical Supplies and Devices. Charges for supply items required for patient care.	
• General Classification (MED-SUR SUPPLIES)	270
• Nonsterile Supply (NON-STER SUPPLY)	221
3. Other Imaging Services.	
• General Classification (IMAGE SVS)	400
• Diagnostic Mammography (DIAG MAMMOGRAPHY)	401
• Ultrasound (ULTRASOUND)	402
4. Hospice Service. Charges for hospice care services for a terminally ill patient. The patient would need to elect these services in lieu of other services for a terminal condition.	
• General Classification (HOSPICE)	650
• Routine Home Care (HOSPICE/RTN HOME)	651
• Continuous Home Care (HOSPICE/ CTNS HOME)	652
5. Home Health Aide (Home Health). Charges made by a home health agency for personnel who are primarily responsible for the personal care of the patient.	
• General Classification (AIDE/ HOME HEALTH)	570
• Visit Charge (AIDE/HOME HLTH/ VISIT)	571
• Hourly Charge (AIDE/HOME HLTH/HOUR)	572

Item 53, Assignment of Benefits

This assignment of benefits will not allow you to release information regarding the patient. A written authorization to release information, signed by the patient or patient representative, is needed (see Item 53). Please note the certification procedure on the back of the UB-92 before completing this item.

Although the UB-92 eliminates the need to send an assignment of benefits to accident and health insurers, hospitals may wish to be extremely careful in the way in which they handle claims involving property and casualty insurers. Property and casualty insurers may not be familiar with the UB-92 and may not be aware that the wording on the back of the UB-92 is sufficient notification of assignment of benefits. Hospitals may wish to send a copy of the assignment on auto accident and similar non-health-oriented insurance carrier claims.

Hospital Billing Procedures

Most of us have been in a hospital at least once in our lives. At the end of a hospital stay, a bill for services is usually received. Hospital billing can be confusing if you do not understand how the process works. However, with basic knowledge and training, competently billing for hospital services should be easily accomplished.

There are two main forms used for billing insurance carriers: the CMS-1500 and the UB-92. Both claim forms are used in a hospital setting.

UB-92 Billing

Services rendered by a hospital or hospital employed personnel are billed on the UB-92. This includes all room and board, medications, operating room charges, supplies used by the patient, x-ray fees (for the equipment, supplies, and room, although not necessarily for the radiologist, etc.).

Many hospitals use bar-coded stickers to assist in billing. A **bar code** is a number that is assigned to a specific item. This number is often represented by a series of thin and fat vertical lines.

In the hospital setting, items will often have a peel-off bar code affixed to them when they are received by the hospital. The bar code is different for each item.

When a patient uses an item, the item is removed from the supply area. The bar code is then peeled off and placed on a special billing page of the patient's chart. If the patient uses two items, two separate bar codes are peeled off and affixed to the patient chart.

When billing is performed, the item numbers from each bar code are entered into the computer. This often is done using a bar-code scanner like the ones seen in many retail and grocery stores. Each number that is entered generates a line item charge on the patient's bill.

Sometimes it can be difficult to determine which charges to put on which form. Some hospitals will even combine the charges and place them on a single form. For example, the hospital may generate one all-inclusive charge for an x-ray. This charge will include not only the equipment, supplies, and the room, but also the services of the radiologist.

When bills with all-inclusive charges are submitted to the insurance carrier for payment, the insurance carrier may insist that the charges be itemized according to charges for the facility (equipment, supplies, and room) and charges for professional services (the provider).

Itemized Bills

Many hospitals provide their patients with an **itemized bill**. This type of bill lists each item, service, or supply on an individual line and shows the cost for that one item. Many patients prefer to receive an itemized bill so that they can understand exactly what they are being billed for. Additionally, facilities in many states are required to provide an itemized bill to any patient who requests one.

Some hospitals will routinely include an itemized bill when billing patients. The markup (the difference between what the hospital pays for an item and what they charge the patient for that same item) can be very high. It is not uncommon for a hospital to charge a patient $10 for a single aspirin.

The increased charge helps to cover the cost of the nurse speaking with the doctor, getting approval for the drug, notating the patient's chart, going to the pharmacy or drug cabinet, placing the required dosage into a paper cup, and then dispensing it to the patient. Additionally, there may be other charges included such as shipping and handling, charges for labeling and inventorying the item, the time it takes for someone to put the information into the computer system, and also the amount of time needed to bill for the item.

Some insurance carriers also will request itemized billings. This allows them to be sure that there are not any noncovered services or items included in the bill.

Personal Items

Personal items are those items that are primarily for the comfort of the patient and are not medically necessary. The following items are considered to be personal items and are not usually covered by a plan. These charges may need to be coded separately, or they may be combined with other ancillary charges. However, patients should be warned at the time they request such items that they are not usually covered by an insurance carrier.

Most hospitals automatically issue an admission kit to incoming patients. An **admission kit** usually includes an emesis basin, carafe, cup, lotion, tissue, and mouthwash. Some plans administratively allow for one kit. Additional kits are usually not covered. This type of kit also may be called a maternity kit, Ob-Gyn kit, hygiene kit, patient comfort kit, or another name.

On the Job Now

Directions: Answer the following questions without looking back at the material just covered. Write your answer in the space provided.

1. Which form would be used to bill services rendered by a hospital or hospital-employed personnel?

_____

2. Why do many patients prefer to receive an itemized bill? _____

_____

Practice Pitfalls

These are a few examples of personal items that are not considered medically necessary and are often excluded by the insurance carrier.

- Barber expenses.
- Personal hygiene kit.
- Videotaping of birth.
- Birth certificate, photos.
- Cot rental.
- Room transfer requested.
- Lotion.
- Television.
- Telephone.
- Toothbrush, toothpaste.
- Guest trays.
- Mouthwash.
- Gift shop expenses.
- Slippers.

DRGs

In the early days of health insurance, providers were reimbursed for each procedure they performed. There was no incentive to limit the procedures.

Diagnosis Related Groups (DRGs) were introduced as a means of cost control for insurance carriers (especially Medicare). The idea was to encourage hospitals to help limit some of the costs associated with certain illnesses.

Not all illnesses that a patient receives treatment for are part of a DRG. There is a specific list of DRGs that have been identified by Medicare and also by some other insurance carriers.

When a patient receives treatment for a DRG illness, the claim is handled differently than if the patient is not being treated for a DRG illness. Under a DRG, the insurance carrier (including the Medicare insurance carrier) will pay a set amount for the total care for the treatment. Even if the hospital costs are above this amount, they will only receive this set amount. They cannot balance bill the patient for any amount that is not covered by the DRG set amount.

However, if the hospital's charges are less than the set amount, they will still receive the set amount from the carrier. They are allowed to keep the full amount.

It is important for the hospital to note those illnesses that are covered under DRGs. Although this notation should not drastically alter patient care, it may remind doctors not to order services or procedures that are questionable.

Ambulatory Patient Classifications

Ambulatory Patient Classifications (APCs) are similar to DRGs but are for patients who receive services on an outpatient basis. As with DRGs, a set amount is allowed for the procedure, all ancillary services, and any necessary follow-up care.

APCs are used as part of the Medicare Outpatient **Prospective Payment System (PPS)**. This is a system set up by Medicare that pays hospitals under APCs rather than on a fee-for-service basis.

It is important for billers to realize that the services provided by a hospital may cover more than

On the Job Now

Directions: Answer the following questions without looking back at the material just covered. Write your answer in the space provided.

1. What does DRGs stand for and why were they introduced? _____

_____

2. What is the difference in the handling of a claim by the insurance carrier for a DRG illness? _____

_____

one APC, and multiple APCs may be included on a single claim.

Many of the services covered under Medicare Part B are grouped under APCs. These include radiation therapy, clinic visits, ER visits, diagnostic tests and services, surgical pathology, cancer chemotherapy, and so on.

Medicare patients who are covered by Part B but not by Part A may have certain additional services covered under APCs.

When billing using APCs, it is important to remember that the single APC code covers all facility charges and services. However, the professional services of physicians are paid as a separate expense. These providers should continue to bill using a separate CMS-1500 form.

Medicare often will use fiscal intermediaries to group the procedures on a hospital bill into the APC groups. For examples of APC groups, look at the C Codes section of the HCPCS.

Excluded Services

Certain services are excluded from APC grouping. These services include ambulance, physical and occupational therapy, speech-language pathology, clinical diagnostic laboratory, durable medical equipment, and nonimplantable prosthetic and orthotic devices. These services will be reimbursed at the separate fee-for-service rate.

Additionally, physicians and nonphysician practitioners continue to be reimbursed under the fee-for-service basis. Nonphysician practitioners include physician's assistants, nurse practitioners, certified nurse midwives, and psychologists.

APCs are only for outpatient care. Thus, services that require the patient to be admitted to the hospital are not covered under the PPS system.

Most hospitals are automatically included in the PPS system. This includes rural hospitals with fewer than 100 beds, certain cancer hospitals, and children's hospitals. However, these types of hospitals may be exempt from some reductions in their Medicare payments.

Chargemaster Descriptions

In previous years, patients were not expected to understand all the items included on their hospital bill. Many of the items were listed by code number, supply number, or by a medical term that was difficult to understand.

Recent legislation has mandated that the information contained on a hospital billing be written in everyday language. This allows the patient to double-check their bill and to reconcile the statement they receive from the hospital with the explanation of benefits received from the insurance carrier. Thus, hospital billing departments are now required to include descriptions on their line item bills that are written in easily understood language. All patients must be charged uniformly for the same service delivered in the same setting.

To comply with this new regulation, each provider is required to have a **Chargemaster Description List (CDL)**. The chargemaster is a list that includes all hospital procedures, services, supplies, and drugs that are billed on the UB-92. A complete service listing includes each of the following components:

Department Name. The name of the department in which the charge originated. Each department should have an abbreviated code that designates the department where the code originates from. For example, the Cardiac Intensive Care Unit might be designated CICU.

Department Number. Each department should be assigned their own number. This allows you to verify quickly the department where the charges originated.

Charge Description Number. Each charge should be given its own individual reference number. This is a unique number assigned by the provider. Charges that originate in a single department often receive similar numbers.

Revenue Code. This is the code that normally appears on the UB-92. (For more information, see the UB-92 chapter.)

Description. A description of the charge or service. This description should be specific enough for the patient to understand the service or item they are being charged for.

CPT® Code. If the service has an appropriate CPT® code associated with it, that code should be listed in this field.

HCPCS Code. If the service or item has an appropriate HCPCS code associated with it, that code should be listed in this field.

Charge. The charge for the service. This should be the normal fee that the provider charges for this service.

Descriptions, codes, and other parts of the CDL should be checked on a regular basis to ensure that they are still accurate and complete. Additionally, the medical biller should become aware of any charges for which the insurance-allowed amount is greater than the billed amount. This may indicate a need to increase the amount charged by the provider in order to receive maximum reimbursement from insurance carriers. This information will be included on an Explanation of Benefits (EOB), which is provided by the insurance carrier on reimbursement of the claim. It is often attached to the check and indicates how the insurance carrier determined the appropriate payment amount.

Providers also need to create an itemized billing form that lists these items. This will allow the patient to see exactly what they are being charged for and what the cost is.

As a medical biller, you may be responsible for choosing the right charge description for billing the patient and for creating itemized patient statements for those patients that request them. You may even be responsible for entering new charge descriptions into the master list.

It is important to watch the CDL as you are using it so that you can spot any errors or items that might seem to be overbilled or underbilled. These errors should be brought to your supervisor's attention immediately.

Entering Charges

There are many people who deal with a patient in a hospital setting. Each of these people may be providing goods or services that need to be billed to the patient. For example, a patient may request pain medication from a nurse. The nurse will contact the doctor with the request. The doctor will prescribe the drugs, and often will be the one to make a note on the patient's chart. The health unit coordinator may be responsible for ordering the dosage of medication from the pharmacy. However, a nurse may be responsible for actually handing the drug to the patient.

In these cases, there must be a specific policy for the recording of information in the patient's chart. If you are responsible for hospital or facility billing, it is important to understand and follow the guidelines for billing patients. Without such a policy, there is a chance that many of the drugs or other items dispensed will not be charged to the patient.

There are several common methods for ensuring that patients are billed for the services and supplies they use.

Bar Coding—Some hospitals place bar codes on every item that they receive into inventory (if the item does not already have a bar code attached). This bar code contains a unique number, and each type of item will receive a different bar code number. A computer billing and inventory system is set up that contains the information to correspond with that bar code number. For example, one number will be used to designate an admit kit and the common charge of $25 for that kit.

When a patient requests or is prescribed an item, the bar code for that item will be scanned into their account. The charge will then appear on their account record in the same way that scanning a bar code rings up your charges in a supermarket.

Some items are too small to receive a bar code (i.e., individual capsules or pills). In these cases, the bar code is placed on the outside of the bottle or on a set of labels nearby. When medicine is dispensed, the appropriate bar code is scanned and the information entered into the patient's account.

Some hospitals choose to use peel-off bar codes. When an item is dispensed, the bar code will be peeled off the item and placed on the patient's chart.

Then, at a later date, all of the items in the patient chart will be scanned in at the same time. After this is done, the page will be replaced with a new blank page. This prevents scanning an item twice and potentially double-billing the patient. In some hospitals, the job of scanning items will fall to the health unit coordinator or a nurse. In other hospitals, it may be the job of the billing department.

Coding from charts—Some hospitals have billers create claims from the information contained in the patient chart. This information can be in the form of triage reports, operative reports, patient history reports, and the day-to-day treatment reports for the patient. It is the responsibility of the hospital biller to obtain the information from the chart regarding the goods and services that were provided.

Combined bar code and chart method—Some hospitals will have some items handled by bar code; other items will need to be obtained from the patient chart. For example, the goods delivered to the patient may be covered by the bar coding method, but other items such as room and board charges will need to be entered by the biller.

Other methods—Although these situations cover many facilities, other facilities may have their own methods for keeping track of goods and services used by the patient. Therefore, it is important to verify the proper billing procedures with your supervisor before billing hospital claims.

Regardless of the type of billing method used, it is the job of the biller to bill claims in a timely manner. This usually means billing patients as soon as their hospital stay is completed. If a patient is receiving extended care, interim billings may need to be created.

Interim Billings

An **interim billing** is a periodic billing for services before the patient is discharged from the hospital.

When creating interim billings, it is important to include all charges through a specified date of service on a single claim form. Subsequent claim forms should cover dates after the closing date of the earlier interim bill. It is important to include all charges in order to reduce the possibility of confusion for an insurance carrier. If the carrier receives more than one bill with the same date of service, some or all of the charges may be denied as duplicate. For example, if a patient received the same medication at two different times during the day, but each medication is billed on a separate claim, the insurance carrier may determine that the second medication charge is merely a duplicate billing of the first one.

How Billing Affects Other Departments

It is important for billers to realize that the information that they enter for patient charges will affect many other hospital departments as well. Each year, hospitals will determine their budgets based on the services and billing of the year before. If billing has been done improperly, a department might have a lower budget than it needs to maintain proficiency.

Additionally, staffing is often allocated based on the amount of services provided and revenues generated by a specific department. Incorrect billing might cause a specific department to be over- or understaffed for the upcoming year.

Supplies also are ordered based on billing charts. Many computer programs have inventory programs tied to them. These programs will indicate when a certain supply is low and may need to be reordered. If items are billed incorrectly, there is the possibility that the facility may run out of an item needed for patient care. This can lead to extra charges incurred from having to rush-order the items or even lead to a lower level of patient care.

Because of these factors, it is vitally important that billers pay close attention to the details of the items being billed. Be sure you are choosing the correct code for the service or item provided.

Preauthorization, Precertifications, and Utilization Reviews

One of the most common jobs of the biller is to handle the preauthorization and precertification of services. Many insurance carriers require the hospital to precertify services before or within a certain period of receiving the services. Without the proper precertification or preauthorization, the insurance carrier may reduce benefits on a claim or refuse to pay for the services altogether.

For more information on completing precertification and preauthorization, see the Managed Care chapter. However, you should be aware that managed care insurers are not the only plans that may require preauthorization, precertification, or utilization review.

Ambulatory Surgical Centers

Ambulatory surgical centers (surgi-centers) are centers equipped to allow for the performance of surgery on an outpatient basis. These centers may be freestanding or affiliated with a major acute care facility. Surgi-centers provide financial savings by eliminating the need for admission into an inpatient facility. An ambulatory surgical facility is a specialized facility that meets all eight of the professionally recognized standards:

1. Provides a setting for outpatient surgeries.

2. Does not provide services or accommodations for overnight stays.

3. Has at least two operating rooms and one recovery room; all the medical equipment needed to support the surgery being performed; x-ray and laboratory diagnostic facilities; and emergency equipment, trays, and supplies for use in life-threatening events.

4. Has a medical staff that is supervised full time by a physician and a registered nurse when patients are in the facility.

5. Maintains a medical record for each patient.

6. Has a written agreement with a local acute care facility for the immediate transfer of patients who require greater care than can be provided on an outpatient basis.

7. Complies with all state and federal licensing and other legal requirements.

8. Is not an office or clinic for any physician.

Usually, plans provide benefits on a global basis, covering the facility room usage charge and supplies (i.e., anesthesia gases, medications, trays) on the same basis as inpatient hospital services.

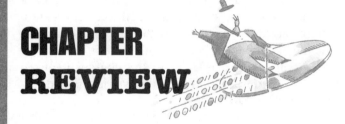

CHAPTER REVIEW

Summary

- The UB-92 is the claim form used when billing for hospital services. It was created by the National Uniform Billing Committee to allow for the necessary information to be inserted on a single form, thus eliminating the need for attachments.

- You should familiarize yourself with the form and know the necessary information. Completely and accurately filling out the UB-92 will help to ensure proper claim payments without unnecessary delays.

- Billing in a hospital setting has several differences from billing in a medical office. Although medical offices often bill using only a CMS-1500, hospitals may use a CMS-1500 for professional services and a UB-92 for facility charges. Additionally, an itemized bill may be used to provide patients with a list of all goods and services received.

- Hospitals often will charge for each individual item received by a patient. Billing is done using a bar code method, using information from a patient chart, a combination of these two methods, or some other method. Regardless of the method used, it is important for the biller to ensure that all items used and all services received by the patient are billed.

- In an effort to manage costs, Medicare and other insurance carriers are implementing payment by DRGs and APCs. Payments made under DRG or APC provisions reimburse the hospital a set amount for the total cost of treatment for a specified condition rather than paying for each individual item or service.

Assignments

Complete the Questions for Review.
Complete Exercise 12–1 through 12–4.

Questions for Review

Directions: Answer the following questions without looking back at the material just covered. Write your answers in the space provided.

1. What is the UB-92 billing form used for? _____

   _____

2. What does Item 17 indicate? _____

   _____

3. What are occurrence codes and occurrence span codes, and what is the difference between them? _____

   _____

   _____

4. What would the code 20 indicate in Item 21 on the UB-92? _____

   _____

5. What would the code 03 indicate in Item 72 on the UB-92? _____

   _____

6. On the UB-92, what is a "Medicare Provider Number"? _____

   _____

7. How would you write the following times on a UB-92?

   1. 9:55 A.M. _____   **6.** 2:48 P.M._____

   2. 10:25 P.M._____   **7.** 5:56 P.M._____

   3. 1:18 A.M. _____   **8.** Noon _____

   4. 8:01 P.M._____   **9.** Midnight _____

   5. 12:23 A.M. _____   **10.** 6:06 P.M._____

8. What does a "Y" in the "Release Information" item denote? _____

   _____

9. A patient entered the hospital on 12/01/CCYY with chest pains. He was diagnosed as having a heart attack and admitted. On 12/05/CCYY the patient developed pneumonia. On 12/10/CCYY the patient expired because of causes associated with pneumonia. On 12/12/CCYY you bill the insurance company for services rendered through 12/04/CCYY. What is the proper diagnosis for the patient? _____

10. Are the sources of admission codes the same for a newborn baby as they are for an adult? _____

11. What is a PPS? _____

_____

_____

12. What is a DRG and how does it work? _____

_____

_____

13. What is the most common claim form used to bill for hospital services? _____

14. What is an APC and to what type of facility does it apply? _____

_____

_____

If you are unable to answer any of these questions, refer back to that section in the chapter, and then fill in the answers.

Exercise 12-1

Directions: Complete a hospital admission form and a UB-92 for the following scenarios. In all cases, the hospital is Provider Medical Center. Refer to the Patient Data Table and Provider Data Table in Appendix C for information.

Upon completion of the UB-92, use an Insurance Claims Register (located in Appendix B) and list all claims that have been fully prepared and are ready for submission to the insurance carrier for payment. Enter the date that you created the UB-92 in the **Date Claim Filed** column.

1. Abby Addison was brought into the ER on 3/7/CCYY after losing consciousness at home. Her condition has progressed from influenza to pneumonia. Annette Adams, M.D. was the attending physician. Dr. Adams's UPIN number is A00720.

Additional information is as follows:

Patient Control #:	PMC97917
Medical Record #:	BA4907
Admit Time:	9:00 A.M.
Discharge Time:	4:20 P.M.
Discharged To:	Home

The following hospital charges were incurred:

Item	# Days or Units	Cost	Total Charge
Room and Board	3	$395.00	$1185.00
Pharmacy	23		845.00
IV Therapy	21		386.15
Med-Surg Supplies	18		224.25
Laboratory	36		727.00
Respiratory Services	3		269.35
EKG/ECG	1		161.53
SUBTOTAL			**$3,798.28**
PAYMENTS/ADJUSTMENTS			**$ 0.00**
BALANCE DUE			**$3,798.28**

2. Bobby Bumble entered the hospital on 3/30/CCYY with a ruptured appendix. Brett Barron, M.D. was the attending physician Dr. Barron's UPIN number is B47921.

Additional information is as follows:

Patient Control #:	PMC71721
Medical Record #:	OB4263
Admit Time:	10:30 A.M.
Discharge Time:	3:45 P.M.
Discharged To:	Home
Procedure Performed:	Appendectomy
Date Procedure Performed:	3/30/CCYY

The following hospital charges were incurred:

Item	# Days or Units	Cost	Total Charge
Room and Board	4	$395.00	$1,580.00
Pharmacy	42		1,567.50
Laboratory	23		983.30
IV Therapy	14		561.50
Med-Surg Supplies	39		1,937.25
Pathology Lab	10		110.50
Dx X-Ray	12		898.90
OR Services	8		977.50
Anesthesia	1		882.25
Respiratory Services	2		74.75
Recovery Room	1		241.45
SUBTOTAL			**$9,814.90**
PAYMENTS/ADJUSTMENTS			**$ 500.00**
BALANCE DUE			**$9,314.90**

3. Cathy Crenshaw entered the hospital emergency room on 4/1/CCYY for treatment of a fractured arm. Cathy fractured her arm when she fell from a stool at home. Carol Carpenter, M.D. was the attending physician. Dr. Carpenter's UPIN number is C12761.

Additional information is as follows:

Patient Control #:	PMC69623
Medical Record #:	AC1616

Procedure Performed: Closed treatment of ulnar shaft fracture without manipulation

Date Procedure Performed: 4/1/CCYY

The following hospital charges were incurred:

Item	# Days or Units	Cost	Total Charge
ER	1		$250.00
Pharmacy	2		75.25
X-Ray	4		147.50
SUBTOTAL			**$472.75**
PAYMENTS/ADJUSTMENTS			**$ 0.00**
BALANCE DUE			**$472.75**

4. Daisy Doolittle entered the hospital for treatment of acute pelvic inflammatory disease on 4/1/CCYY. Deborah Davidson, M.D. was attending physician. Dr. Davidson's UPIN number is D70007.

Additional information is as follows:

Patient Control #:	PMC47898
Medical Record #:	AD7431
Admit Time:	12:15 P.M.
Discharge Time:	9:30 A.M.
Discharged To:	Home

The following hospital charges were incurred:

Item	# Days or Units	Cost	Total Charge
Room and Board	3	$395.00	$1,185.00
Pharmacy	31		321.50
Laboratory	9		314.25
Med-Surg Supplies	19		783.15
Path Lab	11		652.70
IV Therapy	4		89.60
Ultrasound	2		685.20
SUBTOTAL			**$4,031.40**
PAYMENTS/ADJUSTMENTS			**$ 0.00**
BALANCE DUE			**$4,031.40**

5. Edward Edmunds entered the hospital for surgery on his shoulder on 3/10/CCYY. Edward had tendonitis with calcium deposits on his shoulder that restricted movement. Dr. Paul Provider was the attending physician.

Additional information is as follows:

Patient Control #:	PMC56962
Medical Record #:	DE9892
Admit Time:	6:40 A.M.
Discharge Time:	10:20 A.M.
Discharged To:	Home
Procedure Performed: Removal of subdeltoid calcareous deposits, open	
Date Procedure Performed:	3/10/CCYY

The following hospital charges were incurred:

Item	# Days or Units	Cost	Total Charge
Room and Board	2	$395.00	$790.00
Pharmacy	12		567.50
Laboratory	6		483.30
IV Therapy	3		361.50
Med-Surg Supplies	37		937.25
Pathology Lab	7		95.50
Dx X-Ray	6		298.40
OR Services	1		928.50
Anesthesia	1		875.25
Respiratory Services	4		74.75
Recovery Room	1		236.45
SUBTOTAL			**$5,648.40**
PAYMENTS/ADJUSTMENTS			**$ 0.00**
BALANCE DUE			**$5,648.40**

Exercise **12-2**

Directions: Find and circle the words listed below. Words can appear horizontally, vertically, diagonally, forward, or backward.

1. Admission Kit
2. Ambulatory Surgical Centers
3. Charge Master Description List
4. Interim Billing
5. Prospective Payment System

```
T Y U H D E H K D H R K B C T V Z X A S I Y C N U Y F
Z S B F C F U V I V J E Z X L J M J H R F Y H W V N N
Q L I D O D J L T K F B Q W O X Q L O E C V U A S H W
R C G L Y T G X M O R I P S J M H Z I T J J O L R U Y
W A C W N R F A X J T S A N C A U D O N V A F C K A H
S C Y H E O P E J X U R V D V N S V E I L Z V S O N
Q T Y C L I I O G J W L R M E I R J C C N W J J Z S N
A Z A I G F A T G I A R I M S E R C B L T O J T X V M
Z A Q T V U K Z P I W S O R K P D L N A E E R K D D Q
B T W B U D S O M I S W Y V Y S O R O C R M U R U M G
G K A L H S R J I I R E M N J X B P R I I J U L N B E
D B Z J G D I S O M A C Q Y S W Y Z E G M C M Q J C X
M T J B E L G N Q A M O S S B A Q V X R B X Q D N Q Y
W O H D A H K Z D U G X F E Y H T C J U I D A A P X R
F S U O G I U E T I X I E G D G Z H W S L X S I J R V
T V K U T Z H Y R C C R O L Y R Y P B Y L E K D A T K
E F S F W V A F H P W A F Z O A E D J R I K Q V U X E
J F Z N G A C N G F I S T C N G T T D O N U A S O R F
V N H Z W M D J B D A P C O E O J C S T G N W S H M U
X F L X Q C S F L Q N W M Q R J E M I A P U V S H K F
F G J C O K S Y W J L D D E E S Q W O L M R P W B Z J
L T U Q W Z T Y X O I H R Z Y E A A A U W E Q O P Q U
S F S J E R Z T S O L J Y O M K Q I Q B M W G O P Z O
C H I N O L S F B F X L G E L Q P P Z M V W T R A Q W
Q S R P C Z F G U A S A W W F R N G N A S X V T A L O
P R O S P E C T I V E P A Y M E N T S Y S T E M M H G
S P B Q N Q D D A I B Y U N U A X O V R F Z D B F D C
```

Exercise **12-3**

Directions: Complete the crossword puzzle by filling in a word from the keywords that fits each clue.

Across

5. A one-digit code indicating how the patient was referred to the facility.

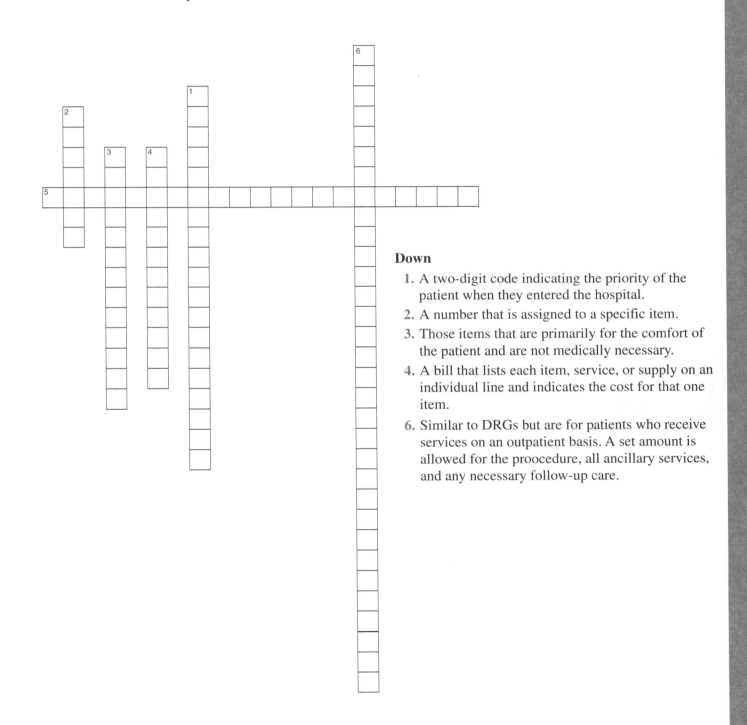

Down

1. A two-digit code indicating the priority of the patient when they entered the hospital.
2. A number that is assigned to a specific item.
3. Those items that are primarily for the comfort of the patient and are not medically necessary.
4. A bill that lists each item, service, or supply on an individual line and indicates the cost for that one item.
6. Similar to DRGs but are for patients who receive services on an outpatient basis. A set amount is allowed for the proocedure, all ancillary services, and any necessary follow-up care.

Exercise 12-4

Directions: Match the following terms with the proper definition by writing the letter of the correct definition in the space next to the term.

1. _____ Condition Codes

2. _____ Occurrence Codes

3. _____ Occurrence Span Codes

4. _____ Revenue Codes

5. _____ Uniform Bill-1992

6. _____ Value Codes

a. Two-digit codes used to identify conditions relating to this bill that may affect payer processing.

b. Codes that identify a specific accommodation, ancillary service, or billing calculation.

c. Codes and associated dates defining a significant event relating to this bill that may affect payer processing.

d. A form used by hospitals or other hospital-type facilities for inpatient and outpatient billing.

e. Codes and the related dates that identify an event relating to the payment of the claim. These codes identify occurrences that happened over a span of time.

f. Codes and the related dollar amounts that identify data of a monetary nature that is necessary for processing the claim.

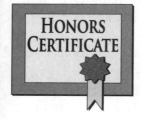

Honors Certification™

The certification challenge for this chapter will be a written test of the information contained in this chapter. Each incorrect answer will result in a deduction of up to 5% from your grade. You must achieve a score of 85% or higher to pass this test. If you fail the test on your first attempt, you may retake the test one additional time. The items included in the second test may be different from those in the first test.

13

Abstracting, Billing, and
Coding from Medical Reports

After completion of this chapter
you will be able to:

- Explain how medical reports relate to billing forms.

- Recognize a triage report, an operative report, a diagnostic report, and a medical history report, and explain their uses.

- Properly create a claim using a medical report.

Keywords and Concepts
you will learn in this chapter:

- Diagnostic Testing Reports
- Operative Reports
- Triage
- Triage Reports

Medical reports are required for virtually every procedure and for all laboratory and radiology examinations. Medical billers often use medical reports to extract the information needed to complete the billing forms. Virtually all the information needed on a claim form is included in the medical reports and the patient's medical record.

Of the numerous types of medical reports, the most common that are used by medical billers include triage reports, operative reports, and diagnostic testing reports.

Abstracting from Medical Records

The medical biller often will be required to create a claim from medical records contained in the patient's chart. The biller will need to abstract the information from medical reports. Triage reports, operative reports, and diagnostic test reports are just a few of the reports that may be included in a patient's chart.

Triage Reports

Triage is a screening system used by medical personnel to determine patient treatment priority in cases when there are more patients needing treatment than there are medical personnel and resources available. This system is designed to maximize the number of patients treated, and in extreme cases, the number of survivors. Triage reports are generated to help in allocating treatment resources to patients on the basis of need.

Triage reports are generated at the scene of accidents, in emergency rooms, and in urgent care clinics. For each patient, the emergency staff performs a rapid physical assessment, takes vital signs, and a brief patient history. This information is detailed on a triage report, which is used throughout the emergency encounter with the patient. These reports are usually handwritten rather than typed, as often the speed and accuracy of accumulating the information are more important than appearance.

When assessing the need for patient care, first priority is given to establishment of an airway and basic life-support measures. Second priority is given to bleeding, neurological trauma, and traumatized bones (i.e., fractures, sprains) and tissue (i.e., open wounds, contusions). Patients are reassessed frequently to determine any change of status.

Operative Reports

Operative reports are generated for most surgical procedures performed. The information contained in these reports often is the sole means of information for medical billers. Therefore, it is important that the medical biller understand the basics of an operative report and how to use it to perform medical billing.

Diagnostic Testing Reports

Diagnostic testing often is performed by an independent laboratory, pathologist, or radiologist. **Diagnostic testing reports** are the "readings" or the interpretation of tests performed.

Medical billers need to familiarize themselves with the terminology contained within the reports to understand the procedures that were rendered.

Medical History and Physical Examination Reports

Whenever a patient is examined by a physician, a brief history of that exam is kept as part of the patient's permanent file. This history should include the following:

- Date of service.
- Symptoms and complaints.
- Past medical, social, and family history.
- Review of systems.
- Current medications.
- Diagnosis.
- Laboratory and x-ray examinations ordered or other referrals.
- Other miscellaneous medical data.

A complete physical examination is often performed with the initial office visit, the initiation of a major surgical procedure, and admission to a healthcare facility. A complete physical examination and thorough check of all body systems are undertaken, and the results are documented in the medical record.

The physician is allowed to bill for the service of compiling a medical history and performing a complete examination on a patient. This code would be considered an E/M (Evaluation and Management) code, as it is not a surgical procedure.

CHAPTER REVIEW

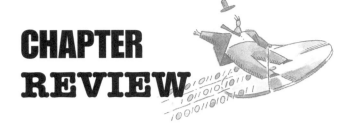

Summary

- The four most common medical reports that medical billers use for billing charges are triage reports, operative reports, diagnostic reports, and medical history and physical examination reports.

- Medical billers should familiarize themselves with these reports and understand how the information relates to the standard medical billing forms.

Assignments

Complete the Questions for Review.
Complete Exercises 13–1 through 13–22.
The reports in Exercises 13–1 through 13–20 follow a patient through a single episode of care. Charge amounts and other varied information are not normally included on the various reports. However, to provide all of the information needed to properly complete these exercises, charge amounts and other information have been included on these reports. The providers for all of these exercises Accept Medicare Assignment, and have an Authorization to Release Information and an Assignment of Benefits signed and on file.

Questions for Review

Directions: Answer the following questions without looking back at the material just covered. Write your answers in the space provided.

1. What are triage reports? _____

   _____

2. What are operative reports? _____

   _____

3. What are diagnostic reports? _____

   _____

4. List six items included on a patient history.

   1. _____

   2. _____

   3. _____

   4. _____

   5. _____

   6. _____

5. In what way does a medical biller use these reports? _____

   If you are unable to answer any of these questions, refer back to that section in this chapter, and then fill in the answers.

Triage Reports

Directions: Complete the appropriate billing form for the following triage reports.

Step 1
Determine the correct billing form to use. These reports are for hospital services.

Step 2
Transfer the information from the triage report to the billing form. Go through the billing form field by field and identify the information that is needed to complete each field.

Step 3
Determine the correct revenue code(s) or CPT® code(s) and the amount charged for the service(s) performed.

Step 4
Transfer the information from the triage report to the billing form. Refer to the Patient Data Table in Appendix C for additional information.

Exercise 13-1

<table>
<tr><td colspan="2">

Arcadia Medical Center
8000 Another Street
Anytown, USA 12345
(765) 555-5555
TIN: 61-0507820

DATE: 01/13/CCYY
</td><td colspan="3">

EMERGENCY SERVICE REPORT
ALLERGIES
NKA

CURRENT MEDS:
NONE

MEDICAL RECORD # 33299-08/Patient Control # 08-99233

PATIENT INFORMATION

Abby Addison
5678 Any Avenue, Anytown, USA 12345
(765) 555-4321
</td></tr>
</table>

ARRIVED VIA: Ambulance	ACCOMPANIED BY: Friend	P.M.D.	TEL. #	NOTIFIED ☐
TRIAGE TIME 14:09 T 98 P 110 R 23 BP 115/82		TIME T P R BP		
LAST TET. TOX. DATE		SIGN:		

25 y/o white female with severe abd pain and nausea beginning 1-12-CCYY. Hematemesis this a.m.
Pt was hospitalized on 1-6-CCYY with epigastric pain. Pt s/p ERCP on 1-10-CCYY stone removed. D/C home 1-11-CCYY.

Pos – dizziness and lightheadedness
Neg – c/p, dyspnea
Neg – dysuria

EMERG ROOM	$205.00
MED-SURG SUPPLIES	$ 54.60
LABORATORY	$172.24
ULTRASOUND	$225.07

DOCTORS ORDERS

TIME	INIT	RESULTS
		RUA:
		CBC: HGB/HCT 10.2/30
		WBC OTHER 14.4
		DIFF: P B M
		E B L
		LYTES:
		Na 140 K 4.5
		CO2 CL
		GLU:126
		BUN:23
		CREAT:0.6
		OTHER LAB
		Beta HCg
		ChL 100
		HCO3 25
		ABG:
		FI02 BE
		PCO2 PO2
		%SAT pH
		X-RAY:
		U/S gallbladder and Upper Abd
		EKG:

COMMUNICATION LOG

CONSULT	CALLED	COMMENTS

DISCHARGE IMPRESSION	DR. ORDERS	TIME	SITE	SIGNATURE
	Discharged to home			

DRAW WOUND IN DIAGRAM WOUND LENGTH_____ ☐ COMPLEX ☐ SIMPLE ☐ PLASTIC DEPTH _____	INVOLVEMENT DISTAL ROM _____OK DISTAL SENS _____OK DISTAL CIRG _____OK TENDONS _____OK	TREATMENT TIME OUT: ☐ Y ☐ N BET. PREP ☐ Y ☐ N IRREG ☐ Y ☐ N ANESTH. 1% XYLOC. DRESSING_____ ☐ Y ☐ N SUTURES ☐ Y ☐ N SPLINT	☐ CHARGES ☐ VALUABLES LISTED ☐ NURSES NOTES ☐ AFTER CARE INSTR. GIVEN

PLAN _ Esophagogastroduodenoscopy

CONDITION: ☐ GOOD   X FAIR   ☐ POOR
DISPOSITION: ☐ HOME   ☐ LEFT WITHOUT BEING SEEN   X ADMIT
                    ☐ LEFT AGAINST MEDICAL ADVICE   ☐ EXPIRED
                    ☐ TRANSFER TO _____   RET TO WORK

Ann Anderson M.D. Attending M.D.	Other M.D.	Alfred Ackerman M.D. Other M.D.
Ann Anderson M.D. PRINT NAME	A79797 UPIN	PRINT NAME	UPIN	Alfred Ackerman M.D. PRINT NAME	A32908 UPIN

Exercise 13-2

Bronson Brothers Medical Center **9876 Bright Lane** **Anytown, USA 12345** **(765) 555-4121** **TIN: 26-0907221** DATE: 06/16/CCYY	**EMERGENCY SERVICE REPORT**

ALLERGIES
NKA

CURRENT MEDS:
NONE

MEDICAL RECORD # 9888-0009

PATIENT INFORMATION

Bobby Bumble
93485 Bumpkiss Court, Anytown, USA 12345
(765) 555-4756

ARRIVED VIA: Ambulance	ACCOMPANIED BY: Friend	P.M.D.	TEL. #	NOTIFIED ☐
TRIAGE TIME 09:37 T 97.5 P 83 R 23 BP 122/81		TIME T P R BP		
LAST TET. TOX. DATE		SIGN:		

49 y/o male w/injury to Rt wrist. Pt states he was running to catch a bus when his Rt ankle gave way. Pt fell to pavement injuring Rt wrist.

Neg – L.O.C.
Neg – head trauma
Neg – dizziness or lightheadedness
Pos – multiple excoriation Rt hand

EMERG ROOM	$205.00	
MED-SURG SUPPLIES	$119.16	
DX XRAY	$272.72	

DOCTORS ORDERS

TIME	INIT	RESULTS
		RUA:
		CBC: HGB/HCT
		WBC OTHER
		DIFF: P B M
		E B L
		LYTES:
		Na K
		CO2 CL
		GLU:
		BUN:
		CREAT:
		OTHER LAB
		ABG:
		FI02 BE
		PCO2 PO2
		%SAT pH
		X-RAY: Rt wrist AP & Lat
		Rt ankle AP & Lat
		EKG:

COMMUNICATION LOG

CONSULT	CALLED	COMMENTS

DISCHARGE IMPRESSION	DR. ORDERS	TIME	SITE	SIGNATURE
Sprain, Rt wrist	F/U with Bill Blake M.D. re: wrist injury			

DRAW WOUND IN DIAGRAM	INVOLVEMENT	TREATMENT	TIME OUT:18:01	
WOUND LENGTH_____ ☐ COMPLEX ☐ SIMPLE ☐ PLASTIC DEPTH_____	DISTAL ROM _____OK DISTAL SENS_____OK DISTAL CIRG_____OK TENDONS_____OK	☐ Y ☐ N BET. PREP ☐ Y ☐ N ANESTH. 1% XYLOC. DRESSING_____ ☐ Y ☐ N SUTURES	☐ Y ☐ N IRREG ☐ Y ☐ N SPLINT	☐ CHARGES ☐ VALUABLES LISTED ☐ NURSES NOTES ☐ AFTER CARE INSTR. GIVEN

PLAN: Splint Applied

CONDITION: X GOOD   ☐ FAIR   ☐ POOR
DISPOSITION: X HOME   ☐ LEFT WITHOUT BEING SEEN   ☐ ADMIT
☐ LEFT AGAINST MEDICAL ADVICE   ☐ EXPIRED
☐ TRANSFER TO _____   RET TO WORK

Bruno Ball M.D. M.D.		M.D.		M.D.
Bruno Ball M.D. PRINT NAME	B26921 UPIN	PRINT NAME UPIN	PRINT NAME UPIN	

Exercise 13-3

Canyon City Hospital
4440 Center Drive
Anytown, USA 12345
(765) 555-8972
TIN: 08-1218240

EMERGENCY SERVICE REPORT

ALLERGIES:
NKA

CURRENT MEDS:
NPH Insulin, 50U, Glucotrol, Lithium,

MEDICAL RECORD # 8779-09

PATIENT INFORMAITON

Cathy Crenshaw
9876 Cranbury Lane, Anytown, USA 12345
(765) 555-3579

DATE: 11/1/CCYY

ARRIVED VIA: Car	ACCOMPANIED BY: self						P.M.D.		TEL. #		NOTIFIED ☐
TRIAGE TIME 07:00	T 98	P 102	R 24	BP 170/90			TIME	T	P	R	BP
LAST TET. TOX.		DATE					SIGN:				

50 y/o female with c/o N/V x 1.5 wks.

Neg – dizziness
Pos – lightheadedness
Neg – L.O.C.
Pos – icterus

EMERG ROOM	$205.00
MED-SURG SUPPLIES	$ 37.02
ULTRASOUND	$225.07

DOCTORS ORDERS

TIME	INIT	RESULTS
		RUA:
		CBC: HGB/HCT
		WBC OTHER
		DIFF: P B M
		E B L
		LYTES:
		Na K
		CO2 CL
		GLU:
		BUN:
		CREAT:
		OTHER LAB
		ABG:
		FI02 BE
		PCO2 PO2
		%SAT pH
		X-RAY:
		U/S Gallbladder/ABD
		EKG:

COMMUNICATION LOG

CONSULT	CALLED	COMMENTS

DISCHARGE IMPRESSION	DR. ORDERS	TIME	SITE	SIGNATURE
Jaundice R/O Bile Duct Obstruction	F/u with Dr. Callahan			

DRAW WOUND IN DIAGRAM
WOUND LENGTH_____
☐ COMPLEX ☐ SIMPLE
☐ PLASTIC DEPTH _____

INVOLVEMENT
DISTAL ROM
_____OK
DISTAL SENS _____OK
DISTAL CIRG _____OK
TENDONS _____OK

TREATMENT
☐ Y ☐ N BET. PREP
☐ Y ☐ N ANESTH. 1% XYLOC.
DRESSING_____
☐ Y ☐ N SUTURES

TIME OUT:14:22
☐ Y ☐ N IRREG

☐ Y ☐ N SPLINT

☐ CHARGES
☐ VALUABLES LISTED
☐ NURSES NOTES
☐ AFTER CARE INSTR. GIVEN

PLAN _____
_____

CONDITION: ☐ GOOD   X FAIR   ☐ POOR
DISPOSITION: X HOME   ☐ LEFT WITHOUT BEING SEEN   ☐ ADMIT
☐ LEFT AGAINST MEDICAL ADVICE   ☐ EXPIRED
☐ TRANSFER TO _____   RET TO WORK

Chris Campbell M.D.					
	M.D.		M.D.		M.D.
Christopher Campbell M.D. PRINT NAME	C29561 UPIN	PRINT NAME	UPIN	PRINT NAME	UPIN

Exercise 13-4

	EMERGENCY SERVICE REPORT		
	ALLERGIES NKA		
Duncan Day Hospital **4499 Door Way** **Anytown, USA 12345** **(765) 555-0196** **TIN: 38-6915703**	**CURRENT MEDS:** NONE		
	Medical Record # 88290499		
	PATIENT INFORMATION Daisy Doolittle 2345 Daffy Lane, Anytown, USA 12345 (765) 555-4311		
DATE: 11/26/CCYY			

ARRIVED VIA: Ambulance Greenlight Ambulance	ACCOMPANIED BY: Self	P.M.D.	TEL. #	NOTIFIED ☐
TRIAGE TIME 07:03 T 97 P 92 R 25 BP 125/85		TIME T P R BP		
LAST TET. TOX. DATE		SIGN:		

DOCTORS ORDERS

		34 y/o Hispanic female, LMP 02/20/CCYY	TIME	INIT	RESULTS
					RUA: 1.008SG
		c/o Vag discharge with bleeding x 1wk. Pt feels she is pregnant, but didn't pass tissue.			
					CBC: HGB/HCT
		Neg – dizzy, lightheadedness			WBC OTHER RBC = 1-2
		Pos – palpable pelvic masses, white vaginal discharge			1-2
					DIFF: P B M
					E B L
					LYTES:
					Na K
					CO2 CL
					GLU:
					BUN:
					CREAT:
					OTHER LAB GC, Wet mount
					Beta HCg
					Gram Stain
					ABG:
		EMERG ROOM $205.00			FI02 BE
		MED-SURG SUPPLIES $ 37.02			PCO2 PO2
		LABORATORY $ 54.04			%SAT pH
		DX XRAY $220.22			X-RAY: Pelvic/low abd
					EKG:

COMMUNICATION LOG

		CONSULT	CALLED	COMMENTS

DISCHARGE IMPRESSION	DR. ORDERS	TIME	SITE	SIGNATURE
Dysfunctional uterine bleeding				

DRAW WOUND IN DIAGRAM WOUND LENGTH_____ ☐ COMPLEX ☐ SIMPLE ☐ PLASTIC DEPTH_____	INVOLVEMENT DISTAL ROM _____OK DISTAL SENS_____OK DISTAL CIRG_____OK TENDONS_____OK	TREATMENT ☐ Y ☐ N BET. PREP ☐ Y ☐ N ANESTH. 1% XYLOC. DRESSING_____ ☐ Y ☐ N SUTURES	TIME OUT: ☐ Y ☐ N IRREG ☐ Y ☐ N SPLINT	☐ CHARGES ☐ VALUABLES LISTED ☐ NURSES NOTES ☐ AFTER CARE INSTR. GIVEN

PLAN D/C home. 1.) F/U with Dr. David Day this week.
2.) Use condoms

CONDITION:	X GOOD	☐ FAIR	☐ POOR
DISPOSITION:	X HOME	☐ LEFT WITHOUT BEING SEEN	☐ ADMIT
	☐ LEFT AGAINST MEDICAL ADVICE		☐ EXPIRED
	☐ TRANSFER TO _____		RET TO WORK

Doris Dean M.D. M.D.		M.D.	M.D.
Doris Dean M.D. PRINT NAME	D85264 UPIN	PRINT NAME UPIN	PRINT NAME UPIN

Exercise 13-5

EMERGENCY SERVICE REPORT		

Eastwood Community Medical Center
7854 East Road
Anytown, USA 12345
(765) 555-8989
TIN: 12-3123152

ALLERGIES
Penicillin

CURRENT MEDS: None

Medical Record # 098-000-432EE

PATIENT INFORMAITON

Edward Edmunds
8888 Every Lane, Anytown, USA 12345
(765)555-7890

DATE: 05/09/CCYY

ARRIVED VIA:	ACCOMPANIED BY: Self	P.M.D.	TEL. #	NOTIFIED ☐
Red Alert Ambulance				

TRIAGE	TIME 06:07	T 97	P 84	R 23	BP 120/80	TIME	T	P	R	BP

LAST TET. TOX.	DATE	SIGN:

66 y/o white male with gunshot wound to both knees.
Pt drove to store. While walking into entrance was struck by bullet
which crossed Lt knee and entered Rt knee.

Neg – L.O.C.
Minimal pain
Minimal bleeding.

DOCTORS ORDERS

TIME	INIT	RESULTS
		RUA:
		CBC: HGB/HCT
		WBC OTHER
		DIFF: P B M
		E B L
		LYTES:
		Na K
		CO2 CL
		GLU:
		BUN:
		CREAT:
		OTHER LAB
		ABG:
		FI02 BE
		PCO2 PO2
		%SAT pH
		X-RAY L and R Knee:
		EKG:

EMERG ROOM	$205.00
PHARMACY	$104.08
MED-SURG SUPPLIES	$ 52.07
DX XRAY	$227.00

COMMUNICATION LOG

CONSULT	CALLED	COMMENTS

DISCHARGE IMPRESSION	DR. ORDERS	TIME	SITE	SIGNATURE
Gunshot wound to knee bilaterally	Cirpo 750 Mg	06:30		

DRAW WOUND IN DIAGRAM	INVOLVEMENT	TREATMENT	TIME OUT:2:58	
WOUND LENGTH_____1"_____ ☐ COMPLEX X SIMPLE ☐ PLASTIC DEPTH _____	DISTAL ROM _____OK DISTAL SENS _____OK DISTAL CIRG _____OK TENDONS _____OK	☐ Y ☐ N BET. PREP ☐ Y ☐ N ANESTH. 1% XYLOC. DRESSING_____ ☐ Y ☐ N SUTURES	☐ Y ☐ N IRREG ☐ Y ☐ N SPLINT	☐ CHARGES ☐ VALUABLES LISTED ☐ NURSES NOTES ☐ AFTER CARE INSTR. GIVEN

PLAN D/C to home. Pt to F/U with Dr. Esther Edelman
tomorrow

CONDITION:	X GOOD	☐ FAIR	☐ POOR	
DISPOSITION:	☐ HOME	☐ LEFT WITHOUT BEING SEEN	X ADMIT	
	☐ LEFT AGAINST MEDICAL ADVICE		☐ EXPIRED	
	☐ TRANSFER TO _____		RET TO WORK	

Eric Ericson M.D.	Evelyn Elliot, M.D.	Ester Edelman, M.D.
M.D.	M.D.	M.D.
Eric Ericson M.D.	E17429	Evelyn Elliot M.D.	E98745	Ester Edelman M.D.	E52352
PRINT NAME	UPIN	PRINT NAME	UPIN	PRINT NAME	UPIN

Operative Reports

Directions: Complete the appropriate billing form for the following operative reports.

Step 1
Determine the correct billing form to use. These reports are for surgical and anesthesiologist services.

Step 2
Transfer the information from the operative report to the billing form. Go through the billing form field by field and identify the information that is needed to complete each field.

Step 3
Determine the correct revenue code(s) or CPT® code(s) and the amount charged for the service(s) performed.

Step 4
Transfer the information from the operative report to the billing form. Refer to the Patient Data Table in Appendix C for additional information.

Exercise 13-6

PATIENT NAME:	Abby Addison	PATIENT'S ACCOUNT NUMBER: 33299-08
SURGEON:	Albert Adler, M.D.	UPIN: A37520
	4753 Apple Lane	
	Anytown, USA 12345	EIN: 34-9600711
PLACE OF SERVICE:	Arcadia Medical Center	
	8000 Another Street	
	Anytown, USA 12345	

DATE OF PROCEDURE: 1-13-CCYY

PREOPERATIVE DIAGNOSIS: Upper gastrointestinal bleed.

POSTOPERATIVE DIAGNOSIS: Most likely cause of the patient's gastrointestinal bleeding was a Mallory-Weiss tear.

NAME OF PROCEDURE: Upper gastrointestinal endoscopy. ($524)

PROCEDURE IN BRIEF: Status post informed consent, the patient was premedicated with Demerol 50 and Versed 2. At this point, an upper GI endoscope was advanced through the esophagus, stomach, and duodenum.

FINDINGS INCLUDED THE FOLLOWING: Normal esophagus, normal stomach, and normal duodenum. There was a slightly raised streak at the GE junction, which was exudative. This was approximately 1 mm × 3 mm. This was consistent with possible Mallory-Weiss tear. No other lesions were appreciated throughout the entire examination. It was also noted that the patient had some mild gastritis consistent with NG tube trauma but no evidence of bleeding.

The overall procedure was tolerated well. The patient was extubated.

ALBERT ADLER, M.D.

AA:AA443
d: 1-14-CCYY
t: 1-14-CCYY
Document: 448800.aaa

Exercise 13-7

DATE:	8/20/CCYY	PATIENT:	Bobby Bumble

PATIENT'S ACCOUNT NUMBER: 9888-0009

PATIENT DOB: 1/1/44

SURGEON:	Ben Bennett, M.D.	UPIN:	B34567
	9810 Brock Lane	PHONE:	(765) 555-9973
	Anytown, USA 12345	SSN:	005-67-8910

ASSISTANT:	Brian Bradley, M.D.	UPIN:	B18976
	5678 Bastion Way	PHONE:	(765) 555-9974
	Anytown, USA 12345	SSN:	566-12-3456

PLACE OF SERVICE: Bronson Brothers Medical Center
9876 Bright Lane
Anytown, USA 12345

PRE-OP DX: Chronic Anterior and Lateral Instability of the Right Ankle

POST-OP DX: Same

PROCEDURE: Anterior Lateral Ligamentous Reconstruction of the Right Ankle Using the Peroneus Brevis Tendon ($672) (assistant surgeon $135)

ANESTHESIOLOGIST:	Bertha Blues, M.D.	UPIN:	B31659
	7654 Bluefield Drive	PHONE:	(765) 555-9975
	Anytown, USA 12345	EIN:	58-6143285

ANESTHESIA: Epidural ($255)

PROCEDURE: The patient was brought into the room and placed in the sitting position. Dr. Blues did an epidural anesthesia without difficulty. Patient was then placed in the supine position. A lift was placed under the right buttock and a sandbag was placed at the foot area when the knee was bent 90°. The entire right lower extremity was then prepped and draped in the usual fashion. A pneumatic tourniquet was used during the initial stages of the case for 22 minutes. This was during the isolation and dissection of the tissues. A long incision was made over the peroneal tendons halfway up the calf, carried behind the lateral malleolus down to the base of the fifth metatarsal. It was dissected through skin and subcutaneous tissue. The sural nerve was not visualized and was felt to be protected by the posterior skin flap. The sheath of the peroneal tendon was then incised its entire length. The peroneus brevis tendon was isolated from the peroneus longus tendon. The brevis tendon was quite small and therefore decision was made during surgery to use the entire tendon rather than the usual half of the tendon. Muscle tissue was dissected from the tendon at the proper length. After measurement for the eventual coursing of the graft, an incision was made across the tendon. The peroneal brevis tendon was then pulled distally and a Bunnell-type suture was placed into the tendon with a double armed 2-0 Ethibond suture. The needles were then cut and a tag was placed. The dissection of the anterior flap was done so that the anterior talofibular area was dissected free. There was a lot of scarring in this area. Hemostasis was obtained by means of cautery. The tourniquet was deflated at this point.

Further dissection was done into the ankle joint so that it was viewed. It was felt to be fairly normal. A small drill hole was placed on the anterior aspect of the fibula and drilled posteriorly. This was widened with a larger drill. The pin was passed through this tunnel from anterior to posterior and was held quite tightly with the foot in neutral position of dorsiflexion plantar flexion and just slight eversion. It was not maximally everted. Sutures were then placed in the tendon and through the bone with #2 Ethibond.

Once this was secured, sutures were placed into the posterior aspect of the tunnel also with 2-0 Ethibond. The peroneal brevis tendon was then further dissected from its sheath and dislodged from its normal groove and carried anterior so the dissection on the calcaneus could occur. The ridge of the calcaneus was identified, and periosteum was stripped using an elevator. The same drill holes were then made keeping the ridge between the two holes and the distance between the holes was approximately 1 cm. The hole was then widened to the same hole as the fibular hole and the graft was passed from posterior to anterior in the calcaneal tunnel. This was done with the suture ligature passer. This was pulled in quite nicely. There was enough graft to suture the remaining part of the graft back into the position of the anterior talar fibular ligament which was done again with #2 Ethibond.

Once wound was all secured with proper sutures, the drawer sign was negative and patient had slight inversion and could be further everted.

The wound was then irrigated with copious amounts of antibiotic solution. Prior to any drill holes, the superior portion of the wound was closed so that the rest of the tendon that was exposed would not dry out. During the procedure, the tendons were kept constantly moistened with antibiotic irrigation fluid. 2-0 Vicryl was then used for the deep subcutaneous tissue, 3-0 Vicryl for the superficial subcutaneous tissue and staples for the skin. The limb was then dressed sterilely and placed into a Jones compression dressing using cotton and fore and aft plaster splints with bias cut and Ace wrap.

The patient tolerated the procedure from an anesthetic standpoint and was transferred to the RR with stable vital signs under the direction of Dr. Blues. Time under anesthesia: 1 hour, 20 min.

BB: BB77   Dictated and authenticated by: BEN BENNETT, M.D.
dt: 8-20-CCYY
t: 8-20-CCYY
Job#:   8112.B

Exercise 13-8

PATIENT NAME: Cathy Crenshaw   PATIENT'S ACCOUNT NUMBER: 8779-09

SURGEON: Chung Choi, M.D.   DATE OF PROCEDURE: 11/12/CCYY
4512 Charley Chan Way   UPIN: C08734
Anytown, USA 12345   EIN: 74-5386738
(765) 555-8196

PLACE OF SERVICE: Canyon City Hospital
4440 Center Drive
Anytown, USA 12345

PREOPERATIVE DIAGNOSIS: Rule out cause of obstructive jaundice in this patient with a recent cholecystec-tomy in March 19YY and now with obvious jaundice.

POSTOPERATIVE DIAGNOSIS: No evidence of obvious stones. Stricture at the distal common bile duct, con-sistent with benign versus malignant disease. Stent placed without difficulty. The patient's pathology report will be reviewed to determine if this is a periampullary carcinoma versus a benign stricture.

NAME OF PROCEDURE:
1. Endoscopic retrograde cholangiopancreatography with biopsy of the ampulla ($346)
2. Cytologic specimens from the pancreatic duct
3. Sphincterotomy ($406)
4. Placement of an internal stent, common bile duct and the duodenum ($410)

PROCEDURE IN BRIEF: Status post informed consent, the patient was premedicated with a total of 150 mg of Demerol, 9 mg of Versed, and 2.5 mg of Glucagon.

At this point, a Pentax upper GI endoscope was advanced through the esophagus into the duodenum and also into the ampulla. The ampulla appeared somewhat erythematous and consistent with the possibility of an infiltrating periampullary carcinoma. A cholangiogram was obtained showing dilatation of the common bile duct with a narrow stricture involving the distal common bile duct. A sphincterotomy was completed at this time and a pancreatogram was also obtained. The pancreatogram appeared normal without any pathology.

A cytologic brush was used to obtain specimens from the pancreatic duct, from the mid body to the ampulla. At this point, with a marked amount of difficulty, the common bile duct was recannulated and a guide wire was advanced into the secondary radicles and a one-step stent was advanced into the common bile duct. This stent was noted to lie between the common hepatic duct and the duodenum with good positioning and good drainage.

The patient also had a biopsy of the ampulla which appeared abnormal, consistent with possible periampullary carcinoma.

CHUNG CHOI, M.D.

CC: CC33
d: 11-12-CCYY
t: 11-12-CCYY
Document: 777.ccc

Exercise 13-9

PATIENT: Doolittle, Daisy   PATIENT'S ACCOUNT NUMBER: 88290499

DATE OF SURGERY: 12/7/CCYY   DOB: 08/01/59

SURGEON: Donald Denny, M.D.*   ASSISTANT: Diana Dorman, M.D.*
4499 Door Way, Ste. 600   4499 Door Way, Ste. 600
Anytown, USA 12345   Anytown, USA 12345
UPIN: D56255   UPIN: D98005
EIN: 62-1368210   EIN: 12-6661243

ANESTHESIOLOGIST: Debbie Donovan*   ANESTHESIA: ($265)   General
4499 Door Way, Ste 600
Anytown, USA 12345
UPIN: D25645
EIN: 22-0709262

PLACE OF PROCEDURE: Duncan Day Hospital
4499 Door Way
Anytown, USA 12345

PRE-OPERATIVE DX: Carcinoma of the Cervix   POST-OP DX: Same

PROCEDURE: Radical Abdominal Hysterectomy, Bilateral Total Pelvic Lymph Node Dissection ($1,713) (assistant surgeon $343), Sigmoidoscopy Removal of Tumor(s) ($546) (assistant surgeon $110), Cystourethroscopy, Ejaculatory Duct Catheterization ($265) (assistant surgeon $53).

FINDINGS: On examination under anesthesia, the vaginal vault was clear. The cervix showed signs of cancer that was biopsied but it seemed to be confined to the cervix and not into the parametrium. Sigmoidoscopy to 20 cm was clear. The bladder was entirely normal with no evidence of problems. Both urethral orifices were clear. The entire abdominal cavity was explored. Liver and gallbladder were normal. The appendix was absent. There was no evidence of any other diseases within the pelvis. No lymph nodes were palpable in the periaortic common iliac and pelvic lymph nodes. The uterus was anterior freely moveable. Both tubes and ovaries appeared normal. There was a corpus luteum cyst on the left ovary and no evidence of any disease once we opened up the parametrium. Superior vesical space and perirectal spaces were clear.

PROCEDURE: Routine prepping and draping of the perineum, inhalation anesthesia. First, examination was carried out using a disposable sigmoidoscope. We examined the rectum to 20 cm. Finding no disease in that area, the bladder was examined using 30° water cystoscopy unit. Finding no disease in that area, the Foley catheter was placed within the bladder and the abdomen was prepped and draped in the usual manner and opened through a transverse incision through skin and subcutaneous tissue and fascia, muscle and peritoneum. Once the peritoneum was opened, and bleeding was controlled with the Bovie, the above findings were noted.

Some peritoneal washings were obtained. The bowel was packed off by means of laparotomy sponges and Balfour retractor was placed within. The uterus was lifted by Carmalt clamps along the broad ligament. The round ligaments were bilaterally clamped, cut, and ligated with stick ties of 0 Vicryl suture. Retroperitoneal space was then opened exposing the ureter and the external iliac vessels. The ureter was dissected down to the tunnel. The infundibulopelvic ligaments were isolated, doubly ligated and cut. Posterior peritoneum was cut down to the ureter. Bladder flap was developed by sharp dissection to the middle third of the vagina. The tissue of this area was dissected off. Lymph node dissection was carried down to the common iliac, external iliac, obturator fossa and hypogastric vessels bilaterally. Lymph nodes on the right side were suspicious for tumor and so were obtained for frozen section.

The entire area was dissected out and bleeding was contained with the Bovie or with clips. The webb was then taken down by first clamping, cutting, and ligating the uterine vessels and part of the webb was taken down with large Weck clips. Once this was accomplished, our attention was directed to the ureter. The ureter was dissected out of its tunnel, the uterine vessels and parametria being taken over it until we could see the ureter from the pelvic brim down to the bladder. The entire webb was taken down with Bovie or hemoclips. Free ties of 2-0 silk suture.

At this point, the posterior peritoneum was cut. The uterosacral ligaments were taken as far laterally as possible. This was taken down with either large Weck clips or stick ties of 0 Vicryl suture until they were entirely free. The rectum was entirely separated from the vagina. The cardinal and uterosacral ligaments were clamped, cut, and ligated with stick ties of 0 Vicryl suture.

The vaginal vault was then entered and the upper third of the specimen was removed. The vaginal vault was closed with interrupted figure 8 of 0 Vicryl suture. Angles were placed with interrupted 0 Vicryl suture. No bleeding was noted from any of the pedicles. The entire pelvis was irrigated with saline. Retroperitoneal drains were then placed with Jackson-Pratts and these were stitched into the skin with 0 silk suture. Retroperitoneal space was closed with 0 Vicryl suture. Sponge and needle counts were reported as correct. The peritoneum was closed with running 0 Vicryl suture. The fascia was closed with interrupted 0 Vicryl suture. Estimated blood loss was 900 cc.

Total time under anesthesia, 2 hr, 15 min.

DONALD DENNY, M.D.

DD:DD333
d: 12/7/CCYY
t: 12/7/CCYY
Document: 5556.dd

*On staff at Duncan Day Hospital

Exercise 13-10

PATIENT NAME:	Edward Edmunds	PATIENT'S ACCOUNT NUMBER:	098-000-432EE

PHYSICIAN:　　　Evelyn Elliot, M.D.　　　ASSISTANT:　　　Ernie Escalante
　　　　　　　　7854 East Road, Ste. 412　　　　　　　　　7854 East Road, Ste. 412
　　　　　　　　Anytown, USA 12345　　　　　　　　　　Anytown, USA 12345
　　　　　　　　UPIN: E98745　　　　　　　　　　　　UPIN: E56123
　　　　　　　　EIN: 09-1605122　　　　　　　　　　EIN: 57-9520009

PLACE OF SERVICE:　　Eastwood Community Medical Center
　　　　　　　　　　7854 East Road
　　　　　　　　　　Anytown, USA 12345

DATE OF OPERATION:　5-10-CCYY

PREOPERATIVE DX:　　Punctate wounds L knee. FB embedded distal R femur, D/T gunshot wound.

POSTOPERATIVE DX:　　Same

ANESTHESIA:　　　　General

OPERATION: Diagnostic and operative arthroscopy, removal of loose and foreign bodies, right knee ($538) (assistant surgeon $108) meniscectomy, right knee medial ($607) (assistant surgeon $122).

PROCEDURE: The patient was prepped and draped in the usual aseptic manner under adequate general anesthetic with the patient in the supine position on a flat operating table with a knee post in place. The arthroscope was introduced into the joint through the anteriolateral portal and the arthroscope was passed into the joint and visualization was started in the medial compartment of the joint. The medial meniscus appeared to be intact with ragged frayed edges but none of which appeared to be a significant tear of the meniscus. The intercondylar notch was found to have and intact anterior cruciate ligament. There was an attached loose body in the anterior portion of the intercondylar notch region along the medial eminence at the base of the anterior cruciate ligament. The lateral compartment was then visualized in its entirety and was found to have no loose bodies. The lateral meniscus was found to have a tear at its anterior to middle third junction. With the aid of basket forceps and motorized incisor shaver, this portion of the meniscus was carefully removed, taking care to leave behind a stable rim of meniscus for support of the patient's knee structures. Following this removal, the loose body in the anterior aspect of the knee was carefully removed with the aid of a pituitary rongeur, and a shaver also was used in this region. Visualization was then turned to the posterior compartments of the knee and in the lateroposterior compartment, there was found a penduculated attached loose body in this region, which was carefully removed in a piecemeal fashion with the pituitary rongeur and with a curved motorized suction incisor blade. Following complete removal of this loose body, a small portion was found to have been detached from the main body of this structure and this was carefully removed with the pituitary rongeur. Attention was then turned to the distal right femur. The foreign body was removed with the aid of a pituitary ronguer and a curved motorized suction incisor blade. Following this, all areas were copiously irrigated. Visualization was carried out in the suprapatellar pouch. There were found no loose bodies in this region. The patient's knee was then carefully flushed of all extraneous fragments and debris and then the puncture incisions were closed with 3-0 nylon suture. Following closure of these punctures, three in total, in the anteromedial, anterolateral as well as the suprapatellar area, the joint was then injected with 25 cc of Marcaine with epinephrine for postop analgesia.

Attention was then turned to the left knee. The arthroscope was introduced through the anteriolateral portal and passed into the joint and visualization was started in the medial compartment of the joint. The medial meniscus appeared to be intact with no significant damage. All areas were copiously irrigated, followed by closure of the punctate wounds (four). The joint was then injected with 25 cc of Marcaine with epinephrine for postop analgesia. Peripheral pulses were checked prior to removing the patient from the operating room. The pulses were adequate and commensurate with the level they were prior to surgery. The patient tolerated this well and was removed from the operating room in satisfactory condition.

EVELYN ELLIOT, M.D.

EE:EE56
d: 5/10/CCYY
t: 5/10/CCYY
Document: 77-997.ee

Diagnostic Reports

Directions: Complete the appropriate billing form for the following diagnostic reports.

Step 1

Determine the correct billing form to use. These reports are for radiology and pathology services.

Step 2

Transfer the information from the operative report to the billing form. Go through the billing form field by field and identify the information that is needed to complete each field.

Step 3

Determine the correct revenue code(s) or CPT® code(s) and the amount charged for the service(s) performed.

Step 4

Transfer the information from the diagnostic report to the billing form. Refer to the Patient Data Table in Appendix C for additional information.

Exercise **13-11**

RADIOLOGY CENTER

PATIENT: Abby Addison   PATIENT'S ACCOUNT NUMBER: 33299-08

REFERRING M.D.:   Ann Anderson, M.D.   DATE: 1-13-CCYY

PROCEDURE: Complete Abdominal Ultrasound, image documentation ($125)

PLACE OF SERVICE: Arcadia Medical Center
                       8000 Another Street
                       Anytown, USA 12345

Scans of the upper abdomen were performed using 3.5 MHz transducer.

The liver is normal in size, contour, and echogenicity. The pancreatic head appears normal in size and echogenic texture. Both kidneys are normal in size, shape and position with a normal echogenic relationship to the liver. The common bile duct measures 4 mm in size, which is well within normal limits, but is inflamed.

INTERPRETATION: Relatively normal gallbladder and upper abdomen.

   Al Alexander, M.D.
   8020 Another Street
   Anytown, USA 12345
   (765) 555-7201
   TIN: 763-76-3763
   UPIN: A96354

AA:AA91
d: 1-13-CCYY
t: 1-14-CCYY
Document: 77738.aa

Exercise 13-12

PATIENT'S NAME: Bobby Bumble   PATIENT'S ACCOUNT NUMBER: 9888-009

PLACE OF SERVICE: Bronson Brothers Medical Center
                              9876 Bright Lane
                              Anytown, USA 12345

X-RAY NUMBER: 80090

ROOM NUMBER: Emergency Room

REFERRING PHYSICIAN: Bruno Ball, M.D.

DATE OF EXAM: 6-19-CCYY

PROCEDURE: X-RAY AP & LAT R ANKLE ($35), X-RAY AP & LAT R WRIST ($37):

INDICATION: Chronic instability R ankle, injury R wrist

FINDINGS:

R ankle: There is no evidence of fx or dislocation. There is evidence of tissue swelling.

R wrist: There is no evidence of fx or dislocation. There is evidence of tissue swelling.

INTERPRETATION: Right ankle: Evidence of tissue swelling. Study limited. Suggest additional studies to correlate physical findings. Suggest MRI to assess tissue damage.

Right wrist: Evidence of tissue swelling.

    Beth Brown, M.D.
    Staff Radiologist
    9876 Bright Lane, Ste. 710
    Anytown, USA 12345
    UPIN: B64820
    EIN: 88-6205121

BB:BB95
d: 6-19-CCYY   1300
t: 6-19-CCYY   1405
Document: 111122.bbb

Exercise **13-13**

RADIOLOGY CENTER

PATIENT: Cathy Crenshaw   PATIENT'S ACCTOUNT NUMBER: 231 010

REFERRING M.D.:   Christopher Campbell

DATE: 11-1-CCYY

PROCEDURE: Complete Abdominal Ultrasound ($125)

PLACE OF SERVICE: Canyon City Hospital
                       44402 Center Drive
                       Anytown, USA 12345

Scans of the upper abdomen were performed using 3.5 MHz transducer.

The liver is normal in size, contour, and echogenicity. The pancreatic head appears normal in size and echogenic texture. Both kidneys are extremely small consistent with renal failure. There is stricture at the distal common bile duct with some inflammation consistent with benign versus malignant disease.

INTERPRETATION: Stricture of the distal common bile duct. Rule out benign versus malignant disease.

> Christine Caplan, M.D.
> 1010 Capital Court
> Anytown, USA 12345
> (765) 555-8450
> SSN 060-10-0601
> UPIN: C05608

CC:CC80
d: 11-1-CCYY
t: 11-1-CCYY
Document: 5566.cc

Exercise **13-14**

PATIENT'S NAME: Daisy Doolittle   PATIENT'S ACCOUNT NUMBER: 88290499

X-RAY NUMBER: 22097222   ROOM NUMBER: Emergency Room

REFERRING PHYSICIAN: Doris Dean, M.D.   DATE OF EXAM: 11/26/CCYY

PLACE OF SERVICE: Duncan Day Hospital
                            4499 Door Way
                            Anytown, USA 12345

SITE: Abdomen X-ray, Single Anteroposterior View ($35)

INDICATION: Dysfunctional uterine bleeding

FINDINGS: Numerous small masses uterus, cervix & vaginal canal

IMPRESSION: Carcinoma of the cervix

     Dave Davis, M.D.
     Staff Radiologist
     4499 Door Way, Ste. 649
     Anytown, USA 12345
     (765) 555-1891
     TIN: 31-3253253
     UPIN: D80908

DD:DD55
d: 11/26/CCYY   1130
t: 11/26/CCYY   1205
Document: 111122.ddd

Exercise 13-15

PATIENT'S NAME:	Edward Edmunds	PATIENT'S ACCOUNT NUMBER: 512555655	
X-RAY NUMBER:	89898003876	ROOM NUMBER:	Emergency Room
REFERRING PHYSICIAN:	Eric Ericson, M.D.	DATE OF EXAM:	5/9/CCYY

PLACE OF SERVICE: Eastwood Community Medical Center
7854 East Road
Anytown, USA 12345

PROCEDURE: X-RAY AP & LAT R & L KNEES: ($32 left) ($32 right)

INDICATION: Gunshot wound to both knees

FINDINGS:
L knee: No evidence of fracture, dislocation or other significant bone or joint pathology
R knee: FB embedded distal R femur, bone fragments in joint space

IMPRESSION: Gunshot wound to both knees. Bullet in distal right femur

Eve Ellis, M.D.
2929 Earle Court
Anytown, USA 12345
SSN: 865-86-5865
UPIN: E76485

EE: EE66
d: 5/9/CCYY
t: 5/9/CCYY
Document: 333322.eee

Medical History and Physical Examination Report

Directions: Complete the appropriate billing form for the following medical reports.

Step 1
Determine the correct billing form to use. These reports are for physician services.

Step 2
Transfer the information from the operative report to the billing form. Go through the billing form field by field and identify the information that is needed to complete each field.

Step 3
Determine the correct revenue code(s) or CPT® code(s) and the amount charged for the service(s) performed.

Step 4
Transfer the information from the medical report to the billing form. Refer to the Patient Data Table in Appendix C for additional information.

Exercise **13–16**

DATE:	1-13-CCYY
PATIENT NAME:	Abby Addison
PATIENT'S ACCOUNT NUMBER:	33299-08
PHYSICIAN:	Alfred Ackerman 3329 Angels Street Anytown, USA 12345 SSN: 332-93-2933 UPIN: A32908
PLACE OF SERVICE:	Arcadia Medical Center 8000 Another Street Anytown, USA 12345
CHIEF COMPLAINT:	Nausea with hematemesis

HISTORY AND PHYSICAL ($75)

HISTORY OF PRESENT ILLNESS: This 25-year-old female, who was discharged from Arcadia Medical Center 2 days ago, is readmitted after severe abdominal pain and nausea, followed by hematemesis today. The patient had been hospitalized on 1/6/CCYY with epigastric pain due to gallbladder disease. There was also evidence for common bile duct obstruction. The patient underwent a laparoscopic cholecystectomy without complications. A gallstone that was blocking the common bile duct could not be retrieved at that time. The patient underwent ERCP on 1-10-CCYY by Dr. Albert Adler, who successfully removed the obstructing stone. The patient felt relief of abdominal symptoms almost immediately. She was discharged home on 1-11-CCYY. The next day, the patient began to experience nausea. She had several episodes of vomiting without evidence of hematemesis. However, on 1-13-CCYY, her abdominal pain worsened and the patient was brought to the hospital by the paramedics. While in transport, the patient vomited bright red blood. She also notes that her stool had been black after hospital discharge. The patient is now admitted and has an NG tube in place.

PAST MEDICAL HISTORY: The patient was hospitalized at Arcadia Medical Center one week ago with gallbladder disease and common bile duct obstruction, as described in the previous section. There is no history of hypertension, diabetes mellitus or heart disease. There are no known allergies.

REVIEW OF SYSTEMS:

CENTRAL NERVOUS SYSTEM: The patient has felt dizzy during the past 24 hours.

CARDIOVASCULAR, RESPIRATORY: There has been no dyspnea or chest pain.

GASTROINTESTINAL: The patient has had severe nausea with vomiting and hematemesis, as described in the history.

GENITOURINARY: There has been no dysuria.

MUSCULOSKELETAL: There have been no joint disturbances.

VITAL SIGNS: Temperature 97.5, pulse 108, respirations 22, and blood pressure 110/80.

PHYSICAL EXAMINATION:

GENERAL: Well-nourished, well-developed female, alert, somewhat apprehensive. NG tube in place draining coffee-ground material.

HEENT: Pupils are equal, round and reactive to light and accommodation. Extraocular muscles are intact. Fundi are poorly visualized.

NECK: Thyroid not palpable. No jugular venous distention.

CHEST: Breath sounds clear to auscultation bilaterally.

HEART: Regular rate and rhythm. No murmurs.

ABDOMEN: Soft, nontender. Punctate wound, secondary to laparoscopic procedure last week.

EXTREMITIES: No pitting edema.

LABORATORY RESULTS IN THE EMERGENCY ROOM: WBC 14.4, hemoglobin 10.2, hematocrit 30.1. Sodium 140, potassium 4.5, chloride 100, bicarbonate 25, BUN 23, creatinine 0.6. Random glucose 126.

ASSESSMENT:
1. Upper gastrointestinal bleed; rule out secondary to Mallory-Weiss tear, rule out complications stemming from Problem No. 2.
2. Status post ERCP (endoscopic retrograde cholangiopancreatography) 3 days ago due to Problems 3 and 4.
3. Status post hospitalization last week with gallstones and common bile duct obstruction, secondary to retained stone.
4. Status post laparoscopic cholecystectomy last week, secondary to problem No. 3.

PLAN:
1. Admit.
2. NG tube to low suction.
3. Upper endoscopy by Dr. Albert Adler.
4. Follow-up.

ALFRED ACKERMAN, M.D.

AA:AA89
d: 1-13-CCYY
t: 1-14-CCYY
Document: 5555.aa

Exercise **13-17**

BILL BLAKE DOCTOR'S OFFICE
9000 Broadway Street
Anytown, USA 12345

PATIENT:	Bobby Bumble
	93485 Bumpkiss Court,
	Anytown, USA 12345
DATE OF BIRTH:	01-01-44
PATIENT'S ACCOUNT NUMBER:	44444
PLACE OF SERVCE:	Dr. Blake's Office
ATTENDING:	Bill Blake, M.D.
DATE:	8-18-CCYY

HISTORY AND PHYSICAL ($65)

HISTORY OF PRESENT ILLNESS: The patient is a 49-year-old white male with chronic instability of the right ankle. Patient states that 2 months ago he was running to catch a bus and the R ankle collapsed underneath him. He fell to the pavement injuring his R ankle and R wrist. He was transported to Bronson Brothers Medical Center. X-rays showed no evidence of fracture or dislocation to either the ankle or wrist. Patient states that he has had chronic instability of the ankle for "a number of years," possibly relating to a college football injury.

PAST MEDICAL HISTORY: Non contributory.

REVIEW OF SYSTEMS:

CARDIO: There has been no history of chest pain, palpitations.

PULMONARY: No shortness of breath.

MUSCULO: Pain right lower extremity and right hand.

CNS: No dizziness, or lightheadedness or paresthesia.

PHYSICAL EXAMINATION:

GENERAL: Cooperative, pleasant middle aged male who appeared in no acute distress.

HEENT: Mouth—pharynx not injected. Neck—supple without mass or tenderness.

CHEST: Clear with equal breath sounds bilaterally. There was no chest wall discomfort demonstrable on compression.

HEART: Normal S1 and S2 without murmur.

ABDOMEN: Benign.

EXTREMITIES: No clubbing, cyanosis. There is non pitting edema to the right ankle. Limited range of motion. Pain with flexion. Right lower extremity is positive for drawer test and inversion test.

ASSESSMENT: Chronic instability, right ankle.

PLAN:
  1. Admit patient to Bronson Brothers Medical Center.
  2. Consultation orthopedic specialist; Ben Bennett M.D. for evaluation and surgical intervention.

     Bill Blake, M.D.
     9000 Broadway Street
     Anytown, USA 12345
     (765) 555-0022
     SSN: 081-89-3081
     UPIN: B44554

BB: BB46
d: 8-18-CCYY
t: 8-18-CCYY
Document: 77788.bb

Exercise **13-18**

DATE: 11-6-CCYY

PATIENT'S ACCOUNT NUMBER: Cathy Crenshaw

PLACE OF SERVICE: Canyon City Hospital
                                            4440 Center Drive
                                            Anytown, USA 12345

HISTORY AND PHYSICAL ($158)

HISTORY OF PRESENT ILLNESS: Patient is a middle-aged female who is presently hospitalized with jaundice over the past two weeks. The patient has had a long history of medical problems, which include: (1) Adult-onset diabetes mellitus, (2) Hypertension, (3) ESRD, (4) Congestive heart failure, and (5) Pneumonia.

The patient's recent medical history started in March, when she presented with gangrene of the left foot. She underwent a left BK amputation, which was eventually converted to a left AK amputation in April. Subsequently, the patient developed cholecystitis in the same hospitalization and underwent a cholecystectomy.

Additional surgical history includes small bowel resection two years ago. Multiple vascular surgeries on the legs, left and right, and she is also status post hysterectomy. Patient discontinued tobacco last year and she has never abused alcohol. Patient was noted to have jaundice in April of this year, but this resolved and she states that she has been tested for Hepatitis B and C at the Dialysis Center and this is now positive.

REVIEW OF SYSTEMS: HEENT: Patient does wear glasses.

CARDIOPULMONARY: Positive for pneumonia, and congestive heart failure related to fluid overload.

SOCIAL HISTORY: History is positive for patient socially being a teacher and she is now retired because of the multiple medical problems. She does occasional part-time work for Creative Creations Corp. making small handicrafts. She has had periodic diarrhea and constipation and also vomiting has started over the past couple of weeks.

PHYSICAL EXAMINATION:	Reveals a well-developed, fairly well-nourished female.
PULSE:	88
BLOOD PRESSURE:	150/90
RESPIRATION:	18
WEIGHT:	132 pounds
HEENT:	Atraumatic and normocephalic. Obvious scleral icterius is noted.
LUNGS:	Clear
CARDIAC:	Normal S1 and normal S2
ABDOMEN:	Soft, benign, nontender
EXTREMITIES:	Without clubbing, cyanosis or edema
NEUROLOGIC:	Grossly normal

The patient does not have all of her medications, so we are unable to review all of her medications.

ASSESSMENT: The patient has jaundice, quite possibly obstructive. Would suggest CBC, PT, PTT, Hepatitis panel to evaluate for the possibility of Hepatitis. Possibility for drug induced vs. viral induced hepatitis. Other considerations include obstructive jaundice, possibly related to common bile duct stone vs. stricture of the common bile duct. Also a possibility that patient may have a neoplasm via periodic jaundice in April and now November. Would therefore also suggest ultrasound, endoscopic retrograde cholangiopancreatography.

Impressions:

1. Jaundice; rule out common bile duct obstruction, rule out pancreatic tumor.
2. Leukocytosis; possibly secondary to #1.
3. End-stage chronic renal failure with hemodialysis.
4. Adult-onset diabetes mellitus.
5. Peripheral vascular disease.
6. Left above-knee amputation, four months ago secondary to #5.
7. Hypertension.
8. Pregangrenous changes, right foot.
9. Status post aortofemoral bypass graft surgery, two years ago.
10. Pulmonary embolism during hospitalization.
11. History of asthma.
12. Surgical correction of small bowel obstruction, 10 years ago.
13. History of polio in childhood with bilateral foot deformities.
14. History of multiple podiatric procedures, secondary to #13.
15. History of recurrent perianal abscesses.
16. History of multiple hospitalizations for psychiatric disorders.

Treatment plan:

1. Surgical evaluation and probable intervention for obstructive jaundice.
2. Laboratory profile.
3. Adjust insulin regimen.
4. Hemodialysis.

> Carl Callahan, M.D.
> 4440 Center Drive, Ste. 210
> Anytown, USA 12345
> (765) 555-2288
> TIN: 12-7658432
> UPIN: C66005

CC:CC999
d: 11-6-CCYY
t: 11-7-CCYY
Document: 9900099.cc

Exercise **13-19**

DAVID DAY M.D.
4508 DOOR WAY
Anytown, USA 12345

PATIENT NAME:	Daisy Doolittle	PATIENT'S ACCOUNT NUMBER:	009998
PHYSICIAN:	David Day, M.D.	DATE:	11/30/CCYY
PLACE OF SERVICE:	Duncan Day Hospital		
	4499 Door Way		
	Anytown, USA 12345		

HISTORY AND PHYSICAL ($158)

Pt to have surgery at Duncan Day Hospital, 12/7/CCYY. Procedure to be performed by Donald Denny, M.D.

CHIEF COMPLAINT: Dysfunctional uterine bleeding, carcinoma of the cervix.

HISTORY OF PRESENT ILLNESS: Pt went to Duncan Day Hospital on 11/26/CCYY complaining of abnormal vaginal discharge & bleeding for one week. LMP 02/20/CCYY. Abd. x-ray taken. Numerous small masses were found in the uterus, cervix & vaginal canal.

PAST MEDICAL HISTORY: Four NSVD, 2 prior abortions Feb 92, Nov 92. 1 miscarriage requiring extraction, 03/20/CCYY.

VITAL SIGNS: BP 120/70, Pulse 90, Resp 23, Temp 99.0

PHYSICAL EXAMINATION:

GENERAL: Well-nourished, well-developed 34 y/o H female, cooperative, nervous.

HEENT: Pupils equal, round and reactive to light and accommodation. Extraocular muscles are intact.

NECK: Thyroid not palpable. No jugular venous distention.

CHEST: Breath sounds good to auscultation bilaterally.

HEART: Regular rate and rhythm, no murmurs.

ABDOMEN: Soft, nontender. Positive multiple non-tender palpable masses in RLQ and LLQ.

PELVIC: Vaginal vault clear, cervix showed signs of cancer that was biopsied.

EXTREMITIES: Normal, with good reflexes.

ASSESSMENT: Probable Carcinoma of the cervix.

PLAN: Surgical procedure by Dr. Donald Denny.

David Day M.D.
(765) 555-7710
TIN: 11-3093109
UPIN: D13093

DD: DD98
d: 11/30/CCYY
t: 11/30/CCYY
Document: 999440.ddd

Exercise 13-20

ESTHER EDELMAN, M.D.
5993 Erlich Street
Anytown, USA 12345
(765) 555-6699

PATIENT NAME: Edward Edmunds   PATIENT'S ACCOUNT NUMBER: 685947-465

DATE: 5-9-CCYY

PLACE OF SERVICE: Eastwood Community Medical Center
                   7854 East Road
                   Anytown, USA 12345

HISTORY AND PHYSICAL ($158)

The patient is to have surgery on 5/10/CCYY, to be performed by Dr. Evelyn Elliot, orthopedic surgeon.

CHIEF COMPLAINT: Gunshot wound to both knees

HISTORY OF PRESENT ILLNESS: This 66-year-old male suffered a gunshot wound that traversed the left knee and entered the right knee, on the morning of 5/9/CCYY. There is a bullet lodged in the distal right femur. Apparently wounds to both lt and rt knee were caused by the same projectile. The patient had driven to a store. While walking from his car to the store entrance he was struck by the bullet. The patient saw no one near who appeared to be responsible.

The patient was seen today in the Eastwood Community Medical Center ER by myself and Dr. Eric Ericson. An orthopedic surgical consultant, Evelyn Elliot, M.D., was called in to discuss possible surgical intervention. Dr. Elliot reviewed the x-ray films. She has recommended surgical intervention to remove the bullet from the distal right femur. Apparently there are bone fragments in the joint space. Since suffering the gunshot wound, the patient has not had severe pain or bleeding. He has been treated with Cipro 750 mg p.o. b.i.d. The patient has not been febrile.

PAST MEDICAL HISTORY: The patient takes no medication on a regular basis. He is not being treated for hypertension, but the patient was given diuretics for about a 2-month period in 19YY. Blood pressure apparently had been elevated at that time. Subsequent measurements of blood pressure have been within normal limits. There is no history of diabetes mellitus. The patient has no frank history of heart disease, but he had an abnormal EKG last year. The record of 3/16/CCYY, reveals normal sinus rhythm with some nonspecific ST and T wave changes. The patient was seen at that time because of dyspepsia. He has had no chest pain in the past. There has never been dyspnea on exertion, and the patient has not been treated for heart disease. The patient has never previously been hospitalized.

PHYSICAL EXAMINATION:

GENERAL: Well-nourished, older aged male, alert, cooperative.

HEENT: PERRLA. Extraocular muscles intact. Fundi poorly visualized.

NECK: Thyroid not palpable. No jugular venous distention.

CHEST: Breath sounds clear to auscultation bilaterally.

HEART: Regular rate and rhythm, no murmurs.

ABDOMEN: Soft, nontender.

RECTAL: Prostate normal size and symmetrical. Stool brown in color.

EXTREMITIES: Right knee with puncture wound medial aspect; moderate edema. 1+ pitting right lower leg edema. Punctate gunshot wounds on the anterior and medial left patellar area.

ASSESSMENT:
1. Gunshot wound right and left knees with projectile embedded in distal right femur.
2. History of abnormal EKG, nonspecific ST and T wave changes, unchanged since March.
3. History of dyspepsia.
4. Allergy to penicillin.

PLAN:
1. Admit to Eastwood Community Medical Clinic.
2. Surgical intervention by orthopedic surgeon, Evelyn Elliot.

    Ester Edelman M.D.
    TIN: 523-52-3523
    UPIN: E52352

EE:EE77
d: 5/9/CCYY
t: 5/9/CCYY
Document: 12345678.eee

Exercise **13-21**

Directions: Upon completion of Exercises 13–1 through 13–20, use an insurance claims register and list all claims that have been fully prepared and are ready for submission to the insurance carrier for payment. Enter the date that you created the CMS-1500 or UB-92 in the **Date Claim Filed** column.

Exercise **13-22**

Directions: Find and circle the words listed below. Words can appear horizontally, vertically, diagonally, forward, or backward.

1. Diagnostic Testing Report
2. Operative Report
3. Triage
4. Triage Report

```
X U C M S M T L K E Z T J C V X Y S K G A J T Z Z
U H Q D E P J B H V H S R H G C J M T T J R R S L
N R N U H E W I L X O C Z I T N T K O F O R W U Z
L Z S U M Q R K D D T T P V A T K O J P B U T X C
X A S J G P K I Q W K R X G B G T M E C E V A I K
V J H L A C O M M E G I C D F M E R L V W M A Y K
I C Y T O B L K O M H A Z N P E G R X L G F B L U
X F M J K G Z K Y U A G L N F N S C E W P P I P J
S A T R N O M N F E Y E R J I V N H V P C I I O Q
W P F I Z X Q O O P E R A T I V E R E P O R T C G
P S Q T Z Z S I D F D X S I L O T P D Z H R A E J
U T T T O T Q H M T U E T K A A I H X A L C T M Q
Y K B N U Y P P L L T Y K A X F D N U W G A X S F
S D F O S P Z A C C B U G S P M L M L L I T E B O
E Z P C H O H C I H S Q W W S Z C K M L L P O U G
Y N Y O V Q N T K S V P J O P W F M T W A V Q R K
H M S C K A S R O E M C D E Q T H N D O D Q I P B
Q B P A M O S F M D U F F Z I I W Q C N B Q J W R
A Q B J N M B R F F K K W F T V J F R V I U V S R
D X J G E F B D P E V D Z A F E O P A R O L K A J
N R A A G Q L Q S J X D R J M E Q M M M B O K L E
J I B K T Q J O P M X T S D G E E Q E I C D G I P
D I S K Q X J Q J N F C H C T Z K Y Z C P P K W M
Q J B G W P D W O D Y O I H F P W C U B C U U F Q
Q C V I D G A G D G C S P D V X K D U D I T H D K
```

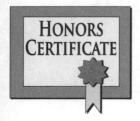

Honors Certification™

The certification challenge for this chapter will be a written test of the information contained in this chapter. Each incorrect answer will result in a deduction of up to 5% from your grade. You must achieve a score of 85% or higher to pass this test. If you fail the test on your first attempt, you may retake the test one additional time. The items included in the second test may be different from those in the first test.

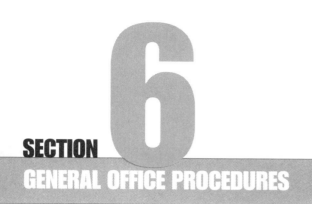

SECTION 6

GENERAL OFFICE PROCEDURES

CHAPTER 14 BASIC OFFICE FUNCTIONS
AND COMMUNICATIONS

14

Basic Office Functions and
Communications

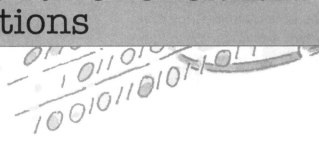

After completion of this chapter
you will be able to:

- Explain how to handle incoming mail.
- Explain how to handle outgoing mail.
- Explain special shipping services that are available.
- List the main types of office equipment and explain their use.
- Describe a tickler file and explain its use.
- List the three basic components of effective written communications.
- Write an effective letter and memo.

- Discuss the importance of a first impression.
- List the primary customer service and patient relations functions in the medical billing arena.
- List 10 items that are important to the art of listening.
- List and describe the steps necessary for problem resolution.
- List and explain the guidelines for dealing with irate or angry customers/patients.

Keywords and Concepts
you will learn in this chapter:

- Binding Machines
- Body
- Certified Mail
- Clarity in Writing
- Closed-Ended Question
- COD
- Coherence in Writing
- Collate
- Complimentary Close
- Correspondence
- Customer Service

- Effectiveness in Writing
- Empathy
- Enclosures
- Facsimile Machine (more commonly referred to as the fax machine)
- Heading
- Inside Address
- Listening
- Memo
- Multiline Phones

- Open-Ended Question
- Opening
- Return Receipt Requested
- Salutation
- Signature
- Standing Appointments
- Summary
- Tickler Files
- Transitional Thought
- Verification

A number of basic procedures need to be followed to help an office run smoothly and to facilitate the organized management of services. Without organization, precious time is lost searching for information or other items. In addition, an unorganized office and unskilled personnel create difficulty and add to the stress level of the patient, since they must wait longer to receive services. The patient may worry that your lack of concern for the office also reflects a lack of concern for them.

Mail

Mail can be separated into two types: incoming mail and outgoing mail. Each has its own set of procedures.

Incoming Mail

In any office, it is imperative that the mail be handled properly and routed to the correct person. Generally, one person is designated to handle the incoming mail. Of course, every office has its own preferences, so check with your supervisor to see what handling procedures have been established for the company where you are employed.

1. Separate mail according to the department or person to whom it is addressed. When separating mail, take note of any mail that was delivered incorrectly to your address. Separating the mail before opening it will allow you to return incorrectly delivered mail in the same condition in which it arrived.

2. If mail is to be opened before it is distributed, slit the envelope neatly across the top. Do not tear or destroy the envelope, so that any needed information can be preserved. This may include the postmark date, return address, or the city from which the envelope was mailed.

3. Many offices date stamp their mail on receipt. If this is the case with your company or organization, there are several steps that you should follow:

   a. Be sure the date on the stamp is accurate. This may be very important when certain pieces of correspondence need to arrive in a timely manner (i.e., billing department mail when interest or late fees are charged on overdue accounts).

   b. Stamp the date stamp on a piece of scratch paper to ensure that it has enough ink and that the impression is clear. If the impression is faint, stamp several more times on the ink pad (if it is used) or on a piece of paper (if the stamp is self-inking). This should start the ink flowing again.

   c. When you stamp a piece of correspondence, place the date in an area where it will not cover any writing.

   d. Stamp down once, firmly and securely. Wiggling the stamp back and forth can cause an unclear impression.

   e. Do not stamp checks, business cards, legal documents, or order forms unless your office specifically requests it. Date stamping such items can result in difficultly processing checks, ordering, or complying with legal requirements.

   f. If you have a choice of ink colors, black is best. Other colors are more difficult to photocopy or may cause a negative impression. This is especially true of red, as most people associate red ink with a warning.

4. If you receive checks in the mail, be sure they are securely attached to any additional papers (i.e., invoices, statements) that are included. These papers may be the only clue as to which account the check should be credited. Some offices prefer that the account number be immediately written on the check. This ensures that the check will be credited to the proper account even if it is separated from its attached documentation.

   If no documentation is attached, check the envelope for additional clues. If the name and address on the check do not match the name and address on the envelope, attach the envelope to the check. This may assist the billing department in locating the correct account.

   Some offices request that the person who opens the checks make an adding machine tape and total the day's receipts. You should always run the tape twice, ensuring that the total is the same each time. Then, take an extra minute to double-check your figures. Often numbers will become transposed, and once a number is in your mind, it is easy for the transposition to occur a second time.

5. When distributing the mail, put urgent-looking correspondence on top of the stack. Also be sure

to put the mail in a place where the recipient will be sure to see it.

6. If correspondence is received that is marked "Personal and Confidential," leave the envelope sealed and deliver it to the intended recipient unopened.

7. If you receive a document in a "next day" or "urgent" envelope, it should be delivered immediately. This type of document should never sit on your desk for more than five minutes.

Although handling mail may seem like a minor task, it is important to do it properly and efficiently. Mail is the lifeblood of many offices. Without it, checks and revenues may be lost, patients may not be served, and communication usually breaks down.

Signing for Mail

Some incoming mail requires a signature on delivery. Before signing, know exactly what you are signing for. Most shipping companies include a notation in fine print stating that your signature is verification that the package was received in good condition and that the contents were not damaged. Also note the number of packages you are signing for. Your signature across four lines of the receipt column is stating that you received four packages. Be sure that the order is complete before signing for it, or you or your practice may be held liable for any merchandise or shipments not received.

It is impossible to tell if the contents are undamaged without opening the box. Take the time to look at the boxes before signing. If the box appears to be damaged, insist on opening it and checking the contents before signing. The delivery person will attempt to have you sign immediately so that he or she can get to the next delivery, but if you do sign, the damaged goods often will not be replaced or paid for by the shipper.

If the contents of the package appear to be damaged, you should note this on the receipt right next to your signature.

Be sure you are authorized to sign for a package. In many offices, the authority to sign for packages is limited to a few people, not to just anyone in the office.

Returned Mailings

In any company there will be mail that is returned because of improper addressing, lack of postage, or the inability of the postal service to locate the intended recipient.

Mail will usually only be forwarded for one year from the date of the recipient's move. After that time, a sticker will be placed on the envelope indicating the new address and the article will be returned to the sender. If a piece of mail is returned because a forwarding address has expired, and the postal service has indicated the new address, the mail should be placed in a new envelope, addressed with the new address and remailed. Be sure to keep the old envelope so that you can update your records.

If a piece of mail is returned with no forwarding address indicated, be sure to delete the name and address from your records. If there is an outstanding balance on an account that has mail returned, be sure the patient's records also are updated. If an outstanding balance or a current patient history does not exist, do not delete the record. Take the time to contact the patient by phone and attempt to locate their new address.

Outgoing Mail

The condition of your outgoing mail is a direct reflection on your office. Therefore, it is imperative that your mail be handled properly. You can imagine the response of a patient who receives a letter bearing bad news that also has been stamped by the postal service "Postage Due."

The first thing is to make sure the mail has been packaged properly. Be sure that the envelope is of adequate size for the material. If there are more than five pages in a document, a #10 (standard-sized) envelope should not be used. The thickness of the pages can cause the envelope to become jammed in the postal service's automated equipment. This may result in tearing and loss of the contents. To ensure that envelopes mailed in larger packages arrive in good condition, a thin sheet of cardboard can be placed in the envelope to add resilience.

Before sealing a box, place a letter or other item inside that lists the company's and the recipient's address. This will allow the package to be delivered even if the address shown on the outside is removed or becomes obliterated. Boxes should be sealed with strong packing tape, not with string.

All shipping companies, including the postal service, have weight and size limits for the packages they will ship. Most will have a weight limit of 70 pounds per box. The combined length and girth should not exceed 108 inches. To determine the measurement, wrap a tape measure once around the box, then add to the resulting measurement the length of the box. Before shipping, contact the carrier and be sure that you know the exact weight and measurement limits they will allow.

Special Shipping Services

Most companies offer numerous shipping services. These include certification (proof of delivery), return receipt requested, **COD (cash on delivery)**, insurance, overnight delivery, and two- or three-day delivery. Additional charges, above and beyond the normal shipping charges, are added for each of these services. Keep any receipts issued to you by the shipper. Without these documents, it is very difficult to trace lost articles or to make a claim for services not delivered.

Certified mail (see Appendix B Forms) is a package or envelope that must be signed for on delivery. This provides you with a record of when the item was delivered and the name of the person who signed for it. To send an envelope by certified mail, fill out the certified mail slip provided by the shipping company. The basic information requested is the name and address of the recipient, and postage must be paid. Calculate the total postage for the item being sent. The total postage amount will include two components; the regular postage fee and the certified mailing fee. The regular postage fee will vary depending on the size and weight of the item being sent. The certified postage fee can be obtained by contacting the United States Postal Office. This tag is attached to the envelope or package to the right of the return address. The tag has a tracking number printed on it. The top portion of the tag is torn off at the perforation and kept as a receipt. If the envelope or package does not arrive, a tracer can be put on it by using the tracking number.

With **return receipt requested** (see Appendix B Forms), on delivery, a receipt is issued and mailed back to the sender of the package. This allows the sender to have proof of the delivery and the name of the person who signed for it. This procedure is usually used with certified mail. The recipient's name and address are placed on one side of the card. The sender's name and address are placed on the reverse of the card. The card is then attached to the envelope or package on the front, or, if there is not sufficient room, on the back. When the article is delivered, the recipient signs the card and the date of delivery is listed. If requested (and if an additional fee is paid), the recipient's address will be provided. The sender also may choose to restrict delivery only to the person or persons to whom the article is addressed.

On the Job Now

Directions: Read and complete the following exercise.

Dr. Paul Provider hands you a letter and a patient chart. He explains that they have agreed that Edward Edmund's medical records would be released to another provider. Mr. Edmund and Dr. Provider have signed all forms necessary for the medical records.

Please fill out the necessary forms to send a copy of Mr. Edmund's medical record by certified mail to Earl Eagle, M.D., 1122 Elephant Avenue, Anytown, USA 12345. Refer to the Patient Data Table and Provider Data Table in Appendix C.

When mailing a shipment of merchandise that the recipient must pay for, COD often is requested. This means that the shipper will collect payment for the item at the time of delivery. When shipping COD (see Appendix B Forms), you must specify whether cash, check, or either is acceptable and the amount to be collected. Add any shipping charges to the amount if the recipient is to pay for shipping.

On the Job Now

Directions: Read and complete the following exercise. Refer to the Patient Data Table and Provider Data Table in Appendix C.

Bobby Bumble would like more information on diabetes and has requested a copy of "How to Cope with Diabetes." Dr. Paul Provider sells these books in his office. Mr. Bumble would like the book shipped immediately and says he will pay for the book as soon as it arrives.

Please fill out the necessary PPS Express COD forms to ship the book to Bobby Bumble. Ship the book PPS Priority overnight; PPS Pak; the COD amount to be collected by the carrier is $ 24.95.

You may wish to purchase insurance for items being shipped. This insurance will pay for lost or damaged items. Many shippers include the first $100 of insurance in the cost of shipping a package. Any amount over this must be requested and paid for before shipping. The fee is usually nominal, between $.50 and $.75 for every $100 of insurance.

If you need an envelope or package to arrive overnight, it is possible to request this service. Articles can be scheduled for either an afternoon delivery or, for an additional charge, a morning delivery. The delivery area is limited, usually to within the continental United States. In addition, articles must be picked up or delivered to the shipper before a specified time to qualify for next-day delivery. This time varies according to your location and the shipper. You also must complete special address labels that request the sender's and receiver's name, address, and phone number, as well as the specific services requested. Many carriers require you to use special packaging and may provide this packaging free of charge on request.

There is also a special charge for two- or three-day delivery, and delivery is usually limited to the continental United States. There also are similar labels and packaging requirements. Check with your shipper for specific details.

In large cities, it is possible to have a package delivered by courier or messenger. The courier comes to your office, picks up the article, and hand-delivers it to the recipient. These services are expensive and are used only for important documents.

On the Job Now

Directions: Read and complete the following exercise.

Abby Addison came to Dr. Paul Provider's office for a recheck visit on 4/15/CCYY. After Ms. Addison left the office, the nurse noticed that Ms. Addison left her blood pressure monitor in the exam room. Dr. Provider asks you to send the monitor to Ms. Addison's home.

Please fill out the necessary forms to ship this item back to Ms. Addison using PPS Ground; PPS Standard overnight; PPS Pak; bill to Dr. Provider's account number 1030-5689-6. Refer to the Patient Data Table and Provider Data Table in Appendix C.

Office Machines

In every office, you will use a number of machines nearly every day. These include the telephone, fax machine, and copy machine.

The Telephone

Virtually every company in existence has a telephone and uses it extensively during the working day. The telephone is often more important than the mail in communicating with customers and helping with the running of the office. Therefore, it is important that you understand how to properly use the telephone.

Most companies have **multiline phones**. This means that there is more than one telephone line into the office. However, the number of these phone lines is limited. If all of the lines are being used, the customer or caller will hear a busy signal and their call will not be connected. For this reason, you should keep your call as brief as possible.

Multiline phones often work similarly to single-line phones, with a few exceptions. Most multiline phones have a single number (i.e., 555-1234), with each additional line numerically increased by one (i.e., line two is 555-1235; line three is 555-1236). The caller needs only to dial the original number (555-1234) and, if that line is busy, the call will automatically roll over to the first available line.

When placing an outgoing call on a multiline phone, many times you will need to choose a line by pushing a button. Before picking up a line, make sure that it is available. Usually, a small lighted button indicates whether the line is currently in use.

Multiline phones often give you the option of placing callers on hold by depressing a hold button. When transferring a call, speaking with a co-worker or interrupting a conversation for any reason, it is best to put the caller on hold rather than to hold your hand over the mouthpiece or set the phone down.

Different types of phones and phone systems have different ways of transferring calls and returning to a held call. These procedures will need to be described to you by someone who is familiar with the phone system. It is important to know these procedures before needing them so that you do not delay or disconnect a caller.

The Facsimile Machine

The **facsimile machine (more commonly referred to as the fax machine)** is a machine that transmits pictures over the phone lines by transmitting a series of dot messages. This allows for nearly instantaneous transmission of a letter, picture, or other document from one place to another.

The invention of the fax machine has made life easier in offices and has taken some of the stress out of having to mail documents early so that they can be received on time. Although the fax machine is a wonderful invention, it is not perfect. Documents can be lost in transmission and they are generally not as clear as printed material. The special paper used in many fax machines is thinner than normal paper, and an imprint can be left on it. For these reasons, it is important that you always follow up a faxed copy with a hard copy of the document sent through the mail.

The ease of transmitting using the fax machine has led to using it for nonessential situations. Always remember that a fax transmission is not as clear, and, therefore, not as professional-looking as something that is printed directly from a typewriter or printer. Also, remember that when transmitting long distances, you are using a phone line. Therefore, a charge will appear on the telephone bill just as if you had spoken over the phone.

If the company you are faxing to has several different departments, there may be several fax machines. A fax cover sheet should always be included with the fax. A cover sheet should include the following information:

- The date and time the fax is being sent.
- The name and telephone number of the person sending the fax.
- The name of the person to whom the fax is directed and his/her department or company.
- The number of pages being sent.
- Sufficient space for messages to be conveyed to the receiver.

The Copy Machine

The copy machine is possibly one of the most widely used office machines. There are always numerous reasons for needing a second copy of a document.

Copy machines can be one of the easiest machines to operate if you understand the basic principles. The first item of importance is the placement of the original. The original should be placed face down on the glass. The exact placement is usually indicated by markings running along the left-hand side of the glass or the bottom. The cover should be closed before making a copy.

To begin the copy process, push the button marked start. Do not lift the cover or remove the original until the copying is complete. To do so will cause a blurred or darkened image on the copy.

Many copiers have special features, such as reduction or enlargement of the original, special paper sizes or types, and collation of the copies. To **collate** copies means to place them in order. For example, if you are making two copies of a document that is three pages long, the machine will turn the pages out in the order of 1, 2, 3, 1, 2, 3. In documents that are not collated, the pages would be done in order of 1, 1, 2, 2, 3, 3.

These special features are usually selected by the push of a button.

Because copiers vary according to style and brand name, it is important that you be shown the exact features and the correct operating procedures for the copier that your company uses.

Other Office Machines

A number of other machines may be used in a medical office setting. These can include the postage meter, postage scale, binding machines, folding machines, coffee makers, and vending machines.

Binding machines bind several pages of a document together, often with a strip down the left-hand side of the document. There are numerous types of binding machines, and numerous brands for each type. Generally, the bindings fall into one of three categories: comb binders (have a plastic strip with projecting teeth), spiral binders (have a curved plastic strip with rounded teeth forming an enclosed circle), and spiral wire binders (have a single continuous piece of wire wound through successive holes from top to bottom of the document).

Folding machines are used to fold numerous pieces of paper. The folding guides can be adjusted to various lengths to handle different sizes of paper and different folds. Because of the strength and speed of most folding machines, care should be taken that jewelry, loose clothing, and long hair are not allowed to enter the machine.

Many offices provide free or low-cost cups of coffee to their employees. However, the responsibility often falls to one or more of the employees to keep the pots filled. All coffee machines require the addition of fresh coffee grounds, and some require the addition of water. Care should be taken to keep the pots cleaned on a regular basis. Also, never set an empty or near-empty glass pot on a heated burner. The glass will shatter when it reaches a certain temperature.

Vending machines are available in many offices. Most are stocked and serviced by outside vending companies that are also in charge of handling the monies received. Many vending companies return a portion of the proceeds to the company that has allowed space for the machine, and the vending company should be called if the machine has run out of items or if service is needed.

Tickler Files

The tickler file system is used by a number of people in numerous office settings. **Tickler files** are often expanding file folders that help you remember items that need to occur on a specific date. Basically a tickler file helps tickle your memory.

A tickler file usually consists of the following folders:

- 12 folders labeled with each month of the year.
- 31 folders labeled with the numbers 1 through 31.

To use a tickler file, place the folders numbered 1 through 31 into the folder for the current month (i.e., if today's date is May 5th, place all the numbered folders inside the May folder). Place all folders in front of the current month (i.e., January through April) behind the December folder at the back of the group. Then place all numbered folders for the days before the current one into the folder following the current month (i.e., if the date is May 5th, the numbered files for days 5–31 would be in the May folder and the folders for days 1–4 would be in the June folder). Now your tickler file is ready to use.

To use your tickler file, simply file each item into the folder for the day it needs to occur on. For example, if you need to sign up the provider for a conference by June 1, then place the information on the conference in the folder numbered 1, which should be in the June folder.

On each day, simply look in the folder for that day. Those are the items that you need to accomplish before the day is out.

If you have items that require your attention several months in the future, simply place them in the folder for that month. At the beginning of each month, take the items in that month's folder and insert them into the proper folder for the day of the month they need to be taken care of.

As each day passes, place the folder for that day into the folder for the next month.

By using a tickler file, you can always remember to accomplish the things that require your attention in the future. You will always be reminded of that call you were supposed to return when someone returned from vacation or that conference to sign up for, and so on.

Tickler files can be especially important in a medical office if you are requesting information or items from outside vendors or providers. For example, if the provider needs to have lab results returned to the office before the patient's next scheduled visit, place a note in the correct folder several days before the appointment. If the lab results have not been received at that time, contact the lab and ask them to forward the results to you. Be sure to place the reminder to contact the lab in the folder for several days ahead of the appointment. That will provide sufficient time for the lab to finish running the results in case they have not done so yet.

Practice Communication

Correspondence is written communication between two people and it has become an integral part of the business world. Without effective written communication, it is almost impossible for a company to succeed. Written communications have permeated every aspect of the business world, from interoffice memos to correspondence with clients, and from filed reports to e-mail messages.

Therefore, one of the most important skills that a medical biller can have is the ability to write clearly and effectively. No one wants to read a dull, boring letter, no matter how short. The dullest subject can be made inviting and exciting with effective writing techniques. Remember that the reader will judge you and your company by the type of correspondence received. Learn to use effective language that is clear, concise, and interesting. Your correspondence also should be grammatically correct and properly punctuated.

Effectiveness in writing means being able to evoke the type of response you want your reader to have, whether you want the reader to call to schedule an appointment or pay a bill. Before beginning to compose a letter, ask yourself the following questions:

1. Is this correspondence really necessary? If the answer is no, eliminate it.

2. Could this information be easily expressed over the phone? Would it save time? If the answer is yes, pick up the phone and call.

3. Has this information been expressed in previous correspondence? If so, perhaps a copy of the previous material or a short note referencing it will suffice.

4. Is it vital that the information be written "for the record?" If so, it must be written.

No one wants to waste time reading through information that is not necessary or that has already been covered. Too many communications of this sort may cause your reader to pay less attention when an important piece of correspondence arrives. If the information must be written, follow these points:

1. Determine what you want to say before you begin to write.

2. Determine what action or response you are seeking from the reader.

3. After the correspondence has been written, proofread it carefully for clarity, proper spelling, and proper grammar.

4. Finally, make sure that the correspondence conveys the message you intended.

Practice
Pitfalls

One trick is to read the correspondence aloud. This helps to identify punctuation and grammar errors that might not have otherwise been caught. You are accustomed to speaking, and passages that are awkward to say aloud usually signal that something is wrong with the way they are written.

There is no prescribed length for a letter. It should be long enough to say what you need in clear and concise language and short enough that your reader does not get lost among the words. When you have completed your idea and made it clear to the reader, your correspondence is complete. Do not delete information just because you want to keep the correspondence brief. If the subject matter is pertinent and has been presented in an interesting manner, it will be read regardless of the length.

Let your writing reflect your personality. The most effective way to write correspondence is to write the way you speak. It provides a human link between the writer and the reader. Be concise, simple, direct, and professional, but be yourself.

The Opening

The first paragraph and the first sentence of your correspondence are critical. You must gain your reader's attention, interest him in reading further, and make the reader receptive to your ideas. Without the reader's attention, you cannot hope to gain the response you are seeking.

Remember that your reader's first interest is usually him- or herself. The reader automatically defines the correspondence according to the personal benefits it will bring. Therefore, you must involve the reader or you run the risk of losing him or her.

The two principal purposes of the **opening** are to attract attention and to develop interest. Therefore, do not try to say too much in the opening. To be successful, the opening must invite sufficient interest to draw the reader into the body of the correspondence.

The Body

The **body** of the correspondence is where you present the purpose of the communication. Here, you let the reader know what you wish to obtain, if anything. If it is succinct enough, any additional information that is needed to verify the request or purpose also should be included here. If it is not, a copy of the information should be attached and a reference should be included in the body of the letter (e.g., see accompanying account statement).

Be sure to provide enough information for the reader to understand your purpose, but not so much that it is overwhelming. Keep the information concise and move the correspondence forward.

Clarity and Coherence

Clarity in writing means exactness of language. It results in the reader understanding what you intended to say. If the meaning is not clear, the entire message has failed, no matter how eloquently it was stated. Remember that your reader cannot respond appropriately if he cannot figure out what you want.

After writing a piece of correspondence, take a moment to put yourself in the reader's place and read the letter as if you were seeing it for the first time. Ask yourself, "Does this say what I intended it to say?" If not, it needs to be rewritten.

Coherence means "sticking together." **Coherence in writing** means that the letter or information flows logically from one idea to the next. Being coherent re-

quires that you do not cram too many ideas into a single piece of correspondence. Eliminate any ideas that are not necessary.

If all the information is necessary and the correspondence is still lengthy, consider inserting headings to help the reader determine when you are moving from one thought to another. If your document is not clear and coherent, you will have failed in your attempt to get a message across to your reader and it is not worth sending.

Grammar, Sentence Structure, and Paragraphs

Make sure your grammar and sentence structure are accurate. The impression your letter creates will be a reflection of you and the provider for whom you work. The last thing you want is your patients thinking that they are attending an unprofessional facility.

Paragraphs should be kept short and to the point. A paragraph should end when a thought is complete. The only exception is when you add a transitional thought to the end of the final sentence. A **transitional thought** segues into the topic of the next paragraph.

The Closing

The **closing** should be a brief summary of the major points contained in the body of the correspondence. Also include a congratulatory or consolatory note if the body of the letter contains good or bad news. Your closing should be fresh, and state in a new and interesting way what the recipient should do, thus enticing him to carry out your wishes.

Correspondence Containing Negative Content

When writing letters that contain negative content (i.e., letters of denial), say "no" as graciously as possible. Your success in keeping this person as a client depends on your saying "no" nicely. Use positive words and phrases to develop a positive feeling within your reader.

Never give bad news in the first paragraph. The reader may stop reading without understanding the reasoning behind the decision. You will have lost the reader without getting the reasons and rationale across in a manner that creates mutual understanding.

Clearly state the reasons for the decision and, if possible, refer the reader to any applicable information to support the provider's decision (i.e., a copy of the contract provisions, a statement of her account). If appeals procedures are applicable, include all the necessary information regarding appeals in your correspondence. This will eliminate unnecessary phone calls at a later date.

Because of time constraints and financial considerations, it may be necessary to respond to your client with a form letter. If the form letter is written in a pleasing tone and uses specific references, you reduce the chances that your reader will think of it as just another form letter. If the letter has been photocopied and is obviously a form letter, consider adding a personal note to the margin that will soften the message.

Format of the Letter

For correspondence to be taken seriously, it is important for it to look professional. There are numerous books available that show various styles and formats for letters. Each company has a preferred style, and this style should be used for all correspondence.

There are three main styles of letters: block style, modified block style, and semiblock style **(see Figures 14–1 through 14–3)**. Each of these styles has specific rules regarding formatting of the letter. It is not considered acceptable to mix two or more styles in a single letter or communication.

Business Letter Envelope Components

This sample business letter envelope **(see Figure 14–4)** includes formal components, some of which are optional for typical, employment-related business letters.

Memos

If a message needs to be communicated to a number of people within a company, a memo is often written. A **memo** (short for memorandum) is a letter intended for distribution within a company **(see Figure 14–5)**.

Companies often write memos to share information internally, such as a change of policy or a new method of performing a task. However, memos can be written about any subject.

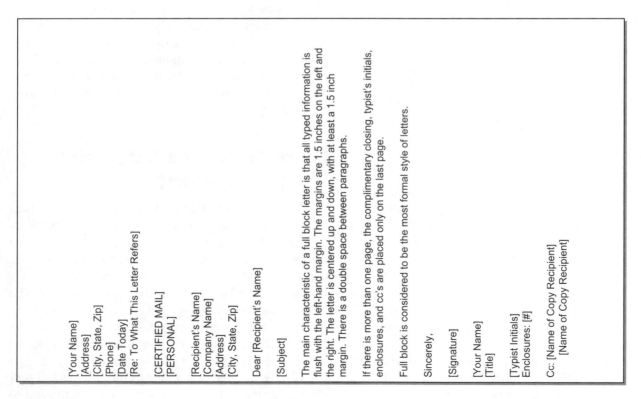

[Your Name]
[Address]
[City, State, Zip]
[Phone]
[Date Today]
[Re: To What This Letter Refers]

[CERTIFIED MAIL]
[PERSONAL]

[Recipient's Name]
[Company Name]
[Address]
[City, State, Zip]

Dear [Recipient's Name]

[Subject]

The main characteristic of a full block letter is that all typed information is flush with the left-hand margin. The margins are 1.5 inches on the left and the right. The letter is centered up and down, with at least a 1.5 inch margin. There is a double space between paragraphs.

If there is more than one page, the complimentary closing, typist's initials, enclosures, and cc's are placed only on the last page.

Full block is considered to be the most formal style of letters.

Sincerely,

[Signature]

[Your Name]
[Title]

[Typist Initials]
Enclosures: [#]

Cc: [Name of Copy Recipient]
[Name of Copy Recipient]

■ **Figure 14–1** Block Style Letter

[Your Name]
[Address]
[City, State, Zip]
[Phone]
[Date Today]
[Re: To What This Letter Refers]

[CERTIFIED MAIL]
[PERSONAL]

[Recipient's Name]
[Company Name]
[Address]
[City, State, Zip]

Attention [Recipient's Name]

Dear [Recipient' Name]

[Subject]

The main characteristic of a modified block letter is that all typed information is flush with the left-hand margin. The margins are 1.5 inches on the left and the right. The letter is centered up and down, with at least a 1.5 inch margin. There is a double space between paragraphs.

If there is more than one page, the complimentary closing, typist's initials, enclosures, and cc's are placed only on the last page.

Modified block letter is not as formal as full block letter.

Sincerely,

[Signature]

[Your Name, Title]

[Typist Initials]
Enclosures: [#]

Cc: [Name of Copy Recipient]

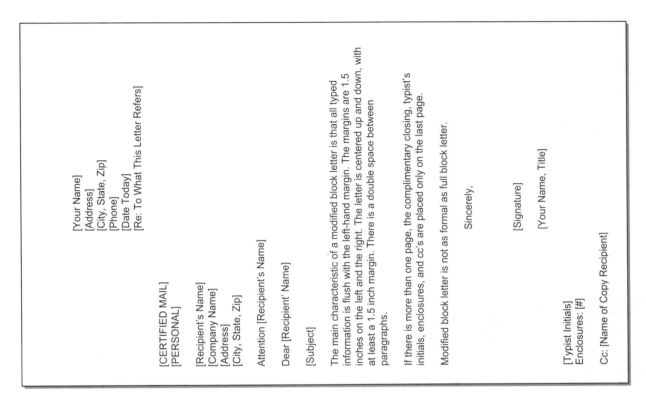

Figure 14–2 Modified Block Style Letter

[Your Name]
[Address]
[City, State, Zip]
[Phone]
[Date Today]
[Re: To What This Letter Refers]

[CERTIFIED MAIL]
[PERSONAL]

[Recipient's Name]
[Company Name]
[Address]
[City, State, Zip]

Attention [Recipient's Name]

Dear [Recipient' Name]

[Subject]

Modified semi-block letters are similar to modified block letters. The only difference is that the paragraphs are indented. Modified semi-block letters are not as formal as full block letters.

If there is more than one page, the complimentary closing, typist's initials, enclosures, and cc's are placed only on the last page.

Sincerely,

[Signature]

[Your Name, Title]

[Typist Initials]
Enclosures: [#]

Cc: [Name of Copy Recipient]
[Name of Copy Recipient]

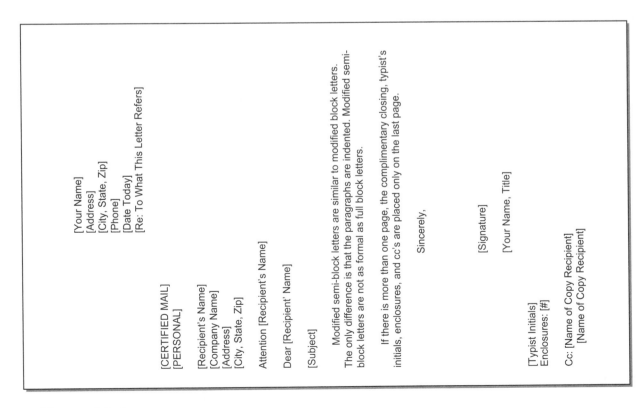

Figure 14–3 Semiblock Style Letter

Practice Pitfalls

Use the following tips when writing letters:

1. Replace the text in brackets [ ] with the component indicated. Do not type the brackets.

2. Try to keep your letters to one page.

3. How many blank lines you add between lines that require more than one depends on how much space is available on the page.

4. The same applies for margins. The standard for margins is one and one-half inch (108 points) for short letters and one inch (72 points) for longer letters. If there is a letterhead, its position determines the top margin.

5. If you do not type one of the more formal components, do not leave space for them. For example, if you do not type the **Reference Line (3)**, **Special Mailing Notations (4)**, and **On-Arrival Notations (5)**, type the **Inside Address (6)** four lines below the **Date (2)**.

On the Job Now

Directions: Write a letter for each of the following scenarios. Refer to the patient chart or Patient Data Table and Provider Data Table in Appendix C for additional information.

1. Write to Abby Addison's insurance company and request her individual deductible amount and coinsurance limit.

2. Write a letter to Bobby Bumble's insurance carrier to inquire as to whether biofeedback is covered under his plan.

3. You have not received payment from Cathy Crenshaw for services on 11/6/CCYY for a history and physical. The charge for the service is $125. Write a letter to Cathy to request payment.

4. Daisy Doolittle did not bring in verification of her Medicaid eligibility. She had surgery on 12/7/CCYY. You need her to bring in or mail a copy of her Medicaid card for December. Let her know that if she does not provide the requested information she will have to personally pay for the services.

5. Edward Edmunds has asked you to write Medicare to find out if removal of a birthmark is a covered service.

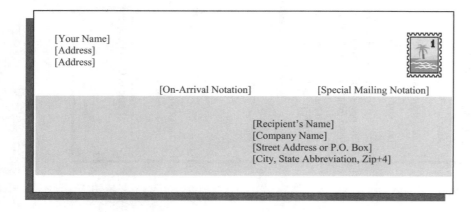

■ **Figure 14–4** Sample Business Letter Envelope

Practice
Pitfalls

Use the following tips when creating envelopes:

1. Replace the text in brackets [ ] with the component indicated. Do not type the brackets.

2. If your envelope does not have a preprinted return address, type it in the upper left-hand corner, in an area not to exceed 50% of the length and 33% of the height of the envelope. Leave a little space between your return address and the top and left edges. How much space will depend on the margin limitations of your printer or typewriter. For example, laser printers typically require margins of at least $\frac{1}{8}$ inch (9 points). However, $\frac{1}{4}$ inch (18 points) to $\frac{1}{2}$ inch (36 points) looks good.

3. Type the **Special Mailing Notation** under the postage area. It does not have to line up perfectly with the stamp as shown, but it looks professional. Type the notation in all uppercase characters, if appropriate. Examples include:

   • SPECIAL DELIVERY

   • CERTIFIED MAIL

   • AIRMAIL

4. Type the **On-Arrival Notation** so that its right edge lines up with the left edge of the recipient's address. This is not a post office requirement but, rather, standard formatting. Type the notation in all uppercase characters, if appropriate. You might want to include a notation on private correspondence, such as when mailing a resignation letter. Examples include:

   • PERSONAL

   • CONFIDENTIAL

5. The gray shaded area is where the OCR (optical character reader) at the post office scans for the recipient's address. Type the recipient's address within the shaded area, below other information. Do not type anything to the left, right, or below the recipient's address. It is a good idea to include a line or two of space below nonaddress information (such as the notations shown), before typing the recipient's address. This makes it easier for the OCR to distinguish the address.

6. You need special software to print a bar code. It is not required for typical, employment-related letters, but if you want to get fancy, and have a later version of Microsoft Word® or WordPerfect®, they will print bar codes.

On the Job Now

Directions: Write a letter and prepare an envelope for each of the following scenarios. Be sure to use appropriate style, structure, and grammar. Refer to the patient chart or Patient Data Table and Provider Data Table in Appendix C.

1. Write a block style letter to your instructors commending them on their excellent teaching skills.

2. Write a semiblock style letter for your boss, Mr. Harry Hamlet, 555 Hughes Hwy, Hanger, HI 05052, to Medical Billing Supply Warehouse, 2323 Kenneth Road, Kriers, KY 54541. The letter should ask whether the store carries patient billing forms, and if so what is the cost. Specifically, inquire as to whether they carry the CMS-1500 and UB-92 forms.

COMPANY LETTERHEAD

TO: ALL EMPLOYEES

FROM: ANNA ABLEBODY

RE: COMPANY DINNER

DATE: JANUARY 2, 2005

****

I would like to take this opportunity to express my appreciation to all those who helped put together a wonderful New Year's Eve party for the company.

I'm sure you all agree that the Food Committee, consisting of Ginny Gourmet and Terri Tidbit did an excellent job of finding a superb caterer and choosing a wonderful menu.

The decorations created by Winnie Wallpaper, Daniel Décor and Orville Ornaments made the lunchroom an enticing place to be and created a festive atmosphere that set the tone for a wonderful party.

The exciting program, which I'm sure we all enjoyed, was prepared and performed by Rita Recital, Patty Presentation, Peter Performance, Annie Appearance and Sally Staging.

And of course we can't forget the much-appreciated efforts of the cleanup crew: Wally Wiper, Betty Broom and Tracy Trash.

Without the efforts of each and every one of these people we would not have enjoyed such a wonderful party. Please take a moment to thank each of these people personally.

■ **Figure 14–5** Sample Memo

There are usually three main reasons for disseminating a memo:

1. It is easier to reach a large number of people with a memo, especially if some of them are out of the office. A memo can be left on a desk, ensuring that more people will see it, rather than relying on word of mouth.

2. A memo contains information that a number of recipients need to read (such as a policy change), or information that they may need to refer to at a later time.

3. A memo provides a tangible medium of communication in a documented form.

Although typing a memo may seem like a minor part of a medical biller's day, memos can be an important part of keeping a company running smoothly.

Many companies will set or change company policies, then notify the personnel by creating a memo and circulating it among the office employees. Employees are then expected to read and follow the new guidelines. If necessary, the memo should be filed with other important papers so the employee may refer to it at a later date.

For these reasons it is important that memos be written in a clear and easy to understand manner. Be careful of the tone you use when writing a memo, as memos often become a permanent part of a company's or an individual's record.

Additionally, morale can be boosted by a well-written, positive memo, or significantly lowered by a negative one. In fact, a memo praising a certain group of employees and sent to all other employees in the company is one of the easiest and least expensive ways to make people feel important.

Writing a memo of praise lets people know you appreciate their work. It also can motivate others to become involved in future projects.

Memo Format

Most companies have a specific format for their memos. This usually consists of printing them on company letterhead, beginning with a header, then the body of the memo.

The Header

The header usually consists of four items: TO, FROM, SUBJECT, and DATE.

TO: The TO header is usually typed in capital letters. The name of the recipients also may be in capital letters, or may be in upper and lower case, depending on the policy of the company. Often company memos are addressed to groups of people rather than to individuals. For example, a memo may be designated "TO: All Managers." When a memo is for several people who are not of a designated group (i.e., all managers), the names of the recipients are typed one after another with a comma and space separating the names. Often these people are listed in order of rank (i.e., partners, managers, general staff), or in alphabetical order.

FROM: The FROM header is also typed in capital letters, with the name of the person creating the memo in either all uppercase or uppercase and lowercase letters, depending on company policy. Usually if one item (i.e., TO, FROM, or SUBJECT) is in all uppercase, then all items will be in all uppercase letters. As with the TO field, this field also may be from a single person or from a group of people (i.e., The Partners).

SUBJECT: The SUBJECT header is typed in all capital letters (also written as RE, short for regarding) and is a one line sentence or topic for the memo. Since memos are often filed among other company papers, two or more subjects of importance are not often covered in the same memo. Instead two (or more) separate memos are issued. This allows people to file the memo according to the subject matter, which then makes it much easier to locate and retrieve when necessary.

DATE: The DATE header is also typed in all capital letters. The date should be given as the date the memo will be distributed. This allows people to track the memos and determine which is the most recent. This can be especially important with memos that alter a company policy or institute a new company policy.

The Body

On most memos, a line or a row of asterisks follows the header information. This separates the header from the body of the memo.

The body of the memo is then typed without a salutation (i.e., Dear Managers), or closing (i.e., Sincerely, The Partners).

Be sure to write clearly and concisely, including all pertinent information. However, extraneous information, which is often included in a formal letter, is not included (i.e., How are you?). Memos usually state the important facts in as few lines as possible. It is very rare for a memo to be longer than one page unless it covers a major policy change.

Once the memo has been typed the person who initiated the memo should approve it. Their approval is usu-

ally given by having them initial the original next to their name in the header section. This initialed original is then photocopied and copies are given to each person to whom the memo is addressed. If you issue two or more conflicting memos regarding the same subject on a single day, the subject line should include information that this memo changes or alters the previous memo issued.

In addition, if more than two memos are issued in a single day with conflicting instructions or changes, the time of the second memo should be placed next to the date. For example, if you issue a memo, then realize you forgot the word "not" in the sentence "On Thursday you should park in the parking garage." The second memo should include the time next to the date. Additionally, the subject line should read something like "Correction of memo re: Parking" to indicate that something on the original memo has been changed.

Patient Relations

Customer service, which is to service the customer or patient, is the most vital function your office will provide. Without it, the facility may lose customers and patients. Without customers or patients, the facility may cease to exist.

Whenever you speak with a customer or patient, either on the phone or in person, or write to them, you are performing a customer service function. Many times the medical biller is the only contact that the person will have with the facility. Therefore, to that person you are the company. The image you convey will be what the person believes is the facility's attitude toward them. Accounts have been won and lost based solely on a customer/patient's experience with customer service personnel. Even a single encounter can be enough to win or lose a customer/patient. The following sections are designed to help the medical biller in developing a more professional and positive approach to customer/patient relationships.

To respond appropriately to the needs of your customers/patients, you must be able to look beneath the surface or the behavior they exhibit to examine the factors that motivate their actions.

When dealing with customers/patients, bear in mind that their primary concern is that their needs are met. If you assist them in meeting their needs in a pleasant and friendly way, their opinion of you, and thus, the company, will be greatly enhanced. Likewise, if you allow their reaction to a situation to influence you in a negative manner, their opinion of the facility will be a negative one.

Every time you have contact with someone you are, in effect, recognizing this person. This recognition can be verbal or nonverbal (such as nodding or smiling at someone).

First Impressions and Image

First impressions are a vital part of determining how a customer/patient feels about a person, company, or facility. This impression is usually formed within four minutes of the first meeting. Four minutes is not a long time, but it is long enough for someone to form an impression that may remain with him throughout the life of the relationship.

The kind of first impression a person makes on another person is often made without anyone recognizing it. Everything communicates something. For example, the first thing people use to form an impression about you is your appearance. This consists not only of your clothing and general appearance but also of your posture, gestures, facial expressions, and the way you move.

The next largest impact is made by your vocal communication. This includes your tone of voice, the volume and pitch, and the speed at which you speak.

Last is your verbal communication. This includes not only the words you speak but also the terminology you use and the way you speak. It is important to use terminology that will be understood by the person to whom you are speaking and to speak distinctly and clearly.

Ways to Make a Good First Impression

If your experiences are typical, you will meet approximately 10,000 people in your lifetime. This is a lot of chances to make a terrific first impression. Next time you meet someone new, use some of the following gestures:

- Extend your hand and give a firm handshake.
- Smile and make eye contact.
- Learn and use the other person's name.
- Be a good listener.

Another point to remember is that when meeting new people in a busy situation (such as at a restaurant networking function), avoid letting your gaze wander around the room while others speak. Focus your attention on the individual, and listen for details that you can use to promote conversation.

Characteristics of Client Relations

It is vital to keep customer service and patient relations a high priority. The personnel who deal with customers and patients must possess highly disciplined personality characteristics. The following characteristics should be demonstrated in each and every client interaction in order to be good at customer service and patient relations:

- Thorough job knowledge.
- Good telephone techniques.
- Knowledge of privacy guidelines and their importance.
- A positive attitude.
- The ability to listen well.
- Knowledge of the business and its practices.

Customer Service Job Functions

As a medical biller, your primary customer service and patient relations functions include, but may not be limited to, the following:

1. Using computerized or manual files to answer inquiries from customers and patients or potential ones. These inquiries may include numerous topics, such as the dispensation of an order, contractual interpretations, or general questions regarding the facility.

2. Promoting positive customer and patient relationships through positive interaction.

3. Handling written correspondence. Strong letter-writing skills are required to articulate the facility's position.

4. Meeting with walk-in customers and patients and handling their questions concerning services and costs.

5. Detecting and handling the initial investigation of potentially fraudulent activities.

6. Advising supervisors of adverse trends or issues noted through contact with customers and patients, client representatives, and others, and maintaining an accurate activity log that documents these trends or issues.

7. Recording comments and reactions (both positive and negative) of customers and patients regarding the services provided.

The Art of Listening

Listening is one of the most important skills a person can learn, especially in the area of customer service. **Listening** is defined as making an effort to hear. Without effort, true listening does not occur. This means that your entire focus should be on what the person is saying, not on any errands you may have to run, other items you may have to get done, or people you would rather be with. Whether you are speaking with a patient who is unprepared, long-winded, tearful, or difficult and irate, the following 10 ideas will help you resolve the patient's problem:

Limit your own talking. It is almost impossible to talk and listen at the same time.

Try to put yourself in the customer's/patient's place. Their problems and needs are important to them and should, therefore, be important to you. You can understand and retain their concerns better if you listen to their point of view.

Ask questions. If you do not understand something or if you need clarification, there is nothing wrong with asking questions. In fact, asking relevant questions helps the customer/patient to feel you are listening closely.

Do not interrupt. A pause does not always mean the person has finished speaking. Very often, people pause when they are trying to formulate a sentence in their mind. Do not rush them. If you allow a pause of at least five seconds between sentences, it will give the person time to add any other points they wish to make.

Concentrate. Focus your mind on the conversation, shutting out all outside distractions. If you find your mind wandering, get it back on track.

Take notes. This will help you remember important points in the conversation. However, do not try to write down every word. Note only key words that are relevant to the problem and that will help you to remember the issues at a later time.

Interjections. An occasional "Yes," "I see," or "I understand" shows the person that you are still tuning in to their words. Just be careful not to overdo it. Too many interjections will make the person feel you are constantly interrupting.

Keep your words and thoughts concise. Personal concerns and stories of what happened to you or someone else waste time and may confuse the person. In addition, it does not help to

move the conversation toward resolution of the person's problem.

React to the problem or concern, not to the person. Do not allow yourself to become irritated at things the person says or the way in which he says them.

Do not jump to conclusions. Do not assume you know what the person is about to say. Also, do not finish their sentences, either mentally or verbally. Let the person finish completely before you offer a solution or suggestion.

Listening with Empathy

Empathy means being able to participate in another person's feelings or perceptions, and to try to sense and understand how another person is feeling and what he is experiencing. In customer service and patient relations, this is a critical part of the listening process.

Empathetic listening, on its own, may resolve your customer's or patient's problem. Giving people a chance to verbally express their problem may clarify their understanding of the situation. It also often provides emotional release and allows them to gain a more logical point of view. Because it gives people a chance to voice their opinions, it can reduce tension and hostility. When people feel you are truly interested in them as well as their problems, thoughts, and opinions, they respect you and are more willing to cooperate with you toward a resolution of problems. Thus, empathetic listening promotes communication, which is essential in the business world. Communication often breaks down because neither party is willing to listen.

Irate or Angry Customers/Patients

Remember the following 10 guidelines in dealing with irate or angry customers/patients:

Remain calm. Remember that the customer/patient is angry at the situation, not you. If you become upset, the discussion will become an argument.

Ask questions. Direct, open-ended questions help to define the problem. However, questions that begin with "Why" are best avoided since they can sometimes be construed as threatening.

Listen carefully to what the person is saying. Do not try to match wits with the person. Allow the person time to vent his feelings. Even angry people will give you valuable information by what they say and how they say it. Let the person know you are listening and are interested by saying "I see" or "Yes, sir." If you are speaking with the person face to face, maintain good eye contact, nod, and keep an attentive facial expression and an open body position.

Be prepared. Be well informed regarding your company and your department. If a person is upset about a policy that cannot be changed, explain how the policy was designed to protect them, you, or the company.

Avoid giving customers/patients the runaround. Try to avoid transferring them to someone else. If at all possible, resolve the problem yourself.

Accept criticism without becoming angry. People who are angry are often looking for a fight to justify their anger. Your pleasant demeanor can be disarming to an angry person.

Agree with the person. Find something in the person's remarks with which you can agree. This will help them to feel you are an ally rather than an enemy. However, never agree to anything that can be misconstrued as a promise of what you or the company will do. Do not place blame. You do not want them to like you and dislike the company.

Avoid defensive behavior. Do not make excuses such as "We are short-staffed," "I am new here," or "It is not my job."

Offer choices. Whenever possible, allow them to choose a plan of action by offering several options. Or ask them how they would like you to resolve the problem. This way, they will feel in control of the situation and will take responsibility for the outcome.

Be personal. Introduce yourself and learn the person's name. Say the name as often as it is appropriate during the conversation.

Remember that the more friendly, pleasant, and helpful you are, the more helpful, responsive, and satisfied your customers/patients will be.

Problem Resolution

Listening skills are used throughout the entire problem resolution process. However, there are also specific steps that will bring you and the customer/patient to the resolution of a problem or concern. Following are the six basic steps necessary for a resolution:

- Greet the person.
- Acknowledge the problem.

- Question the person to determine the best way to proceed toward a resolution of the problem.
- Verify the information received from the person and any further actions agreed on.
- Counsel the person regarding the steps he or she will need to take toward a resolution of the problem.
- Close the conversation.

Greet the Customer/Patient

The way you greet a person and begin a conversation sets the tone for the entire encounter. This depends not so much on the words you say but on the tone of your voice and the way you say the words. A pleasant greeting can defuse an angry customer/patient and improve the outlook of their concern. Your voice should communicate pleasantness, caring, and concern from the first word.

To better prepare yourself for customer or patient calls, practice greeting them in a pleasant, happy voice. Before you answer the phone or turn toward a customer/patient, take a moment for a quick breath and a smile. Focus your attention on them, not on the task in front of you or any other thoughts. If your mind is not focused, the person will hear your distraction in the tone of your voice.

When a customer or patient enters the office, it is important to greet them as soon as you see them. If you are on the phone or are unable to give your full attention, smile and say, "I'll be with you in just a moment." Then get to them as quickly as you can.

Acknowledge the Problem

Acknowledging your customer's or patient's concern or problem opens the line of communication and lets them know that you are interested in helping to find a solution. It also lets them know that they are important. They will recognize that you empathize with their concern, and that you want to resolve the problem or prevent it from occurring again.

Example:
Medical Biller: "This is John Doe. How may I help you?"
Customer/Patient: "I just got a notice from your office saying that I haven't paid my bill and it is 90 days past due. I paid this bill three months ago."
Medical Biller: "I can understand why you might be upset, sir. If I can ask you a few questions, we can resolve this quickly."

Notice that the response should not be an apology or an admission of error. It also should not accuse or place the blame on the customer/patient. Your primary goal is to acknowledge that a problem or situation exists and that you are willing to work with the person to find a solution. Your voice should remain soft and slow, not allowing the person's anger to seep into your own voice.

Question the Customer/Patient

Questioning is a learned skill. It is used to clarify the reason for an inquiry and to gain information needed to work toward a resolution of the person's concern. There are two kinds of questions: open-ended and closed-ended.

On the Job Now

Directions: In the following exercise, choose the statement that best reflects complete acknowledgment.

1. _____ It's no problem to issue you another statement. Let me get your full name and address so I can send it right out.
2. _____ Well, you can't pay your bill if you don't know how much it is, can you?
3. _____ We'll have to give you a new statement. Hopefully you won't lose this one as well.

Open-ended questions are those that cannot be answered with a "yes," "no," or other brief response. These questions encourage people to respond freely. They usually begin with words such as "tell me," "why," or "what." Examples of open-ended questions include:

- "Why were you sent here?"
- "What kind of problem do you have?"
- "What happened that you feel that way?"

Closed-ended questions limit or restrict the client's response, usually to a yes or no answer or other brief response. These types of questions usually begin with words like "who," "are," "did," "what," and "which." Therefore, a closed-ended question brings about a specific, narrow response.

Closed-ended questions should be used when you need specific information, need to take more control of the conversation, or need to confirm or verify your understanding of the situation. Examples of closed-ended questions include:

- "What is your account number?"
- "When did you come in for treatment?"
- "Was the item purchased at a pharmacy?"

Both types of questions are usually necessary in a conversation. They will allow you to resolve the problem quickly while retaining the best possible interrelationship. Too many closed-ended questions may make the person feel as if he is being interrogated. Too many open-ended questions may allow the conversation to wander. Regardless of the type of questions used, listen carefully for the answer in order to resolve the situation. Think through the meaning of the answer before you consider what your next step or your next question should be.

Verify the Information

Verification means repeating the information and asking if you have understood it correctly. It is important to make sure that you have understood the person's concerns and the answers to your questions, especially when you are speaking to someone with an accent. Minor mispronunciations in language can lead to big misunderstandings. For example, consider the ramifications of misunderstanding the following two sentences: "Call me tonight," and "Kill me tonight." As you can see, a mispronounced vowel can change the meaning of a statement.

By using verification, you can make sure that you and the person are saying the same thing and have the same understanding of the situation. Verification also builds a stronger rapport with the person, since the person will realize that you are trying to understand and are truly listening to what she is saying. Verification sentences often begin with phrases such as:

- "If I understand you correctly . . . "
- "May I repeat this back to you to make sure I understand?"
- "So you mean . . . "
- "Then you want us to . . . "

If you believe the person does not understand, question him or her to find out what is unclear. For example:

- "You seem unsure, Mr. Brown; what concerns you?"
- "Specifically, what part is unclear to you, Mrs. Hall?"
- "Is there anything that you would like explained again, sir?"

When repeating information for a second time, it is often better to rephrase it than to repeat it word for word. If there still seems to be a problem, try using examples.

It also might be helpful to offer any resource material that is available. This may include pamphlets, copies of documents, or other materials.

Counsel the Customer/Patient

Now you are ready to move on to the counseling step. Counseling may not be necessary in all encounters. When a short or simple answer is required, just answer the question and conclude the conversation. For example:

- "Yes, Mrs. Minor, we have your appointment listed at two o'clock on Tuesday."
- "Yes, Mr. Sampson, the check for that account was received Monday."

However, counseling can be invaluable when the response is lengthy or complex. For example:

- "According to our records we never received payment for Dr. Jordan's claim. May I suggest you talk with the insurance carrier and find out when the claim was paid? If it has been longer than two weeks, ask them if they would like us to resubmit the claim."

Counseling is also helpful when the response requires that you take further action. For example:

- "I need to check our records to see if your account has been paid. Are you able to hold a moment while I pull up the file?"

Finally, counseling assists when the response requires a delay before the problem can be resolved.

- "I need to contact the corporate office for a copy of the records. It will probably take a few days. When I receive it, I'll call you back. You should hear from us by Monday, Mr. Smith."

Counseling entails explaining the situation and then explaining both what the person should do next and what you will do next. In the previous examples, the following could be seen:

- The patient was expected to contact the insurance carrier's office and you would wait for their response.
- You would check the records and the client would hold.
- You would contact the corporate office and the customer would expect your call by Monday.

Counseling allows a clear picture of the situation and the actions to be taken. In this way, each person is clear about what the next step should be in helping to bring the situation to a successful resolution.

Close the Conversation

Once a plan of action has been agreed on or the person's questions have been answered, it is time to close the call. The important thing to bear in mind is that the encounter should not be considered finished until the person is as satisfied as possible.

When you feel the person is satisfied, use the following steps to close the call:

1. **Summarize the outcomes.** A **summary** is a brief statement reminding the person of what you have agreed to and how it will help or solve his concern. It needs to be clear and concise, and stated in a positive way. Make sure that your caller is satisfied and fully understands before closing a conversation. For example:
   - "Good, then I'll send that report out right away, Mrs. Phillips, and if you have any questions about it, just give me a call."
   - "So, you'll call the corporate office at the toll-free number I just gave you and find out why they've rejected your application. You'll also ask them what they need to review in your application. If you still have a concern after you've

talked to them, just give us a call. Thank you for calling. Good-bye, Mrs. Smith."

2. **Thanking the customer/patient.** Do not forget to thank the customer/patient. If people feel unappreciated they may take their business elsewhere. The two words "thank you" may be the easiest and one of the most important ways to keep your customers and patients and your job.

Occasionally, a customer or patient may want to continue to chat after a resolution has been reached. In such a case, summarizing the agreed-on actions in a succinct way will send the message that the conversation is concluding. With determined persons, it may be necessary to firmly but kindly let them know that you have other matters that need your attention. You can explain that although you would love to chat, you need to get back to work.

The use of these basic steps in problem resolution will bring positive results and will help your customer/patients to feel important and appreciated. This is what customer service and patient relations are all about.

On the Job Now

Directions: Answer the following questions and write your answers in the space provided.

1. Of the 10 steps covered in "The Art of Listening," which is your strongest? _____

2. Which of these steps do you need to pay more attention to? List all that apply. _____

3. Specifically, list three actions that you can take to improve your techniques listed in question 2. _____

Maintaining an Appointment Calendar

A well-maintained appointment calendar can make the difference between having a chaotic or calm day. By simply looking at your calendar at the beginning and end of each day, you will know where your free time slots are. If you practice the habit of keeping an orderly calendar, you can decide when the best time would be to do your various tasks. Following are a few tips on how to maintain a calendar.

Put the day and date on the calendar. Make sure the day and date are prominently displayed at the top of each page. With most appointment calendars this information is preprinted. However, if you are using a weekly or monthly planner, the day and date may be displayed anywhere on the page.

A person's name should be on the calendar. If you have calendars for more than one person, put the name of the person the calendar applies to prominently on the top of the calendar. This will help prevent you from writing an appointment on the wrong calendar.

Give your boss a copy of the calendar. If you keep a calendar for your boss, on a periodic basis put a copy of their calendar for the upcoming day or week on their desk. This allows them to know when they need to arrive in the morning, and to plan out their day.

Keep your old calendars. Invariably there will come a time when you are filling out your expense report or other documentation and someone asks "On what date were you in Dallas?" or "When did you meet with so-and-so?" By keeping the old appointment calendars, you can find this information quickly and easily. The rule of thumb is to keep old calendars for at least 18 months. This allows the information to be available for preparing tax returns or for other purposes. However, if the calendar is the only source for obtaining or verifying information that was used for a tax return, the calendar should be kept for at least four years.

Appointment Setting

Medical billers often are asked to set appointments for their supervisors. They are sometimes handed an appointment calendar, and the request is made, without the biller having any idea of how to go about the task.

Appointment setting is easy if you follow a few basic rules; however, not following these rules can cause a lot of trouble. Here are some of the main appointment setting rules to keep in mind.

Insert standing appointments. Start by putting in any standing appointments. **Standing appointments** are any appointments that happen on a regular basis (i.e., board meeting every second Tuesday at 8 A.M.). Block out the hours you (or the person the calendar pertains to) are usually not in the office, and also any regularly scheduled lunch hours. Many appointment calendars have extended hours, indicating the way work is often done. They may start with space for 6 A.M. or 7 A.M. appointments. If the person you are setting an appointment for usually reaches the office at 9 A.M., shade out the hours before 9 A.M. A gray or dull-colored highlighter often works well for this. If you need to schedule appointments for these times, you can write over the highlighter and still see the information.

Set appointments during a time that is beneficial to your schedule. Unless you want to start meeting people from the first moment you walk in the door, try not to schedule anything for the first half hour after you arrive. This will allow you to make or return phone calls, get a cup of coffee, take off your jacket, and so on. It also allows time for you to look over those things that may have been placed on your desk after you left the previous day, and allows you a buffer in case you come in later than expected.

Additionally, a half-hour of downtime immediately after lunch for your boss can solve a multitude of problems and also can help you catch up if you are running late.

Most people like to organize everything and clean off their desk before leaving for the night. If possible, block out a half-hour at the end of the day for this.

By not making appointments at these times, you can relieve some of the stress on yourself.

Write appointments down. Write an appointment in the calendar as soon as you receive it. Do not put it off to do later, regardless of how busy you are. Appointment information is often written on small pieces of paper that are easily lost. Be sure to include the name of the appointment, the location, and the phone number of the person whom the appointment is with. Then shade out or draw a vertical line through any remaining lines corresponding to the time of the appointment. For example, if your calendar has a line for each quarter-hour, and Mrs. Smith wants a meeting for two hours, write her name, phone number, and the location of the appointment on the first three lines, and then draw a vertical line through the remaining five lines to indicate that the appointment will continue through that time.

Differing appointment times on the calendar. If appointment times differ from the preprinted lines on the calendar, indicate the time of the appointment in parentheses (i.e., if the appointment calendar has a line for every 15 minutes and someone wants a 20 minute appointment). This can prevent you from overlapping the appointments and causing you to fall behind.

List phone numbers with appointments. Put any phone numbers with the appointments. Then, if you need to cancel an appointment or reschedule, you do not have to go hunting all over to try and find a phone number. This can be very important if you suddenly have an emergency and you ask someone else to cancel all your appointments. This would not be the time to stop and locate the phone numbers for all of your afternoon appointments.

Do not schedule appointments without the calendar. Do not schedule an appointment if you are not able to verify that the time requested is available. You may think you know what times are open, but, without the calendar in front of you, you may not be aware of changes that have been made.

Do not schedule appointments that have not been approved. Do not schedule any appointments if you are not told to do so. This is especially important if you are scheduling appointments for your boss. You do not want to find that someone else has a second calendar or, even worse, that you have scheduled an appointment for someone the boss refuses to see.

Be on time. Be on time for all of your appointments. If you schedule a meeting, set a time to visit with a client, or tell a friend you will meet them for a working breakfast, you must be there at the time you set or you may lose their respect. Being on time is just a common courtesy, and it will really help you or your employer to maintain a professional relationship.

By following these simple rules, appointment setting can be accomplished easily and with a minimum of hassle. However, not following the rules can lead to stressful problematic situations.

On the Job Now

Directions: Read the following statements and rate yourself on how you feel you handle customers. Be honest. This is the only way you can recognize your strengths and weaknesses and work toward improving your weaknesses. Use the following numbers to answer the questions:

1 = Never, 2 = Seldom, 3 = Sometimes, 4 = Often, 5 = Always.

1. _____ I want the service I provide to leave an excellent impression, so I constantly look for ways to improve it.

2. _____ I put the customer's needs first as (s)he is my ultimate boss.

3. _____ I accept people without judging them.

4. _____ I am aware that my attitudes and moods affect the way I respond to customers.

5. _____ I show patience and courtesy regardless of the customer's behavior.

6. _____ I do not allow myself to become irritated or lose my composure when dealing with angry customers.

7. _____ I have developed the habit of following up on all complaints that are brought to my attention.

8. _____ I understand the customer and see his/her problem as most important, and I do all I can to resolve it.

9. _____ I treat all customers equally, regardless of their position, rank, color, clothes, accent, or other distinguishing features.

10. _____ I recognize it is perceptions that count when dealing with customers, so I do not allow my frustrations or irritations to show.

11. _____ If something the customer says offends me, I focus on what the client is feeling, not on getting even.

12. _____ I use professional language in my dealings with customers.

13. _____ I use proper telephone techniques and always identify myself to the caller.

14. _____ I make sure the customer is satisfied before terminating the conversation.

15. _____ I do not transfer a call unless it is absolutely necessary to resolve the customer's problem.

_____ Total

Scoring: Add the total for each question and then compute your score. The following scale gives an analysis of your client service quotient.

68–75	Excellent! Your behavior and attitudes set examples for others to follow.
59–67	Good. You have a high awareness of how important your role is in customer service.
50–58	Moderate. You may be allowing your own biases and feelings to affect your customer service.
41–49	Needs definite improvement. Time to get in touch with the obstacles between you and the quality service you should be providing.
Below 40	Poor. You need to make a concentrated effort to turn your attitudes and values around. Change may be slow.

CHAPTER REVIEW

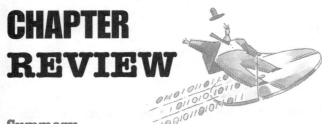

Summary

- Although each office has its own procedures to follow, it is important to understand the basic procedures that govern incoming mail, outgoing mail, special shipping services, and dealing with office machines. Without basic knowledge of the equipment and how to use it, it is impossible for medical billers to do their job properly.

- Correspondence is written communication between two people. Regardless of the content of the letter or the response you wish to evoke, the main purpose of correspondence is to communicate your thoughts, ideas, and desires to another person. To achieve this, be sure that the correspondence is necessary, formulate your ideas before beginning to write, and determine the action you wish the recipient to take.

- Written correspondence should always contain an opening, a body, and a closing. It should also be clear, concise, coherent, and grammatically correct. Combining all these elements will help to achieve effective written communications.

- A memo is a way of communicating important information within a company as quickly and easily as possible. Memos usually follow a specified format, with a header including TO, FROM, SUBJECT, and DATE headings.

- Customer service and patient relations are some of the most vital functions that medical billers perform. Without good service customers and patients may go elsewhere. Although it takes hard work, patience, and a good disposition to perform good customer service functions, it is well worth the time and effort.

- Here are the most important customer service topics discussed in this chapter, and they should always be kept in mind when dealing with your clients:
  - Greet the customer/client promptly.
  - Identify yourself by giving your name and title.
  - Write down the customer/patient's name and account number as soon as identification is provided.
  - Be professional in voice and choice of words.
  - Listen to what the person has to say. If the person is angry, let her get the anger out.
  - Do not react to a person's hostility with hostility of your own.
  - Give out accurate information. If you do not know the answer to a question, take the caller's name and phone number and tell them that you will investigate the matter and will call them back.
  - Stay informed concerning all policies and procedures and know the procedures of the company for which you work.
  - Be patient with the customer/patient. She/he might not be familiar with your procedures.
  - Always be supportive of your peers and your company. Acknowledge when a mistake has been made but do not make derogatory remarks about other personnel or company policies or procedures.
  - Be empathetic.
  - When necessary, use appropriate disclaimers.

Assignments

Complete the Questions for Review.
Complete Exercises 14–1 through 14–3.

Questions for Review

Directions: Answer the following questions without looking back at the material just covered. Write your answers in the space provided.

1. What is the best ink color to use when date-stamping incoming mail? _____

2. (True or False?) When signing for receipt of a package, your signature certifies that the contents were received undamaged and in good condition. _____

3. Name five special shipping services that you can purchase.

  1. _____

  2. _____

  3. _____

  4. _____

  5. _____

4. When dialing out on a multiline phone, what is the first thing you should check before picking up the phone?

_____

5. Before you begin writing a piece of correspondence you should _____

_____

6. What is the purpose of the opening in a letter? _____

_____

7. The body of the letter explains the _____

_____

8. If information must be written in the form of a letter, what four points should be followed?

  1. _____

  2. _____

  3. _____

  4. _____

9. If you are writing a letter of denial, should you give the bad news in the first paragraph? _____

10. What are the three main reasons for disseminating a memo? _____

_____

_____

_____

11. What is the usual format for a memo? _____

_____

12. What four items does the header section usually consist of? _____

_____

13. (True or False?) Headers are usually typed in lowercase letters. _____

14. (True or False?) Approval of a memo is given by signing one's name at the bottom of the memo. _____

15. What are the six basic steps that will bring you and the client to the resolution of a problem or concern?

   1. _____

   2. _____

   3. _____

   4. _____

   5. _____

   6. _____

If you are unable to answer any of these questions, refer back to that section in the chapter, and then fill in the answers.

Exercise **14-1**

Directions: Find and circle the words listed below. Words can appear horizontally, vertically, diagonally, forward, or backward.

1. Certified Mail
2. Closed-Ended Question
3. Coherence in Writing
4. Effectiveness in Writing
5. Facsimile Machine
6. Multiline Phones
7. Return Receipt Requested

```
G G A W C G D L W U E M G N V J L V I P W D
K N M Z F O W S S B K D T Q C A J Z M S E F
Q H I D T B H O Y S K D Q O I K C U Q T E A
C C J T Q W K E X A Z N L A K J L S S T U C
U Y W D I Q Z D R N M X R G D T M E I E Y S
L L G X K R K I E E K G I V I T U P M Y S I
T Z W A B S W Q Z R N M U L N Q I D L X K M
J M A Q I C V N I X O C I D E Q W G I K Q I
X V U Y B M R Y I A C N E R W Q P P V J P L
E M Q I Q O G D G S E Q T I Q T Q E H G X E
A U V H Z U I Q T P S P I K N M A K V H U M
Y W S G P C O J H K I E L O H W B M Q O Y A
X J W E G O U O V E Z M N E R S R S H W T C
Y P B X L Q N V C J B B C E D L F I B J N H
O G J G T E W E H K Q H T Y V U B B T H Z I
V E H F S P R P Y U O S R T U I G T K I E N
D D K A K N G R L L H B G T Q Q T Z J O N E
W I C F R T R S T Y U O X R D D P C N A H G
X P G U K F W Z X W V T B P K S X S E E M T
D O T S I Y Q F X B X L B G Q X D D Z F A O
X E W G T V L I A M D E I F I T R E C P F K
R C L O S E D E N D E D Q U E S T I O N D E
```

Exercise 14-2

Directions: Complete the crossword puzzle by filling in a word from the keywords that fits each clue.

Across

1. To service the customer or patient.
3. Bind several pages of a document together, often with a strip down the left-hand side of the document.
5. Short for memorandum, it is a letter intended for distribution within a company.
6. Being able to participate in another person's feelings or perceptions.

Down

2. Any appointment that happens on a regular basis.
4. Exactness of language.
7. Expanding file folders that help you remember items that need to occur on a specific date.

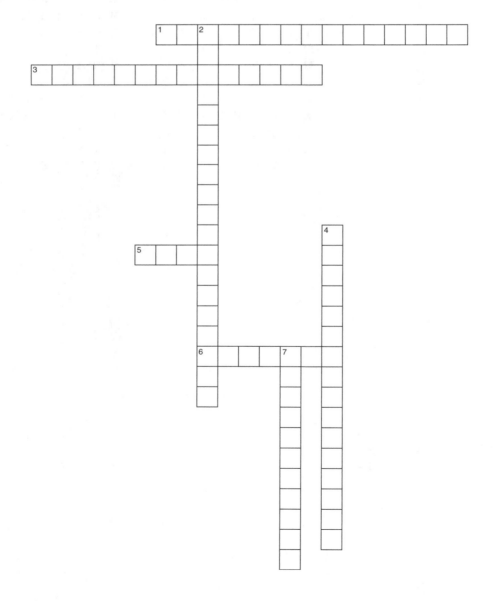

Exercise **14-3**

Directions: Match the following terms with the proper definition by writing the letter of the correct definition in the space next to the term.

1. _____ Body

2. _____ Correspondence

3. _____ Open-ended Question

4. _____ Summary

5. _____ Verification

a. A question that cannot be answered with a "yes," "no," or other brief response.

b. A brief statement of information covered.

c. The place in a correspondence in which you present the purpose of the communication.

d. Repeating information and asking if you have understood it correctly.

e. Written communication between two people.

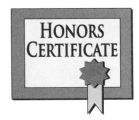

Honors Certification™

The certification challenge for this chapter will be a written test of the information contained in this chapter. Each incorrect answer will result in a deduction of up to 5% from your grade. You must achieve a score of 85% or higher to pass this test. If you fail the test on your first attempt, you may retake the test one additional time. The items included in the second test may be different from those in the first test.

Letters

The certification challenge for this section consists of a written test. The instructor will give you a topic along with sender and receiver addresses and ask you to compose a letter in block, modified block, or semiblock style. You must create and print out a letter in the correct style, as well as create an envelope. Spelling, grammar, and punctuation count, as well as correct style. The letter should have no errors in it. Each error will result in a deduction of up to 5% from your grade, depending on the type of error. You must receive a score of 85% or higher to pass this test. You are not allowed to use any reference materials when taking the test.

If you fail the test on your first attempt, you may retake the test one additional time. The addresses, subject matter, and style may be changed for the second test.

Memos

The certification challenge for this section consists of a written test. You will be required to create a memo in the correct format using the header information and topic supplied to you by your instructor. Spelling, grammar, and punctuation count, as well as correct style. The memo should have no errors in it. Each error will result in a deduction of up to 5% from your grade, depending on the type of error. You must receive a score of 85% or higher to pass this test. You are not allowed to use any reference materials when taking the test.

If you fail the test on your first attempt, you may retake the test one additional time. The items included in the second test may be different from those in the first test.

Person to Person Customer Service and Patient Relations

The certification challenge for this section consists of a role-play situation. You will be asked to role play a situation, providing good service to a customer who may not always be friendly or polite. The number of times you raise your voice, say something inappropriate, or react in a negative manner will be recorded. You must have less than three inappropriate responses to the customer's behavior.

If you fail the test on your first attempt, you may retake the test one additional time. The items included in the second test may be different from those in the first test.

CHAPTER 15 JOB SEARCH PREPARATION

15

Job Search
Preparation

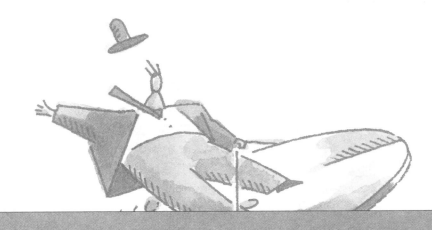

After completion of this chapter
you will be able to:

- Explain the keys and functions of the calculator.
- Properly use the calculator to add, subtract, multiply, and divide numbers.
- Gain speed and accuracy in using the calculator.
- List and describe the items that will help to make you faster and more accurate when using the computer.
- Describe the three different machines that make up a computer.
- Describe the keyboard and its five components: Typewriter Keys, Numeric Keys, Editing and Cursor Control Keys, Function Keys, and Status Lights.
- List and describe the eight techniques that can help you achieve frustration-free computing.
- Recognize and define computer terms.

- List the tips for properly maintaining your computer files.
- Determine your marketing objectives.
- List and discuss the five items that should be included on a résumé.
- Prepare a top-notch résumé.
- List and describe the five things to avoid when preparing a résumé.
- Exhibit proper interviewing techniques and appropriate mannerisms and dress.
- Write an effective cover letter requesting a job.
- List and describe the four basic components to the interview process.
- Describe the most common misconceptions regarding how a salary should be determined.

Keywords and Concepts
you will learn in this chapter:

- Brightness Control
- Calculator
- Central Processing Unit (CPU)
- Computer Disk Drive

- Computer Monitor
- Contrast Control
- Cover Letter
- Cursor

- Hard Drive
- Keyboard
- Power Switch
- Résumé

After having learned the necessary information to work in your chosen field, it is time to look for employment. In order to get the job you want, it is essential to have the job-hunting skills that will allow you to find the best position for you, and then to successfully get hired. As part of the job search preparation, it is important to become proficient in the use of calculators and computers. These tools are widely used in most businesses, and health claims examiners use them to do much of their work.

Calculator Basics

A **calculator** is a machine that computes numbers. It is used to add, subtract, multiply, and divide numbers, as well as compute percentages, square roots, and other mathematical calculations.

Working as a medical biller you will probably use a calculator every day. Often, there are charges that need to be totaled and amounts that need to be figured. Calculating these sums manually would take many hours. Therefore, it is vital that a medical biller master the use of the calculator.

Key Descriptions

Following are the keys most commonly found on a calculator and a description of their functions.

 PAPER ADVANCE KEY—Advances the paper tape without affecting your calculations.

C **CLEAR KEY**—Clears the display and the independent add register, pending operations and error/overflow conditions. Reactivates the calculator after an automatic power down.

% **PERCENT KEY**—Completes multiplication and division operations and shows the result as a decimal.

CE **CLEAR ENTRY KEY**—Clears the last entry only, thus enabling you to enter another number in its place without clearing out all previously entered numbers.

÷ **DIVIDE KEY**—Instructs the calculator to divide the number in the display by the next value entered.

= **EQUAL KEY**—Completes any pending operation.

X **MULTIPLY KEY**—Instructs the calculator to multiply the number in the display by the next value entered.

→ **BACKSPACE KEY**—Deletes the right-most digit in the display and shifts the remaining digits one place to the right.

0-9, 00 **NUMBER KEYS**—Enter numbers containing up to 10 digits. For numbers between one and negative one, a zero automatically precedes the decimal, allowing a maximum of nine digits to the right of the decimal.

. **DECIMAL POINT KEY**—Enters a decimal point. Most calculators have a floating decimal point which allows you to automatically set the decimal point at a given location in the number.

- **SUBTRACT KEY**—Subtracts the number in the display from the independent add register.

+ **ADD KEY**—Adds the number in the display to the independent add register.

D/# **DATE/NON-ADD KEY**—Prints a reference number or date without affecting calculations in progress.

/S **SUBTOTAL KEY**—Displays and prints the subtotal in the independent add register. Pressing this key does not affect the contents of the add register.

*/T **TOTAL KEY**—Displays and prints the total in the independent add register, then clears the register.

MT **MEMORY TOTAL KEY**—Displays and prints the value in memory, then clears the memory.

MS **MEMORY SUBTOTAL KEY**—Displays and prints the value in memory without clearing the memory.

M- **SUBTRACT FROM MEMORY KEY**—Prints the number in the display and subtracts it from the value in memory. If a pending multiplication or division operation has been entered, this key completes the operation and subtracts the result from memory.

M+ **ADD TO MEMORY KEY**—Prints the number in the display and adds it to the value in memory. If a pending multiplication or division operation has been entered, this key completes the operation and then adds the result into memory.

On the Job Now

Directions: Fill in the blank spaces without looking back at the text just covered.

1. The _____ instructs the calculator to divide the number in the display by the next value entered.
2. The Percent Key completes _____ and division operations and shows the result as a decimal.
3. The Backspace Key deletes the _____ digit in the display and shifts the remaining digits one place to the right.
4. The _____ prints a reference number or date without affecting calculations in progress.
5. The Memory Subtotal Key _____ and prints the value in memory without clearing the memory.

Printer Tape Symbols

Multiple symbols may be printed on printer tapes during calculations. Usually, these symbols will appear to the right of tape entries. Symbols not indicated should be explained in the specific calculator manual.

Symbol	Meaning or Explanation
+	Addition operation
–	Subtraction operation
<>	Subtotal of additions and subtractions
*	Total after "=," "%," or "*/T" is pressed
x	Multiplication operation
÷	Division operation
=	Completion of an operation
%	Percentage
+ *	Percentage add-on
– *	Percentage discount
#	Reference number or date printed in the center of the printer tape
C	Clear key erases all entries
M *	Addition to memory
M–	Subtraction from memory
M <>	Memory subtotal
M *	Memory total
E	Error/overflow condition
IC	**Item Counter Symbol.** When the printer switch is in the IC position, the number of additions to and subtractions from the independent add register is printed above each total or subtotal. The item counter for the independent add register is reset when "*/T" is pressed.

Computer Basics

As with most other industries, the majority of businesses are automated. The computer has, therefore, become an indispensable tool.

Only time and usage will make the medical biller accurate and fast on the computer. However, the following information may assist you when entering data:

Familiarity. Become familiar with the processing program you are using. If you know the fields (spots where specific information is entered), input rates will significantly increase because less verification and decision making will be required.

Visual Coordination. When learning to use the computer, watch either the video screen or the document you are inputting. Every effort should be made not to watch your fingers, as it is a difficult habit to break.

Preparation. Prepare your documents so that less shuffling of papers is required (i.e., unstaple, arrange by date).

Comfort. A comfortable chair that is adjusted to the correct height decreases fatigue.

Hands Free of Objects. Both hands should be free for typing in data. Pens, pencils, and other tools should not be held when entering data.

The computer is actually a combination of three different machines; the central processing unit (CPU), the monitor, and the keyboard.

The Computer

The **central processing unit (CPU)** is the rectangular box that houses the memory and functional components of the computer. A tremendous amount of studying is required to understand all the inner workings of the computer. However, you should become familiar

Practice
Pitfalls

Following are several tips for maintaining your computer files:

1. Make sure your paper systems are uncluttered and well structured by adhering to the following:

    a. Throw out old or marginally useful information.

    b. Divide remaining paper files into three classes: working, reference, and archives. Arrange the working files to be nearest you, and the archives to be out of your office.

    c. Create a subject filing structure for each of these classes of paper by mapping out your key functions.

2. Now go into your computer system and set up the same filing structure for your electronic documents. The closer your paper and electronic systems parallel each other, the easier it will be to remember where to file things and where to search for them.

3. If you use e-mail, especially in a corporate environment, you may have hundreds, or in extreme cases even thousands, of messages in your inbox. Begin deleting messages that are no longer needed, starting with the oldest.

4. Messages you want to save should be put into the electronic folders or directories you set up in step 2.

5. Now do the same with word processing or spreadsheet files.

6. If you need to recapture space on your hard drive, organize your electronic archive system with the same categories you established in step 1 and transfer your files from your hard drive to floppies or another storage medium.

7. Go through your hard drive and determine if there are any programs you are not using. If so, delete or transfer these to another storage medium.

8. If you are in a corporate environment or on the Internet and are being swamped with messages, remove yourself from these distribution lists.

9. Go through your documentation and clear out manuals for programs you are no longer using.

10. In the future, establish a certain time each day to process both your paper and e-mail. Do it daily so that your files do not build up in your system.

---

with a few components, such as the power switch, the reset button, and the disk drives.

The power switch is the on/off switch for the computer. It can be located anywhere on the computer, but it often is found toward the back.

The reset button often is found on the front of the computer. Pressing this button clears the screen and "reboots" or restarts the system. In other words, it achieves the same function as turning the computer off and then on again. Use caution with this button. If you do not save your data before pressing this button, it may be lost.

A **computer disk drive** is simply a place for the storage of information. Usually, a computer contains a "hard drive" within it. The **hard drive** provides space (memory) for information to be stored within the computer itself.

If there is insufficient memory in the hard drive or if there is a need to make data transportable to another

computer or to make a copy of the data, you may record the information on disks.

In the front of most computers is a slot (or several slots). These are alternate floppy disk drives. If the data you are using is stored on a disk, slide the disk into the slot to retrieve it.

At no time should a medical biller be required to repair the computer (unless this is part of their job). If something is wrong with the equipment, a computer repair technician should be called for on-site repair or the computer should be returned or taken to a computer service center. However, first make sure that all connections are in place at the back of the unit. This is similar to making sure that a television set is plugged in before calling a repairman.

There are a number of connections between the computer and its various components, the power source, and peripheral units (i.e., modems, fax machines). To ensure that all connections are in place,

On the Job Now

Directions: Add each of the following columns of numbers, then subtract the numbers from your total to arrive at zero. Clear the entries from your calculator and subtract the following columns of numbers and total, then add the numbers to your total to arrive at zero. Use the printer tape to check accuracy.

54659	46181	645.25	54.65
54165	35164	618.46	.12
41579	87319	614.79	2.76
45126	63453	641.76	78.11
56421	34150	123.08	457.12
20131	78455	469.61	3894.94
78991	23459	849.25	845.79
54164	89925	456.57	209.46
77986	24875	172.85	568.78
12094	23459	501.36	1056.23
12323	57847	841.43	347.51
71014	56748	051.65	351.91
71952	80893	540.71	6519.19
13671	10781	211.65	5056.20
24563	80974	549.93	645.51
63541	43729	635.45	345.48
0.168	89174	333.01	470.00
48567	39874	514.45	456.47

turn off the computer, and simply look at the back of the computer. If any cords or cables are disconnected, they may be the source of the problem. However, be sure that you know where to plug in the cable before attempting to slide it into any of the slots. Plugging in a cord or cable incorrectly can destroy your machine, your programs, or the machines and programs of others whose computers are attached to yours.

The Monitor

The **computer monitor** is the screen that is connected to the computer. It is this screen that allows you to see the programs and the data you are working with. There are four items you should be familiar with on the computer monitor: the power switch, the contrast control, the brightness control, and the cursor.

There is a **power switch** on the monitor like the one on the computer, which turns the monitor on and off. When the monitor is not in use for an extended period of time, the power switch should be turned off to prevent the image from burning into the screen. Be aware that turning off the monitor does not turn off the computer. Therefore, the data and information you were working on are still there. You just cannot see it.

The **contrast control** turns the contrast up and down between varying fields. This control usually is used to provide more or less contrast between those sections in a document that have been bolded or highlighted and those that have not.

The **brightness control** changes the brightness of the image on the screen. Adjust this knob so that you can read the screen without difficulty or glare.

The **cursor** is the small lighted symbol on the monitor screen that indicates where you are in the program or document. Depending on the system, this symbol may look like a bright straight line, a bright blinking line, or a blinking or solid box.

The Keyboard

The **keyboard** is your primary means of communicating with your computer. The input commands and data are typed in through the keyboard. Its layout roughly resembles that of an ordinary typewriter. To describe the keyboard more clearly, we will divide it into six parts, each with its own function:

- Keyboard angle adjustment.
- Typewriter keypad with control keys.
- Numeric keypad.
- Editing and cursor control keys.
- Function keys.
- Three status lights.

Keyboard Angle Adjustment

You can adjust your keyboard to two different positions for your typing comfort. To adjust, push on the adjustable leg handles on both sides and turn them to the desired position.

Typewriter Keypad with Control Keys

The typewriter area of the keyboard looks and behaves a lot like a standard typewriter keyboard. Like a typewriter, the Shift key produces capital letters. To type the special characters shown above the numbers on the number keys, hold down the Shift key and press the appropriate number key. For example, the Shift key with the number 1 produces an exclamation mark (!).

The computer keyboard also includes several special control keys specifically associated with computer operations, including Esc, Ctrl, Alt, and Enter. Here is a brief explanation of some important keyboard and control key functions:

CAPS LOCK—With this key, you can type uppercase letters without holding down the Shift key. When Caps Lock is engaged, the indicator light in the upper-right-hand corner of the keyboard lights up. The Caps Lock key only affects the 26 letters of the alphabet. To type special symbols, you still need to press the Shift key.

ENTER—This key acts as both the Return key and the Enter key. As the Return key, it ends the line being typed and advances the cursor to the next line. As the Enter key, it is used to execute commands you have typed.

SHIFT—For uppercase letters, punctuation, or symbols, either one of the two Shift keys can be pressed. When the Caps Lock key is engaged, the Shift key acts as an "Un-Shift" key, allowing you to type lowercase letters.

SPACE BAR—Moves the cursor one position to the right. It also will erase characters to the right, replacing them with blanks if the computer is in the typeover mode instead of insert mode.

BACKSPACE—This key erases one character to the left of the cursor.

On the Job Now

Directions: Fill in the blank spaces with the correct word without looking at the material just covered.

1. There are four items you should be familiar with on the computer monitor: the power switch, the _____, the brightness control, and the cursor.

2. There is a _____ on the monitor like the one on the computer that turns the monitor on and off.

3. The cursor is a _____ symbol on the monitor screen that indicates where you are in the program or document.

4. The keyboard is your _____ means of communicating with your computer.

5. The _____ changes the brightness of the images on the screen.

TAB—Moves the cursor to the next tab stop. In some programs the Tab key will act as a margin release to the left if the Shift key is depressed, or will move the cursor one tab spot to the left.

ESC—The Escape key has different functions depending on the program.

ALT—Like the Shift key, Alt performs no function on its own. It is used in combination with other keys. The function of Alt varies depending on the application being used.

CTRL—This key performs no function on its own. Like the Shift and Alt keys, the control key (Ctrl) is used only in combination with other keys. Ctrl performs many different functions depending on the application being used.

Pressing two or three keys simultaneously can be used to perform a series of unique program control and screen control functions as shown in the following:

KEYS	FUNCTION DESCRIPTION
Ctrl/Break	Terminates the execution of a program and identifies the line where it stops.
Ctrl/Alt/Del	This function resets the computer.
Shift/Print	Causes all data on the screen only to be printed.

To produce the function indicated, press and hold down the first (and second if it is a series of three) key(s) and press the last key. This is by no means a comprehensive list of the functions available.

Numeric Keypad

The numeric keypad is located separately from the alphabetic keys. It is usually on the right-hand side of a computer keyboard. The keypad performs a dual function.

With the Num Lock key engaged (indicated by the status light in the upper-right-hand corner of some keyboards), the keypad can be used for the rapid data entry of numbers. With Num Lock disengaged, the keypad can be used to move the cursor or to perform special editing features.

A 101-key-enhanced keyboard provides a separate keypad for cursor control and editing (located immediately to the left of the numeric keypad). For this reason, most users will find it convenient to leave the Num Lock key on, thus allowing for the rapid entry of numbers. If your keyboard is not a 101-enhanced keyboard, you will probably not want to leave the Num Lock key on.

The following keys operate the same regardless of whether or not the Num Lock key is on or off:

ENTER   Works the same as the Enter key on the typewriter keypad.

+   Displays the Plus symbol.

−   Displays the Minus symbol.

*   Displays the Asterisk, used for multiplication.

/   Displays the Slash, used for division.

The following keys perform differently depending on whether the Num Lock key is turned on or off.

KEY	NUM LOCK ON	NUM LOCK OFF
1 End	1	END—Moves the cursor to the end of the line.
2 ↓	2	↓ —Moves the cursor down.
3 Pg Dn	3	Pg Dn—Moves the cursor down one page, or 25 lines.
4 ←	4	← —Moves the cursor to the left.
5	5	No function.
6 →	6	→ —Moves the cursor to the right.
7 Home	7	HOME—Moves the cursor to the beginning of the line.
8 ↑	8	↑ —Moves the cursor up.
9 Pg Up	9	Pg Up—Moves the cursor up one page, or 25 lines.
0 Ins	0	INS—This key toggles (turns on and off) between Insert and Typeover mode.

. Del Decimal DEL—(Delete) Erases one character at the position of the cursor.

Editing and Cursor Control Keys

The 101-key-enhanced keyboard contains a separate set of editing keys usually located between the Typewriter and Numeric keypads.

HOME—Moves the cursor to the first character of the line.

CURSOR UP—Moves the cursor up one line for each keystroke.

CURSOR DOWN—Moves the cursor down one line for each keystroke.

CURSOR RIGHT—Moves the cursor to the right one character position for each keystroke.

CURSOR LEFT—Moves the cursor to the left one character position for each keystroke.

END—Moves the cursor to the right of the last character on the current line.

DELETE—Deletes characters at the cursor. All characters to the right will be moved left. If this key is held down, it will erase each character as it reaches the cursor.

INSERT/TYPEOVER—On "Insert," characters typed will be inserted before previously typed text, pushing the existing text to the right. On "Typeover," existing characters will be typed over.

PAGE UP—Moves the cursor up one page, or 25 lines.

PAGE DN—Moves the cursor down one page, or 25 lines.

SCROLL LOCK—When the Scroll Lock key is pressed, the Scroll Lock light will be illuminated on the keyboard. Once the Scroll Lock light is on, it can be turned off by pressing the Scroll Lock key again, which also will turn off the Scroll Lock mode of operation. Refer to the computer application program manual for more details on this key.

PRINT SCREEN—When the Print Screen key is pressed, the data displayed on the screen will be printed (if the computer is connected to a printer). If the Ctrl key is pressed and held while this key is pressed, the printer function will be disabled or enabled.

PAUSE BREAK—This key suspends the program execution until another key is pressed. When used with the Ctrl key, the program being run will be terminated.

Function Keys

Along the top half of the keyboard or on the left side of some keyboards are 12 function keys that allow complex program commands to be performed with a single keystroke.

Different software programs use function keys for different purposes. Therefore, to properly use these keys, the program-specific user's guide must be referred to. It is highly advisable not to use the function keys without referring to the program instructions, as they may delete data or cancel parts of a program.

Three Status Lights

The three status lights are usually located in the upper-right-hand corner of the keyboard. They are labeled NUM LOCK, CAPS LOCK, and SCROLL LOCK. The **Num Lock** light, when lit, signifies the Num Lock function is engaged, thus causing the keys on the numeric keypad to act as numbers rather than cursor movement keys.

When the **Caps Lock** light is on, it signifies that all letters typed on the keyboard will appear as capital letters.

Scroll Lock is a feature that only works with some computer programs. When the **Scroll Lock** is used in these applications, the cursor is locked onto whatever line it is on when the Scroll Lock button is pushed, and the entire page will move around it. For example, if your cursor is halfway down the page when you hit the Scroll Lock button, your cursor will remain halfway down the page. When you hit the arrow down key, the entire document will move up one line, but the cursor will remain in the center of the screen.

Computer Terms

There are a number of terms used in the computer industry that can be confusing to those who have never dealt with computers. The following terms are those most commonly used by medical billers and other computer users.

Bit—(Contraction for binary digit) a single binary digit, either 0 or 1. A bit is the smallest unit of data stored in a computer; all other data must be coded into a pattern of individual bits.

Boot (or bootstrap)—the process of starting up a computer.

CD-ROM—a compact disc format used to hold text, graphics and hi-fi stereo. Basically, it is like an audio CD, but it uses a different format for data. You will need a CD-ROM drive for most

Practice
Pitfalls

According to Murphy's Law, anything that can go wrong will go wrong. However, a number of techniques will help to eliminate the frustration of losing computer-stored information. The following eight techniques should be learned and should become a daily part of your computer life:

1. Save your data often and make backup copies while working on it. A second copy of the data should be saved to a second file when you are finished. A power surge or brief break in the power supply can erase your entries in less than one second.

2. Keep a backup copy in a different location. A second copy of important data should be stored in a different room or, if possible, a different building. This preserves the data in case of fire, destruction of the building, or water damage.

3. Always date the copies of your files so that you can retrieve the latest disk easily.

4. Use permanent disks or tapes to store copies of financial and confidential records and keep them in a secure fireproof location.

5. Maintain a notebook or log that shows what you have stored in the computer and the file name it is located under.

6. Set up a system for naming documents so that they will be easily accessible even if you do not have the log.

7. Handle data diskettes properly. This includes:

   a. Never touch the magnetic media housed inside the plastic cover. There is a hole in the plastic through which the computer reads the information. On the 3.5-inch disk, this hole is covered by a piece of sliding metal.

   b. Store all disks inside plastic or paper covers to protect them from damage. Insert and remove the disk carefully from the cover to prevent scratching the magnetic media.

   c. Never fold, spindle, or mutilate your disk.

   d. Keep diskettes stored at temperatures between 50° and 125° F. Never leave a data disk exposed to sunlight.

   e. Keep all magnets away from your data disks. Information stored on a magnetic medium can be erased when it comes in contact with a magnet. This includes the magnet contained in office supplies, such as paper clip holders.

   f. Before touching a data disk, discharge any static electricity you may have picked up by touching a piece of metal or an antistatic mat. Static electricity also demagnetizes and can erase the data contained on a disk.

   g. When carrying disks across a carpeted area, place the disk inside its protective sleeve and inside another object such as a disk storage box or between the pages of a book. This will prevent erasure by any static electricity that you may pick up by walking across the carpet.

   h. To prevent any changes to information stored on a data disk, slide the button on the disk designed for this purpose. To change the data at a later date, simply slide the button back to the original position.

   i. Do not write on a disk label with a ballpoint pen or pencil; use a felt-tip marker. The pressure applied when writing with a pen or pencil may cause indentations on the magnetic media, which may damage the diskette.

8. If you accidentally delete or are unable to retrieve information, immediately remove the disk from the computer. Do not save anything on the disk. Many computer files can be reconstructed with the proper programs but only if the information has not been written over.

Remember that it is far easier to retrieve data that has been stored properly than to recreate it. Taking proper care of your data will ensure that it will be retrievable when you need it.

new software, as it is a lot easier and quicker for developers to distribute and for you to install software in this format.

Chip or **Silicon Chip**—another name for an integrated circuit, a complete electronic circuit on a slice of silicon crystal only a few millimeters square.

Computer Graphics—use of computers to display and manipulate information in pictorial form.

Central Processing Unit (CPU)—the CPU or processor is considered the brain of the computer. The CPU makes everything else perform, and it is one of the major factors that determine the computer's overall speed. The faster the CPU, the faster the computer can execute your instructions.

Data—facts, figures, and symbols, especially as stored in computers. The term is often used to mean raw, unprocessed facts, as distinct from information, to which a meaning or interpretation has been applied.

Database—a structured collection of data, which may be manipulated to select and sort desired items of information.

Desktop Publishing—use of microcomputers for small-scale typesetting and page makeup.

Disk—a common medium for storing large volumes of data. A magnetic disk is rotated at high speed in a disk-drive unit as a read-write (playback or record) head passes over its surfaces to record or read magnetic variations that encode the data.

Download—to load a file from the Internet or another source onto your computer.

DOS—acronym for disk operating system, a computer operating system specifically designed for use with disk storage; also used as an alternate name for a particular system, MS-DOS.

Electronic Mail—or e-mail, is a system that enables the users of a computer network to send messages to other users.

Gigabyte—a measure of memory capacity, equal to one billion bytes. It is also used, less precisely, to mean 1,000 megabytes.

Hacking—unauthorized access to a computer, either for fun or for malicious or fraudulent purposes.

Hard Drive—the storage place on a computer. It stores information in your computer. You will need a lot of hard drive space to hold all the information you want on your computer.

Hardware—the mechanical, electrical, and electronic components of a computer system, as opposed to the various programs that constitute software.

Interface—the point of contact between two programs or pieces of equipment.

Joystick—an input device that signals to a computer the direction and extent of displacement of a hand-held lever.

Keyboard—an input device resembling a typewriter keyboard, used to enter instructions and data.

Laptop Computer—a portable microcomputer, small enough to be used on the operator's lap.

Light Pen—a device resembling an ordinary pen, used to indicate locations on a computer screen.

Megabyte—a unit of memory equal to 1,024 kilobytes. It is sometimes used, less precisely, to mean one million bytes.

Memory—the part of a system used to store data and programs either permanently or temporarily. There are two main types: immediate access memory and backing storage. Random Access Memory (RAM) is what your computer and operating system uses to perform functions. RAM is considered a temporary storage area for particular pieces of information required by the computer at any given moment. The more RAM you have, the faster your computer will perform.

Microprocessor—complete computer central processing unit contained on a single integrated circuit, or chip.

Modem—(acronym for modulator/demodulator) device for transmitting computer data over telephone lines.

Mouse—an input device used to control a pointer on a computer screen.

Operating System—a program that controls the basic operation of a computer.

Printer—an output device for producing printed copies of text or graphics.

Procedure—a small part of a computer program that performs a specific task, such as clearing the screen or sorting a file.

Screen or Monitor—an output device on which the computer displays information for the benefit of the operator.

Software—a collection of programs and procedures for making a computer perform a specific task, as opposed to hardware, the physical components of a computer system.

Speech Recognition—or voice input, any technique by which a computer can understand ordinary speech.

Spreadsheet—a program that mimics a sheet of ruled paper, divided into columns and rows.

Touch Screen—an input device allowing the user to communicate with the computer by touching a display screen.

Virtual Memory—a technique whereby a portion of the computer-backing storage memory is used as an extension of its immediate-access memory.

Virtual Reality—advanced form of computer simulation, in which a participant has the illusion of being part of an artificial environment.

Virus—a piece of software that can replicate itself and transfer itself from one computer to another without the user being aware of it. Some viruses are relatively harmless, but others can damage or destroy data.

Word—a group of bits that a computer's central processing unit treats as a single working unit.

Word Processing—storage and retrieval of written text by computer. Word processing software packages enable the writer to key in text and amend it in a number of ways.

Workstation—high-performance desktop computer with strong graphics capabilities, traditionally used for engineering, scientific research, and desktop publishing.

Zip Drives—like floppy disk drives, except they hold the equivalent of about 80 floppy disks. You also could use a zip drive for backup purposes.

Job Search Preparation

Regardless of the career path you have chosen, all the education in the world is worthless if you do not have good job-hunting skills. Without them, you may never gain employment.

Gaining successful employment requires you to look for a job, and also to market yourself. This works for direct mail advertising companies around the world, and it can work for you, too. It is important to start with a set of written objectives, know what separates you from the competition, and familiarize yourself with your target audience.

Job Search Objectives

First, determine your job search objectives. What responsibilities do you want in the position you are looking for? Is there a specific title for such responsibilities? What type of work environment do you desire (i.e., office, hospital, restaurant, outdoor work)? What can you reasonably expect, both in the way of title and salary? Writing down your objectives can help to solidify them in your mind and help you formulate a plan of action.

Uniqueness

Most available job openings have numerous people applying for the position. You need to emphasize your uniqueness and the talents that you can bring to the job. What sets you apart from your competitors? Do you have a special talent or area of expertise? Call attention to it. What about a skill you can share with other employees? Highlight it. Let prospective employers know how you can help to train co-workers, saving the company time and money while helping the operation run smoothly. Do you have contacts in a particular industry that might allow your employer to expand? Tell prospective employers these details to set you apart from the competition.

Target Audience

Success at finding the right job depends not only on the previous two areas discussed but also on looking in the right place. You would not go to a restaurant to find a job as a typist. Likewise, you would not go to a typing pool to find a job as a waiter. Much depends on where you look for a job.

After deciding on the particular organizations offering the best opportunities, find out who the decision makers are. Who would be the best person for you to contact regarding employment? Get the person's title and name. Find out as much as you can about the person who makes the decisions at the companies you are targeting. What are their professional affiliations (i.e., AFL-CIO, AMA)? What is their career background? What are their job-related concerns and corporate responsibilities? The answers to these questions will help you establish rapport with the person and help you bring out your commonalities.

Build Your Database

Once you have established your target audience, make an organized collection of information about the companies and possible job prospects. Your collection needs to keep track of potential employers, professional contacts, and resources.

Keep detailed and well-organized notes on everyone you speak with that can help you reach your objectives. Always write down the person's name, title, the company or organization name, address, phone and fax numbers, any professional affiliations, the date you spoke or met, how you reached them, what follow-up you should make, and any other relevant information.

Build a file on each company from all the resources available to you. This can include job banks, trade publications, executive search firms, civic groups, alumni associations, social networks, colleagues or co-workers, former employers, and anyone else who can help you. You will be surprised at how many people you know when you start to write them down.

The Résumé

Now you are ready to develop your résumé and cover letter. Think of these items as sales materials for your career. The cover letter should invite and interest your target audience enough that they will read your résumé. Your **résumé** is a summary of employment experience and qualifications, essentially the marketing brochure that gets you in the door. Both need to proclaim the benefits you offer to an employer. Sample résumés can be found at the end of this chapter.

A First-Class Résumé

A résumé can be your best friend or your worst enemy. A first-class résumé is one of the most important items you can have in your job search and can open doors for you. A bad résumé will slam them shut. In essence, a résumé is your personal representative. It tells the company not only who you are but also the type of person you are. No one would welcome an employee who is sloppy and disorganized. Likewise, your résumé should not be full of errors or difficult to read. Your résumé is a direct reflection of you. Its goal is to get you an interview and help you to land that great job.

The initial screening of a résumé occurs very quickly; sometimes it is merely scanned for a few seconds. Your format should keep this in mind. The purpose of this quick scan is to weed out the résumés that

have obvious typographic errors, are poorly organized, or are substandard in reproduction. If the author of a résumé was not careful enough to proofread and correct his own résumé, why should an employer think the person would be any more conscientious at work? If your résumé is hard to read or difficult to file (because of odd-shaped paper), it will undoubtedly end up in file 13, also known as the trash can.

Before you write your résumé, do a little research. Find a current book on résumé writing. This type of book will give you a wealth of information and good résumé samples.

The Basics

Your résumé should typically be no longer than one page. It should be printed on white or off-white 8.5 × 11 inch paper. Do not use bright or fancy colors. Professionals in the Human Resources area prefer one-page résumés. One-page résumés are easier to read and yet provide enough information to introduce you and your experience. Do not jeopardize your job opportunities by being long-winded or by listing every minute detail about your professional history.

Always be concise and do not abbreviate any words. The chance of being misunderstood is not worth saving the space.

The following five items should be included on your résumé:

1. **Name, address, and telephone number:** you would be surprised at how many people leave off one or more pieces of this vital information. Make sure that all the information is correct. Do not cut corners. Your address should include an apartment number and the zip code, and your phone number should include the area code. The easier it is for an employer to contact you, the better.

2. **Objective statement:** some employers and résumé writers consider an objective statement to be optional. However, if you have a specific direction, include it. It lets the prospective employer know what your goals are. If you are interested in several different jobs, you might want to replace the objective statement with a qualifying statement. In this way, you will not have to prepare separate objective statements (and résumés) for each job title. Make sure that your résumé shows that you have some direction. Your cover letter also should reinforce this.

3. **Qualifying statement:** a qualifying statement is a way to toot your own horn. It sells you as a

potential employee and lists your abilities and experiences. You can get ideas for your qualifying statement in the want ads. See what skills and characteristics are desired (i.e., excellent written and verbal communication skills, ability to handle a variety of tasks, and excellent organizational ability). These are exactly the types of statements that should go into your qualifying statement.

4. **Work experience:** there are a variety of ways to state your experience. The most common approach is to list your employment history in reverse chronological order, putting your most recent job first. However, if you have had numerous job changes or a gap in employment, you do not necessarily want to emphasize this. Therefore, you might consider using the functional format résumé. This lists together all related experiences rather than listing according to date.

5. **Education:** if you have education or training beyond the high school level you will want this fact to stand out. Find a way to highlight this so that, even when your résumé is scanned quickly, additional education can be noticed. The simplest format is to list the degree or certificate, followed by your major or course of study. Follow this with the name and location of the school and year in which you graduated (i.e., Certificate of Completion, Medical Billing, Los Angeles College, Los Angeles, CA, 2001). Education and training should be listed in reverse chronological order. See sample résumés at the end of this chapter.

Optional information, if you have room at the bottom, should include special skills, personal notes, hobbies, and references.

Professional Services

If you need additional help, a number of professional résumé services are available. It is essential that your résumé look professional. This includes the use of a word processor and a letter-quality printer. If you do not have access to this type of equipment, it may be a good investment to hire someone to type and print it for you.

Edit and Proofread

You must edit and proofread your résumé very carefully. Remember that this single sheet of paper can either help or hurt you in getting a job. It is a direct reflection on you. Before you send it to a potential employer, get a friend to check it for errors and content. Another person can often spot things that you have missed.

What to Avoid

Some of these items may seem obvious, but a surprising number of people make these errors on their résumés. The following seven items are things to avoid when you are composing your résumé:

1. Never send a carbon copy or an inferior quality copy of your résumé to a prospective employer.
2. Never use abbreviations; this includes the term "etc." Anything important enough to be stated should be written out. Write it out or leave it out.
3. Do not waste time and space detailing mundane, entry-level jobs that have no bearing on your present job search.
4. Do not list a desired salary. Discussions of this sort should be saved for the interview. If you ask for too high of a salary, you may not be granted an interview. If you ask for too little, a prospective employer may wonder what you are worth.
5. Consider the importance of salary, job location, and position desired before you limit yourself. Ask yourself if any of these are more important than a chance for advancement.
6. Do not include information on your age, marital status, religion, or race.
7. Do not put "References available on request," as this just annoys prospective employers.

Words to Use in Your Résumé

Use an active voice in your résumé. Action verbs and specific nouns are best when describing your job duties and accomplishments. Following are words to use in your résumé:

Accomplish	Achieve	Act
Adapt	Administer	Advertise
Advise	Aid	Analyze
Apply	Approach	Approve
Arrange	Assemble	Assess
Assign	Assist	Attain
Budget	Build	Calculate
Catalog	Chair	Clarify
Collaborate	Communicate	Compare
Compile	Complete	Conceive
Conciliate	Conduct	Consult
Contract	Control	Cooperate
Coordinate	Correct	Counsel

Create	Decide	Define
Delegate	Demonstrate	Design
Detail	Determine	Develop
Devise	Direct	Distribute
Draft	Edit	Employ
Encourage	Enlarge	Enlist
Establish	Estimate	Evaluate
Examine	Exchange	Execute
Exhibit	Expand	Expedite
Facilitate	Familiarize	Forecast
Formulate	Generate	Govern
Guide	Handle	Head
Hire	Identify	Implement
Improve	Increase	Index
Influence	Inform	Initiate
Innovate	Inspect	Install
Institute	Instruct	Integrate
Interpret	Interview	Introduce
Invent	Investigate	Lead
Maintain	Manage	Manipulate
Market	Mediate	Moderate
Modify	Monitor	Motivate
Negotiate	Obtain	Operate
Order	Organize	Originate
Oversee	Perceive	Perform
Persuade	Plan	Prepare
Present	Preside	Process
Produce	Program	Promote
Propose	Provide	Publicize
Publish	Qualify	Raise
Recommend	Reconcile	Record
Recruit	Rectify	Redesign
Reduce	Regulate	Relate
Renew	Report	Represent
Reorganize	Research	Resolve
Review	Revise	Scan
Schedule	Screen	Select
Sell	Serve	Settle
Solve	Speak	Staff
Standardize	Stimulate	Summarize
Supervise	Support	Survey
Synthesize	Systematize	Teach
Train	Transmit	Update
Write		

The Cover Letter

Your résumé provides a potential employer with your qualifications. The **cover letter** is an introduction to your résumé. It invites the potential employer to read further. Your cover letter should be concise and to the

Practice
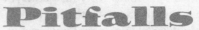

The following tips will help you to create a top-notch résumé:

Put a brief description of yourself at the top that highlights your strengths. For example, "A seasoned veteran that is responsible for overseeing three branch offices in three states." Most employers spend only a few seconds on each résumé, so get your selling points up front.

Try several different formats. Do not limit yourself to a standard chronological format. Experiment with a functional format, grouping your past activities under headings such as "Team Coordination" or "Supervisory Activities" with applicable experience listed under each. If you have a strong specialty that a prospective employer may need, this format may highlight that trait more effectively than a list of jobs held.

Stick to one or two fonts. Do not try to show off your computer skills by including a multitude of fonts in your résumé. This often ends up looking messy and disjointed.

point. What you are really trying to say with the cover letter is that you are enclosing your résumé and are available for an interview at the prospective employer's convenience. The cover letter should be neatly typed on white or off-white 8.5 × 11 inch paper. See a sample cover letter at the end of this chapter.

Letter Writing Do Nots

The following are items you should avoid when writing your cover letter:

1. Do not include anything in your letter that cannot be substantiated in your interview.
2. Do not try to force an interview by using sympathy or any sense of urgency.
3. Do not load your cover letter with unnecessary information; just present the important facts. The cover letter should be an addendum to your résumé.
4. Do not address your letter to a company or a title. Find out the name of the person who holds that title and address it to that person. If you cannot, address it to the department or division that will supervise your work.

On the Job Now

Directions: Answer the following questions without looking back at the material just covered. Write your answers in the space provided.

1. Why should you make sure that your résumé is no longer than one page? _____
   _____
   _____

2. List the five items that should be included on your résumé.

   1. _____
   2. _____
   3. _____
   4. _____
   5. _____

3. List the seven items to avoid when you are composing your résumé.

   1. _____
   2. _____
   3. _____
   4. _____
   5. _____
   6. _____
   7. _____

5. Do not mail a résumé without a cover letter.
6. Do not forget to request an interview in your cover letter.
7. Do not forget to proofread your cover letter, checking for appearance, grammar, and spelling errors.

Marketing Yourself

When marketing your skills, keep in mind the following things:

- Segment your audience.
- Prepare your portfolio.
- Professionally market yourself.

Let's discuss each item individually.

People respond to various things differently. Salespeople know this and segment their audience accordingly. You also need to segment your audience to be sure you are presenting the right benefit (talent) to the right market in the right tone. This often means you have to write several different résumés and cover letters. It is worth it if you want to get the right job. Just be sure your objectives, experience, and message are appropriate to the segment you are trying to sell.

You also might consider creating a portfolio on yourself. This portfolio could include your résumé, letters of reference, graphs or charts supporting your accomplishments, samples of previous work, and other informational material. Present the information neatly. A handsome presentation folder conveys a stronger impact than a cover letter and résumé alone. Its very size commands more attention. Be careful to not overload it with too much extraneous information. Present only the best of what you have to offer.

Depending on the situation, it can often be best to present your portfolio during the interview rather than including it with your résumé.

Searching for a job is not enough. Instead, you must professionally market yourself. Take charge of the situation and of your career. Job hunters take what comes along; marketing yourself means more. It means going out and searching for the job you want, then selling yourself until you get it.

Develop a plan that will make things happen. Assemble your resources. Present yourself with purpose, professionalism, and positive energy. Not only is this more effective, but also it is better for your morale than just starting another dreaded job search!

The Job Interview

The job interview can be one of the most frightening experiences a potential employee faces. Add to this the knowledge that most working adults make an average of 10 career changes in their lifetime, each requiring a number of job interviews. That is a lot of stress to go through, but with knowledge can come the power to take control of the interview and turn fear into success.

Part of being prepared for an interview is having your directions, questions, interview agenda, and information about the company before the interview, so do your homework! If prepared properly, you (the applicant) will know exactly where you stand and how you did by the end of the interview.

Keep in mind that the key to getting hired is chemistry. If someone likes you, they will go out of their way to make you fit.

Your goal should be to get a job offer or at the very least get to the next step, which is another interview. Remember you can turn any offer down but not if you do not have it!

Dress

How you dress and present yourself is also very important. Men should wear a gray or dark blue suit, a white shirt with contrast tie, and polished black shoes. Women should wear a conservative suit with a plain blouse that has a conservative neckline, and low-heeled shoes. Both men and women should make sure their hair is neat and trimmed, and that their hands and nails are clean. Wear little or no jewelry, and no perfume or cologne; you never know what the interviewer might be sensitive to. Give a firm handshake, smile, and make eye contact. Display interest, energy, and confidence.

The Application

When you arrive, you may be given an application to fill out. This application is very important because whatever information you put on it is what the employer will be verifying (i.e., salary, reasons for leaving, education). Remember, keep it simple. Take a black pen to fill out your application. This color of ink photocopies well.

In the section for "Salary Desired" write the word "open" or "negotiable." NEVER write a dollar amount!

Remember when filling out the area "Reasons for Leaving" that once you put this information on an application it becomes a permanent record. You have signed to have this information verified by the potential employer. Companies do not typically give information beyond salary, start and end dates, and voluntary or involuntary termination (involuntary could be layoff or fired). Whatever you write should be as positive as possible. Employers look for patterns (i.e., job changes because of disagreement with boss, laid off more than once, conflict with other employees, disagreements with management decisions, etc.). When found, good or bad, they feel they get the picture of the applicant. Although you want to be honest, you also want to keep these reasons neutral if possible.

Be accurate with your education. State the correct degree you earned and the year you received it. This is the easiest information on your application to verify.

Interviewing

Interviewing research indicates that there are four basic components to the interview process:

- The first four seconds.
- The next five minutes.
- The main portion.
- The end or closing.

It is important to fully understand each of these components so that you can control them and reap the best rewards from the interview process.

The First Four Seconds

First impressions are very important. They can put you off to a good start, or they can strike a mark against you that will be hard to erase if an interviewer forms a negative impression.

Eighty percent of a first impression is based on your appearance. For that reason, it is suggested that you dress more formally than you might dress on the job. Keep your appearance conservative; flashy styles can be risky.

The handshake is a symbolic gesture of trust. A firm, brief handshake and direct eye contact indicate self-confidence and trustworthiness.

The Next Five Minutes

The next five minutes of an interview can often determine whether you get a job offer or not. Studies reveal that interviewers often form an opinion within this five-minute period. They then seek information that will validate this initial impression. Thus, their opinion influences their decision to either hire or reject the candidate. If the impression was negative, one study reveals, 90% of the time the applicant was not hired. If the opinion was positive, the candidate received a job offer 75% of the time.

Therefore, your primary goal during this time should be to make sure the initial impression is positive. The following suggestions have been found to be the most important:

1. Keep the tone of your voice calm but interested. You should be careful to speak clearly in a voice that is loud enough to be heard, but not so loud that it is annoying.

2. Make direct eye contact with the interviewer. It gives the impression that you are open and honest and have nothing to hide. Eye contact can actually be equal in power to the sound and tone of the voice.

3. Your posture conveys a large message when you are sitting as well as standing. Remaining straight and tall with shoulders back will convey confidence. Leaning forward slightly in your chair will convey interest.

4. Never underestimate the power of a smile for opening the lines of communication.

The Main Portion

After the important amenities have been taken care of, the general questioning will begin. Listen carefully to the questions and focus your answers on the job requirements and on highlighting your strengths. Look for any specific problems that the organization may have. Highlight your skills and work history as they relate to the employer's needs. Remember that if they did not have a need, they would not be interviewing you. Make them believe they need you.

Try to find out as much as possible about the company, the job, and the people. A good interview is a two-way, give-and-take situation. Interviewers expect you to ask questions. Therefore, strong well-directed questions help to create a positive impression. Be sure to listen carefully to the response, and use the information to strengthen your position.

The personality trait that attracts an interviewer the most is enthusiasm. If you like what you have heard about this company, or what you are hearing in the interview, do not be afraid to let the interviewer know. Be comfortable about revealing your personality and the kind of person you are, but do it with interest, awareness, and energy. Many studies have indicated

that individuals often are hired based more on their personality than on their skills.

The middle portion of the interview can present some of your greatest difficulty. Be aware of the hidden agenda behind each question. Is the interviewer trying to find out about your skills, your education, or your background?

If an interviewer continually returns to a specific topic, especially in your past, they are unconsciously telling you that they are questioning the response or that they discern a weakness. Remember to control your responses. Frame your experiences in a positive light and focus on the positive aspects that will most benefit the company.

There is probably at least one situation in your history that you would rather not have come out in the open. This may be a termination, a misdemeanor or felony conviction, or a similar problem.

First, determine whether the information will come up during the normal course of the interview, or during the background check. Most companies run a preliminary check on their prospective employees. This may include a brief phone call to previous employers and a check of police records.

Research has shown that negative aspects are seen much more negatively when they are revealed bit by bit. The impression is that you may have other things wrong if they ask the right questions to bring them out.

Take control of this situation by disclosing any negative information briefly and forthrightly before you are asked. In this way you can place the best possible light on the situation. Even a termination can be turned from a negative into a positive by sincerely and honestly discussing what you have learned from the experience and what you will do differently, if you are given the opportunity.

The End or Closing

Finally, you have reached the closing moments of the interview. Many people begin to lose concentration and relax at this point. Do not! Keep yourself focused. A strong finish may be the difference between you and someone else in a tight race. Show the interviewer you are still excited about the job, especially now that you know more about it and the company.

Make a strong final note by succinctly summarizing your positive points as they relate to the job. There is nothing wrong with asking when a decision on the candidates will be made. When you have the answer, show your enthusiasm by letting the interviewer know that you will call back the afternoon of the decision.

On the Job Now

Directions: Answer the following questions without looking back at the material just covered. Write your answers in the space provided.

1. List four items you will need to be prepared for an interview.

    1. _____

    2. _____

    3. _____

    4. _____

2. List the four basic components to the interview process.

    1. _____

    2. _____

    3. _____

    4. _____

3. What portion of the interview can be the most difficult and why? _____

_____

_____

Interviewing is much like a game. If you make all the right moves, you will win the job. If you make errors, you will not. In the end, it is all up to you and the way you play.

Getting Paid What You Are Worth

The issue of salary will undoubtedly come up, either during the interview or before. Salary is probably the most important issue among workers today. Nevertheless, the way in which salary is determined is often one of the least understood aspects when it comes to evaluating your worth. Far too many people see their salary as an extension of themselves and how much they are worth. Often, their point of view is totally unrealistic according to the marketplace.

Let's review four of the most common misconceptions regarding how a salary should be determined:

1. **Seeing your monetary compensation as a reflection of your worth as a person.** It is not. Your salary is based on your objective value in the marketplace. If your skills are in high demand, you will be paid more than if they are not. This is perhaps the single most common mistake

employees make. Their pride tells them that they are too good to work for such meager pay. If you are one of these people, you need to face the fact that the laws of supply and demand determine your market worth, not you. If everyone were able to set their own salary, inflation would increase drastically. You would be making $450 per hour, but a loaf of bread would cost $50.

Bear in mind that when supply and demand chooses a market value for your work, at least it is an objective value, not a subjective one determined by others. So do not take it personally.

2. **Expecting your pay to be determined by your needs.** This is the second most common complaint, and we have all heard it. Employees making comments like: "My partner is out of work, and we cannot pay our bills on my salary alone." "I'm a single parent with children to feed." "I have to put my children in private school." "This salary barely covers the cost of rent and bills every month. What am I supposed to eat on?"

The fact is that no employer can afford to pay an employee based on their needs. People are funny characters. When they have money, they tend to spend it. In the end, you will probably always need more money than you earn. Keep your

440

professional dignity by never basing a request for a raise on these types of appeals.

3. **Expecting the length of your employment to determine your market value.** No matter how long you have worked at a particular position, if you can offer nothing more than the person who has worked at the job for a year, then both of you will be paid at approximately the same level. Many employees expect automatic annual raises. This works fine until a company decides that it is less expensive to terminate the older employee and hire a new one at a lower salary. Then the policy does not sound so good anymore.

Recognize that your pay reflects the value of the work you do. Granted, more experience usually leads to a higher quality of employee, and often the pay reflects this. However, the box boy in the supermarket, no matter how great a box boy he is, will never earn as much as the supervisor of a department.

4. **Expecting your pay to go up as the company's profits go up.** This idea ignores a fundamental concept: Employees are not shareholders. They are not taking risks with their money. Those who expect their pay to increase when the company's profits increase almost never suggest that they should take a pay cut when the company has a bad year. Yet, one is exactly the same as the other. If an employee wishes to share in a company's profits and if the company is publicly held, the employee should purchase company stock. However, these employees, like the current shareholders, will then run the risk of losing their money if profits fall.

If you, as an employee, recognize these misconceptions about salary, you are less likely to base your request for a raise on unsound reasons. Take into consideration what would be a valid reason for requesting a raise.

First and fundamentally, you need to make some personal decisions. Ask yourself: "Am I in the right job?" "Do I enjoy what I am doing?" Regardless of your answer, the next question should be, "Is it more important for me to have money or to be happy?" The truth is that it takes a lot of money to compensate someone for being miserable. And if you are miserable in your job, you are probably not putting forth your best effort. Lack of effort is definitely not going to get you the raises you would like. So what do you do? First, find the right job.

The next important principle is that the laws of supply and demand will prevail. If you want to increase your market value, you must increase your worth to the company, usually by increasing your skills and abilities.

The following suggestions can help you increase your value to the company:

1. Adopt an active mentality, not a passive one. No one is going to increase your skills and abilities for you; you have to do it yourself and it takes work.

2. Never stop learning. Do not be satisfied with knowing your job inside and out. After you have mastered that, begin learning the other jobs in the company, preferably those of the next step up the ladder. Ask questions, read books, or take classes. Make sure that you become a valuable asset to the company and that you are ready for advancement and promotion when the opportunity arises.

3. Make long-range plans rather than waiting for life to just happen to you. Those who sit around rarely go anywhere.

4. Finally, realize that very often a significant change in salary comes from changing jobs, either within your present company or by moving to a different employer. We have all heard comments such as, "If I were working at the company down the street, I could make more than this!" The obvious response is, "If that is true, then why don't you work at that company?" If the bosses hear you make such a comment, they may assist your transfer to the company down the street by firing you.

Many employees cannot accept the fact that it is either true that their current pay is below market or it is not. If it is true, why not move on? If it is not, change your market value.

CHAPTER REVIEW

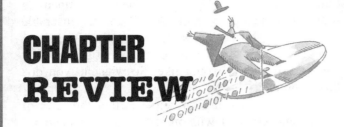

Summary

- Proficient use of the calculator is essential for the medical biller. Learning the functions of each of the keys and how to use the calculator to achieve the desired results takes practice.

- Computers have infiltrated all aspects of business life. Using the computer saves time and produces neater and cleaner reports, reduces errors, and allows for the electronic submission of data.

- Learning to use a computer program quickly and accurately and learning the proper means of storing information will provide the medical biller with a valuable skill.

- To find the right job takes more than just a passive look at the classified ads. You must first determine your objectives, your uniqueness, and your target audience. With these topics firmly in mind, write an effective résumé and cover letter that will introduce you to a prospective employer.

- When you have been granted an interview, keep in mind that the first four seconds are the most critical, followed by the next five minutes. However, the body of the interview and the closing also are important in determining whether you get a second interview or a job offer.

- When it comes to salary, your pay is based on your worth to the marketplace. The higher the demand for your skills, the more value that will be placed on them and the higher the salary you will be paid. Salary is not determined by your worth as a person, your needs, your length of employment, or the company's profits.

Assignments

Complete the Questions for Review.

Complete Exercises 15–1 through 15–6.

Practice gaining speed and accuracy by repeating Exercises 15–1 and 15–2 until you have mastered the feel of the keys.

The more prepared you are, the better your job interview will be.

Questions for Review

Directions: Answer the following questions without looking back at the material just covered. Write your answers in the space provided.

1. The _____ key completes multiplication and division operations and shows the results as a decimal.

2. What function does the divide key perform? _____

   _____

3. The _____ key completes any pending operations.

4. What is the function of the total key? _____

   _____

5. The memory total key displays and prints the value currently in _____, then clears the

   _____.

6. The numeric keypad is used for the _____ when the Num Lock is on.

7. The space bar performs two functions. What are they?

   1. _____

   2. _____

8. What two functions does the Enter key perform?

   1. _____

   2. _____

9. Function keys perform what function? _____

   _____

10. The cursor is _____

    _____.

11. What three points should your written marketing plan cover?

    1. _____

    2. _____

    3. _____

12. To determine your _____, consider the responsibilities you want on your next job, the industry in which you want to work, and what you can reasonably expect in the way of title and salary.

13. Your _____ lets the employer know what your goals are.

14. What is your résumé? _____

15. (True or False?) Never use an active voice or concise phrasing in your résumé. _____

16. A _____ is a way to toot your own horn.

17. (True or False?) Do not put anything in your cover letter that you cannot substantiate in an interview.

18. You should not job-hunt but instead _____ yourself.

19. Working adults normally make how many career changes in a lifetime? _____

20. (True or False?) The only way to achieve a significant increase in pay is to change jobs. _____

    If you are unable to answer any of these questions, refer back to that section in the chapter, and then fill in the answers.

Exercise 15-1

Directions: Add each of the following columns of numbers and then subtract the numbers from your total to arrive at zero. Clear the entries from your calculator and subtract the following columns of numbers and total; then add the numbers to your total to arrive at zero. Use the printer tape to check accuracy.

71459	12181	128.49	12.89
28695	57926	321.67	.92
13579	71349	014.89	7.16
58246	02763	906.76	18.21
69021	75396	741.08	267.93
54321	74185	529.63	1234.56
67891	29630	369.25	892.10
83214	36925	801.47	809.13
47986	80147	753.85	693.21
32694	42569	102.36	5679.32
15723	00147	564.12	137.14
38014	73528	321.65	432.78
98752	60413	498.70	6789.50
20361	13311	321.65	1090.17
13979	21769	789.93	578.15
02031	24989	456.89	692.00
11484	67400	999.01	780.29
25763	09121	847.03	566.17

Exercise **15–2**

Directions: Perform the function indicated for each list of numbers. Try not to watch your hands. Speed is not important at the beginning of performing these exercises. It will come later as you become more familiar with the keys.

1. Add the following numbers.

A.	12	B.	65	C.	44	D.	334
	24		70		69		781
	67		49		26		456
	41		52		73		241
	92		100		84		908
	34		99		35		528
	72		34		21		803

E.	295	F.	4576	G.	54	H.	32.514
	630		8493		835		8.123
	816		90.56		046		61.54
	902		3809		516		123.64
	517		9238		943		543.55
	703		12.98		.0015		999.83
	491		540.5				

2. Enter the first number, then subtract the following numbers.

A.	9999	B.	7654	C.	4329
	45		11		649
	66		92		42
	90		561		631
	1504		341		42
	3535		940		792
	901		52		406

D.	1000.00	E.	564.000	F.	410014
	10.00		.630		.123
	.20		.920		654.456
	341.00		162.000		84.25
	1.78		.789		67.48
	.78		231.000		138.03
	592.00		501.000		486.381

Exercise 15-3

Directions: Perform the function indicated for each list of numbers. Try not to watch your hands. Speed is not important at the beginning. It will come later as you become more familiar with the keys.

1. Multiply the following.

A. 231 $\times 42$	B. 5482 $\times 61$	C. 7602 $\times 201$	D. 891 $\times 23.61$
E. 43.92 $\times .639$	F. 24.51 $\times 70\%$	G. 903.45 $\times 85\%$	H. 2503.99 $\times 90\%$
I. 492.67 $\times 75\%$	J. 29.16 $\times 55\%$	K. 564465 $\times 21\%$	L. 654.21 $\times 75\%$

2. Divide the first number by the second number in the following equations.

A. 5634 51	B. 56348 543	C. 999999 .99	D. 3541 66
E. 1000 . 01	F. 65430 125	G. 514623 1523	H. 5100 45

Exercise 15-4

Directions: Complete the following items.

1. Fill out the Résumé Questionnaire on the following pages.

2. Using the résumés on the following pages as examples, create your own résumé.

3. Using the following cover letter as an example, create your own cover letter.

Résumé Questionnaire

First Name _____ M.I. _____ Last Name _____

Street _____

City _____ State _____ Zip _____

Day Phone _____ Eve. Phone _____ Soc. Sec. # _____

Position Objective: In the spaces below, enter the Occupational Titles of those positions which you feel you would be best qualified to fill. Opposite each position, enter the total years experience you have. Then indicate your minimum acceptable annual salary. "OPEN" is unacceptable. (Salary information is for your use and should not be included on an application.)

Occupational or Professional Title(s)	Years Experience	Desired Annual Salary
_____	_____	$_____
_____	_____	$_____
_____	_____	$_____
_____	_____	$_____

Experience Summary: Please summarize briefly your overall experience and accomplishments.

_____
_____
_____

Education: Type of Degree, Diploma, Certificate, or Years completed: (i.e., HS Diploma, # year(s) College, AA/BA) Highest Level: Type: _____ Major _____

Name of School, College, or University _____

Additional Courses/Seminars Taken and/or Awards: _____
_____

U.S. Citizenship: Yes _____ No _____

Type of Employment: _____ Full Time _____ Part Time _____ Temp _____ Contract _____

Geographic Area: _____ Open to Any Area   Area Desired _____

Skills/Abilities: Include any skills and abilities that may be of benefit to an employer. _____
_____
_____
_____
_____

Work History: Under each position title, describe your duties, responsibilities, and accomplishments. Be sure to list your present or last employer first.

From/To (Mo/Yr) _____ Company Name _____

Location (City & State) _____

Position Title _____ Salary $ _____

Type of Firm or Industry _____

Responsibilities/Accomplishments: _____

_____

From/To (Mo/Yr) _____ Company Name _____

Location (City & State) _____

Position Title _____ Salary $ _____

Type of Firm or Industry _____

Responsibilities/Accomplishments: _____

_____

From/To (Mo/Yr) _____ Company Name _____

Location (City & State) _____

Position Title _____ Salary $ _____

Type of Firm or Industry _____

Responsibilities/Accomplishments: _____

_____

Other Experience/Accomplishments: List briefly any additional experience or accomplishments that you would consider significant. _____

_____

_____

Industry Experience: Please indicate the industries in which you have experience and specify type(s) (i.e., agriculture, construction). _____

_____

_____

_____

Foreign Language(s): _____

I hereby certify that all of the information contained herein is complete and accurate and I agree to report any changes promptly.

Signature: _____ Date: _____

SALLY STUDENT
12345 SUMMER STREET
SANDY, SC 20000
(803) 555-1234

Sample Résumé #1

OBJECTIVE:

To obtain a position in the medical industry which will enable me to use my billing and communications background, supervisory experience, administrative skills, and creative talents.

QUALIFYING STATEMENT:

I am hardworking and have excellent verbal and communication skills in both English and Spanish. I also have the ability to handle a variety of tasks and have good organizational skills.

EXPERIENCE:

Medical Biller/Receptionist—Spring Street Medical Offices, 1234 Spring Street, Sandy, SC, 20001. Duties included: Billing for services using HCFA-1500 and UB-92 billing forms, billing Medicare and Medicaid patients, maintaining medical records, setting appointments, answering phones, typing correspondence, greeting clients, ordering supplies. Job was an internship for completion of requirements for Medical Billing Certificate from The Suburban School. 2/02–present

Waitress—The Scrumptious Supper, 4567 Sister Street, Sandy, SC 20030. Duties included: Taking orders, serving customers, cashiering, assisting with making of desserts and other items, bussing tables, acting as hostess. 9/00–2/02

Cook/Server—McStephens Fast Hamburgers, 98765 Stale Street, Sandy, SC 20002. Duties included: Taking orders, serving customers, receiving moneys, keeping an accurate cash drawer, cooking foods (including hamburgers and fries), preparing and maintaining salad bar and condiments bar. 4/98–9/00

EDUCATION:

Medical Billing Certificate, The Suburban School, 8765 Sullen Street, Sandy, SC 20022. Maintained a 3.95 GPA and graduated among the top in the class.

Sandy Adult Community School, 84756 Seashore Street, Sandy, SC 20007. Took classes and seminars in Computer Basics, Creative Writing, Working with DOS, Windows, and Word.

Diploma. Sandy High School, 3456 Sunset Street, Sandy, SC 20012. GPA 3.75 Perfect attendance certificate, 1995, 1994. Also took two business courses.

SKILLS:

Computer literate in PowerPoint, Word, Quicken, type (50 wpm), 10 key (6,000 kph), understand medical terminology, knowledgeable in proper business correspondence. Speak and write in both English and Spanish. Hobbies include writing and learning computer programs.

RÉSUMÉ

Sample Résumé #2

NAME: Holly Hopeful

ADDRESS: 4536 Hammer Way
Hollywood, CA 90611

PHONE: (818) 555-1772

EDUCATION: Certificate—Administrative Assisting 2004, Success School

EXPERIENCE: 2003–present—Program Assistant. In charge of data entry, answering telephones, typing, and creating files, flyers and circulars. I also took care of sign-in logs and scheduling appointments.

2002–2003—Office Manager for Sam's Shoe Store. Assisted with running the office, hiring and firing duties and maintained and ordered the stock/inventory. I also scheduled employees and handled financial records.

2000–2002—Sales Clerk for Sarah's Sweet Shoppe. I assisted customers, maintained the cash drawer, and maintained and ordered stock. I also handled customer service and dealt with returns and dissatisfied customers.

Ivana Job
4646 Jessup Court
Jacobs, IL 60911
(815) 555-0101

Sample Résumé #3

OBJECTIVE:	A challenging position utilizing my administrative assisting skills and experience.
QUALITIES:	Excellent organizational and problem-solving abilities. Effectively handle multiple priorities and working under pressure. Skilled with people. Computer literate. Intelligent, accurate, goal-oriented, and self-motivated. Superior work ethics.
SUMMARY OF EXPERIENCE:	Over 15 years experience in accounting and office work with an emphasis in managing personnel for a large drug store and pharmacy.
WORK HISTORY: 2003–Present	STORE MANAGER: Responsible to CEO for overall operation of drug store. Administered all human resource functions including hiring, employee relations, payroll and work scheduling. Supervised and set operating procedures for numerous departments. Assisted accounting department with accounts payable, accounts receivable, general ledger, and collections. Responsible for multi-account bank reconciliations, tax returns and monthly financial statements. Wrote employee policy and training manual.
2002–2003	BUYER: Extensive purchasing and merchandising responsibilities including vendor negotiations, inventory controls and setting displays. Handled advertising, sales and promotions. Improved level of customer service.
1998–2002	PHARMACY TECHNICIAN: Assisted pharmacists in fulfilling prescriptions. Coordinated activities of pharmacy personnel. Obtained broad technical knowledge of drugs and medical terminology. Voted employee of the month three times.
EDUCATION, LICENSES:	Certificate, Administrative Assisting. Savemore School, Sandy, SC State of SC Pharmacy Technician License #TCH 000000

Holly Hopeful   **Sample Cover Letter #1**
4536 Hammer Way
Hollywood, CA 90611
(818) 555-1772

January 2, CCYY

Steve Springer
Personnel Supervisor
Stupendous Supports
102938 Sports Street
Sandy, SC 20020

Dear Mr. Springer:

Please consider me for an administrative assistant position with your firm.

I recently completed my education at The Suburban School, where I received a certificate in administrative assisting. I completed the course with a 3.95 grade point average and was among the top students in my class. The course covered everything an administrative assistant should know, including using reference books, time management skills, legal issues, general office procedures, computer basics, calculator basics, typing, speedwriting, proofreading, correspondence writing, Word, PowerPoint, basic office accounting, customer service, event planning, and travel arrangements. I am familiar with the use of Quicken Accounting and Billing, type 50 words per minute, and can enter 6,000 keystrokes per hour on the ten key.

I also completed a three-month internship at Spring Street Offices in conjunction with this course, which utilized the knowledge that I had learned. During this internship I completed administrative assistant, billing and receptionist duties for an office that staffed eight professionals and had over 7,500 customers.

I am a conscientious, enterprising person who works very hard to turn in a good performance. I enjoy being creative and industrious. I learn quickly and am more than willing to take on the challenge of learning new things. I am dependable and loyal, and have had perfect attendance at my jobs for the past three years. I also get along well with co-workers and supervisors.

Thank you for taking the time to consider my résumé. I would be happy to interview with you at your convenience.

Sincerely,

Holly Hopeful
Holly Hopeful

Exercise **15-5**

Directions: Find and circle the words listed below. Words can appear horizontally, vertically, diagonally, forward, or backward.

1. Calculator
2. Computer Disk Drive
3. Cover Letter
4. Hard Drive
5. Power Switch

```
B I D T C R S J U L X W R A W E F
C N I E O K E R J J E J H X X V K
Q N F H M V Q C B Q J R L J J I D
V C C K P Q B J O T N W S Q C R U
E J B O U C P V D W U W O O D D L
P L S M T R M E V M U O V Q I D X
P U F I E J O P Q N K E B A O R D
J Z K S R P O T Z A R R H Z Y A R
K M U B D T I E A L O K B A C H B
W S W F I E V Z E L Y T P B V G F
D V M Y S B B T J S U P D E T P D
N T N V K H T B X Z G C G R A D T
Z Y B A D E A K D T I E L C K E S
O W G D R J Q U H Z Y N D A M L I
M Q R T I U C L F I C W Y O C H V
Q V S A V A G F Q W R A X F L O K
V P L Y E U H C T I W S R E W O P
```

Exercise 15-6

Directions: Complete the crossword puzzle by filling in a word from the keywords that fits each clue.

Across

3. A summary of employment experience and qualifications.
4. A knob that turns the contrast up and down between varying fields.
5. The primary means of communicating with your computer.
6. The rectangular box that houses the memory and functional components of the computer.

Down

1. The small lighted symbol on the monitor screen that indicates where you are in the program or document.
2. A knob that changes the brightness of the image on the screen.

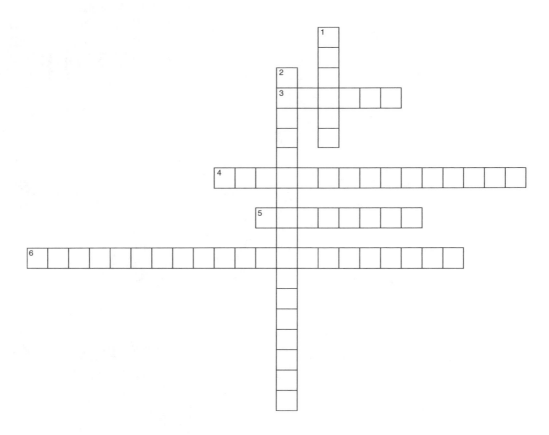

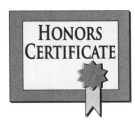

Honors Certification™

The Honors Certification Challenge™ for this section is a timed test. You will be given several tests with problems similar to those found in Exercises 15–1 through 15–6 and will be asked to complete the problems and write in your answers. Each incorrect keystroke will result in a 2% deduction from your grade. You must achieve a score of 85% or higher to pass this test. If you fail the test on your first attempt, you may take the test one additional time. The items included in the second test may be different from those included in the first test.

There also will be a five-minute timed test to determine your average keystrokes per minute. You must achieve a speed of 200 keystrokes per minute in order to pass this test. If you fail the test on your first attempt, you may take the test one additional time. The items included in the second test may be different from those included in the first test.

Résumé and Cover Letter

Create a perfect résumé and cover letter. This is a pass/fail item. You must be sure that there are no errors in either the cover letter or the résumé. If any errors are found, you must correct them before this item will be considered complete. When finished, your résumé and cover letter should be printed on nice paper. You may take as long as necessary to complete this challenge.

Interview

You will be interviewed by your teacher or one of your classmates. The interview will take place in front of your class. You must dress appropriately for the interview and conduct yourself as you would in a real interview situation. This is a pass/fail situation. Whether you pass or fail will be determined by whether a majority of your classmates would give you a job based on your interview. If 85% of the class would hire you, you pass.

If you fail the test on your first attempt, you may retake the test one additional time. However, 90% of the students must give you a passing score on the second interview.

SECTION
APPENDICES

Appendix A

Provider and Medical
Abbreviations

Table of Contents

Provider Abbreviations

CA—Certified Acupuncturist. Usually required for other than an MD or DO. Provider must have this certification to provide acupuncture treatments.

Clinical Psychologist—Licensed to perform psychological testing and therapy. Referral by an MD is usually not required.

CRNA—Certified Registered Nurse Anesthetist. Certified to administer anesthesia under the direction of an MD.

DC—Doctor of Chiropractic. Performs manual manipulations of the spine and other musculoskeletal areas. Licensed for office visits, x-rays, nutritional supplements, manipulations, ultrasound, and physical therapies. All other services should be questioned. Cannot draw blood or perform surgery.

DDS—Doctor of Dental Surgery. Licensed to perform all dental care, including dental surgeries and surgeries to the face and jaw.

DMD—Doctor of Medical Dentistry. Licensed to perform dental care, including dental surgeries and surgeries to the face and jaw. The only difference between a DDS and a DMD is the school attended; the training and licensing authorizations are the same.

DO—Doctor of Osteopathy. Licensed to perform any service that an MD can perform. Training is essentially the same as an MD.

DPM—Doctor of Podiatry Medicine. Licensed for the care, treatment, and surgery of the feet.

DSC—Doctor of Surgical Chiropody. The same as a podiatrist; deals with foot surgeries. DSC is an old licensing designation that is seldom seen today.

EdD —Doctor of Education. An educational degree, not a licensing. The licensing needs to be obtained. Without appropriate licensing, services by this provider would not usually be covered.

EMT—Emergency Medical Technician. Licensed to administer emergency procedures such as CPR. Cannot perform tracheotomies. Usually works in an ambulance.

LCSW—Licensed Clinical Social Worker. Licensed to provide psychological counseling. Referral from an MD is usually required.

LPN—Licensed Practical Nurse. Equivalent to an LVN. LVNs are in California, whereas LPNs are from other states.

LVN—Licensed Vocational Nurse. Lower level (usually a two-year program) nurse, not certified to perform IV-Push (injecting medications directly into a vein) and cannot be a charge nurse on a floor.

MD—Medical Doctor. Licensed to perform any and all medical care/procedures.

MFCC—Marriage, Family, Child Counselor. Licensed to provide psychological counseling and marriage and family counseling. Usually requires a referral from an MD.

Midwife—Licensed as a registered nurse and certified as a nurse midwife. Usually handles routine maternity cases. Must be associated with an MD or a DO to handle emergency cases.

MSW—Master of Social Work. Licensed to provide family and psychological counseling. Referral from an MD is usually required.

MT—Medical Technologist. Usually works in a laboratory and can draw blood and perform lab testing. An MT also can administer injections and perform EKGs.

Myofunctionist —Licensed to perform myofunctional speech therapy. This involves the reeducation of the facial muscles needed to speak and breathe.

NA—Nurse's Aide. Licensed to assist patients not requiring skilled nursing care. Normally employed in skilled nursing facilities, nursing homes and home health agencies. (Also known as a CNA—Certified Nurse's Aide.)

NP—Nurse Practitioner. A nurse practitioner is a registered nurse (RN) who has completed advanced education and training in the diagnosis and management of common medical conditions. They provide some of the same care provided by physicians and maintain close working relationships with physicians.

OD—Doctor of Optometry. An optometrist. Not licensed to perform surgery. Most commonly performs eye refractions, dispenses glasses, and contacts.

OT—Occupational Therapist. Licensed to perform occupational therapy. Occupational therapy is the retraining of muscles and nerves, usually in the hands and arms, necessary for the performance of routine daily movements (i.e., learning to feed oneself, brush hair, and other activities of daily living).

PA—Physician Assistant. Physician Assistants are healthcare professionals licensed to practice medicine with physician supervision. PA responsibilities include conducting physical exams, diagnosing and treating illnesses, ordering and interpreting tests, counseling on preventive health care, assisting in surgery, and writing prescriptions. PA-C stands for Physician Assistant-Certified; the person that holds the title has taken a national certification examination.

Paramedic—Licensed to administer emergency care. Has more extensive training than an EMT. Normally works in an ambulance or for a fire department.

PhD—An educational degree (doctorate) not a licensing. Services by this provider would be covered only when there is also appropriate licensing.

RN—Registered Nurse. Registered nurses provide direct patient care. This level of nursing is higher than an LVN/LPN.

RPT—Registered Physical Therapist. Licensed to perform physical (muscle) therapy when services are prescribed by an MD or DO.

Medical Abbreviations

AA	Aortic aneurysm
ABD	Abdomen
ABG	Arterial blood gas
ACTH	Adrenocorticotropic hormone
ADI	American Drug Index
ADL	Activities of daily living
ADR	Adverse drug reaction
AFIB	Atrial fibrillation
AFO	Ankle-foot orthosis
AG	Antigen
AGGLUT	Agglutination
AGL	Acute granulocytic leukemia
AHS	Allied Health Services
AIDS	Acquired immunodeficiency syndrome
AK	Above knee
AKA	Above-knee amputation
AL	Aluminum
ALK	Alkaline
ALS	Amyotrophic lateral sclerosis
AMA	Against medical advice
AMI	Acute myocardial infarction
ANS	Autonomic nervous system
AODM	Adult-onset diabetes mellitus
APP	Application
AR	Accounts receivable
AROM	Active range of motion

ASBD	Arteriosclerotic brain disease
ASC	Ambulatory surgical center
ASCHD	Arteriosclerotic coronary heart disease
ASCVD	Arteriosclerotic cardiovascular disease
ASD	Atrial septal defect
ASHD	Arteriosclerotic heart disease
AVF	Arteriovenous fistula
AVR	Aortic valve replacement
AZT	Azidothymidine
BBB	Bundle branch block
BILI	Bilirubin
BK	Below knee
BKA	Below-knee amputation
BLS	Basic life support
BMR	Basal metabolic rate
BOM	Bilateral otitis media
BP	Blood pressure
BR	By report
BS	Blood sugar
BSO	Bilateral salpingo-oophorectomy
BUN	Blood urea nitrogen
BX	Biopsy
C&S	Culture and sensitivity
CA	Cancer
CABG	Coronary artery bypass graft
CABP	Coronary artery bypass
CAD	Coronary artery disease
CAPD	Chronic ambulatory peritoneal dialysis
CBC	Complete blood count
CBS	Chronic brain syndrome
CCF	Congestive cardiac failure
CCPD	Continuous cycling peritoneal dialysis
CCU	Coronary care unit
CF	Cystic fibrosis
CHB	Complete heart block
CHD	Coronary heart disease
CHF	Congestive heart failure
CL	Chloride
CM	Centimeter
CNS	Central nervous system
COPD	Chronic obstructive pulmonary disease
CP	Cerebral palsy
CPAP	Continuous positive airway pressure
CPK	Creatine phosphokinase
CPR	Cardiopulmonary resuscitation
CRD	Chronic renal disease
CRF	Chronic renal failure
CRIF	Closed reduction internal fixation
CSF	Cerebrospinal fluid
CT	Computed axial tomography
CTS	Carpal tunnel syndrome

CU	Cubic	HBEAB	Hepatitis be antibody
CV	Cardiovascular	HBEAG	Hepatitis be antigen
CVA	Cerebrovascular accident	HBP	High blood pressure
CVD	Cardiovascular disease	HCT	Hematocrit
CXR	Chest x-ray	HEENT	Head, eyes, ears, nose, and throat
D&C	Dilation and curettage	HIV	Human immunodeficiency virus
D&E	Dilation and evacuation	HKAF	Hip, knee, ankle, foot
D/T	Due to	HKAFO	Hip knee ankle foot orthosis
DHS	Department of Health Services	HOSP	Hospital
DJD	Degenerative joint disease	HR	Hour
DM	Diabetes mellitus	HX	History
DME	Durable medical equipment	I&D	Incision and drainage
DNR	Do not resuscitate	IBS	Irritable bowel syndrome
DOA	Dead on arrival	ICF	Intermediate care facility
DOS	Date of service	ICP	Intracranial pressure
DPT	Diphtheria, pertussis, and tetanus	ICU	Intensive care unit
DT	Delirium tremens	IDDM	Insulin-dependent diabetes mellitus
DTT	Diphtheria tetanus toxoid	IH	Infectious hepatitis
DVT	Deep vein thrombosis	IHD	Ischemic heart disease
DX	Diagnosis	IM	Intramuscular
EAC	Estimated acquisition cost	IP	Inspiratory pressure
EBV	Epstein-Barr virus	IPD	Intermittent peritoneal dialysis
ECF	Extended-care facility	IPPB	Intermittent positive-pressure breathing
ECG	Electrocardiogram	IUD	Intrauterine device
EDC	Expected date of confinement	IUP	Intrauterine pregnancy
EEG	Electroencephalogram	JODM	Juvenile-onset diabetes mellitus
EGD	Esophagogastroduodenoscopy	JRA	Juvenile rheumatoid arthritis
EKG	Electrocardiogram	KAF	Knee, ankle, and foot
EMG	Electromyogram	KO	Knee orthosis
ENT	Ear, nose, and throat	KUB	Kidney ureter bladder
EOB	Explanation of benefits	L/S	Lumbosacral
EOMB	Explanation of Medicare benefits	LAD	Left anterior descending
EPSDT	Early periodic screening, diagnosis, and treatment	LB(S)	Pound(s)
		LBBB	Left bundle branch block
ER	Emergency room	LBP	Low blood pressure
ESRD	End-stage renal disease	LCA	Left coronary artery
EST	Electroshock therapy	LE	Lower extremity
EUA	Examination under anesthesia	LFT	Liver function tests
EUD	Etiology undetermined	LGI	Lower gastrointestinal
F/U	Follow-up	LLL	Left lower lobe
FB	Foreign body	LLQ	Left lower quadrant
FBS	Fasting blood sugar	LMP	Last menstrual period
FSH	Follicle-stimulating hormone	LOC	Loss of consciousness
FUO	Fever of undetermined origin	LP	Lumbar puncture
FX	Fracture	LSO	Lumbar sacral orthosis
GE	Gastroesophageal	LTC	Long-term care
GI	Gastrointestinal	LUL	Left upper lobe
GTT	Glucose tolerance test	LUQ	Left upper quadrant
GU	Genitourinary	MEDS	Medications
GYN	Gynecologic	MG	Milligram
H&P	History and physical	MI	Myocardial infarction
H/O	History of	MIN(S)	Minute(s)

MM	Millimeter
MMIS	Medicaid Management Information System
MMR	Measles, mumps, and rubella
MONO	Mononucleosis
MRI	Magnetic resonance imaging
MS	Multiple sclerosis
MVA	Motor vehicle accident
MVP	Mitral valve prolapse
NA	Sodium
NEC	Not elsewhere classified
NH	Nursing home
NKA	No known allergies
NKDA	No known drug allergies
NM	Nuclear medicine
NOC	Not otherwise classified
NOS	Not otherwise specified
NP	Nasopharyngeal
NSR	Normal sinus rhythm
NSVD	Normal spontaneous vaginal delivery
O2	Oxygen
OM	Otitis media
OPD	Obstructive pulmonary disease
OPV	Oral poliovirus
OU	Both eyes
OV	Office visit
OZ	Ounce
PAP	Papanicolaou
PC	Professional component
PDR	Physicians' Desk Reference
PERLA	Pupils equal, react to light and accommodation
PHP	Prepaid health plan
PID	Pelvic inflammatory disease
PIN	Physician Identifier Number
PKG	Package
PO	By mouth
POE	Proof of Eligibility
POS	Place of Service
PPN	Peripheral parenteral nutrition
PRN	As occasion requires
PRO	Professional Review Organization
PROM	Passive range of motion
PTT	Partial thromboplastin time
PUD	Peptic ulcer disease
PVD	Peripheral vascular disease
QD	Every day
QID	Four times a day
R/O	Rule out
RA	Rheumatoid arthritis
RA	Remittance Advice
RBC	Red blood cell
RDS	Respiratory distress syndrome

REM	Rapid eye movements
RF	Rheumatoid factor
RHD	Rheumatic heart disease
RLL	Right lower lobe
RLQ	Right lower quadrant
RML	Right middle lobe
RO	Rule out
RT	Right
RUL	Right upper lobe
RUQ	Right upper quadrant
RV	Right ventricular
RVS	Relative value studies
RX	Prescription
S/P	Status post
SBO	Small bowel obstruction
SED	Sedimentation
SEWH	Shoulder, elbow, wrist, and hand
SI	Sacroiliac
SIDS	Sudden infant death syndrome
SLR	Straight leg raising
SMA	Schedule of maximum allowances
SNF	Skilled nursing facility
SOB	Shortness of breath
SOC	Share of cost
SQ	Subcutaneous
SSA	Social Security Administration
SSI/SSP	Supplemental Security Income/State Supplemental Program
SSN	Social Security Number
STD	Sexually Transmitted Disease
T&A	Tonsillectomy and adenoidectomy
TAB	Therapeutic abortion
TAH	Total abdominal hysterectomy
TAR	Treatment Authorization Request
TB	Tuberculosis
TD	Tetanus diphtheria
TMJ	Temporomandibular joint
TOS	Type of service
TPL	Third party liability
TSH	Thyroid-stimulating hormone
TV	Total volume
UA	Urinalysis
UE	Upper extremity
UGI	Upper gastrointestinal
UNI	Unilateral
URI	Upper respiratory infection
UTI	Urinary tract infection
UV	Ultraviolet
VA	Veterans Administration
VC	Vital capacity
VD	Venereal disease
VDRL	Venereal Disease Research Laboratory

Appendix B
Forms

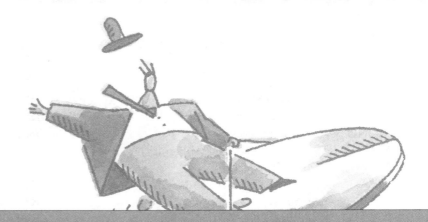

Table of Contents

Paul Provider, M.D.
5858 Peppermint Place
Anytown, USA 12345
(765) 555-6768

PATIENT INFORMATION SHEET

INSURED'S INFORMATION

Patient Account No.: _____ Assigned Provider: _____ Birth Date: _____

Name: (Last, First, Middle) _____ Gender: _____

Address: (Inc City, State, Zip) _____

Home Phone: _____ Marital Status: _____ Social Security #: _____

Employer Name: _____ Work Phone: _____

Employer Address: _____

Employment Status: _____ Referred By: _____

Allergies/Medical Conditions: _____ Email Address: _____

Primary Ins Policy: _____ Address: _____

Member's ID #: _____ Group #: _____ Insured's Name: _____

Secondary Ins Policy: _____ Address: _____

Member's ID #: _____ Group #: _____ Insured's Name: _____

SPOUSE'S INFORMATION

Patient Account No.: _____ Assigned Provider: _____ Birth Date: _____

Name: (Last, First, Middle) _____ Gender: _____

Social Security #: _____ Employment Status: _____

Employer Name: _____ Work Phone: _____

Employer Address: _____

Allergies/Medical Conditions: _____ Student Status: _____

Primary Ins Policy: _____ Address: _____

Member's ID #: _____ Group #: _____ Insured's Name: _____

Secondary Ins Policy: _____ Address: _____

Member's ID #: _____ Group #: _____ Insured's Name: _____

CHILD #1

Patient Account No.: _____ Assigned Provider: _____ Birth Date: _____

Name of Minor Child: _____ Social Security #: _____

Gender: _____ Marital Status: _____ Relationship to Insured: _____

Allergies/Medical Conditions: _____ Student Status: _____

Primary Ins Policy: _____ Insured's Name: _____

Secondary Ins Policy: _____ Insured's Name: _____

CHILD #2

Patient Account No.: _____ Assigned Provider: _____ Birth Date: _____

Name of Minor Child: _____ Social Security #: _____

Gender: _____ Marital Status: _____ Relationship to Insured: _____

(continues on next page)

Allergies/Medical Conditions: _____ Student Status: _____

Primary Ins Policy: _____ Insured's Name: _____

Secondary Ins Policy: _____ Insured's Name: _____

CHILD #3

Patient Account No.: _____ Assigned Provider: _____ Birth Date: _____

Name of Minor Child: _____ Social Security #: _____

Gender: _____ Marital Status: _____ Relationship to Name: _____

Allergies/Medical Conditions: _____ Student Status: _____

Primary Ins Name: _____ Insured's Name: _____

Secondary Ins Name: _____ Insured's Name: _____

CHILD #4

Patient Account No.: _____ Assigned Provider: _____ Birth Date: _____

Name of Minor Child: _____ Social Security #: _____

Gender: _____ Marital Status: _____ Relationship to Insured: _____

Allergies/Medical Conditions: _____ Student Status: _____

Primary Ins Name: _____ Insured's Name: _____

Secondary Ins Name: _____ Insured's Name: _____

EMERGENCY CONTACT

Name: _____ Home Phone: _____ Other Phone: _____

Address: (Inc City, State, Zip) _____

ACKNOWLEDGMENT AND AUTHORITY FOR TREATMENT AND PAYMENT

Initial

_____ I consent to treatment as necessary or desirable to the care of the patient(s) named above, including but not restricted to whatever drugs, medicine, performance of operations and conduct of laboratory, x-ray, or other studies that may be used by the attending doctor, his/her nurse or qualified designate:

_____ I also acknowledge full responsibility for the payment of such services and agree to pay for them upon demand, in full, AT THE TIME OF SERVICE. If the physician must use a collection agency/attorney or court to collect its charges, then I will pay reasonable attorney fees and costs incurred in collecting same, regardless of insurance coverage.

_____ I hereby authorize payment directly to Paul Provider, M.D. of the medical expense benefits otherwise payable to me but not to exceed my indebtedness to said physician on account of the enclosed charge.

_____ I hereby authorize any medical practitioner, medical or medically related facility, insurance or reinsuring company, consumer reporting agency, or employer having information with respect to any physical or mental condition and/or treatment of me or my minor children and any other non-medical information of me and my minor children to give to the group policyholder, my employer, or its legal representative, any and all such information.

_____ I understand the information obtained by the use of the Authorization will be used to determine eligibility for insurance, and eligibility for benefits under any existing policy. Any information obtained will not be released by/to any organization EXCEPT to the group policyholder, my employer, reinsuring companies, the Medical Information Bureau, Inc., or other persons or organizations performing business or legal services in connection with my application, claim, or as may be otherwise lawfully required or as I may further authorize.

_____ I further agree that a photographic copy of this Authorization shall be valid as the original. This Authorization shall be valid for one year from the date shown below.

Signature of Insured: _____ Date: _____

Signature of Spouse: _____ Date: _____

(continued)

Paul Provider, M.D.
5858 Peppermint Place
Anytown, USA 12345
(765) 555-6768

Insurance Coverage Form

INSURED: _____ BIRTH DATE: _____

SSN: _____ EFFECTIVE DATE: _____

INSURANCE POLICY: _____

ADDRESS: _____

ID/MEMBER #: _____ GROUP #: _____

DEPENDENT AGE LIMIT: _____

_____

INDIV. DEDUCTIBLE AMOUNT: _____ 3 MO CARRYOVER:_____

FAMILY DEDUCTIBLE: _____AGGREGATE/NONAGGREGATE

STANDARD COINSURANCE _____ LIFETIME MAXIMUM _____

COINSURANCE LIMIT _____

_____

BENEFITS PAID AT OTHER THAN THE STANDARD COINSURANCE % [Including benefit, coinsurance amount and special circumstances (i.e., SSO allowed at 100%, required for hysterectomy, coronary bypass, etc.)]:

_____

_____

PREAUTHORIZATION REQUIRED FOR: _____

_____

_____

ACCIDENT BENEFIT AMOUNT: _____ TREATMENT TO BE RECEIVED WITHIN _____ DAYS

OTHER NOTES/COMMENTS: _____

_____

Total Payments (CCYY)

Indicate below the names of the insured and their dependents. When any of the following information is received, write it in pencil followed by the date. This will help you to realize when a patient's deductible has been met and if they are nearing any maximum benefit.

	INSURED	DEPENDENT	DEPENDENT	DEPENDENT	DEPENDENT
NAME:	_____	_____	_____	_____	_____
DEDUCTIBLE:	_____	_____	_____	_____	_____
COINS PD:	_____	_____	_____	_____	_____
LIFETIME:	_____	_____	_____	_____	_____

DOCTOR'S FIRST REPORT OF OCCUPATIONAL INJURY OR ILLNESS

Within 5 days of your initial examination, for every occupational injury or illness, send two copies of this report to the employer's workers' compensation insurance carrier or the insured employer. Failure to file a timely doctor's report may result in assessment of a civil penalty. In the case of diagnosed or suspected pesticide poisoning, send a copy of the report to Division of Labor Statistics and Research, P.O. Box 555555, Anytown, USA 12345-6789, and notify your local health officer by telephone within 24 hours.

	PLEASE DO NOT USE THIS COLUMN
1. INSURER NAME AND ADDRESS	
2. EMPLOYER NAME	Case No.
3. Address: No. and Street City Zip	Industry
4. Nature of business (e.g., food manufacturing, building construction, retailer of women's clothes.)	County
5. PATIENT NAME (first name, middle initial, last name) 6. Sex ☐Male ☐ Female 7. Date of Mo. Day Yr. Birth:	Age
8. Address: No. and Street City Zip 9. Telephone number ( )	Hazard
10. Occupation (Specific job title) 11. Social Security Number - -	Disease
12. Injured at: No. and Street City County	Hospitalization
13. Date and hour of injury Mo. Day Yr. Hour or onset of illness _____ a.m. _____ p.m. 14. Date last worked Mo. Day Yr.	Occupation
15. Date and hour of first Mo. Day Yr. Hour examination or treatment _____ a.m. _____ p.m. 16. Have you (or your office) previously treated patient? ☐Yes ☐No	Return Date/Code

Patient please complete this portion, if able to do so. Otherwise, doctor please complete immediately. Inability or failure of a patient to complete this portion shall not affect his/her rights to workers' compensation under the California Labor Code.

17. **DESCRIBE HOW THE ACCIDENT OR EXPOSURE HAPPENED.** (Give specific object, machinery or chemical. Use reverse side if more space is required.)

18. **SUBJECTIVE COMPLAINTS** (Describe fully. Use reverse side if more space is required.)

19. **OBJECTIVE FINDINGS** (Use reverse side if more space is required.) A. Physical examination B. X-ray and laboratory results (State if non or pending.)

20. **DIAGNOSIS** (if occupational illness specify etiologic agent and duration of exposure.) Chemical or toxic compounds involved?   ☐Yes   ☐ No
ICD-9 Code ___ ___ ___ - ___ ___

21. Are your findings and diagnosis consistent with patient's account of injury or onset of illness?   ☐Yes   ☐No   If "no," please explain.

22. Is there any other current condition that will impede or delay patient's recovery?   ☐Yes   ☐No   If "yes," please explain.

23. **TREATMENT RENDERED** (Use reverse side if more space is required.)

24. If further treatment required, specify treatment plan/estimated duration.

25. If hospitalized as inpatient, give hospital name and location   Date   Mo.   Day   Yr.   Estimated stay admitted

26. WORK STATUS -- Is patient able to perform usual work?   ☐Yes   ☐No
If "no," date when patient can return to: Regular work ____/____/____
Modified work ____/____/____   Specify restrictions _____

Doctor's Signature _____   License Number _____
Doctor Name and Degree (please type) _____   IRS Number _____
Address _____   Telephone Number _____

FORM 5021 (Rev. 4)

Any person who makes or causes to be made any knowingly false or fraudulent material statement or material representation for the purpose of obtaining or denying workers' compensation benefits or payments is guilty of a felony.

Lien Letter

TO: Attorney _____

_____

_____, Confusion

RE: Medical Reports and Insurance Carrier Lien

FOR_____

    I do hereby authorize the above insurance carrier to furnish you, my attorney, with a full report of any records and resultant payments of myself in regard to the accident in which I was involved.

    I hereby authorize and direct you, my attorney, to pay directly to said insurance carrier such sums as may be due and owed for payment of medical services rendered me or the provider of services both by reason of this accident and by reason of any other bills that are due, and to withhold such sums from any settlement, judgment or verdict as may be necessary to adequately protect said insurance carrier. And I hereby further give a lien on my case to said insurance carrier against any and all proceeds of any settlement, judgment or verdict which may be paid to you, my attorney, or myself as the result of the injuries for which I have been treated or injuries in connection therewith.

    I fully understand that I am directly and fully responsible for reimbursement of any payments for all medical bills submitted for services rendered and that this agreement is made solely for said insurance carrier's additional protection and in consideration of its awaiting payment. And I further understand that such payment is not contingent on any settlement, judgment or verdict by which I may eventually recover said fee.

Dated: _____   Patient's Signature: _____

    The undersigned being attorney of record for the above patient does hereby agree to observe all the terms of the above and agrees to withhold such sums from any settlement, judgment or verdict as may be necessary to adequately protect said insurance carrier named above.

Dated: _____   Attorney's Signature: _____
Mr./Ms. Attorney: Please sign, date, and return one copy to our office at once.

Keep one copy for your records.

Lien Form

WORKERS' COMPENSATION APPEALS BOARD

STATE OF CONFUSION

CASE NO. _____

NOTICE AND REQUEST FOR ALLOWANCE OF LIEN

_____

LIEN CLAIMANT   ADDRESS
VS.

_____

INJURED WORKER   ADDRESS

_____

EMPLOYER   ADDRESS

_____

INSURANCE CARRIER   ADDRESS

The undersigned hereby requests the Workers' Compensation Appeals Board to determine and allow as a lien the sum of

_____ dollars ($_____) against

any amount now due or which may hereafter become payable as compensation to _____
                                                                                                                    INJURED WORKER

on account of injury sustained by him/ her on _____.
                                                                              DATE

This request and claim for lien is for: (Mark appropriate box)
- ❑ The reasonable expense incurred by or on behalf of said injured worker for medical treatment to cure or relieve from the effects of said injury; or
- ❑ The reasonable medical expense incurred to prove a contested claim; or
- ❑ The reasonable value of living expenses of said injured worker or of his dependents, subsequent to the injury, or
- ❑ The reasonable living expenses of the wife or minor children, or both, of said injured worker, subsequent to the date of injury, where such injured worker has deserted or is neglecting his family; or
- ❑ The reasonable fee for interpreter's services performed on _____.
                                                                                                      DATE

NOTE: ITEMIZED STATEMENTS MUST BE ATTACHED
The undersigned declares that he delivered or mailed a copy of this lien claim to each of the above-named parties on

_____

ATTORNEY FOR LIEN CLAIMANT   DATE

_____

ADDRESS OF ATTORNEY FOR LIEN CLAIMANT   LIEN CLAIMANT

INJURED WORKER'S CONSENT TO ALLOWANCE OF LIEN

I consent to the requested allowance of a lien against my compensation.

_____

ATTORNEY FOR INJURED WORKER   INJURED WORKER

DEPARTMENT OF INDUSTRIAL RELATIONS
DIVISION OF INDUSTRIAL ACCIDENTS

Paul Provider, M.D.
5858 Peppermint Place
Anytown, USA 12345
(765) 555-6768

INSURANCE TRACER

Date: _____

Dear Insurance Carrier:

We sent a claim to you over six weeks ago and have not heard back from you.
Patient:
Insured:
Address:
SSN/Birth Date:
Group Number:
Claim Amount:
Date Billed:
Date of Services:
Date of Illness or Injury:
Diagnosis:
Employer:
Address:

Please supply the following information on the above named claim within ten days. Payment on this claim is overdue and we would like to avoid involving the patient and the state insurance commissioner in a reimbursement complaint.

Claim pending because:_____
_____
Payment in progress. Check will be mailed on:_____
Payment previously made. Date: _____
To whom:_____
Check #: _____ Payment Amount: _____
Claim denied. Reason: _____
_____
Patient notified: Yes   No
Remarks: _____

Thank you for your assistance.

Completed by: _____

Encounter Form

Date: _____

Paul Provider, M.D.
5858 Peppermint Place ● Anytown, USA 12345 ● (765) 555-6768

Provider Information

Name: _____
Address: _____
City: _____ State: _____ Zip Code: _____
Telephone#: _____
Fax#: _____
Tax ID #: _____
Medicaid ID #: _____
Medicare ID #: _____

Provider's Signature: _____ Date: _____

Patient Information

Name: _____
Address: _____
City: _____ State: _____ Zip Code: _____
Telephone#: _____
Patient Account #: _____
Date of Birth: _____
Gender: _____
Relationship to Guarantor: _____
Marital Status: _____
SSN #: _____

Appointment Information

Appt. Date: _____ Time: _____
Request Next Appt. Date: _____ Time: _____
Date of First Visit: _____
Date of Injury: _____
Referring Physician: _____

Guarantor Information

Name: _____
Insurance ID#: _____
Insurance Plan Name: _____
Insurance Plan Group#: _____
Employer Name: _____
Employer Address: _____
City: _____ State: _____ Zip Code: _____
SSN #: _____

Authorization

☐ Authorization to Release Information
☐ Authorization for Assignment of Benefits
☐ Authorization for Consent for Treatment
☐ I understand that my insurance will be billed as a courtesy to me but that there may be a patient responsibility remaining on account.

Signature: _____ Date: _____

Insurance Type: ☐ Private ☐ Medicare ☐ Medicaid ☐ Workers' Compensation ☐ Other _____

Clinical Information

	Date of Service	Place of Service	CPT Code/Description	ICD-9 Code/ Description	Fee
1.					
2.					
3.					
4.					
5.					
6.					
7.					
8.					

Billing Instructions

Notes: _____

Special Instructions: _____

Statement of Account Information

Previous Balance: $ _____   Payment: $ _____
Today's Fee: $ _____   Received by:
Copay: $ _____   ☐ Cash
Adjustment: $ _____   ☐ Check
☐ Credit Card
New Balance: $ _____   ☐ Other

Patient Receipt

RECEIPT Date _____ CC _____ No.

Received From _____

Address _____

_____ **Dollars $** _____

For _____

ACCOUNT			HOW PAID		
AMT OF ACCOUNT			CASH		
AMT PAID			CHECK		
BALANCE DUE			MONEY ORDER		

By _____

PAUL PROVIDER, M.D. 5858 Peppermint Place Anytown, USA 12345

RECEIPT Date _____ CC _____ No.

Received From _____

Address _____

_____ **Dollars $** _____

For _____

ACCOUNT			HOW PAID		
AMT OF ACCOUNT			CASH		
AMT PAID			CHECK		
BALANCE DUE			MONEY ORDER		

By _____

PAUL PROVIDER, M.D. 5858 Peppermint Place Anytown, USA 12345

RECEIPT Date _____ CC _____ No.

Received From _____

Address _____

_____ **Dollars $** _____

For _____

ACCOUNT			HOW PAID		
AMT OF ACCOUNT			CASH		
AMT PAID			CHECK		
BALANCE DUE			MONEY ORDER		

By _____

PAUL PROVIDER, M.D. 5858 Peppermint Place Anytown, USA 12345

Paul Provider, M.D.
5858 Peppermint Place
Anytown, USA 12345
(765) 555-6768

Ledger Card/Statement of Account

RESPONSIBLE PARTY: _____

ADDRESS: _____

TELEPHONE #: _____

PATIENT NAME: _____ PATIENT ACCOUNT #: _____

SPECIAL NOTES: _____
_____

Date	Description of Service	Charge	Payments	Adjustments	Remaining Balance

Paul Provider, M.D.
5858 Peppermint Place
Anytown, USA 12345
(765) 555-6768

Day Sheet/Daily Journal

Date	Name	Description of Service	Charge	Payments	Adjustments	Remaining Balance

Deposit Slip/Ticket

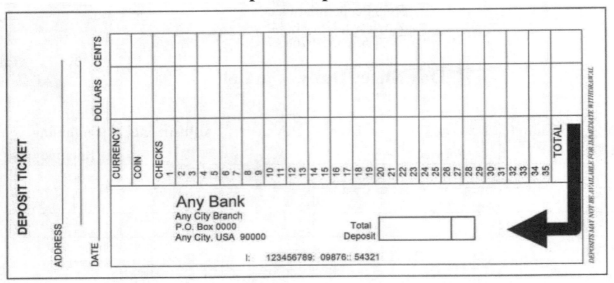

Patient Claim Form

Information must be printed or typewritten. Claim form must be completed and returned to us at the indicated address.

TO BE COMPLETED BY MEMBER

1. Information Pertaining To Member

Name: Last, First, M.I.		Gender:	Date Of Birth	Member ID #
Home Address: Street	City	State Zip		Telephone Number
Marital Status	Name Of Spouse	Spouse's Date Of Birth		Member ID #
Is Spouse Employed?	If Yes, Name And Address Of Employer			Employer Phone Number

2. Information Pertaining To Patient

Patient Name: Last, First, M.I.		Sex	Date Of Birth	Member ID #
Home Address: Street	City	State Zip		Telephone Number
Is Patient Employed? Full-Time Part Time No	Relationship To Employee?	If Dependent Child Over 19, Name Of School Where Full-time Student		

3. Information Regarding Current Treatment

Related To Illness?	Related To Pregnancy?	Related To Work?	Description Of Illness Or Injury
Date Of Accident	Where It Happened?	Describe Accident	

4. Information Regarding Insurance

Are You, Your Spouse or Dependent Children Covered By Any Other Insurance?	Name Of Insured
If Yes, Name And Address Of Insurance	Insurance Phone Number

Patient's Or Guardian's Signature

I certify that the above information is true and correct and I authorize the release of any medical information necessary to process this claim.

Signed: Date:

Assignment of Benefits:

I assign payment of benefits to the following provider:

Address: Street	City	State Zip	Telephone Number

(continues on next page)

TO BE COMPLETED BY PHYSICIAN

Patient's Name: Last, First, M.I.					

Home Address: Street	City	State	Zip	Telephone Number

Is Condition Due To Illness?	Injury?	Work Related?	Pregnancy?	If Yes, Date Of Last Menstrual Period

Diagnosis Or Nature Of Illness Or Injuries. Give Description And ICD-9 Code.

_____

_____

Date Of Service	Place Of Service	Description Of Medical Services Or Supplies Provided	CPT Code	ICD-9 Code	Charge

Date Of First Symptoms	Date Of Accident	Date Patient First Seen		Total Charges	
Dates Patient Unable To Work From To	If Still Disabled, Date Patient Should Return To Work			Amount Paid	
Patient Still Under Care For This Condition?	Date Of Same Or Similar Illness Or Condition		Does Patient Have Other Health Coverage?		

Under Section 6019 Of The Internal Revenue Code, Recipients Of Medical Payments Must Provide Identifying Numbers To Payors Who Must Report Such Payments To The Internal Revenue Service.   Taxpayer ID Number: _____ Social Security Number: _____

Physician's Name: _____ Signature: _____

_____

Street Address	City	State	Zip

INFORMATION REGARDING THIS CLAIM FORM

A Separate Claim Must Be Filed For Each Different Injury Or Illness.

A Claim Must Be Filed Within 90 Days of The Date Of Service Or Claim Benefits May Be Reduced.

If Patient Is Medicare Eligible, Claim Must First Be Submitted To Medicare For Payment. We Cannot Process Claim Without Information Regarding Medicare's Payment.

(continued)

Paul Provider, M.D.
5858 Peppermint Place
Anytown, USA 12345
(765) 555-6768

Superbill/Charge Slip

Date of Service: _____ Account Number: _____

Name (Last, First): _____

X	Code	Description	Fee	X	Code	Description	Fee	X	Code	Description	Fee
Initial				**Established**				**Special Procedures**			
	99202	Expanded Exam	60.00		99211	Minimal Exam	35.00				
	99203	Detailed Low Complexity	100.00		99212	Brief Straightforward Exam	40.00				
	99204	Comp Moderate Complexity Exam	140.00		99213	Expanded Low Complexity Exam	45.00				
	99205	Comp High Complexity Exam	160.00		99214	Detailed Moderate Complexity Exam	60.00				
					99215	Comp High Complexity Exam	90.00				
Consultations				**Laboratory**				**Prescriptions**			
	99244	Comprehensive	150.00		36415	Venipuncture	20.00				
					81000	Urinalysis	30.00				
					82948	Glucose Fingerstick	18.00				
					93000	EKG	55.00				

X	Code	Diagnosis	X	Code	Diagnosis	X	Code	Diagnosis
	466	Bronchitis, Acute		401	Hypertension		460	Upper Resp Tract Infection
	428	Congestive Heart Failure		414	Ischemic Heart Disease		599.0	Urinary Tract Infection
	431	CVA		724.2	Low Back Syndrome		616	Vaginitis
	250.0	Diabetes Mellitus		278.0	Obesity		490	Bronchitis
	625.3	Dysmenorrhea		715	Osteoarthritis		244	Acquired Hypothyroidism
	345	Epilepsy		462	Pharyngitis. Acute		**ICD-9**	**Other Diagnosis**
	0009.0	Gastroenteritis		714	Rheumatoid Arthritis			

Remarks/Special Instructions	New Appointment	Statement of Account	
		Old Balance	
		Today's Fee	
Referring Physician	Recall	Payment	
		New Balance	

CPT® codes, descriptions, and two-digit numeric modifiers are copyrighted by the American Medical Association. All Rights Reserved.

PAUL PROVIDER, M.D.
5858 Peppermint Place
Anytown, USA 121345
(765) 555-6768

Insurance Claims Register

Page No. _____

Date Claims Filed	Patient Name	Name of Insurance Policy	Place Claim Sent	Claim Amount	Follow-Up Date	Paid Amount	Remaining Balance

APPROVED OMB-0938-0008

CARRIER

| | PICA | | HEALTH INSURANCE CLAIM FORM | PICA | | |

| 1. MEDICARE | MEDICAID | CHAMPUS | CHAMPVA | GROUP HEALTH PLAN | FECA BLK LUNG | OTHER | 1a. INSURED'S I.D. NUMBER (FOR PROGRAM IN ITEM 1) |
| (Medicare #) | (Medicaid #) | (Sponsor's SSN) | (VA File #) | (SSN or ID) | (SSN) | (ID) | |

2. PATIENT'S NAME (Last Name, First Name, Middle Initial)

3. PATIENT'S BIRTH DATE MM | DD | YY   SEX   M | F

4. INSURED'S NAME (Last Name, First Name, Middle Initial)

5. PATIENT'S ADDRESS (No., Street)

6. PATIENT RELATIONSHIP TO INSURED   Self | Spouse | Child | Other

7. INSURED'S ADDRESS (No., Street)

CITY | STATE

8. PATIENT STATUS   Single | Married | Other

CITY | STATE

ZIP CODE | TELEPHONE (Include Area Code) ( )

Employed | Full-Time Student | Part-Time Student

ZIP CODE | TELEPHONE (INCLUDE AREA CODE) ( )

9. OTHER INSURED'S NAME (Last Name, First Name, Middle Initial)

10. IS PATIENT'S CONDITION RELATED TO

11. INSURED'S POLICY GROUP OR FECA NUMBER

a. OTHER INSURED'S POLICY OR GROUP NUMBER

a. EMPLOYMENT? (CURRENT OR PREVIOUS)   YES | NO

a. INSURED'S DATE OF BIRTH MM | DD | YY   SEX   M | F

b. OTHER INSURED'S DATE OF BIRTH MM | DD | YY   SEX   M | F

b. AUTO ACCIDENT?   PLACE (State)   YES | NO

b. EMPLOYER'S NAME OR SCHOOL NAME

c. EMPLOYER'S NAME OR SCHOOL NAME

c. OTHER ACCIDENT?   YES | NO

c. INSURANCE PLAN NAME OR PROGRAM NAME

d. INSURANCE PLAN NAME OR PROGRAM NAME

10d. RESERVED FOR LOCAL USE

d. IS THERE ANOTHER HEALTH BENEFIT PLAN?   YES | NO   *If yes*, return to and complete item 9 a-d.

READ BACK OF FORM BEFORE COMPLETING & SIGNING THIS FORM.
12. PATIENT'S OR AUTHORIZED PERSON'S SIGNATURE. I authorize the release of any medical or other information necessary to process this claim. I also request payment of government benefits either to myself or to the party who accepts assignment below.

SIGNED _____ DATE _____

13. INSURED'S OR AUTHORIZED PERSON'S SIGNATURE. I authorize payment of medical benefits to the undersigned physician or supplier for services described below.

SIGNED _____

PATIENT AND INSURED INFORMATION

14. DATE OF CURRENT: ILLNESS (First symptom) OR INJURY (Accident) OR PREGNANCY(LMP) MM | DD | YY

15. IF PATIENT HAS HAD SAME OR SIMILAR ILLNESS GIVE FIRST DATE MM | DD | YY

16. DATES PATIENT UNABLE TO WORK IN CURRENT OCCUPATION MM | DD | YY   FROM   TO   MM | DD | YY

17. NAME OF REFERRING PHYSICIAN OR OTHER SOURCE

17a. I.D. NUMBER OF REFERRING PHYSICIAN

18. HOSPITALIZATION DATES RELATED TO CURRENT SERVICES MM | DD | YY   FROM   TO   MM | DD | YY

19. RESERVED FOR LOCAL USE

20. OUTSIDE LAB? $ CHARGES   YES | NO

21. DIAGNOSIS OR NATURE OF ILLNESS OR INJURY. (RELATE ITEMS 1,2,3 OR 4 TO ITEM 24E BY LINE)

1. |____.___   3. |____.___

2. |____.___   4. |____.___

22. MEDICAID RESUBMISSION CODE   ORIGINAL REF. NO.

23. PRIOR AUTHORIZATION NUMBER

24. A. DATE(S) OF SERVICE					B. Place of Service	C. Type of Service	D. PROCEDURES, SERVICES, OR SUPPLIES (Explain Unusual Circumstances) CPT/HCPCS	MODIFIER	E. DIAGNOSIS CODE	F. $ CHARGES	G. DAYS OR UNITS	H. EPSDT Family Plan	I. EMG	J. COB	K. RESERVED FOR LOCAL USE
From MM DD YY	To MM DD YY														
1															
2															
3															
4															
5															
6															

25. FEDERAL TAX I.D. NUMBER   SSN EIN

26. PATIENT'S ACCOUNT NO.

27. ACCEPT ASSIGNMENT? (For govt. claims, see back)   YES | NO

28. TOTAL CHARGE $

29. AMOUNT PAID $

30. BALANCE DUE $

31. SIGNATURE OF PHYSICIAN OR SUPPLIER INCLUDING DEGREES OR CREDENTIALS (I certify that the statements on the reverse apply to this bill and are made a part thereof.)

SIGNED _____ DATE _____

32. NAME AND ADDRESS OF FACILITY WHERE SERVICES WERE RENDERED (If other than home or office)

33. PHYSICIAN'S, SUPPLIER'S BILLING NAME, ADDRESS, ZIP CODE & PHONE #

PIN# _____ GRP# _____

PHYSICIAN OR SUPPLIER INFORMATION

(APPROVED BY AMA COUNCIL ON MEDICAL SERVICE 8/88)   **PLEASE PRINT OR TYPE**   FORM HCFA-1500 (12-90), FORM RRB-1500, FORM OWCP-1500

UB-92 Billing Form

APPROVED OMB NO. 0938-0279

		2		3 PATIENT CONTROL NO.	4 TYPE OF BILL

ST11843 1PLY UB-92

1

5 FED. TAX NO.	6 STATEMENT COVERS PERIOD FROM THROUGH	7 COV D.	8 N-C D.	9 C-I D.	10 L-R D.	11

12 PATIENT NAME		13 PATIENT ADDRESS

14 BIRTHDATE	15 SEX	16 MS	17 DATE ADMISSION	18 HR	19 TYPE	20 SRC	21 D HR	22 STAT	23 MEDICAL RECORD NO.	CONDITION CODES 24 25 26 27 28 29 30	31

32 CODE OCCURRENCE DATE	33 CODE OCCURRENCE DATE	34 CODE OCCURRENCE DATE	35 CODE OCCURRENCE DATE	36 CODE OCCURRENCE SPAN FROM THROUGH	37 A B C

a
b
38

	39 CODE VALUE CODES AMOUNT	40 CODE VALUE CODES AMOUNT	41 CODE VALUE CODES AMOUNT
a			
b			
c			
d			

42 REV. CD.	43 DESCRIPTION	44 HCPCS / RATES	45 SERV. DATE	46 SERV. UNITS	47 TOTAL CHARGES	48 NON-COVERED CHARGES	49
1							
2							
3							
4							
5							
6							
7							
8							
9							
10							
11							
12							
13							
14							
15							
16							
17							
18							
19							
20							
21							
22							
23							

50 PAYER	51 PROVIDER NO.	52 REL INFO	53 ASG BEN	54 PRIOR PAYMENTS	55 EST. AMOUNT DUE	56
A						
B						
C						

57

DUE FROM PATIENT ▶

58 INSURED'S NAME	59 P. REL	60 CERT. - SSN - HIC - ID NO.	61 GROUP NAME	62 INSURANCE GROUP NO.
A				
B				
C				

63 TREATMENT AUTHORIZATION CODES	64 ESC	65 EMPLOYER NAME	66 EMPLOYER LOCATION
A			
B			
C			

67 PRIN. DIAG. CD.	68 CODE	69 CODE	70 CODE	OTHER DIAG. CODES 71 CODE	72 CODE	73 CODE	74 CODE	75 CODE	76 ADM. DIAG. CD.	77 E-CODE	78

79 P.C.	80 PRINCIPAL PROCEDURE CODE DATE	81 OTHER PROCEDURE CODE DATE	OTHER PROCEDURE CODE DATE	82 ATTENDING PHYS. ID

A
B

OTHER PROCEDURE CODE DATE	OTHER PROCEDURE CODE DATE	OTHER PROCEDURE CODE DATE	83 OTHER PHYS. ID

C
D
E

A

84 REMARKS	OTHER PHYS. ID

B

a
b
c
d

85 PROVIDER REPRESENTATIVE	86 DATE
X	

UB-92 HCFA-1450   OCR/ORIGINAL   I CERTIFY THE CERTIFICATIONS ON THE REVERSE APPLY TO THIS BILL AND ARE MADE A PART HEREOF.

Hospital Admission Form

Provider Information

			Admission Information	

Admission Information

Name: _____   Admission Date: _____   Time: _____
Address: _____   Discharge Date: _____   Time: _____
City: _____ State: _____ Zip Code: _____   Attending Phy's ID#: _____
Telephone#: _____ Fax#: _____   Attending Physician: _____
Medicare ID#: _____ UPIN#: _____   Date of Injury: _____
Tax ID #: _____ Accepts Medicare Assignment: ☐
Provider Rep: _____ Date: _____

Patient Information

Name: _____
Address: _____
City: _____ State: _____ Zip Code: _____
Telephone#: _____ Patient Control #: _____
Date of Birth: _____ Gender: _____
Marital Status: _____ Relationship to Guarantor: _____
Student Status: ☐ Full-time ☐ Part-time
Insurance Type: ☐ Pvt ☐ M/care ☐ M/caid ☐ WC ☐ Other _____

Guarantor Information

Name: _____
Address: _____
City: _____ State: _____ Zip Code: _____
Insurance ID #: _____ SSN: _____
Insurance Name: _____
Insurance Group #: _____
Employer Name: _____

Authorization

☐ Authorization to Release Information
☐ Authorization for Assignment of Benefits
☐ Authorization for Consent for Treatment
☐ My insurance will be billed but there may be a balance due.
Signature: _____ Date: _____

Clinical Information

Principal Diagnosis: _____
Other Diagnosis: _____
Surgical Procedure: _____
Other Procedures: _____

Remarks: _____

Previous Balance:	Today's Fee:	Payment:	Adjustment:	New Balance:

Domestic Return Receipt

PROVIDER POSTAL SERVICES

First-Class Mail
Postage & Fees Paid
PPS
Permit No. P-18

●Sender: Please print your name, address, and ZIP+4 in this box●

SENDER: *COMPLETE THIS SECTION*

- Complete items 1, 2, and 3. Also complete item 4 if Restricted Delivery is desired.
- Print your name and address on the reverse so that we can return the card to you.
- Attach this card to the back of the mailpiece, or on the front if space permits.

1. Article Addressed to:

2. Article Number
   (Transfer from service label)

COMPLETE THIS SECTION ON DELIVERY

A. Signature

X

☐ Agent
☐ Addressee

B. Received by (Printed Name) | C. Date of Delivery

D. Is delivery address different from item 1?   ☐ Yes
   If YES, enter delivery address below: ☐ No

3. Service Type
   ☐ Certified Mail   ☐ Express Mail
   ☐ Registered   ☐ Return Receipt for Merchandise
   ☐ Insured Mail   ☐ C.O.D

4. Restricted Delivery? *(Extra Fee)*   ☐ Yes

| PPS Form 2894 | Domestic Return Receipt | 105535-06-P-6211 |

Certified Mail Form

PLACE STICKER AT THE BOTTOM OF THE PACKAGE
FOLD AT DOTTED LINE

Certified Mail

1000   0555   0001   2222   5555

0001   0222   1000   5555   2222

Provider Postal Services-Certified Mail

Sender's Name

Street, Apt. No.; or PO Box No.

City, State, ZIP + 4

	$
Postage	$
Certified Fee	$
Total Postage	$

Recipient's Name (To be completed by mailer)

Street, Apt. No.;

City, State, ZIP + 4

Ground Tracking ID
COD Prepaid

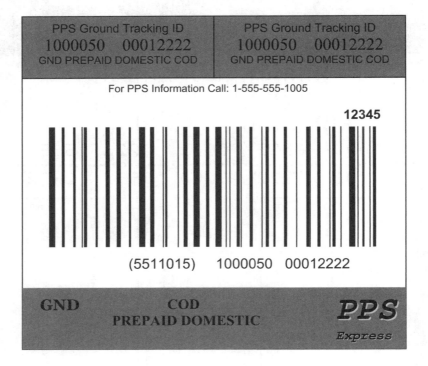

COD Airbill

PPS *Express*   *C.O.D Airbill*   PPS Tracking Number 1005 1222

Form
I.D. No.   **1055**   Sender's Copy

5005

1 From   *Please print and press hard.*

Sender's PPS
Account Number 1005-5505-5

Date

Sender's
Name _____   Phone (   )_____

Company _____

Address _____   Dept./Floor/Suite/Room

City _____   State _____   ZIP _____

2 Your Internal Billing Reference

First 4 characters will appear on invoice.

3 To

Recipient's
Name _____   Phone (   )_____

Company _____

Address _____
To "HOLD" at PPS location, print PPS address.   We cannot deliver to P.O. boxes or P.O. ZIP codes.

Address _____   Dept./Floor/Suite/Room

City _____   State _____   ZIP _____

Questions? Call 1 555 555 1005

4a Express Package Service   *Packages up to 150 lbs.*

☐ PPS Priority Overnight   ☐ PPS Standard Overnight   ☐ PPS First Overnight
Next business morning   Delivery commitment may be later in some areas.   Earliest next business morning
delivery to select locations   Next business afternoon

☐ PPS 2Day   ☐ PPS Express Saver
Second business day   Third business day
PPS Envelope rate not available. Minimum charge: One-pound rate

4b Express Freight Service   *Packages over 150 lbs.*

Delivery commitment may be later in some areas.

☐ PPS 1Day Freight*   ☐ PPS 2Day Freight   ☐ PPS 3Day Freight
Next business day   Second business day   Third business day
*Call for confirmation:

5 Packaging

☐ PPS Envelope*   ☐ PPS Pak*   ☐ Other   Declared value limit $500
Includes Small,
Large and Sturdy Pak

6 Special Handling   [Include PPS address in Section 3]

☐ SATURDAY Delivery   ☐ HOLD Weekday   ☐ HOLD Saturday
at PPS Location   at PPS Location

7 Payment   *Bill to:*   [Enter PPS Acct. No. or Credit Card No. below.]

☐ Sender   ☐ Recipient   ☐ Third Party   ☐ Credit Card   ☐ Cash/Check
Acct. No. in
Section 1 will be billed.

PPS Acct. No.
Credit Card No. _____

Exp.
Date _____

Total Packages   Total Weight   Total Declared Value†

$ _____ .00

PPS Use Only

†Our Liability is limited to $100 unless you declare a higher value.

8 Release Signature   *Sign to authorize delivery without obtaining signature.*

By signing you authorize us to deliver this shipment without obtaining a signature
and agree to indemnify and hold us harmless from any resulting claims.

COD Shipper Receipt

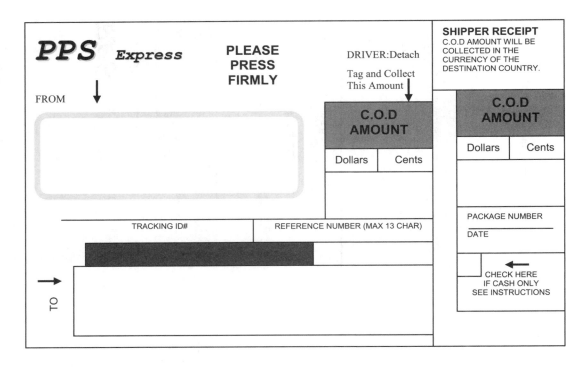

Ground Tracking ID
Prepaid

Airbill

PPS *Express*   *Airbill*   PPS Tracking Number 1005 1222   Sender's Copy

5005

Form I.D. No. **1055**

1 From *Please print and press hard.*

Date

Sender's PPS
Account Number 1005-5505-5

Sender's Name ___ Phone ( )

Company

Address ___ Dept./Floor/Suite/Room

City ___ State ___ ZIP

2 Your Internal Billing Reference
First 4 characters will appear on invoice.

3 To

Recipient's Name ___ Phone ( )

Company

Address ___ Dept./Floor/Suite/Room
To "HOLD" at PPS location, print PPS address.   We cannot deliver to P.O. boxes or P.O. ZIP codes.

City ___ State ___ ZIP

Questions? Call 1 555 555 1005

4a Express Package Service
Packages up to 150 lbs.

☐ PPS Priority Overnight ☐ PPS Standard Overnight ☐ PPS First Overnight
Next business morning   Next business afternoon   Earliest next business morning
delivery to select locations   Delivery commitment may be later in some areas.

☐ PPS 2Day ☐ PPS Express Saver
Second business day   Third business day
PPS Envelope rate not available. **Minimum charge: One-pound rate**

4b Express Freight Service
Packages over 150 lbs.
Delivery commitment may be later in some areas.

☐ PPS 1Day Freight* ☐ PPS 2Day Freight ☐ PPS 3Day Freight
Next business day   Second business day   Third business day
*Call for confirmation:

5 Packaging
Declared value limit $500

☐ PPS Envelope* ☐ PPS Pak* ☐ Other
Includes Small, Large and Sturdy Pak

6 Special Handling
[Include PPS address in Section 3]

☐ SATURDAY Delivery ☐ HOLD Weekday ☐ HOLD Saturday
at PPS Location   at PPS Location

7 Payment   *Bill to:* [Enter PPS Acct. No. or Credit Card No. below.]

☐ Sender ☐ Recipient ☐ Third Party ☐ Credit Card ☐ Cash/Check
Acct. No. in
Section 1 will be billed.

PPS Acct. No.
Credit Card No. ___ Exp. Date

Total Packages | Total Weight | Total Declared Value†
$ ___ .00
PPS Use Only

†Your Liability is limited to $100 unless you declare a higher value.

8 Release Signature   *Sign to authorize delivery without obtaining signature.*

By signing you authorize us to deliver this shipment without obtaining a signature
and agree to indemnify and hold us harmless from any resulting claims.

PAUL PROVIDER, M.D.
Medical Billing Office
5858 Peppermint Place
Anytown, USA 12345
(765) 555-6768

Serving all your medical needs for 20 years

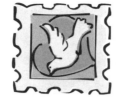

Paul Provider, M.D.
5858 Peppermint Place
Anytown, USA 12345

Appendix C

Tables

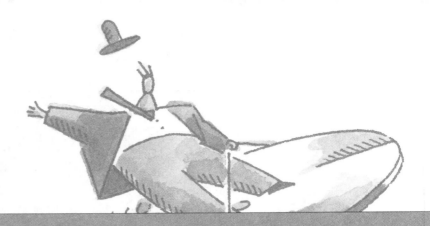

Table of Contents

Patient Data Table

	Abby Addison	Bobby Bumble	Cathy Crenshaw	Daisy Doolittle	Edward Edmunds
Patient Name **Address**	5678 Any Avenue Anytown, USA 12345	93485 Bumpkiss Court Anytown, USA 12345	9876 Cranbury Lane Anytown, USA 12345	1234 Daffy Lane Anytown, USA 12345	8888 Every Lane Anytown, USA 12345
Telephone # **Home** **Work**	(765) 555-4321 (765) 555-4567	(765) 555-4756 (765) 555-6272	(765) 555-3579 (765) 555-1489	(765) 555-4311	(765) 555-7890 (765) 555-7788
Date of Birth	12/12/CCYY-38	1/4/CCYY-62	2/4/CCYY-63	8/1/CCYY-47	1/10/CCYY-79
Social Security #	001-01-0010	002-02-0020	003-03-0030	004-04-0040	508-12-3456
Marital Status/Gender	Single/Female	Married/Male	Single/Female	Married /Female	Widow/Male
Patient Account #	GMBC5509-001	GMBC5509-002	GMBC5509-003	GMBC5509-004	GMBC5509-005
Allergies/Medical Conditions	None/Hypertension	None/Diabetes	None/Chronic Bronchitis	None/Congenital Hypothyroidism	None/Coronary Artery Disease
Insurance Carrier	Rover Insurers, Inc. 5931 Rolling Road Ronson, CO 81369	Ball Ins. Carriers 3895 Bubble Blvd. Ste. 283 Boxwood, CO 85931	No Insurance (Cash patient)	Medicaid P.O. Box 0098 Anytown, USA 12342	Medicare P.O. Box 1234 Anytown, USA 12345
Member's ID #	001-01 RED	002-02 BLUE		004-04 MEDI	508-12-3456A
Group Policy #	41935	98135		Parts A & B	
Policy/Employer	Red Corporation 1234 Nockout Road Newton, NM 88012 (970) 555-0863	Blue Corporation 9817 Bobcat Blvd. Bastion, CO 81319 (970) 555-5432	Creative Creations Corp. 1234 Creature Lane Anytown, USA 12345 (765) 555-5631	None	Retired
Workers' Comp Ins. Carrier	Red Apple Ins. 1234 Abbey Road Anytown, USA 12345 (765) 555-2477	Blueberry Ins. 4662 Beach Blvd. Anytown, USA 12345 (765) 555-6543	None	None	None
Workers' Comp Claim Number	None	25101606	None	None	None
Assigned Provider	Paul Provider, M.D.	Paul Provider, M.D.	Paul Provider, M.D.	Paul Provider, M.D.	Paul Provider, M.D.
Referred By	Friend	Spouse	Friend	Dr. Daniel Dobby	Edith Evan, M.D.
Responsible Party	Self	Self	Self	Self	Self
Person to Contact in Emergency	Alice Avery 8765 Any Avenue Anytown, USA 12345 (765) 555- 4756	Barbara Bumble 93485 Bumpkiss Court Anytown, USA 12345 (765) 555-4756	Carmen Castro 6789 Cranbury Lane Anytown, USA 12345 (765) 555-6954	Danny Doolittle 1234 Daffy Lane Anytown, USA 12345 (765) 555-4311	Edgar Edmunds 7777 Every Lane Anytown, USA 12345 (765) 555-5566

■ **Table AC–1** Patient Data Table

Provider Data Table

Provider Name:	Paul Provider	Provider Medical Group	Laboratory Provider	Provider Medical Center
Address:	5858 Peppermint Place	5858 Peppermint Place	5859 Peppermint Place	6969 Pauly Main Court
City, State Zip	Anytown, USA 12345	Anytown, USA 12345	Anytown, USA 12345	Anytown, USA 12345
Telephone #:	(765) 555-6768	(765) 555-6868	(765) 555-6767	(765) 555-8901
Accepts Medicare Assignment	Yes	Yes	Yes	Yes
Authorization to Release Information on File	Yes	Yes	Yes	Yes
Assignment of Benefits on File	Yes	Yes	Yes	Yes
TIN:	99-1234567	99-2395605	99-9874343	99-7654321
UPIN:	P12345	W12345	000277	000101
PIN:	PP876543	WW876543	2315845	3241896

■ **Table AC–2** Provider Data Table

Order of Benefit Determination

Rule #	Description
1	The plan without a COB provision will be primary to a plan with a COB provision.
2	When a plan does not have OBD rules, and as a result the plans do not agree on the OBD, the plan without these OBD rules will determine the order of payment.
3	The plan that covers an individual as an employee will be primary to a plan that covers that individual as a dependent.
4	If an individual is an employee under two plans, the primary is the one under which the employee has been covered the longest.
5	If an employee is an active employee under one plan and a retiree (or laid off) under another, the active plan will pay as primary.
The parent birthday rule, explained in #6 and #7, affects the OBD for dependent children of parents who are living together and married (not divorced or legally separated).	
6	The plan of the parent whose birthday (based on month and day only) occurs first during the calendar year is the primary plan.
7	When both parents' birthdays are the same (based on month and day), the plan that covered one parent the longest is the primary plan.
For dependents of legally separated or divorced parents and those whose parents have remarried, the order of benefits determination is based on the following rule:	
8	The plan of the parent specified as having legal responsibility for the health care expense of the child is the primary plan.
For dependents of separated parents with no court decree:	
9	The plan of the parent with custody is prime.
10	The plan of the step-parent (if any) with whom the child resides is secondary.
11	The plan of the natural parent without custody is tertiary.
12	The step-parent (if any) who does not reside with the child has no legal right to declare dependency. Therefore, no coordination should be performed because the child is probably not an eligible dependent under the plan.
13	For joint custody, with no additional responsibility designation, the plan of the parent whose coverage has been in effect the longest would be the primary payer. However, this rule may vary by administrator. Some parents pay costs on a 50/50 basis, thereby sharing equally in the health care risk.

■ **Table AC–3** Order of Benefit Determination

Medicare Secondary Payer

If the patient...	And this condition exists...	Then the program pays first...	And this program pays second...
Is age 65 or older, and is covered by a Group Health Plan through a current employer or spouse's current employer...	The employer has less than 20 employees...	**Medicare**	Group Health Plan
	The employer has 20 or more employees, or at least one employer is a multi-employer group that employs 20 or more individuals...	Group Health Plan	**Medicare**
Has an employer retirement plan and is age 65 or older or is disabled and age 65 or older...	The patient is entitled to Medicare...	**Medicare**	Retiree coverage
Is disabled and covered by a Large Group Health Plan from work, or is covered by a family member who is working...	The employer has less than 100 employees...	**Medicare**	Large Group Health Plan
	The employer has 100 or more employees, or at least one employer is a multi-employer group that employs 100 or more individuals...	Large Group Health Plan	**Medicare**
Has end-stage renal disease and Group Health Plan Coverage...	Is in the first 30 months of eligibility or entitlement to Medicare...	Group Health Plan	**Medicare**
	After 30 months...	**Medicare**	Group Health Plan
Has end-stage renal disease and COBRA coverage...	Is in the first 30 months of eligibility or entitlement to Medicare...	COBRA	Medicare
	After 30 months...	**Medicare**	COBRA
Is covered under Workers' Compensation because of job-related illness or injury...	The patient is entitled to Medicare...	Workers' Compensation (for healthcare items or services related to job-related illness or injury)	**Medicare**
Has black lung disease and is covered under the Federal Black Lung Program...	The patient is eligible for the Federal Black Lung Program...	Federal Black Lung Program (for healthcare services related to black lung disease)	**Medicare**
Has been in an auto accident where no-fault or liability insurance is involved...	The patient is entitled to Medicare...	No-fault or liability insurance (for accident-related healthcare services)	**Medicare**
Is age 65 or older OR is disabled and covered by Medicare and COBRA...	The patient is entitled to Medicare...	**Medicare**	COBRA
Has Veterans Health Administration (VHA) benefits...	Receives VHA authorized healthcare services at a non-VHA facility...	VHA	Medicare may pay when the services provided are Medicare-covered services and are not covered by the VHA

■ **Table AC–4** Medicare Secondary Payer

Quick Reference Codes

ORGANIZATION OF VOLUME I	
Number	**Body System/Classification**
00 – 13	Infective and Parasitic Diseases
14 – 23	Neoplasms
24 – 27	Endocrine, Nutritional, Metabolic Diseases
28	Diseases of the Blood and Blood-Forming Organs
29 – 31	Mental/Nervous Disorders
32 – 38	Diseases of the Nervous System and Sense Organs
39 – 45	Diseases of the Circulatory System
46 – 51	Diseases of the Respiratory System
52 – 57	Diseases of the Digestive System
58 – 62	Diseases of the Genito-Urinary System
63 – 67	Complications of Pregnancy, Childbirth and the Puerperium
68 – 70	Diseases of the Skin and Subcutaneous Tissue
71 – 73	Diseases of the Musculoskeletal System and Connective Tissue
74 – 75	Congenital Anomalies
76 – 77	Certain Causes of Perinatal Morbidity and Mortality
78 – 79	Symptoms, Signs and Ill-Defined Conditions
80 – 86	Fractures, Dislocations, Sprains and Internal Injuries
87 – 90	Lacerations
91 – 99	Other Accidents, Poisoning and Violence (nature of the injury)
V0 – Y24	Miscellaneous Informative Codings (a particular diagnosis is not indicated)

SECTIONS OF THE CPT® AND RVS	
Code	**Description**
99201 – 99499	**Evaluation and Management**
CPT® 00100 – 01999 RVS 10000 – 69999 99100 – 99140	**Anesthesia:**
10021 – 69999	**Surgery**
70010 – 79999	**Radiology/Nuclear Medicine**
80048 – 89356	**Pathology and Laboratory Tests**
90281 – 99199 and 99500 – 99602	**Medicine**

EVALUATION AND MANAGEMENT CODES	
Code	**Description**
99201 – 99215	Office or Other Outpatient Services
99217 – 99220	Hospital Observation Services
99221 – 99239	Hospital Inpatient Services
99241 – 99275	Consultations
99281 – 99288	Emergency Department Services
99289 – 99290	Pediatric Critical Care Patient Transport
99291 – 99292	Critical Care Services
99293 – 99296	Inpatient Neonatal and Pediatric Critical Care Services
99298 – 99299	Intensive (Non-Critical) Low Birth Weight Services
99301 – 99316	Nursing Facility Services
99321 – 99333	Domiciliary, Rest Home, or Custodial Care Services
99341 – 99350	Home Services

■ **Table AC–5** Quick Reference Codes *(continues on next page)*

99354 – 99360	Prolonged Services
99361 – 99373	Case Management Services
99374 – 99380	Care Plan Oversite Services
99381 – 99429	Preventive Medicine Services
99431 – 99440	Newborn Care Services
99450 – 9945	Special Evaluation and Management Services
99499	Other Evaluation and Management Services

ANESTHESIA CODES

Code	Description
00100 – 00222	Head
00300 – 00352	Neck
00400 – 00474	Thorax
00500 – 00580	Intrathoracic
00600 – 00670	Spine and Spinal Cord
00700 – 00797	Upper Abdomen
00800 – 00882	Lower Abdomen
00902 – 00952	Perineum
01112 – 01190	Pelvis (Except Hip)
01200 – 01274	Upper Leg (Except Knee)
01320 – 01444	Knee and Popliteal Area
01420 – 01522	Lower Leg
01710 – 01782	Upper Arm and Elbow
01810 – 01860	Forearm, Wrist and Hand
01905 – 01933	Radiological Procedures
01951 – 01953	Burns, Excisions or Debridement
01958 – 01969	Obstetric
01990 – 01999	Other Procedures

SURGERY CODES

Code	Description
10040 – 19499	Integumentary System
20000 – 29999	Musculoskeletal System
30000 – 32999	Respiratory System
33010 – 37799	Cardiovascular System
38100 – 38999	Hemic and Lymphatic System
39000 – 39599	Mediastinum and Diaphragm
40490 – 49999	Digestive System
50010 – 53899	Urinary System
54000 – 55899	Male Genital System
55970 – 55980	Intersex Surgery
56400 – 58999	Female Genital System
59000 – 59899	Maternity Care and Delivery
60000 – 60699	Endocrine System
61000 – 64999	Nervous System
65091 – 68899	Eye and Ocular Adnexa
69000 – 69979	Auditory System
69990	Operating Microscope
93501 – 93553	Cardiac Catheterizations

(continues on next page)

RADIOLOGY CODES

Code	Description
70010 – 76499	Diagnostic Radiology
76506 – 76999	Diagnostic Ultrasound
77261 – 77799	Radiation Oncology
78000 – 79999	Nuclear Medicine

PATHOLOGY CODES

Code	Description
80048 – 80076	Organ or Disease Oriented Panels
80100 – 80103	Drug Testing
80150 – 80299	Therapeutic Drug Assays
80400 – 80440	Evocative/Suppression Testing
80500 – 80502	Consultations (Clinical Pathology)
81000 – 81099	Urinalysis
82000 – 84999	Chemistry
85002 – 85999	Hematology and Coagulation
86000 – 86849	Immunology
86850 – 86999	Transfusion Medicine
87001 – 87999	Microbiology
88000 – 88099	Anatomic Pathology
88104 – 88199	Cytopathology
88230 – 88299	Cytogenic Studies
88300 – 88399	Surgical Pathology
88400	Transcutaneous Procedures
89050 – 89240	Other Procedures
89250 – 89356	Reproductive Medicine Procedures

MEDICINE CODES

Code	Description
90281 – 90399	Immune Globulins
90471 – 90474	Immunization Administration for Vaccines/Toxoids
90476 – 90749	Vaccines/Toxoids
90780 – 90781	Therapeutic or Diagnostic Infusions
90782 – 90799	Therapeutic, Prophylactic or Diagnostic Injections
90801 – 90899	Psychiatry
90900 – 90911	Biofeedback
90918 – 90999	Dialysis
91000 – 91299	Gastroenterology
92002 – 92499	Ophthalmology
92502 – 92700	Special Otorhinolaryngologic Services
92950 – 93799	Cardiovascular
93875 – 93990	Non-Invasive Vascular Studies
94010 – 94799	Pulmonary
95004 – 95199	Allergy and Clinical Immunology
95250	Endocrinology
95805 – 96004	Neurology and Neuromuscular Procedures
96100 – 96117	Central Nervous System Assessments/Tests
96150 – 96155	Health and Behavior Assessment /Intervention

(continues on next page)

96400 – 96549	Chemotherapy Administration
96567 – 96571	Photodynamic Therapy
96900 – 96999	Special Dermatological Procedures
97001 – 97799	Physical Medicine and Rehabilitation
97802 – 97804	Medical Nutrition Therapy
97810 – 97814	Acupuncture
98925 – 98929	Osteopathic Manipulative Treatment
98940 – 98943	Chiropractic Manipulative Treatment
99000 – 99091	Special Services, Procedures and Reports

Place of Service Codes

Place of Service	Description
01	**Pharmacy** (A facility or location where drugs and other medically related items and services are sold, dispensed, or otherwise provided directly to patients).
02	**Unassigned** N/A
03	**School** (A facility whose primary purpose is education).
04	**Homeless Shelter** (A facility or location whose primary purpose is to provide temporary housing to homeless individuals, e.g., emergency shelters, individual or family shelters).
05	**Indian Health Service Free-standing** (A facility or location, owned and operated by the Indian Health Service, which provides diagnostic, therapeutic (surgical and nonsurgical), and rehabilitation services to American Indians and Alaska Natives who do not require hospitalization).
06	**Indian Health Service Provider-based Facility** (A facility or location, owned and operated by the Indian Health Service, which provides diagnostic, therapeutic (surgical and nonsurgical), and rehabilitation services rendered by, or under the supervision of, physicians to American Indians and Alaska Natives admitted as inpatients or outpatients).
07	**Tribal 638 Free-standing Facility** (A facility or location owned and operated by a federally recognized American Indian or Alaska Native tribe or tribal organization under a 638 agreement, which provides diagnostic, therapeutic (surgical and nonsurgical), and rehabilitation services to tribal members who do not require hospitalization).
08	**Tribal 638 Provider-based Facility** (A facility or location owned and operated by a federally recognized American Indian or Alaska Native tribe or tribal organization under a 638 agreement, which provides diagnostic, therapeutic (surgical and nonsurgical), and rehabilitation services to tribal members).
09-10	**Unassigned** (N/A).
11	**Office** (Location other than a hospital, Skilled Nursing Facility [SNF], Military Treatment Facility, Community Health Center, State or Local Public Health Clinic or Intermediate Care Facility [ICF], where the health professional routinely provides health examinations, diagnosis, and treatment of illness or injury on an ambulatory basis).
12	**Home** (Location other than a hospital or other facility where the patient received care in a private residence).
13	**Assisted Living Facility** (Congregate residential facility with self-contained living units providing assessment of each resident's needs and on-site support 24 hours a day, 7 days a week, with the capacity to deliver or arrange for services including some healthcare and other services).
14	**Group Home (non-facility)** (Congregate residential foster care setting for children and adolescents in state custody that provides some social, healthcare, and educational support services and that promotes rehabilitation and reintegration of residents into the community).
15	**Mobile Unit** (A facility/unit that moves from place-to-place equipped to provide preventive, screening, diagnostic, and/or treatment services.)
16-19	**Unassigned**
20	**Urgent Care Facility** (Location, distinct from a hospital emergency room, an office, or a clinic, whose purpose is to diagnose and treat illness or injury for unscheduled, ambulatory patients seeking immediate medical attention.)
21	**Inpatient Hospital** (A facility other than psychiatric, which primarily provides diagnostic, therapeutic (both surgical and nonsurgical) and rehabilitation services by, or under the supervision of, physicians to patients admitted for a variety of medical conditions).
22	**Outpatient Hospital** (A portion of a hospital which provides diagnostic, therapeutic (both surgical and nonsurgical), and rehabilitation services to sick and injured persons who do not require hospitalization or institutionalization.) A patient who is not admitted to a hospital (i.e., one who is under 24-hour supervision) is an outpatient.
23	**Emergency Room -- Hospital** (A portion of a hospital where emergency diagnosis and treatment of illness or injury is provided.) Patients in the emergency room are considered to be facility outpatients. (Remember to also complete box 24I.)

■ **Table AC–6** Place of Service Codes

(continues on next page)

24	**Ambulatory Surgical Center (ASC)** (A freestanding facility other than a physician's office where surgical and diagnostic services are provided on an ambulatory basis.) When this code is used, the facility must be a CMS-approved ASC.
25	**Birthing Center** (A facility other than a hospital's maternity facilities or a physician's office that provides a setting for labor, delivery, and immediate postpartum care as well as immediate care of newborn infants.)
26	**Military Treatment Facility** (MTF) (A medical facility operated by one or more of the Uniformed Services.) MTF also refers to certain former U.S. Public Health Service facilities now designated as Uniformed Service Treatment Facilities (USTF).
27-30	**Unassigned**
31	**Skilled Nursing Facility** (A facility which primarily provides inpatient skilled nursing care and related services to patients who require medical, nursing, or rehabilitative services, and which does not provide the level of care or treatment available in a hospital).
32	**Nursing Facility** (A facility which provides skilled nursing care and related services for the rehabilitation of injured, disabled, or sick persons or on a regular basis health-related care services above the level of custodial care to other than mentally retarded individuals.)
33	**Custodial Care Facility** (A facility which provides room, board and personal assistance services, generally on a long-term basis, and which does not include a medical component.)
34	**Hospice** (A facility, other than a patient's home, in which palliative and supportive care for terminally ill patients and their families is provided.)
35-40	**Unassigned**
41	**Ambulance -- Land** (A land vehicle specifically designed, equipped and staffed for lifesaving and transporting the sick or injured.)
42	**Ambulance -- Air or Water** (An air or water vehicle specifically designed, equipped and staffed for lifesaving and transporting the sick or injured.)
43-48	**Unassigned**
49	**Independent Clinic (non-facility)** (A location, not part of a hospital and not described by any other Place of Service code, that is organized and operated to provide preventive, diagnostic, therapeutic, rehabilitative, or palliative services to outpatients only.)
50	**Federally Qualified Health Center** (A facility located in a medically underserved area that provides Medicare beneficiaries preventive primary medical care under the general direction of a physician.)
51	**Inpatient Psychiatric Facility** (A facility that provides inpatient psychiatric services for the diagnosis and treatment of mental illness on a 24-hour basis, by or under the supervision of a physician.)
52	**Psychiatric Facility-Partial Hospitalization** (A facility for the diagnosis and treatment of mental illness that provides a planned therapeutic program for patients who do not need full-time hospitalization, but who need broader programs than are possible from outpatient visits in a hospital-based or hospital-affiliated facility.)
53	**Community Mental Health Center** (A facility that provides comprehensive mental health services on an ambulatory basis, primarily to individuals residing or employed in a defined area. Includes a physician-directed mental health facility.)
54	**Intermediate Care Facility/Mentally Retarded** (A facility which primarily provides health-related care and services above the level of custodial care of mentally retarded individuals but does not provide the level of care or treatment available in a hospital or SNF.)
55	**Residential Substance Abuse Treatment Facility** (A facility which provides treatment for substance (alcohol and drug) abuse to live-in residents who do not require acute medical care. Services include individual and group therapy and counseling, family counseling, laboratory tests, drugs and supplies, psychological testing, and room and board.)
56	**Psychiatric Residential Treatment Center** (A facility or distinct part of a facility for psychiatric care which provides a total 24-hour therapeutically planned and professionally staffed group living and learning environment.)
57	**Non Residential Substance Abuse Treatment Facility (non-facility)** (A location which provides treatment for substance (alcohol and drug) abuse on an ambulatory basis. Services include individual and group therapy and counseling, family counseling, laboratory tests, drugs and supplies, and psychological testing.)

(continues on next page)

58-59	Unassigned
60	**Mass Immunization Center** (A location where providers administer pneumococcal pneumonia and influenza virus vaccinations and submit these services as electronic media claims, paper claims, or using the roster billing method. This generally takes place in a mass immunization setting, such as a public health center pharmacy or mall, but may include a physician office setting.)
61	**Comprehensive Inpatient Rehabilitation Facility** (A facility that provides comprehensive rehabilitation services under the supervision of a physician to inpatients with physical disabilities. Services include rehabilitation nursing, physical therapy, occupational therapy, speech pathology, social or psychological services, and orthotics and prosthetics services. There are specific licensing requirements for these facilities.)
62	**Comprehensive Outpatient Rehabilitation Facility** (A facility that provides comprehensive rehabilitation services under the supervision of a physician to inpatients with physical disabilities. Services include physical therapy, occupational therapy, and speech pathology services. There are specific licensing requirements for these facilities.)
63-64	Unassigned
65	**End Stage Renal Disease Treatment Facility** (A facility other than a hospital, which provides dialysis treatment, maintenance and/or training to patients or caregivers on an ambulatory or home-care basis.)
66-70	Unassigned
71	**State or Local Public Health Clinic** (A facility maintained by either State or local health departments that provides ambulatory primary medical care under the general direction of a physician. Such facilities must be physician-directed.)
72	**Rural Health Clinic** (A certified facility which is located in a rural medically underserved area that provides ambulatory primary medical care under the general direction of a physician. Qualified facilities do not bill Part B of Medicare for items or services except for DME and orthotics and prosthetics.)
73-80	Unassigned
81	**Independent Laboratory** (A laboratory certified to perform diagnostic and/or clinical tests independent of an institution or a physician's office.) With the exception of hospital inpatients, the place of service for lab tests will be based on where "drawn" instead of where the test is actually performed. If the physician is billing for a lab service performed in his/her own office, then use the appropriate code for provider's office. If an independent laboratory is billing, show the place where the sample is drawn. An independent laboratory drawing a sample in its laboratory shows the code for independent laboratory as the place of service. If an independent laboratory is billing for a test on a sample drawn on a hospital inpatient, then the appropriate code for hospital inpatient is entered as the place of service. If the independent laboratory is billing for a test on a sample drawn in a physician's office, then the appropriate code is for provider's office.
82-98	Unassigned
99	**Other Unlisted Facility** (Other service facilities not identified above.)

Hospital Revenue Codes

Major Category	Subcategory (Standard Abbreviation)
001	**Total Charges.** To reflect the total of all charges on this bill.
01X	**Reserved for internal payer use.**
02X-06X	**Reserved for National Assignment.**
07X-09X	**Reserved for State Assignment.**
10X	**All-inclusive Rate.** Flat fee charge incurred on either a daily basis or total stay basis for services rendered. Charge may cover room and board plus ancillary services or room and board only. 0　All-inclusive room and board plus ancillary (ALL-INCL R&B/ANC) 1　All-inclusive room and board (ALL-INCL R&B)
11X	**Room and Board--Private (Medical or General).** Routine service charges for single-bed rooms. 0　General Classification (R&B/PVT) 1　Medical/Surgical/Gyn (MED-SER-GYN/PVT) 2　OB (OB/PVT) 3　Pediatric (PEDS/PVT) 4　Psychiatric (PSYCH/PVT) 5　Hospice (HOSPICE/PVT) 6　Detoxification (DETOX/PVT) 7　Oncology (ONCOLOGY/PVT) 8　Rehabilitation (REHAB/PVT) 9　Other)OTHER/PVT)
12X	**Room and Board--Semiprivate Two-Bed (Medical or General).** Routine service charges incurred for accommodations with two beds. 0　General Classification (R&B/SEMI) 1　Medical/Surgical/Gyn (MED-SUR-GYN/2 Bed) 2　OB (OB/2 Bed) 3　Pediatric (PED/ 2 Bed) 4　Psychiatric (PSYCH/2 Bed) 5　Hospice (HOSPICE/2 Bed) 6　Detoxification (DETOX/2 Bed) 7　Oncology (ONCOLOGY/2 Bed) 8　Rehabilitation (REHAB/2 Bed) 9　Other (OTHER/2 Bed)
13X	**Semiprivate--Three and Four Beds.** Routine service charges incurred for accommodations with three and four beds. 0　General Classification (R&B/3&4 Bed) 1　Medical/Surgical/Gyn (MED-SUR-GYN/3&4 Bed) 2　OB (OB/3&4 Bed) 3　Pediatric (PED/3&4 Bed) 4　Psychiatric (PSYCH/3&4 Bed) 5　Hospice (HOSPICE/3&4 Bed) 6　Detoxification (DETOX/3&4 Bed) 7　Oncology (ONCOLOGY/3&4 Bed) 8　Rehabilitation (REHAB/3&4 Bed) 9　Other (OTHER/3&4 Bed)

■ **Table AC–7** Hospital Revenue Codes

14X	**Private (Deluxe).** Deluxe rooms are accommodations with amenities substantially in excess of those provided to other patients.
	0 General Classification (R&B/PVT/DLX)
	1 Medical/Surgical/Gyn (MED-SUR-GYN/DLX)
	2 OB (OB/DLX)
	3 Pediatric (PED/DLX)
	4 Psychiatric (PSYCH/DLX)
	5 Hospice (HOSPICE/DLX)
	6 Detoxification (DETOX/DLX)
	7 Oncology (ONCOLOGY/DLX)
	8 Rehabilitation (REHAB/DLX)
	9 Other (OTHER/DLX)
15X	**Room and Board—Ward (Medical or General).** Routine service charge for accommodations with five or more beds.
	0 General Classification (R&B/WARD)
	1 Medical/Surgical/Gyn (MED-SUR-GYN/WARD)
	2 OB (OB/WARD)
	3 Pediatric (PED/WARD)
	4 Psychiatric (PSYCH/WARD)
	5 Hospice (HOSPICE/WARD)
	6 Detoxification (DETOX/WARD)
	7 Oncology (ONCOLOGY/WARD)
	8 Rehabilitation (REHAB/WARD)
	9 Other (OTHER/WARD)
16X	**Other Room and Board.** Any routine service charges for accommodations that cannot be included in the more specific revenue center codes.
	0 General Classification (R&B)
	4 Sterile Environment (R&B/STRL)
	7 Self-Care (R&B/SELF)
	9 Other (R&B/Other)
17X	**Nursery.** Charges for nursing care to newborn and premature infants in nurseries.
	0 General Classification (NURSERY)
	1 Newborn (NURSERY/NEWBORN)
	2 Premature (NURSERY/PREMIE)
	5 Neonatal ICU (NURSERY/ICU)
	9 Other (NURSERY/OTHER)
18X	**Leave of Absence.** Charges for holding a room while the patient is temporarily away from the provider.
	0 General Classification (LOA)
	1 Reserved (RESERVED)
	2 Patient Convenience (LOA/PT CONV)
	3 Therapeutic Leave (LOA THER)
	4 ICF/MR--any reason (LOA/ICF/ MR)
	5 Nursing Home (for hospitalization) (LOA/NURS HOME)
	6 Other Leave of Absence (LOA/OTHER)
19X	**Not Assigned.**
20X	**Intensive Care.** Routine service charge for medical or surgical care provided to patients who require a more intensive level of care than is rendered in the general medical or surgical unit.
	0 General Classification (ICU)
	1 Surgical (ICU/SURGICAL)
	2 Medical (ICU/MEDICAL)
	3 Pediatric (ICU/PEDS)
	4 Psychiatric (ICU/PSYCH)
	6 Post-ICU (POST ICU)
	7 Burn Care (ICU/BURN CARE)
	8 Trauma (ICU/TRAUMA)
	9 Other Intensive Care (ICU/OTHER)

(continues on next page)

21X	**Coronary Care.** Routine service charge for medical or surgical care provided to patients with coronary illness who require a more intensive level of care than is rendered in the general medical care unit. 0 General Classification (CCU) 1 Myocardial Infarction (CCU/MYO INFARC) 2 Pulmonary Care (CCU/PULMON) 3 Heart Transplant (CCU/TRANS-PLANT) 4 Post-CCU (POST CCU) 9 Other Coronary Care (CCU/OTHR)
22X	**Special Charges.** Charges incurred during an inpatient stay or on a daily basis for certain services. 0 General Classification (SPCL CHGS) 1 Admission Charge (ADMIT CHG) 2 Technical Support Charge (TECH SUPPT CHG) 3 UR Service Charge (UR CHG) 4 Late Discharge, Medically Necessary (LATE DISCH/MED NEC) 9 Other Special Charges (OTHER SPEC CHG)
23X	**Incremental Nursing Charge Rate.** Charge for nursing service assessed in addition to room and board. 0 General Classification (NURSING INCREM) 1 Nursery (NUR INCR/NURSERY) 2 OB (NUR INCR/OB) 3 ICU (NUR INCR/ICU) 4 CCU (NUR INCR/CCU) 5 Hospice (NUR INCR/HOSPICE) 9 Other (NUR INCR/OTHER)
24X	**All-Inclusive Ancillary.** A flat rate incurred on either a daily basis or total stay basis for ancillary services only. 0 General Classification (ALL INCL ANCIL) 9 Other Inclusive Ancillary (ALL INCL ANCIL/OTHER)
25X	**Pharmacy.** Charges for medication produced, manufactured, packaged, controlled, assayed, dispensed, and distributed under the direction of a licensed pharmacist. This category includes blood plasma, other components of blood, and IV solutions. 0 General Classification (PHAR) 1 Generic Drugs (DRUGS/GENRC) 2 Nongeneric Drugs (DRUGS/ NONGENRC) 3 Take Home Drugs (DRUGS/ TAKEHOME) 4 Drugs Incident to Other Diagnostic Services (DRUGS/INCIDENT OTHER DX) 5 Drugs Incident to Radiology (DRUGS/INCIDENT RAD) 6 Experimental Drugs (DRUGS/ EXPERIMT) 7 Nonprescription (DRUGS/ NONPSCRPT) 8 IV Solutions (IV SOLUTIONS) 9 Other Pharmacy (DRUGS/OTHER)
26X	**IV Therapy.** Administration of intravenous solution by specially trained personnel to individuals requiring such treatment. 0 General Classification (IV THER) 2 Infusion Pump (IV THER/INFSN PUMP) 3 IV Therapy--Pharmacy Services (IV THER/PHARM/ SVC) 4 IV Therapy/Drug/Supply Delivery (IV THER/DRUG/ SUPPLY DELV) 9 Other IV Therapy (IV THERP/ OTHER) NOTE: Providers billing for home IV therapy should use the HCPCS code that describes the pump in Item 44.
27X	**Medical/Surgical Supplies and Devices.** Charges for supply items required for patient care. 0 General Classification (MED-SUR SUPPLIES) 1 Nonsterile Supply (NON-STER SUPPLY) 2 Sterile Supply (STERILE SUPPLY) 3 Take Home Supplies (TAKE HOME SUPPLY) 4 Prosthetic/Orthotic Devices (PROSTH/ORTH DEV) 5 Pacemaker (PACE MAKER) 6 Intraocular Lens (INTRA OC LENS) 7 Oxygen-Take Home (O2/ TAKEHOME) 8 Other Implants (SUPPLY/ IMPLANTS) 9 Other Supplies/Devices (SUPPLY/ OTHER)

(continues on next page)

28X	**Oncology.** Charges for the treatment of tumors and related diseases. 0 General Classification ONCOLOGY 9 Other Oncology (ONCOLOGY/ OTHER)
29X	**Durable Medical Equipment (Other Than Renal).** Charges for medical equipment that can withstand repeated use (excluding renal equipment). 0 General Classification (DME) 1 Rental (MED EQUIP/RENT) 2 Purchase of new DME (MED EQUIP/NEW) 3 Purchase of used DME (MED EQUIP/USED) 4 Supplies/Drugs for DME Effectiveness (Home Health Agency Only) (MED EQUIP/SUPPLIES/ DRUGS) 9 Other Equipment (MED EQUIP/ OTHER)
30X	**Laboratory.** Charges for the performance of diagnostic and routine clinical laboratory tests. 0 General Classification (LAB) 1 Chemistry (LAB/CHEMISTRY) 2 Immunology (LAB/IMMUNLGY) 3 Renal Patient (Home) (LAB/RENAL HOME) 4 Nonroutine Dialysis (LAB/NR DIALYSIS) 5 Hematology (LAB/HEMAT) 6 Bacteriology & Microbiology (LAB/BACT-MICRO) 7 Urology (LAB/UROLOGY) 9 Other Laboratory (LAB/OTHER)
31X	**Laboratory Pathological.** Charges for diagnostic and routine lab tests on tissues and culture. 0 General Classification (PATH LAB) 1 Cytology (PATHOL/CYTOLOGY) 2 Histology (PATHOL/HYSTOL) 4 Biopsy (PATHOL/BIOPSY) 9 Other (PATHOL/OTHER)
32X	**Radiology--Diagnostic.** Charges for diagnostic radiology services provided for the examination and care of patients. Includes taking, processing, examining, and interpreting radiographs and fluorographs. 0 General Classification (DX X-RAY) 1 Angiocardiography (DX X-RAY/ ANGIO) 2 Arthrography (DX X-RAY/ARTH) 3 Arteriography (DX X-RAY/ ARTER) 4 Chest X-Ray (DX X-RAY/CHEST) 9 Other (DX X-RAY/OTHER)
33X	**Radiology--Therapeutic.** Charges for therapeutic radiology services and chemotherapy that are required for care and treatment of patients. Included therapy by injection or ingestion of radioactive substances. 0 General Classification (RX X-RAY) 1 Chemotherapy--Injected (CHEMOTHER/INJ) 2 Chemotherapy--Oral (CHEMOTHER/ORAL) 3 Radiation Therapy (RADIATION RX) 5 Chemotherapy--IV (CHEMOTHERP-IV) 9 Other (RX X-RAY/OTHER)
34X	**Nuclear Medicine.** Charges for procedures and tests performed by a radioisotope laboratory utilizing radioactive materials as required for diagnosis and treatment of patients. 0 General Classification (NUC MED) 1 Diagnostic (NUC MED/DX) 2 Therapeutic (NUC MED/RX) 9 Other (NUC MED/OTHER)
35X	**CT Scan.** Charges for computed tomographic scans of the head and other parts of the body. 0 General Classification (CT SCAN) 1 Head Scan (CT SCAN/HEAD) 2 Body Scan (CT SCAN/BODY) 9 Other CT Scans (CT SCAN/OTHR)
36X	**Operating Room Services.** Charges for services provided to patients in the performance of surgical and related procedures during and immediately following surgery. 0 General Classification (OR SERVICES) 1 Minor Surgery (OR/MINOR) 2 Organ Transplant--Other than kidney (OR/ORGAN TRANS) 7 Kidney Transplant (OR/KIDNEY TRANS) 9 Other Operating Room Services (OR/OTHER)

(continues on next page)

37X	**Anesthesia.** Charges for anesthesia services in the hospital.
	0 General Classification (ANESTHE)
	1 Anesthesia Incident to Radiology (ANESTHE/INCIDENT RAD)
	2 Anesthesia Incident to Other Diagnostic Services (ANESTHE/ INCDNT OTHER DX)
	4 Acupuncture (ANESTHE/ ACUPUNC)
	9 Other Anesthesia (ANESTHE/ OTHER)
38X	**Blood.**
	0 General Classification (BLOOD)
	1 Packed Red Cells (BLOOD/PKD RED)
	2 Whole Blood (BLOOD/WHOLE)
	3 Plasma (BLOOD/PLASMA)
	4 Platelets (BLOOD PLATELETS)
	5 Leucocytes (BLOOD/ LEUCOCYTES)
	6 Other Components (BLOOD/ COMPONENTS)
	7 Other Derivatives (Cryoprecipitates) (BLOOD/DERIVATIVES)
	9 Other Blood (BLOOD/OTHER)
39X	**Blood Storage and Processing.** Charges for storage and processing of whole blood.
	0 General Classification (BLOOD/ STOR-PROC)
	1 Blood Administration (BLOOD/ ADMIN)
	9 Other Blood Storage and Processing (BLOOD/OTHER STOR)
40X	**Other Imaging Services.**
	0 General Classification (IMAGE SVS)
	1 Diagnostic Mammography (DIAG MAMMOGRAPHY)
	2 Ultrasound (ULTRASOUND)
	3 Screening Mammography (SCRN MAMMOGRAPHY)
	4 Positron Emission Tomography (PET SCAN)
	9 Other Imaging Services (OTHER IMAGE SVS)
	NOTE: High-risk beneficiaries should be noted by the inclusion of one of the following ICD-9-CM diagnosis codes:
	V10.3 Personal History--Malignant neoplasm breast cancer
	V16.3 Family History--Malignant neoplasm breast cancer (mother, sister or daughter with breast cancer)
	V15.89 Other specified personal history representing hazards to health (not given birth prior to 30, a personal history of biopsy proven breast disease). Must be coded to the appropriate 4th or 5th digit.
41X	**Respiratory Services.** Charges for administration of oxygen and certain potent drugs through inhalation or positive pressure and other forms of rehabilitative therapy through measurement of inhaled and exhaled gases and analysis of blood and evaluation of the patient's ability to exchange oxygen and other gases.
	0 General Classification (RESPIR SVC)
	2 Inhalation Services (INHALATION SVC)
	3 Hyperbaric Oxygen Therapy (HYPERBARIC O2)
	9 Other Respiratory Services (OTHER RESPIR SVS)
42X	**Physical Therapy.** Charges for therapeutic exercises, massage, and utilization of light, heat, cold, water, electricity, and assistive devices for diagnosis and rehabilitation of patients who have neuromuscular, orthopedic, and other disabilities.
	0 General Classification (PHYS THERP)
	1 Visit Charge (PHYS THERP/ VISIT)
	2 Hourly Charge (PHYS THERP/ HOUR)
	3 Group Rate (PHYS THERP/ GROUP)
	4 Evaluation or Reevaluation (PHYS THER/EVAL)
	9 Other Physical Therapy (OTHER PHYS THERP)

(continues on next page)

43X	**Occupational Therapy.** Charges for teaching manual skills and independent personal care to stimulate mental and emotional activity on the part of patients. 0 General Classification (OCCUP THERP) 1 Visit Charge (OCCUP THERP/ VISIT) 2 Hourly Charge (OCCUP THERP/ HOUR) 3 Group Rate (OCCUP THERP/ GROUP) 4 Evaluation or Reevaluation (OCCUP THER/EVAL) 9 Other Occupational Therapy (OTHER OCCUP THERP)
44X	**Speech-Language Pathology.** Charges for services provided to persons with impaired functional communications skills. 0 General Classification (SPEECH PATHOL) 1 Visit Charge (SPEECH PATH/ VISIT) 2 Hourly Charge (SPEECH PATH/ HOUR) 3 Group Rate (SPEECH PATH/ GROUP) 4 Evaluation or Reevaluation (SPEECH PATH/EVAL) 9 Other Speech-Language Pathology (OTHER SPEECH PAT)
45X	**Emergency Room.** Charges for emergency treatment to those ill and injured persons who require immediate unscheduled medical or surgical care. 0 General Classification (EMERG ROOM) 9 Other Emergency Room (OTHER EMER ROOM)
46X	**Pulmonary Function.** Charges for tests that measure inhaled and exhaled gases and analysis of blood and for tests that evaluate the patient's ability to exchange oxygen and other gases. 0 General Classification (PULMON FUNC) 9 Other Pulmonary Function (OTHER PULMON FUNC)
47X	**Audiology.** Charges for the detection and management of communication handicaps centering in whole or in part on the hearing function. 0 General Classification (AUDIOL) 1 Diagnostic (AUDIOLOGY/DX) 2 Treatment (AUDIOLOGY/RX) 9 Other Audiology (OTHER AUDIOL)
48X	**Cardiology.** Charges for cardiac procedures rendered in a separate unit within the hospital. Such procedures include but are not limited to heart catheterization, coronary angiography, Swan-Ganz catheterization, and exercise stress test. 0 General Classification (CARDIOL) 1 Cardiac Cath Lab (CARDIAC CATH LAB) 2 Stress Test (STRESS TEST) 9 Other Cardiology (OTHER CARDIOL)
49X	**Ambulatory Surgical Care.** 0 General Classification (AMBUL SURG) 9 Other Ambulatory Surgical Care (OTHER AMBL SURG)
50X	**Outpatient Services.** Outpatient charges for services rendered to an outpatient who is admitted as an inpatient before midnight of the day following the date of service. These charges are incorporated on the inpatient bill of Medicare patients. 0 General Classification (OUTPATIENT SVS) 9 Other Outpatient Services (OUTPATIENT/OTHER)
51X	**Clinic.** Clinic (nonemergency/scheduled outpatient visit) charges for providing diagnostic, preventive, curative, rehabilitative, and education services on a scheduled basis to ambulatory patients. 0 General Classification (CLINIC) 1 Chronic Pain Center (CHRONIC PAIN CL) 2 Dental Clinic (DENTAL CLINIC) 3 Psychiatric Clinic (PSYCH CLINIC) 4 OB-GYN Clinic (OB-GYN CLINIC) 5 Pediatric Clinic (PEDS CLINIC) 9 Other Clinic (OTHER CLINIC)
52X	**Free-Standing Clinic.** 0 General Classification (FR/STD CLINIC) 1 Rural Health--Clinic (RURAL/ CLINIC) 2 Rural Health--Home (RURAL/ HOME) 3 Family Practice (FAMILY PRAC) 9 Other Freestanding Clinic (OTHER FR/STD CLINIC)

(continues on next page)

53X	**Osteopathic Services.** Charges for a structural evaluation of the cranium, entire cervical, dorsal, and lumbar spine by a doctor of osteopathy. 0 General Classification (OSTEOPATH SVS) 1 Osteopathic Therapy (OSTEOPATH RX) 9 Other Osteopathic Services (OTHER OSTEOPATH)
54X	**Ambulance.** Charges for ambulance service, usually unscheduled, to the ill/ injured who require immediate medical attention. 0 General Classification (AMBUL) 1 Supplies (AMBUL/SUPPLY) 2 Medical Transport (AMBUL/MED TRANS) 3 Heart Mobile (AMBUL/ HEARTMOBL) 4 Oxygen (AMBUL/OXY) 5 Air Ambulance (AIR AMBUL) 6 Neonatal Ambulance Services (AMBUL/NEONAT) 7 Pharmacy (AMBUL/PHARMACY) 8 Telephone Transmission EKG (AMBUL/TELEPHONIC EKG) 9 Other Ambulance (OTHER AMBULANCE) NOTE: Units may be either miles or trips. NOTE: On items 55-58, charges should be reported to the nearest hour.
55X	**Skilled Nursing.** Charges for nursing services that must be provided under the direct supervision of a licensed nurse to ensure the safety of the patient and to achieve the medically desired result. This code may be used for nursing home services or a service charge for home health billing. 0 General Classification (SKILLED NURS) 1 Visit Charge (SKILLED NURS/ VISIT) 2 Hourly Charge (SKILLED NURS/ HOUR) 9 Other Skilled Nursing (SKILLED NURS/OTHER)
56X	**Medical Social Services.** Charges for services such as counseling patients, interviewing patients, and interpreting problems of social situation rendered to patients on any basis. 0 General Classification (MED SOCIAL SVS) 1 Visit Charge (MED SOC SERVS/ VISIT) 2 Hourly Charge (MED SOC SERVS/HOUR) 9 Other Medical Social Services (MED SOCIAL SERVS/OTHER)
57X	**Home Health Aide (Home Health).** Charges made by a home health agency for personnel that are primarily responsible for the personal care of the patient. 0 General Classification (AIDE/ HOME HEALTH) 1 Visit Charge (AIDE/HOME HLTH/ VISIT) 2 Hourly Charge (AIDE/HOME HLTH/HOUR) 9 Other Home Health Aide (AIDE/ HOME HLTH/OTHER)
58X	**Other Visits (Home Health).** Charges by a home health agency for visits other than physical therapy, occupational therapy or speech therapy, which must be specifically identified. 0 General Classification (VISIT/ HOME HEALTH) 1 Visit Charge (VISIT/HOME HLTH/ VISIT) 2 Hourly Charge (VISIT/HOME HLTH/HOUR) 9 Other Home Health (VISIT/HOME HLTH/OTHER)
59X	**Units of Service (Home Health).** Revenue code used by a home health agency that bills on the basis of units of service. 0 General Classification (UNIT/ HOME HEALTH) 9 Home Health Other Units (UNIT/ HOME HLTH/OTHER)
60X	**Oxygen Home Health.** Charges by a home health agency for oxygen equipment, supplies, or contents, excluding purchased items. If a beneficiary has purchased a stationary oxygen system, and oxygen concentrator or portable equipment, revenue codes 292 or 293 apply. DME other than oxygen systems is billed under codes 291, 292, or 293. 0 General Classification (O2/HOME HEALTH) 1 Oxygen--Stationary Equipment, Supplies or Contents (O2/STAT EQUIP/SUPPL/CONT) 2 Oxygen--Stationary Equipment or Supplies Under 1 LPM (O2/STAT EQUIP/UNDER 1 LPM) 3 Oxygen--Stationary Equipment or Supplies Over 4 LPM (O2/STAT EQUIP/OVER 4 LPM) 4 Oxygen--Portable Add-on (O2/ PORTABLE ADD-ON)

(continues on next page)

61X	**MRI.** Charges for Magnetic Resonance Imaging of the brain and other parts of the body. 0 General Classification (MRI) 1 Brain (including brain stem) (MRI-BRAIN) 2 Spinal Cord (including spine) (MRI-SPINE) 9 Other MRI (MRI-OTHER)
62X	**Medical/Surgical Supplies.** Charges for supplies required for patient care. This code is an extension of code 27X and allows for the reporting of additional breakdown, if needed. Subcategory 1 is for providers who are not able to bill supplies used for radiology procedures under radiology. Subcategory 2 is for providers who are not able to bill supplies used for other diagnostic procedures under diagnostic procedures. 1 Supplies Incident to Radiology (MED-SUR SUPP/INCDNT RAD) 2 Supplies Incident to Other Diagnostic Services (MED-SUR UPP/INCDNT ODX)
63X	**Drugs Requiring Specific Identification.** Charges for drugs and biologicals requiring specific identification required by the payer. If you are using HCPCS to identify the drug, the HCPCS code should be entered in Item 44. 0 General Classification (DRUGS) 1 Single Source Drug (DRUG/ SNGLE) 2 Multiple Source Drug (DRUG/ MULT) 3 Restrictive Prescription (DRUG/ RSTR) 4 Erythropoietin (EPO) less than 10,000 units (DRUG/EPQ10,000 Units) 5 Erythropoietin (EPO) more than 10,000 units (DRUG/EPQ10,000 Units) 6 Drugs requiring detailed coding (DRUGS/DETAIL CODE) NOTE: Revenue Code 636 relates to a HCPCS code. Therefore, the appropriate HCPCS code should be entered in Item 44. The specific units of services to be reported should be in hundreds (100s) rounded to the nearest hundred.
64X	**Home IV Therapy Services.** Charge for IV drug therapy services that are done in the patient's home. For home IV providers, the appropriate HCPCS code must be entered for all equipment and covered therapy. 0 General Classification (IV THER SVC) 1 Nonroutine Nursing, Central Line (NON RT NURSING/CENTRAL) 2 IV Site Care, Central Line, HCPCS related(IV SITE CARE/CENTRAL) 3 IV Start/Change Peripheral Line (IV STRT/CHNG/PERIPHRL) 4 Nonroutine Nursing Peripheral Line (NON RT NURSING/PERIPHRL) 5 Training Patient/Caregiver, Central Line (TRNG PT/CAREGVR/ CENTRAL) 6 Training Disabled Patient, Central Line (TRNG DSBLPT/CENTRAL) 7 Training Patient/Caregiver, Peripheral Line (TRNG PT/ CAREGVR/PERIPHRL) 8 Training Disabled Patient, Peripheral Line (TRNG DSBLPT/ PERIPHRL) 9 Other IV Therapy Services (OTHER IV THERAPY SVC) NOTE: Units need to be reported in 1-hour increments.

65X	**Hospice Service.** Charges for hospice care services for a terminally ill patient. The patient would need to elect these services in lieu of other services for a terminal condition.
	0 General Classification (HOSPICE)
	1 Routine Home Care (HOSPICE/RTN HOME)
	2 Continuous Home Care (HOSPICE/ CTNS HOME)
	3 RESERVED
	4 RESERVED
	5 Inpatient Respite Care (HOSPICE/ IP RESPITE)
	6 General Inpatient Care (Nonrespite) (HOSPICE/IP NONRESPITE)
	7 Physician Services (HOSPICE/ PHYSICIAN)
	9 Other Hospice (HOSPICE/OTHER)
	    NOTE: There must be a minimum of 8 hours of care (not necessarily continuous) during a 24-hour period to receive the Continuous Home Care rate from Medicare under code 652. If less than 8 hours of care are provided, code 651 should be used. Any portion of an hour counts as an hour.
	    When billing Medicare under code 657, a physician procedure code must be entered in Item 44. Code 657 is used by the hospice to bill for physician's services furnished to hospice patients when the physician is employed by the hospice or receives payment from the hospice for services rendered.

(continues on next page)

66X	**Respite Care.** Charges for hours of service under the Respite Care Benefit for homemaker or home health aide, personal care services, and nursing care provided by a licensed professional nurse. 0 General Classification (RESPITE CARE) 1 Hourly Charge/Skilled Nursing (RESPITE/SKILLED NURSE) 2 Hourly Charge/Home Health Aide/ Homemaker (RESPITE/HMEAID/ HMEMKR
67X	**Not Assigned.**
68X	**Not Assigned.**
69X	**Not Assigned.**
70X	**Cast Room.** Charges for services related to the application, maintenance, and removal of casts. 0 General Classification (CAST ROOM) 9 Other Cast Room (OTHER CAST ROOM)
71X	**Recovery Room.** 0 General Classification (RECOV RM) 9 Other Recovery Room (OTHER RECOV RM)
72X	**Labor Room/Delivery.** Charges for labor and delivery room services provided by specially trained nursing personnel to patients, including prenatal care during labor, assistance during delivery, postnatal care in the recovery room, and minor gynecological procedures if they are performed in the delivery suite. 0 General Classification (DELIVROOM/LABOR) 1 Labor (LABOR) 2 Delivery (DELIVERY ROOM) 3 Circumcision (CIRCUMCISION) 4 Birthing Center (BIRTHING CENTER) 9 Other Labor Room/Delivery (OTHER/DELIV-LABOR)
73X	**EKG/ECG (Electrocardiogram).** Charges for operation of specialized equipment to record electromotive variations in actions of the heart muscle on an electrocardiograph for diagnosis of heart ailments. 0 General Classification (EKG/ECG) 1 Holter Monitor (HOLTER MON) 2 Telemetry (TELEMETRY) 9 Other EKG/ECG (OTHER EKG/ECG)
74X	**EEG (Electroencephalogram).** Charges for operation of specialized equipment to measure impulse frequencies and differences in electrical potential in various areas of the brain to obtain data for use in diagnosing brain disorders. 0 General Classification (EEG) 9 Other EEG (OTHER EEG)
75X	**Gastrointestinal Services.** 0 General Classification (GASTR-INTS SVS) 9 Other Gastrointestinal (OTHER GASTROINTS) NOTE: Use 759 with the procedure code for endoscopic procedure.
76X	**Treatment/Observation Room.** Charges for the use of a treatment room, or observation room charges for outpatient observation services. 0 General Classification (TREATMT/OBSERVATION RM) 1 Treatment Room (TREATMT RM) 2 Observation Room (OBSERV RM) 9 Other Treatment/Observation Room (OTHER TREAT/OBSERV RM)
77X	**Not Assigned.**
78X	**Not Assigned.**
79X	**Lithotripsy.** Charges for using lithotripsy in the treatment of kidney stones. 0 General Classification (LITHOTRIPSY) 9 Other Lithotripsy (LITHOTRIPSY/ OTHER)

(continues on next page)

80X	**Inpatient Renal Dialysis.** A waste removal process that uses an artificial kidney when the body's own kidneys have failed. The waste may be removed directly from the blood (hemodialysis) or indirectly from the blood by flushing a special solution between the abdominal covering and the tissue (peritoneal dialysis). In-unit lab nonroutine tests are medically necessary tests in addition to or at greater frequency than routine tests that are performed in the dialysis unit. 0 General Classification (RENAL DIALY) 1 Inpatient Hemodialysis (DIALY/ INPT) 2 Inpatient Peritoneal (Non-CAPD) (DIALY/INPT/PER) 3 Inpatient Continuous Ambulatory Peritoneal Dialysis (DIALY/ INPT/CAPD) 4 Inpatient Continuous Cycling Peritoneal Dialysis (DIALY/ INPT/CCPD) 9 Other Inpatient Dialysis (DIALY/ INPT/OTHER)
81X	**Organ Acquisition.** The acquisition of a kidney, liver, or heart for use in transplantation. Organs other than these are included in category 89X. Living donor is a living person from whom kidney is obtained for transplantation. Cadaver is an individual who has been pronounced dead according to medical and legal criteria from whom organs have been obtained for transplantation. 0 General Classification (ORGAN ACQUISIT) 1 Living Donor--Kidney (KIDNEY/ LIVE) 2 Cadaver Donor--Kidney (KIDNEY/ CADAVER) 3 Unknown Donor--Kidney (KIDNEY/UNKNOWN) 4 Other Kidney Acquisition (KIDNEY/OTHER) 5 Cadaver Donor--Heart (HEART/ CADAVER) 6 Other Heart Acquisition (HEART/ OTHER) 7 Donor--Liver (LIVER ACQUISIT) 9 Other Organ Acquisition (ORGAN/ OTHER)
82X	**Hemodialysis--Outpatient or Home.** A program under which a patient performs hemodialysis away from the facility using his or her own equipment and supplies. Hemodialysis is the removal of waste directly from the blood. 0 General Classification (HEMO/OP OR HOME) 1 Hemodialysis/Composite or Other Rate (HEMO/COMPOSITE) 2 Home Supplies (HEMO/HOME/ SUPPL) 3 Home Equipment (HEMO/HOME/ EQUIP) 4 Maintenance 100% (HEMO/HOME/ 100%) 5 Support Services (HEMO/HOME/ SUPSERV) 9 Other Outpatient Hemodialysis (HEMO/HOME/OTHER)
83X	**Peritoneal Dialysis--Outpatient or Home.** A program under which a patient performs peritoneal dialysis away from the facility using his or her own equipment and supplies. Waste is removed by flushing a special solution between the tissue and the abdominal covering. 0 General Classification (PERTNL/ OP OR HOME) 1 Peritoneal/Composite or Other Rate (PERTNL/COMPOSITE) 2 Home Supplies (PERTNL/HOME/ SUPPL) 3 Home Equipment (PERTNL/ HOME/EQUIP) 4 Maintenance 100% (PERTNL/ HOME/100%) 5 Support Services (PERTNL/HOME/ SUPSERV) 9 Other Outpatient Peritoneal (PERTNL/HOME/OTHER)
84X	**Continuous Ambulatory Peritoneal Dialysis (CAPD)--Outpatient or Home.** A program under which a patient performs continual dialysis away from the facility using his or her own equipment and supplies. The patient's peritoneal membrane is used as a dialyzer. 0 General Classification (CAPD/OP OR HOME) 1 CAPD/Composite or Other Rate (CAPD/COMPOSITE) 2 Home Supplies (CAPD/HOME/ SUPPL) 3 Home Equipment (CAPD/HOME/ EQUIP) 4 Maintenance 100% (CAPD/HOME/ 100%) 5 Support Services (CAPD/HOME/ SUPSERV) 9 Other Outpatient CAPD (CAPD/ HOME/OTHER)

(continues on next page)

85X	**Continuous Cycling Peritoneal Dialysis (CCPD)--Outpatient or Home.** A program under which a patient performs continual dialysis away from the facility using his or her own equipment and supplies. A machine is used to make automatic exchanges at night. 0 General Classification (CCPD/OP OR HOME) 1 CCPD/Composite or Other Rate (CCPD/COMPOSITE) 2 Home Supplies (CCPD/HOME/ SUPPL) 3 Home Equipment (CCPD/HOME/ EQUIP) 4 Maintenance 100% (CCPD/HOME/ 100%) 5 Support Services (CCPD/HOME/ SUPSERV) 9 Other Outpatient CCPD (CCPD/ HOME/OTHER)
86X	**Reserved for Dialysis (National Assignment).**
87X	**Reserved for Dialysis (National Assignment).**
88X	**Miscellaneous Dialysis.** Charges for dialysis services not identified elsewhere. *Rationale*: Ultrafiltration is the process of removing excess fluid from the blood of dialysis patients by using a dialysis machine but without the dialysis solution. The designation is only used when the procedure is not performed as a part of a normal dialysis session. 0 General Classification (DIALY/ MISC) 1 Ultrafiltration (DIALY/ ULTRAFILT) 2 Home Dialysis Aid Visit (HOME DIALY AID VISIT) 9 Miscellaneous Dialysis Other (DIALY/MISC/OTHER)
89X	**Other Donor Bank.** Charges for the acquisition, storage, and preservation of all human organs (excluding kidneys). 0 General Classification (DONOR BANK) 1 Bone (DONOR BANK/BONE) 2 Organ (other than Kidney) (DONOR BANK/ORGN) 3 Skin (DONOR BANK/SKIN) 9 Other Donor Bank (OTHER DONOR BANK)
90X	**Psychiatric/Psychological Treatments.** Charges for providing treatment for emotionally disturbed patients, including patients admitted for diagnosis and for treatment. 0 General Classification (PSYCH TREATMENT) 1 Electroshock Treatment (ELECTRO SHOCK) 2 Milieu Therapy (MILIEU THER) 3 Play Therapy (PLAY THERAPY) 9 Other (OTHER PSYCH RX)
91X	**Psychiatric/Psychological Services.** Charges for providing nursing care and professional services for emotionally disturbed patients, including patients admitted for diagnosis and those admitted for treatment. 0 General Classification (PSYCH SVS) 1 Rehabilitation (PSYCH/REHAB) 2 Day Care (PSYCH/DAYCARE) 3 Night Care (PSYCH/NIGHTCARE) 4 Individual Therapy (PSYCH/INDIV RX) 5 Group Therapy (PSYCH/GROUP RX) 6 Family Therapy (PSYCH/FAMILY RX) 7 Biofeedback (PSYCH/BIOFEED) 8 Testing (PSYCH/TESTING) 9 Other (PSYCH/OTHER)
92X	**Other Diagnostic Services.** Charges for other diagnostic services not otherwise categorized. 0 General Classification (OTHER DX SVS) 1 Peripheral Vascular Lab (PERI-VASCUL LAB) 2 Electromyogram (EMG) 3 Pap Smear (PAP SMEAR) 4 Allergy Test (ALLERGY TEST) 5 Pregnancy Test (PREG TEST) 9 Other Diagnostic Service (ADDL DX SVS)
93X	**Not Assigned.**

(continues on next page)

94X	**Other Therapeutic Services.** Charges for other therapeutic services not otherwise categorized. 0 General Classification (OTHER RX SVS) 1 Recreational Therapy (RECREA-TION RX) 2 Education/Training (EDUC/TRNG) 3 Cardiac Rehabilitation (CARDIAC REHAB) 4 Drug Rehabilitation (DRUG REHAB) 5 Alcohol Rehabilitation (ALCOHOL REHAB) 6 Complex Medical Equipment--Routine (CMPLX MED EQUIP-ROUT) 7 Complex Medical Equipment--Ancillary (CMPLX MED EQUIP-ANC) 9 Other Therapeutic Services (ADDITIONAL RX SVS) NOTE: Use 930 with a procedure code for plasmapheresis. Use 932 for dietary therapy and diabetes-related services, education, and training.
95X	**Not Assigned.**
96X	**Professional Fees.** Charges for medical professionals that the hospitals or third party payers require to be separately identified. 0 General Classification (PRO FEE) 1 Psychiatric (PRO FEE/PSYCH) 2 Ophthalmology (PRO FEE/EYE) 3 Anesthesiologist (MD) (PRO FEE/ ANES MD) 4 Anesthetist (CRNA) (PRO FEE/ ANES CRNA) 9 Other Professional Fees (OTHER PRO FEE)
97X	**Professional Fees (continued).** 1 Laboratory (PRO FEE/LAB) 2 Radiology--Diagnostic (PRO FEE/RAD/DX) 3 Radiology--Therapeutic (PRO FEE/RAD/RX) 4 Radiology--Nuclear Medicine (PRO FEE/NUC MED) 5 Operating Room (PRO FEE/OR) 6 Respiratory Therapy (PRO FEE/ RESPIR) 7 Physical Therapy (PRO FEE/ PHYSI) 8 Occupational Therapy (PRO FEE/ OCUPA) 9 Speech Pathology (PRO FEE/ SPEECH)
98X	**Professional Fees (continued).** 1 Emergency Room (PRO FEE/ER) 2 Outpatient Services (PRO FEE/ OUTPT) 3 Clinic (PRO FEE/CLINIC) 4 Medical Social Services (PRO FEE/ SOC SVC) 5 EKG (PRO FEE/EKG) 6 EEG (PRO FEE/EEG) 7 Hospital Visit (PRO FEE/HOS VIS) 8 Consultation (PRO FEE/CONSULT) 9 Private Duty Nurse (FEE/PVT NURSE)
99X	**Patient Convenience Items.** Charges for items that are generally considered by the third party payors to be strictly convenience items and, as such, are not covered. 0 General Classification (PT CONV) 1 Cafeteria/Guest Tray (CAFETERIA) 2 Private Linen Service (LINEN) 3 Telephone/Telegraph (TELEPHN) 4 TV/Radio (TV/RADIO) 5 Nonpatient Room Rentals (NONPT ROOM RENT) 6 Late Discharge Charge (LATE DISCH) 7 Admission Kits (ADMIT KITS) 8 Beauty Shop/Barber (BARBER/BEAUTY) 9 Other Patient Convenience Items (PT CONVENCE/OTH)

Hospital Form Locator Codes

Type of Bill Codes (Form Locator 4)

Code	1st Digit: Type of Facility
1	Hospital
2	Skilled nursing facility
3	Home health
4	Christian science (hospital)
5	Christian science (extended care)
6	Intermediate care
7	Clinic
8	Special Facility
Code	**2nd Digit: Bill Classifications (Clinics only)**
1	Rural Health
2	Clinic – Hospital Based or Independent Renal dialysis center
3	Free-standing
4	Other rehabilitation facility
5	Clinic – CORF
6	Clinic – CMHC
9	Other
Code	**2nd Digit – Bill Classifications (Except Clinics & Special Facilities)**
1	Inpatient (including Medicare Part A)
2	Inpatient (Medicare Part B only)
3	Outpatient
4	Other
5	Intermediate Care, Level I
6	Intermediate Care, Level II
7	SubAcute Inpatient
8	Swing Beds
Code	**2nd Digit – Bill Classifications (Special Facilities only)**
1	Hospice (Non Hospital Based)
2	Hospice (Hospital Based)
3	Ambulatory Surgical Center
4	Free Standing Birth Center
5	Critical Access Hospital
6	Residential Facility
9	Other
Code	**3rd Digit: Frequency**
0	Non-Payment/Zero
1	Admit through discharge claim
2	Interim: first claim
3	Interim: continuing claims
4	Interim: last claim
5	Late charge only
6	Reserved
7	Replacement of prior claim
8	Void/cancel of prior claim
9	Final Claim for a Home Health PPS Episode

■ **Table AC–8** Hospital Form Locator Codes   (continues on next page)

Sex Codes (Form Locator 15)

Code	Definitions
M	Male
F	Female
U	Unknown

Marital Status Codes (Form Locator 16)

Code	Definition
S	Single
M	Married
X	Legally separated
D	Divorced
W	Widowed
U	Unknown
P	Life partner

Type of Admission Codes (Form Locator 19)

Code	Definition
1	Emergency
2	Urgent
3	Elective
4	Newborn
5	Trauma Center
9	Information not available

Source of Admission Codes Except Newborns (Form Locator 20)

Code	Definition
1	Physician referral
2	Clinical referral
3	HMO referral
4	Transfer from a hospital
5	Transfer from a skilled nursing facility
6	Transfer from another health facility
7	Emergency room
8	Court/law enforcement
9	Information not available
A	Transfer from a critical access hospital
B	Transfer from another HHA
C	Readmission to same HHA

Additional Source of Admission Codes for Newborns (Form Locator 20)

Code	Definition
1	Normal delivery
2	Premature delivery
3	Sick baby

(continues on next page)

4	Extramural birth
5	Information not available

Patient Status (Form Locator 22)

Code	Definition
01	Discharged to home or self-care (routine discharge)
02	Discharged/transferred to another short-term general hospital
03	Discharged/transferred to a skilled nursing facility
04	Discharged/transferred to an intermediate care facility
05	Discharged/transferred to another type of institution (including distinct parts) or referred for outpatient services to another institution
06	Discharged/transferred to home under care of organized home health service organization
07	Left against medical advice or discontinued care
08	Discharged/transferred to home under care of home IV therapy provider
09	Admitted as an inpatient to this hospital
20	Expired (or did not recover – Christian Science patient)
30	Still a patient or expected to return for outpatient services
31-39	Reserved for National Assignment
40	Expired at home (for hospice care only)
41	Expired in a medical facility such as a hospital, SNF, ICF, or free-standing hospice (for hospice care only)
42	Expired, place unknown (for hospice care only)
43	Discharged/transferred to a Federal Hospital
50	Discharged to a hospice, Home
51	Discharged to hospice, Medical Facility

Condition Codes (Form Locator 24-30)

Code	Definition
02	Enter this code if the patient alleges that the medical condition causing this episode of care is due to environment/event from his/her employment.
03	Indicates that patient/patient representative has stated that coverage may exist beyond that reflected on this bill.
04	Indicates bill is submitted for informational purposes only. Examples would include a bill submitted as a utilization report, or a bill for a beneficiary who is enrolled in a risk-based managed care plan (such as Medicare+Choice) and the hospital expects to receive payment from the plan.
05	Enter this code if you have filed a legal claim for recovery of funds potentially due to a patient or on behalf of a patient.

Release of Information Indicator Codes (Form Locator 52)

Code	Definitions
Y	Yes
R	Restricted or modified release
N	No release

(continues on next page)

Member's Relationship to the Insured Codes (Form Locator 59)
(Date of Service is before October 16, 2003)

Code	Definition
01	Patient is the insured
02	Spouse
03	Natural child/insured has financial responsibility
04	Natural child/insured does not have financial responsibility
05	Stepchild
06	Foster child
07	Ward of the court
08	Employee
09	Unknown
10	Handicapped dependent
11	Organ donor
12	Cadaver donor
13	Grandchild
14	Niece/nephew
15	Injured plaintiff
16	Sponsored dependent
17	Minor dependent of a minor dependent
18	Parent
19	Grandparent
20	Life partner

Member's Relationship to the Insured Codes (Form Locator 59)
(Date of Service is after October 16, 2003)

Code	Definitions
01	Spouse
04	Grandfather or Grandmother
05	Grandson or Granddaughter
07	Niece/nephew
10	Foster Child
15	Ward
17	Stepson or Stepdaughter
18	Self
19	Child
20	Employee
21	Unknown
22	Handicapped dependent
23	Sponsored dependent
24	Dependent of minor dependent
29	Significant other
32	Mother
33	Father
36	Emancipated minor
39	Organ donor
40	Cadaver donor
41	Injured plaintiff

(continues on next page)

43	Child where insured has no financial responsibility
53	Life partner
G8	Other relationship

Valid Employment Status Codes (Form Locator 64)

Code	Definition
1	Employed full-time
2	Employed part-time
3	Not employed
4	Self-employed
5	Retired
6	On active military duty
9	Unknown

State Abbreviations

NAME OF STATE	ABBREVIATION
Alabama	AL
Alaska	AK
American Samoa	AS
Arizona	AZ
Arkansas	AR
California	CA
Colorado	CO
Connecticut	CT
Delaware	DE
District of Columbia	DC
Florida	FL
Georgia	GA
Guam	GU
Hawaii	HI
Idaho	ID
Illinois	IL
Indiana	IN
Iowa	IA
Kansas	KS
Kentucky	KY
Louisiana	LA
Maine	ME
Maryland	MD
Massachusetts	MA
Michigan	MI
Minnesota	MN
Mississippi	MS
Missouri	MO
Montana	MT
Nebraska	NE
Nevada	NV
New Hampshire	NH
New Jersey	NJ
New Mexico	NM
New York	NY
North Carolina	NC
North Dakota	ND
Ohio	OH
Oklahoma	OK
Oregon	OR
Pennsylvania	PA
Puerto Rico	PR
Rhode Island	RI
South Carolina	SC
South Dakota	SD
Tennessee	TN
Texas	TX
Utah	UT
Vermont	VT

■ **Table AC–9** State Abbreviations   *(continues on next page)*

Virginia	VA
Virgin Islands	VI
Washington	WA
West Virginia	WV
Wisconsin	WI
Wyoming	WY

Other Address Abbreviations

OTHER ADDRESS	ABBREVIATION
Alley	Aly
Avenue	Ave
Boulevard	Blvd
Branch	Br
Bypass	Byp
Causeway	Cswy
Center	Ctr
Circle	Cir
Court	Ct
Courts	Cts
Crescent	Cres
Drive	Dr
Expressway	Expy
Extension	Ext
Freeway	Fwy
Gardens	Gdns
Grove	Grv
Heights	Hts
Highway	Hwy
Lane	Ln
Manor	Mnr
Place	Pl
Plaza	Plz
Point	Pt
Post Office	PO
Road	Rd
Rural	R
Rural Route	RR
Square	Sq
Street	St
Terrace	Ter
Trail	Trl
Turnpike	Tpke
Viaduct	Via
Vista	Vis

■ **Table AC–10** Other Address Abbreviations

Appendix D
CMS-1500/1500 Health
Insurance Claim Form

Table of Contents

CMS-1500 Claim Form Matrix

Header—Top of Form   Purpose: Directs the claim to the appropriate payer.

```
PLEASE          ROVER INSURERS INC
DO NOT          5931 ROLLING ROAD
STAPLE          RONSON CO 81369
IN THIS
AREA
□□□ PICA                                              APPROVED MOB-0938-0008
                                                                  PICA □□□
```

HEALTH INSURANCE CLAIM FORM

	Commercial/Private	Medicare	Medicaid	Workers' Compensation
Information to Enter	Enter the name and address of the payer(s) to whom this claim is being sent. Use spaces to separate names. Enter address information as follows: 1st line=Name; 2nd line=First line of address; 3rd line=Second line of address, if necessary; and 4th line=city, state (2 digits) and zip code. Do not use punctuation except "#" and "-." If an attention line is needed place it in the second line.	Required.	Required.	Required.

Block 1—Insurance Coverage Information   Purpose: Shows the type of health insurance coverage applicable to this claim.

```
1. MEDICARE    MEDICAID    CHAMPUS       CHAMPVA      GROUP           FECA          OTHER
                           HEALTH PLAN   BLK LUNG

□ (Medicare #) □ (Medicaid #) □ (Sponsor's SSN) □ (VA File #) ☒ (SSN or ID) □ (SSN) □ (ID)
```

	Commercial/Private	Medicare	Medicaid	Workers' Compensation
Information to Enter	Enter an X in the applicable box.	For an Individual Plan place an X in "OTHER." For a Group Plan place an X in "GROUP."	Enter an X in the "MEDICARE" box.	Enter an X in the "MEDICAID" box.	Enter an X in "OTHER," unless diagnosis is for "FECA BLK LUNG." If FECA, place an X in that box.

Block 1a—Insured's Identification, Policy or Certificate Number and Group Number   Purpose: Identifies the patient to the payer.

```
1a INSURED'S I.D NUMBER          (FOR PROGRAM IN ITEM 1)

001 00 RED
```

	Commercial/Private	Medicare	Medicaid	Workers' Compensation
Information to Enter	Enter the insured's identification number as shown on the insured's health	Required.	Enter the patient's	Enter the	Enter the patient's WC

Table AD–1 CMS-1500 Claim Form Matrix

	Medicare HICN.	patient's Medicaid ID number, complete with any prefixes and suffixes.	claim number if available. If not, enter employer's policy number, or patient's SSN. If a SSN is not available, a driver's license number and jurisdiction, a green card number, a visa number, or passport number can be used.
insurance card for the payer to whom the claim is being submitted. Do not use punctuation.			

Block 2—Patient's Name   Purpose: Identifies the patient.

2. PATIENT'S NAME (Last, First, Middle Initial).
ADDISON ABBY

	Commercial/Private	Medicare	Medicaid	Workers' Compensation
Information to Enter	Required.	Required.	Required.	Required.
Enter the patient's full last name, first name, and middle initial. Use spaces to separate names. If the patient uses a last name suffix (i.e., Jr, Sr) enter it after the last name and before the first name. Do not use punctuation except a "-"; which may be used for hyphenated names.				

Block 3—Patient's Birth Date   Purpose: Identifies the patient; distinguishes persons with similar names.

3. PATIENT'S BIRTH DATE
MM DD YY   SEX
12 12 1968   M ☐ F ☒

	Commercial/Private	Medicare	Medicaid	Workers' Compensation
Information to Enter	Required.	Required.	Required.	Required.
Enter the patient's date of birth. Use the eight-digit numeric date (MM DD CCYY). Use spaces to separate parts of the field. Enter an X in the correct box to indicate the sex of the patient.				

Block 4—Insured's Name   Purpose: Identifies the patient's source of insurance.

4. INSURED'S NAME (Last, First, Middle Initial)

SAME

	Commercial/Private	Medicare	Medicaid	Workers' Compensation
Information to Enter	Required.	If Medicare is the primary carrier, leave empty. If not, list name.	If insured is also the patient, leave empty. If not, list name.	Enter the name of the patient's employer.
Enter the insured's full last name, first name, and middle initial. If the insured uses a last name suffix (i.e., Jr, Sr) enter it after the last name and before the first name. Use spaces to separate names. Do not use punctuation except a "-"; which may be used for hyphenated names. If the patient and insured are the same enter "SAME."				

525

Block 5—Patient's Address Purpose: Further identifies patient; allows contact for questions.

5. PATIENT'S ADDRESS (No., Street)
5678 ANY AVENUE

CITY	STATE
ANYTOWN	USA

ZIP CODE	TELEPHONE (Include Area Code)
12345	(765) 555 4321

Information to Enter	Commercial/Private	Medicare	Medicaid	Workers' Compensation
Enter the patient's mailing address and telephone number. Do not use punctuation except "#" and "-". Use the two-digit state code and if available nine-digit zip code.	Required.	Required.	Required.	Required.

Block 6—Patient's Relationship to Insured Purpose: Identifies patient's source of insurance; also distinguishes patient from insured.

6. PATIENT'S RELATIONSHIP TO INSURED
Self [X] Spouse [] Child [] Other []

Information to Enter	Commercial/Private	Medicare	Medicaid	Workers' Compensation
Enter an X in the correct box to indicate the patient's relationship to the insured. For unmarried domestic partner check the "OTHER" box.	Required.	Use only if block 4 is completed.	Leave empty, unless there is other coverage.	Enter an X in the "OTHER" box.

Block 7—Insured's Address Purpose: Further identifies insured; allows contact for questions.

7. INSURED'S ADDRESS (No., Street)
SAME

CITY	STATE

ZIP CODE	TELEPHONE (INCLUDE AREA CODE)

Information to Enter	Commercial/Private	Medicare	Medicaid	Workers' Compensation
Enter the insured's address and telephone number. Do not use punctuation except "#" and "-". Use the two-digit state code and if available nine-digit zip code. Enter "SAME" if block 4 is completed and the address is the same as block 5.	Required.	Complete only if block 4 is completed.	Complete only if block 4 is completed.	Enter the address and telephone number of the patient's employer.

Block 8—Patient Status   Purpose: Allows determination of liability and COB.

8. PATIENT STATUS

| Single ☐ | Married ☐ | Other ☒ |
| Employed ☒ | Full-Time ☐ Student | Part-Time ☐ Student |

Information to Enter	Commercial/Private	Medicare	Medicaid	Workers' Compensation
Enter an X in the box for the patient's marital status and for the patient's employment or student status. If widowed or divorced select the "Single" box. Use "Other" for domestic partner.	Required.	Required.	Not required.	Enter an X in the "Employed" box.

Block 9—Other Insured's Name   Purpose: Identifies other sources of insurance.

9. OTHER INSURED'S NAME (Last, First, Middle Initial)

Information to Enter	Commercial/Private	Medicare	Medicaid	Workers' Compensation
If item 11d is marked, complete fields 9–9-d, otherwise leave blank. Enter the name of the holder of a secondary or other policy that may cover the patient. Enter the other insured's full last name, first name, and middle initial of the enrollee in another health plan. Use spaces to separate names. Do not use punctuation except a "-", which may be used for hyphenated names. If the patient and insured are the same enter "SAME."	Required.	If Medicare is the primary insurer leave 9–9d empty. If not, enter info.	If Medicaid is the primary insurer leave 9–9d empty. If not, enter info.	Not required unless claim has not been declared WC.

Block 9a—Other Insured's Policy or Group Number   Purpose: Identifies other sources of insurance.

a. OTHER INSURED'S POLICY OR GROUP NUMBER

Information to Enter	Commercial/Private	Medicare	Medicaid	Workers' Compensation
Enter the policy or group number of the other insured as indicated in block 9. Copy the number from the health identification card. Complete only if block 9 is completed.	Required.	Indicate "Medigap" if Medigap insurance is listed.	Required.	Not required unless claim has not been declared WC.

527

Block 9b—Other Insured's Date of Birth   Purpose: Identifies other insurance source. Also used to determine the primary source of insurance.

b. OTHER INSURED'S DATE OF BIRTH
MM   DD   YY   SEX
                 M ☐   F ☐

	Commercial/Private	Medicare	Medicaid	Workers' Compensation
Information to Enter	Required.	Required.	Required.	Not required unless claim has not been declared WC.

Enter the date of birth and sex of the other insured as indicated in block 9. Enter an X in the correct box to indicate the sex of the other insured. Use the eight-digit numeric date (MM DD CCYY). Use spaces to separate parts of the field. Complete only if block 9 is completed.

Block 9c—Employer's Name or School Name   Purpose: Identifies other sources of insurance.

c. EMPLOYER'S NAME OR SCHOOL NAME

	Commercial/Private	Medicare	Medicaid	Workers' Compensation
Information to Enter	Required.	Required.	Required.	Not required unless claim has not been declared WC.

Enter the name of the other insured's employer or school as indicated in block 9. Complete only if block 9 completed.

Block 9d—Insurance Plan Name or Program Name   Purpose: Identifies other sources of insurance.

d. INSURANCE PLAN NAME OR PROGRAM NAME

	Commercial/Private	Medicare	Medicaid	Workers' Compensation
Information to Enter	Required.	Required.	Required.	Not required unless claim has not been declared WC.

Enter the other insured's insurance plan or program name. Complete only if block 9 completed.

Block 10a–10c—Is Patient's Condition Related to Employment?   Purpose: Identifies primary liability for condition.

10.   IS PATIENT'S CONDITION RELATED TO:

a. EMPLOYMENT? (CURRENT OR PREVIOUS)
     ☐ YES   ☒ NO

b. AUTO ACCIDENT?   PLACE (State)
     ☐ YES   ☒ NO

c. OTHER ACCIDENT?
     ☐ YES   ☒ NO

	Commercial/Private	Medicare	Medicaid	Workers' Compensation
Information to Enter				

Enter an X in the correct box to indicate whether one or more of the services described in Item 24 are for a condition or injury that occurred on-the-job or as a result of an automobile or other accident. The state postal code must be shown if "YES" is checked in 10b for "Auto Accident." Any item marked "Yes" indicates that there may be other applicable insurance coverage that would be primary, such as automobile liability insurance.

| Required. | Enter an X in the "No" box. If "Yes," the other payer should be billed as primary, before billing Medicare. | Enter an X in the "No" box. If "Yes," the other payer should be billed as primary, before billing Medicaid. | Enter an X in the "Yes" box for 10a. |

Block 10d—Reserved for Local Use?   Purpose: To be determined by local payer.

10d. RESERVED FOR LOCAL USE

Information to Enter	Commercial/Private	Medicare	Medicaid	Workers' Compensation
Refer to the most current instructions from the applicable public or private payer regarding the use of this field.	Per payer specifications; otherwise leave empty.	Per payer specifications; otherwise leave empty.	Enter the share of cost collected from patient.	Per payer specifications; otherwise leave empty.

Block 11—Insured's Policy Group or FECA Number   Purpose: Identifies insured's policy or group number.

11. INSURED'S POLICY GROUP OR FECA NUMBER:
41935

Information to Enter	Commercial/Private	Medicare	Medicaid	Workers' Compensation
Enter the insured's policy or group number as it appears on the insured's health care identification card. The FECA number is a 9-digit alphanumeric identifier assigned to a patient claiming work-related conditions under FECA.	Required.	If Medicare is the primary insurance carrier, list "NONE" and proceed to block 12. If there is a terminating event with regard to insurance (e.g., insured retired) enter "NONE" and proceed to block 11b.	Not required.	Not required.

Block 11a—Insured's Date of Birth   Purpose: Identifies other sources of insurance. Used to determine the primary source of insurance.

a. INSURED'S DATE OF BIRTH				
MM	DD	YY	SEX	
12	12	1968	M ☐ F ☒	

Information to Enter	Commercial/Private	Medicare	Medicaid	Workers' Compensation

Enter the insured's date of birth (this refers to the insured indicated in block 1a). Enter an X in the correct box to indicate the sex of the insured. Use the eight-digit numeric date (MM DD CCYY). Use spaces to separate parts of the field.

Required.	Not required.	Not required.	Not required.

Block 11b—Employer's Name or School Name   Purpose: Identifies other sources of insurance.

b. EMPLOYER'S NAME OR SCHOOL NAME
RED CORPORATION

	Commercial/Private	Medicare	Medicaid	Workers' Compensation
Information to Enter Enter the name of the insured's employer or school.	Required.	If a change in the insured's insurance status has occurred enter the reason (e.g., RETIRED).	Not required.	Not required.

Block 11c—Insurance Plan Name or Program Name   Purpose: Identifies other sources of insurance.

c. INSURANCE PLAN NAME OR PROGRAM NAME
ROVER INSURERS INC

	Commercial/Private	Medicare	Medicaid	Workers' Compensation
Information to Enter Enter the insured's insurance plan or program name.	Required.	Not Required.	Not required.	Not required.

Block 11d—Is There Another Health Benefit Plan?   Purpose: Identifies other sources of insurance.

d. IS THERE ANOTHER HEALTH BENEFIT PLAN?
☐ YES   ☒ NO   *If yes, return to and complete item 9 a-d*

	Commercial/Private	Medicare	Medicaid	Workers' Compensation
Information to Enter When appropriate enter an X in the correct box, if there is another health benefit plan other than the plan indicated in block 1. If marked "YES" complete blocks 9—9d.	Required.	Required.	Required.	Not required, unless claim has not been declared WC, then enter an X in the "Yes" box and complete 9–9d.

Block 12—Authorization for Release of Medical Information   Purpose: Gives permission to release any medical or other information necessary to process and/or adjudicate the claim.

READ BACK OF FORM BEFORE COMPLETING & SIGNING THIS FORM

12.   PATIENT'S OR AUTHORIZED PERSON'S SIGNATURE I authorize the release of any medical or other information necessary to process this claim. I also request payment of government benefits either to myself or to the party who accepts assignment below.

SIGNED SIGNATURE ON FILE   DATE

Information to Enter	Commercial/Private	Medicare	Medicaid	Workers' Compensation
Enter "Signature on File", "SOF" or legal signature. When a legal signature is provided, enter date signed in the six-digit format (MMDDYY) or eight-digit (MMDDCCYY) format. If there is no signature on file, leave blank or enter "No Signature on File."	Required.	Required.	Not required.	Not required.

Block 13—Authorization for Assignment of Benefits to Provider   Purpose: Gives permission authorizing payment of benefits to the provider of services.

13.   INSURED'S OR AUTHORIZED PERSON'S SIGNATURE I authorize payment of medical benefits to the undersigned physician or supplier for services described below.

SIGNED SIGNATURE ON FILE

Information to Enter	Commercial/Private	Medicare	Medicaid	Workers' Compensation
Enter "Signature on File", "SOF" or legal signature. If there is no signature on file, leave blank or enter "No Signature on File."	Required.	Required.	Not required.	Not required.

Block 14—Date of Illness, Injury, or Pregnancy   Purpose: Helps payers identify benefits.

14.   DATE OF CURRENT: ▼ ILLNESS (1st symptom)
      MM   DD   YY   ▼ INJURY (Accident)
                         PREGNANCY (LMP)

Information to Enter	Commercial/Private	Medicare	Medicaid	Workers' Compensation
Enter the first date of the present illness, injury, or pregnancy. Use the six-digit format (MM DD YY). Use spaces to separate parts of the field. For pregnancy, use the date of the last menstrual period.	Required.	Required.	Not required.	Requires a specific date for the on-the-job illness or injury. The date should be the same as that indicated on the Doctor's First Report.

531

Block 15—If Patient Has Had Same or Similar Illness, Give First Date   Purpose: Allows determination of liability and COB.

15. IF PATIENT HAS HAD SAME OR SIMILAR ILLNESS,
GIVE FIRST DATE   MM DD YY

Information to Enter	Commercial/Private	Medicare	Medicaid	Workers' Compensation
Enter the first date that the patient had the same or a similar illness. Use the six-digit numeric date (MM DD YY). Use spaces to separate parts of the field.	Required.	Not required.	Not required.	Not required.

Block 16—Patient Disability Dates for Current Occupation   Purpose: Identifies dates of disability.

16. DATES PATIENT UNABLE TO WORK IN CURRENT OCCUPATION
    MM DD YY   MM DD YY
FROM   TO

Information to Enter	Commercial/Private	Medicare	Medicaid	Workers' Compensation
If the patient is employed and is unable to work in current occupation, an eight-digit numeric date (MMDDCCYY) must be shown for the "from-to" dates that the patient is unable to work. An entry in this field may indicate employment-related insurance coverage.	Required.	Required.	Not required.	Required.

Block 17—Name of Referring Physician or Other Source   Purpose: Identifies referral source.

17. NAME OF REFERRING PHYSICIAN OR OTHER SOURCE

DOROTHY DOCTOR MD

Information to Enter	Commercial/Private	Medicare	Medicaid	Workers' Compensation
Enter the name (First Name, Middle Initial, Last Name) and credentials of the professional who referred or ordered the service(s) or supply(s) on the claim. Use spaces to separate names. Do not use punctuation except a "-," which may be used for hyphenated names. For services billed by an assistant surgeon or anesthesiologist enter the name and credential of the primary surgeon. For DME claims enter the name of the prescribing provider.	Required.	Required.	Required.	Enter the SSN or EIN of the employer.

Block 17a—I.D. Number of Referring Physician   Purpose: Identifies referral source.

17a. I.D. NUMBER OF REFERRING PHYSICIAN

D45678

Information to Enter	Commercial/Private	Medicare	Medicaid	Workers' Compensation
Enter the identifying number (i.e., NPI, UPIN, MHCP ID numbers) of the referring or ordering physician, or other source. Required when block 17 is completed.	Enter a UPIN, PIN or NPI number.	Enter a UPIN, PIN or NPI number.	Enter a UPIN, PIN or NPI number.	Enter a SSN or EIN number.

Block 18—Hospitalization Dates   Purpose: Identifies services related to an inpatient stay.

18. HOSPITALIZATION DATES RELATED TO CURRENT SERVICES
MM   DD   YY   MM   DD   YY
FROM   TO

Information to Enter	Commercial/Private	Medicare	Medicaid	Workers' Compensation
Enter the inpatient hospital admission date followed by the discharge date (if discharge has occurred). If not discharged, leave discharge date blank. Use the eight-digit numeric date (MM DD CCYY). Use spaces to separate parts of the field. This date is when a medical service is furnished as a result of, or subsequent to, a related hospitalization.	Required.	Required.	Required.	Required.

Block 19—Reserved for Local Use   Purpose: Provides additional information.

19. RESERVED FOR LOCAL USE

Information to Enter	Commercial/Private	Medicare	Medicaid	Workers' Compensation
Refer to the most current instructions from the applicable public or private payer regarding the use of this field.	Per payer specifications; otherwise leave empty.	Per payer specifications; otherwise leave empty.	Per payer specifications; otherwise leave empty.	Per payer specifications; otherwise leave empty.

Block 20—Outside Lab $Charges   Purpose: Identifies purchased laboratory, pathology, or radiology services.

20. OUTSIDE LAB? $ CHARGES
☐ YES   ☒ NO

Information to Enter	Commercial/Private	Medicare	Medicaid	Workers' Compensation
Complete this field when billing for purchased services. Enter an X in the "Yes" box if the reported service(s) were performed by an outside laboratory. If "Yes", enter the purchase price. Do not use a dollar sign. Use	Required.	Required.	Enter an X in the "No" box as outside	Required.

a space to divide the dollars and cents. Enter an X in the "No" box if outside laboratory service(s) are not included on the claim. When "YES" is marked, enter the independent provider's name and address in Block 32.

laboratories must bill Medicaid directly.

Block 21—Diagnosis or Nature of Illness or Injury   Purpose: Supports the reason for the service(s) and provides information necessary to process the claim. The diagnosis must relate to the service(s) performed.

21. DIAGNOSIS OR NATURE OF ILLNESS OR INJURY, (RELATE ITEMS 1,2,3, OR 4 TO ITEM 24E BY LINE)

1. | 401 .
2. | .
3. | .
4. | .

Information to Enter	Commercial/Private	Medicare	Medicaid	Workers' Compensation
Enter the patient's diagnosis/condition. Enter up to four ICD-9CM diagnosis codes. Relate lines 1,2,3,4 to the lines of service in 24E by line number. Use the highest level of specificity. Do not use punctuation.	Required.	Required.	Required.	Required.

Block 22—Medicaid Resubmission   Purpose: Use to identify a resubmission of an incorrectly processed Medicaid claim.

22. MEDICAID RESUBMISSION CODE | ORIGINAL REF. NO.

Information to Enter	Commercial/Private	Medicare	Medicaid	Workers' Compensation
List the original reference number for resubmitted claims. Refer to the most current instructions from the applicable public or private payer regarding the use of this field. Leave empty for all payers except Medicaid.	Not required.	Not required.	Enter the correct Medicaid Transaction Control Number.	Not required.

Block 23—Prior Authorization Number   Purpose: Determines eligibility of the current service(s).

23. PRIOR AUTHORIZATION NUMBER

Information to Enter	Commercial/Private	Medicare	Medicaid	Workers' Compensation
Enter any of the following: prior authorization or precertification number; referral number; or CLIA number; as assigned by the payer for the current service when applicable. Notations such as "Prescription on File" can be noted for DME or pharmacy claims; or "SSO Performed" can be noted for claims which require an SSO to be performed.	Required.	Required.	Required.	Not required.

Block 24A—Date(s) of Service [lines 1-6]   Purpose: Informs the payer of the date(s) of service(s).

24.	A			DATE(S) OF SERVICE		
		From			To	
MM	DD	YY	MM	DD	YY
01	26	YY	01	26	YY

Information to Enter	Commercial/Private	Medicare	Medicaid	Workers' Compensation
Enter date(s) of service, from and to: If one date of service only, enter the date under "From." Leave "To" blank or re-enter "From" date. If grouping services, the place of service, type of service, procedure code, charges, and individual provider for each line must be identical for that service line. The number of days must correspond to the number of units in 24G. Use the six-digit numeric date (MM DD YY). Use spaces to separate parts of the field.	Required.	Required.	Leave "To" date empty. No date ranging allowed.	Required.

Block 24B—Place of Service [lines 1-6]   Purpose: Informs the payer as to where the service(s) were performed.

B
Place of Service
11

Information to Enter	Commercial/Private	Medicare	Medicaid	Workers' Compensation
Enter the two-digit code for the "Place of Service" for each item used or service performed. Refer to the Place of Service list in Appendix C.	Required.	Required.	Required.	Required.

Block 24C—Type of Service [lines 1-6]   Purpose: No longer used.

C
Type
of
Service

	Commercial/Private	Medicare	Medicaid	Workers' Compensation
Information to Enter	Not required.	Not required.	Not required.	Not required.
Leave empty.				

Block 24D—Procedures, Services, or Supplies [lines 1-6]   Purpose: Informs payer as to what services were performed.

D
PROCEDURES, SERVICES, OR SUPPLIES
(Explain Unusual Circumstances)
CPT/HCPS | MODIFIER

99212

	Commercial/Private	Medicare	Medicaid	Workers' Compensation
Information to Enter	Required.	Required.	Required.	Required.
Enter the CPT® or HCPCS codes and modifier(s) (if applicable) from the appropriate code set in effect on the date of service. Use spaces to separate parts of field. Do not use hyphens for modifiers.				

Block 24E—Diagnosis Code [lines 1-6]   Purpose: Informs the payer which diagnosis relates to each procedure.

E
DIAGNOSIS
CODE

1

Information to Enter	Commercial/Private	Medicare	Medicaid	Workers' Compensation
Enter the diagnosis code reference number as shown in block 21 to relate the date of service and the procedures performed to the primary diagnosis. When multiple services are performed, the primary reference number for each service should be listed first, other applicable services should follow. The reference number(s) should be a 1, or 2, or 3, or 4; or multiple numbers as applicable. Do not use punctuation or enter ICD-9-CM codes here. Use spaces to separate line numbers.	Required.	Required.	Required.	Required.

Block 24F—$ Charges [lines 1-6]   Purpose: Informs the payer of the total amount charged for each service line.

F
$ CHARGES
40 : 00

Information to Enter	Commercial/Private	Medicare	Medicaid	Workers' Compensation
Enter the charge for each listed service. Enter numbers right justified in the dollar area of the field. If more than one date or unit is shown in 24G, the dollars shown should reflect the total of the services. Do not use dollar signs. Do not use commas as thousands marker. Use a space to separate parts of field.	Required.	Required.	Required.	Required.

Block 24G—Days or Units [lines 1-6]   Purpose: Informs the payer of the number or quantity of each service provided.

G
DAYS OR UNITS
1

Information to Enter	Commercial/Private	Medicare	Medicaid	Workers' Compensation
Enter the number of days or units for each service line. This field is most commonly used for multiple visits, units of supplies, anesthesia units or minutes, or oxygen volume. If only one service is performed, the number 1 must be entered. For anesthesia, enter the total minutes of anesthesia provided (convert hours to minutes).	Required.	Required.	Required.	Required.

Block 24H—EPSDT / Family Plan [lines 1-6]   Purpose: Indicates whether the services were for Early, Periodic, Screening, Diagnosis and Treatment services.

H
EPSDT Family Plan

Information to Enter	Commercial/Private	Medicare	Medicaid	Workers' Compensation
Leave empty unless Medicaid Claim.	Not required.	Not required.	Enter "E" for EPSDT services, or enter "F" for family planning services.	Not required.

Block 24I—EMG [lines 1-6]   Purpose: Indicates if services were for emergency treatment in a hospital.

I
EMG

Information to Enter	Commercial/Private	Medicare	Medicaid	Workers' Compensation

Information to Enter	Commercial/Private	Medicare	Medicaid	Workers' Compensation
Check with payer to determine if this field is required. If required, enter Y for "YES" or leave blank if "NO."	Per payer specifications; otherwise leave empty.	Per payer specifications; otherwise leave empty.	If services rendered in the ER, enter an "X".	Not required.

Block 24J—COB [lines 1-6]   Purpose: Indicates whether patient has other insurance, and if COB should be applied.

COB

Information to Enter	Commercial/Private	Medicare	Medicaid	Workers' Compensation
Check with payer to determine if this field is required. If required, enter an X if the patient has other insurance, and an EOB is attached.	Per payer specifications; otherwise leave empty.	Per payer specifications; otherwise leave empty.	Per payer specifications; otherwise leave empty.	Not required.

Block 24K—Reserved For Local Use   Purpose: Identifies the specific doctor that performed the services.

K
RESERVED FOR
LOCAL USE

Information to Enter	Commercial/Private	Medicare	Medicaid	Workers' Compensation
If a medical group is the provider listed in block 33 enter the UPIN, PIN or NPI number of the individual provider that performed the services.	Required.	Required.	Required.	Required.

Block 25—Federal Tax I.D. Number Purpose: Identifies the billing provider.

25. FEDERAL TAX I.D. NUMBER   SSN □   EIN ☒

99-1234567

	Commercial/Private	Medicare	Medicaid	Workers' Compensation
Information to Enter Enter the billing provider's federal tax identification number (include hyphen), social security, or employer identification number (include hyphen). Specify type of number by entering an X in the correct box. Use spaces to separate parts of field.	Required.	Required.	Required.	Required.

Block 26—Patient's Account Number Purpose: Identifies the patient.

26. PATIENT'S ACCOUNT NO.

GMBC5509 001

	Commercial/Private	Medicare	Medicaid	Workers' Compensation
Information to Enter Enter the patient's account number assigned by the billing provider.	Required.	Required.	Required.	Required.

Block 27—Accept Assignment? Purpose: Indicates if the provider accepts assignment of Medicare benefits.

27. ACCEPT ASSIGNMENT?
(For govt. claims, see back)
☒ YES   □ NO $

	Commercial/Private	Medicare	Medicaid	Workers' Compensation
Information to Enter Enter an X in the correct box.	Required.	Required.	"Yes" box must be marked.	Not required.

Block 28—Total Charge Purpose: Informs the payer of the total dollars charged for the billed services.

28. TOTAL CHARGE
$ 40 : 00

	Commercial/Private	Medicare	Medicaid	Workers' Compensation
Information to Enter Enter the sum of the charges in column 24F [lines 1-6]. Use a space to divide the dollars and cents. Do not use dollar signs. Do not use commas as thousands marker.	Required.	Required.	Required.	Required.

Block 29—Amount Paid   Purpose: Indicates payments made by other payers or by the patient.

29. AMOUNT PAID
$ | 5 | 00 | $

Information to Enter	Commercial/Private	Medicare	Medicaid	Workers' Compensation
Enter the amount the patient or other payers paid on covered services only. Use a space to divide the dollars and cents. Do not use dollar signs. Do not use commas as thousands marker.	Required.	Required.	Do not enter the Medicaid copayment amount.	Required.

Block 30—Balance Due   Purpose: Indicates the balance due to be paid to the provider of services.

30. BALANCE DUE
$ | 35 | 00

Information to Enter	Commercial/Private	Medicare	Medicaid	Workers' Compensation
Subtract block 29 from block 28 to arrive at the amount to be entered in this block.	Required.	Not required.	Enter the balance due if Medicaid is the secondary payer. Otherwise not required.	Required.

Block 31—Signature of Physician or Supplier Including Degrees or Credentials   Purpose: Identifies the provider of service(s) or supply(s).

31. SIGNATURE OF PHYSICIAN OR SUPPLIER
     INCLUDING DEGREES OR CREDENTIALS
     (I certify that the statements on the reverse
     apply to this bill and are made a part thereof.)

SIGNED Paul Provider MD DATE
0126CCYY

Information to Enter	Commercial/Private	Medicare	Medicaid	Workers' Compensation
Enter the signature of the physician, supplier or representative with the degree, credentials, or title and the date signed. Use the eight-digit numeric date (MM DD CCYY).	Required.	Required.	Required.	Required.

541

Block 32—Name and Address of Facility Where Services Were Rendered   Purpose: Identifies where the service(s) were rendered or supplies provided.

32. NAME AND ADDRESS OF FACILITY WHERE SERVICES
WERE RENDERED (if other than home or office)

Information to Enter	Commercial/Private	Medicare	Medicaid	Workers' Compensation
Enter the name and address, city, state, and zip code of the location where the services were rendered if other than box 33 or patient's home. Suppliers should enter the location where supplies were accepted. Do not use punctuation except "#" and "-." Use two-digit state code and, if available, nine-digit zip code. If block 18 is completed or block 20 contains an X in the "Yes" box enter name and address of facility here.	Required.	Required.	Required.	Required.

Block 33—Physician's/Supplier's Billing Name, Address, Zip Code and Phone Number   Purpose: Identifies the billing provider.

33. PHYSICIAN'S, SUPPLIERS BILLING NAME, ADDRESS, ZIP CODE &
PHONE #

PAUL PROVIDER MD
5858 PEPPERMINT PLACE
ANYTOWN USA 12345
(765) 555 6768

PIN#   P12345   GRP#

Information to Enter	Commercial/Private	Medicare	Medicaid	Workers' Compensation
Enter the billing provider's name, address, city, state, zip code, and telephone number. Enter the PIN, NPI, or Group Number. Do not use punctuation except "#" and "-." Use the two-digit state code and, if available, the nine-digit zip code.	Required.	Required.	Enter the provider's Medicaid number in the Group # field.	Required.

CMS-1500 Sample Claims

Figure AD–1 is a completed CMS-1500 claim for Abby Addison, who has private insurance. The physician has a signed authorization to release benefits and assignment of benefits on file. The provider also accepts Medicare as-signment. The patient was seen by Dr. Provider in the hospital for hypertension. The doctor performed an initial comprehensive hospital visit and examination of moderate complexity. The patient was referred to Dr. Provider by Dr. Doctor. The patient was hospitalized at Provider Medical Center from 05/07/CCYY through 05/09/CCYY.

CMS-1500 Sample Claims

PLEASE DO NOT STAPLE IN THIS AREA

ROVER INSURERS INC
5931 ROLLING ROAD
RONSON CO 81369

APPROVED MOB-0938-0008

□□□ PICA

HEALTH INSURANCE CLAIM FORM

PICA □□□

1. MEDICARE / MEDICAID / CHAMPUS / CHAMPVA / GROUP HEALTH PLAN / FECA BLK LUNG / OTHER	1a. INSURED'S I.D NUMBER (FOR PROGRAM IN ITEM 1)
☐ (Medicare #) ☐ (Medicaid #) ☐ (Sponsor's SSN) ☐ (VA File #) ☒ (SSN or ID) ☐ (SSN) ☐ (ID)	001 01 RED

2. PATIENT'S NAME (Last, First, Middle Initial).	3. PATIENT'S BIRTH DATE	4. INSURED'S NAME (Last, First, Middle Initial)
ADDISON ABBY	MM 12 DD 12 YY 1968 SEX M ☐ F ☒	SAME

5. PATIENT'S ADDRESS (No., Street)	6. PATIENT'S RELATIONSHIP TO INSURED	7. INSURED'S ADDRESS (No., Street)
5678 ANY AVENUE	Self ☒ Spouse ☐ Child ☐ Other ☐	

CITY	STATE	8. PATIENT STATUS	CITY	STATE
ANYTOWN	USA	Single ☒ Married ☐ Other ☐		

ZIP CODE	TELEPHONE (Include Area Code)		ZIP CODE	TELEPHONE (INCLUDE AREA CODE)
12345	(765) 555 4321	Employed ☒ Full-Time Student ☐ Part-Time Student ☐		

9. OTHER INSURED'S NAME (Last, First, Middle Initial)	10. IS PATIENT'S CONDITION RELATED TO:	11. INSURED'S POLICY GROUP OR FECA NUMBER: 41935
a. OTHER INSURED'S POLICY OR GROUP NUMBER	a. EMPLOYMENT? (CURRENT OR PREVIOUS) ☐ YES ☒ NO	a. INSURED'S DATE OF BIRTH MM 12 DD 12 YY 1968 SEX M ☐ F ☒
b. OTHER INSURED'S DATE OF BIRTH MM DD YY SEX M ☐ F ☐	b. AUTO ACCIDENT? PLACE (State) ☐ YES ☒ NO	b. EMPLOYER'S NAME OR SCHOOL NAME RED CORPORATION
c. EMPLOYER'S NAME OR SCHOOL NAME	c. OTHER ACCIDENT? ☐ YES ☒ NO	c. INSURANCE PLAN NAME OR PROGRAM NAME ROVER INSURERS INC
d. INSURANCE PLAN NAME OR PROGRAM NAME	10d. RESERVED FOR LOCAL USE	d. IS THERE ANOTHER HEALTH BENEFIT PLAN? ☐ YES ☒ NO If yes, return to and complete item 9 a-d

READ BACK OF FORM BEFORE COMPLETING & SIGNING THIS FORM
12. PATIENT'S OR AUTHORIZED PERSON'S SIGNATURE I authorize the release of any medical or other information necessary to process this claim. I also request payment of government benefits either to myself or to the party who accepts assignment below.

SIGNED **SIGNATURE ON FILE** DATE

13. INSURED'S OR AUTHORIZED PERSON'S SIGNATURE I authorize payment of medical benefits to the undersigned physician or supplier for services described below.

SIGNED **SIGNATURE ON FILE**

14. DATE OF CURRENT: ◄ ILLNESS (1st symptom) INJURY (Accident) PREGNANCY (LMP) MM DD YY	15. IF PATIENT HAS HAD SAME OR SIMILAR ILLNESS, GIVE FIRST DATE MM DD YY	16. DATES PATIENT UNABLE TO WORK IN CURRENT OCCUPATION MM DD YY MM DD YY FROM TO

17. NAME OF REFERRING PHYSICIAN OR OTHER SOURCE	17a. I.D. NUMBER OF REFERRING PHYSICIAN	18. HOSPITALIZATION DATES RELATED TO CURRENT SERVICES MM DD YY MM DD YY
DOROTHY DOCTOR MD	D45678	FROM 05 07 CCYY TO 05 09 CCYY

19. RESERVED FOR LOCAL USE	20. OUTSIDE LAB? ☐ YES ☒ NO $ CHARGES

21. DIAGNOSIS OR NATURE OF ILLNESS OR INJURY, (RELATE ITEMS 1,2,3, OR 4 TO ITEM 24E BY LINE)	22. MEDICAID RESUBMISSION CODE ORIGINAL REF. NO.
1. 401 . 3.	23. PRIOR AUTHORIZATION NUMBER
2. . 4.	

24. A DATE(S) OF SERVICE From MM DD YY To MM DD YY	B Place of Service	C Type of Service	D PROCEDURES, SERVICES, OR SUPPLIES (Explain Unusual Circumstances) CPT/HCPCS | MODIFIER	E DIAGNOSIS CODE	F $ CHARGES	G DAYS OR UNITS	H EPSDT Family Plan	I EMG	J COB	K RESERVED FOR LOCAL USE
05 07 YY 05 07 YY	21		99222	1	160 00	1				

25. FEDERAL TAX I.D. NUMBER SSN EIN	26. PATIENT'S ACCOUNT NO.	27. ACCEPT ASSIGNMENT? (For govt. claims, see back)	28. TOTAL CHARGE	29. AMOUNT PAID	30. BALANCE DUE
99-1234567 ☐ ☒	GMBC5509 001	☒ YES ☐ NO	$ 160 00	$	$ 160 00

31. SIGNATURE OF PHYSICIAN OR SUPPLIER INCLUDING DEGREES OR CREDENTIALS (I certify that the statements on the reverse apply to this bill and are made a part thereof.)	32. NAME AND ADDRESS OF FACILITY WHERE SERVICES WERE RENDERED (If other than home or office)	33. PHYSICIAN'S, SUPPLIERS BILLING NAME, ADDRESS, ZIP CODE & PHONE #
SIGNED *Paul Provider MD* DATE 05/08/CCYY	PROVIDER MEDICAL CENTER 6969 PAULY MAIN COURT ANYTOWN USA 12345	PAUL PROVIDER MD 5858 PEPPERMINT PLACE ANYTOWN USA 12345 765 555 6768 PIN# P12345 GRP#

(APPROVED BY AMA COUNCIL ON MEDICAL SERVICE 8/88)

PLEASE PRINT OR TYPE

FORM CMS-1500 (12-90)
FORM OWCP-1500   FORM RRB-1500
FORM AMA-OP050591

■ **Figure AD–1** Private Insurance Claim

Figure AD–2 is a completed CMS-1500 claim for Edward Edmunds, who has Medicare coverage. The physician has a signed authorization to release benefits and assignment of benefits on file. The provider also accepts Medicare assignment. The patient was seen in Dr. Provider's office for a recheck for his condition of coronary artery disease.

PLEASE DO NOT STAPLE IN THIS AREA

MEDICARE
555 MEDICARE BLVD SUITE 200
MEDICARE USA 12345

APPROVED MOB-0938-0008

□□□ PICA

HEALTH INSURANCE CLAIM FORM

PICA □□□

| 1. MEDICARE ☒ (Medicare #) | MEDICAID ☐ (Medicaid #) | CHAMPUS ☐ (Sponsor's SSN) | CHAMPVA ☐ (VA File #) | GROUP HEALTH PLAN ☐ (SSN or ID) | FECA BLK LUNG ☐ (SSN) | OTHER ☐ (ID) | 1a. INSURED'S I.D NUMBER (FOR PROGRAM IN ITEM 1) 508 12 3456A |

2. PATIENT'S NAME (Last, First, Middle Initial).
EDMUNDS EDWARD

3. PATIENT'S BIRTH DATE — MM 01 DD 10 YY 1927 — SEX M ☒ F ☐

4. INSURED'S NAME (Last, First, Middle Initial)

5. PATIENT'S ADDRESS (No., Street)
8888 EVERY LANE

CITY ANYTOWN STATE USA

ZIP CODE 12345 TELEPHONE (Include Area Code) (765) 555 7890

6. PATIENT'S RELATIONSHIP TO INSURED
Self ☒ Spouse ☐ Child ☐ Other ☐

8. PATIENT STATUS
Single ☐ Married ☐ Other ☒
Employed ☐ Full-Time Student ☐ Part-Time Student ☐

7. INSURED'S ADDRESS (No., Street)

CITY STATE

ZIP CODE TELEPHONE (INCLUDE AREA CODE)

9. OTHER INSURED'S NAME (Last, First, Middle Initial)

a. OTHER INSURED'S POLICY OR GROUP NUMBER

b. OTHER INSURED'S DATE OF BIRTH — MM DD YY — SEX M ☐ F ☐

c. EMPLOYER'S NAME OR SCHOOL NAME

d. INSURANCE PLAN NAME OR PROGRAM NAME

10. IS PATIENT'S CONDITION RELATED TO:

a. EMPLOYMENT? (CURRENT OR PREVIOUS) ☐ YES ☒ NO

b. AUTO ACCIDENT? ☐ YES ☒ NO PLACE (State)

c. OTHER ACCIDENT? ☐ YES ☒ NO

10d. RESERVED FOR LOCAL USE

11. INSURED'S POLICY GROUP OR FECA NUMBER:
NONE

a. INSURED'S DATE OF BIRTH — MM DD YY — SEX M ☐ F ☐

b. EMPLOYER'S NAME OR SCHOOL NAME

c. INSURANCE PLAN NAME OR PROGRAM NAME

d. IS THERE ANOTHER HEALTH BENEFIT PLAN? ☐ YES ☒ NO If yes, return to and complete item 9 a-d

READ BACK OF FORM BEFORE COMPLETING & SIGNING THIS FORM
12. PATIENT'S OR AUTHORIZED PERSON'S SIGNATURE I authorize the release of any medical or other information necessary to process this claim. I also request payment of government benefits either to myself or to the party who accepts assignment below.

SIGNED SIGNATURE ON FILE DATE _____

13. INSURED'S OR AUTHORIZED PERSON'S SIGNATURE I authorize payment of medical benefits to the undersigned physician or supplier for services described below.

SIGNED SIGNATURE ON FILE

14. DATE OF CURRENT: ◄ ILLNESS (1st symptom) INJURY (Accident) PREGNANCY (LMP) — MM DD YY ◄

15. IF PATIENT HAS HAD SAME OR SIMILAR ILLNESS, GIVE FIRST DATE MM DD YY

16. DATES PATIENT UNABLE TO WORK IN CURRENT OCCUPATION — MM DD YY FROM TO MM DD YY

17. NAME OF REFERRING PHYSICIAN OR OTHER SOURCE

17a. I.D. NUMBER OF REFERRING PHYSICIAN

18. HOSPITALIZATION DATES RELATED TO CURRENT SERVICES — MM DD YY FROM TO MM DD YY

19. RESERVED FOR LOCAL USE

20. OUTSIDE LAB? ☐ YES ☒ NO $ CHARGES

21. DIAGNOSIS OR NATURE OF ILLNESS OR INJURY, (RELATE ITEMS 1,2,3, OR 4 TO ITEM 24E BY LINE)
1. 414 .
2. .
3. .
4. .

22. MEDICAID RESUBMISSION CODE ORIGINAL REF. NO.

23. PRIOR AUTHORIZATION NUMBER

24. A. DATE(S) OF SERVICE From MM DD YY To MM DD YY	B. Place of Service	C. Type of Service	D. PROCEDURES, SERVICES, OR SUPPLIES (Explain Unusual Circumstances) CPT/HCPS MODIFIER	E. DIAGNOSIS CODE	F. $ CHARGES	G. DAYS OR UNITS	H. EPSDT Family Plan	I. EMG	J. COB	K. RESERVED FOR LOCAL USE
04 05 YY 04 05 YY	11		99211	1	35 00	1				

25. FEDERAL TAX I.D. NUMBER SSN EIN
99-1234567 ☐ ☒

26. PATIENT'S ACCOUNT NO
GMBC5509 005

27. ACCEPT ASSIGNMENT? (For govt. claims, see back) ☒ YES ☐ NO

28. TOTAL CHARGE $ 35 00

29. AMOUNT PAID $

30. BALANCE DUE $ 35 00

31. SIGNATURE OF PHYSICIAN OR SUPPLIER INCLUDING DEGREES OR CREDENTIALS (I certify that the statements on the reverse apply to this bill and are made a part thereof.)
SIGNED Paul Provider MD DATE 04/06/CCYY

32. NAME AND ADDRESS OF FACILITY WHERE SERVICES WERE RENDERED (If other than home or office)

33. PHYSICIAN'S, SUPPLIERS BILLING NAME, ADDRESS, ZIP CODE & PHONE #
PAUL PROVIDER MD
5858 PEPPERMINT PLACE
ANYTOWN USA 12345
765 555 6768
PIN# P12345 GRP#

(APPROVED BY AMA COUNCIL ON MEDICAL SERVICE 8/88) **PLEASE PRINT OR TYPE** FORM CMS-1500 (12-90) FORM OWCP-1500 FORM RRB-1500 FORM AMA-OP050591

■ **Figure AD–2** Medicare Claim

Figure AD–3 is a completed CMS-1500 claim for Daisy Doolittle, who is covered under Medicaid. The physician has a signed authorization to release benefits and assignment of benefits on file. The provider also accepts Medicare assignment. The patient was seen in Dr. Provider's office for the first time for family planning services.

Figure AD–3 Medicaid Claim

Figure AD–4 is a completed CMS-1500 claim for Bobby Bumble, for a Workers' Compensation claim. The physician has a signed authorization to release benefits and assignment of benefits on file. The provider also accepts Medicare assignment. The patient was referred by his employer. Dr. Jones performed a physical examination and history, new patient, moderate complexity; x-ray of the skull, 2 views; removal of foreign body from the nose; and irrigation of the eyes. The doctor states that the patient is unable to perform regular work duties from October 10, CCYY to October 30, CCYY.

1500 Health Insurance Claim Form

The NUCC has recommended that the healthcare industry adopt the following timeline for the transition to the new version of the 1500 Health Insurance Claim Form (version 08/05).

- October 1, 2006: Health plans, clearinghouses, and other information support vendors should be ready to handle and accept the revised (08/05) 1500 claim form.
- October 1, 2006–February 1, 2007: Providers can use either the current (12/90) version or the revised (08/05) version of the 1500 Claim Form.
- February 1, 2007: The current (12/90) version of the 1500 Claim Form is discontinued.

These guidelines are recommendations only and the health plan or clearinghouse should be consulted prior to submitting a claim on the revised form.

PLEASE
DO NOT
STAPLE
IN THIS
AREA

BLUEBERRY INSURANCE
4662 BEACH BLVD
ANYTOWN USA 12345

APPROVED MOB-0938-0008

□□□ PICA

HEALTH INSURANCE CLAIM FORM

PICA □□□

1. MEDICARE	MEDICAID	CHAMPUS	CHAMPVA	GROUP HEALTH PLAN	FECA BLK LUNG	OTHER	1a. INSURED'S I.D NUMBER	(FOR PROGRAM IN ITEM 1)
☐ (Medicare #)	☐ (Medicaid #)	☐ (Sponsor's SSN)	☐ (VA File #)	☐ (SSN or ID)	☐ (SSN)	☒ (ID)	25101606	

2. PATIENT'S NAME (Last, First, Middle Initial).	3. PATIENT'S BIRTH DATE				SEX	4. INSURED'S NAME (Last, First, Middle Initial)
BUMBLE BOBBY	MM 01	DD 04	YY 1944	M ☒	F ☐	BLUE CORPORATION

5. PATIENT'S ADDRESS (No., Street)	6. PATIENT'S RELATIONSHIP TO INSURED	7. INSURED'S ADDRESS (No., Street)
93485 BUMPKISS COURT	Self ☐ Spouse ☐ Child ☐ Other ☒	9817 BOBCAT BLVD

CITY	STATE	8. PATIENT STATUS	CITY	STATE
ANYTOWN	USA	Single ☐ Married ☒ Other ☐	ANYTOWN	USA
ZIP CODE TELEPHONE (Include Area Code)		Employed ☒ Full-Time Student ☐ Part-Time Student ☐	ZIP CODE TELEPHONE (INCLUDE AREA CODE)	
12345 (765) 555 4756			12345 (765) 567 8901	

9. OTHER INSURED'S NAME (Last, First, Middle Initial)	10. IS PATIENT'S CONDITION RELATED TO:	11. INSURED'S POLICY GROUP OR FECA NUMBER:
a. OTHER INSURED'S POLICY OR GROUP NUMBER	a. EMPLOYMENT? (CURRENT OR PREVIOUS) ☒ YES ☐ NO	a. INSURED'S DATE OF BIRTH MM DD YY SEX M ☐ F ☐
b. OTHER INSURED'S DATE OF BIRTH MM DD YY SEX M ☐ F ☐	b. AUTO ACCIDENT? PLACE (State) ☐ YES ☒ NO	b. EMPLOYER'S NAME OR SCHOOL NAME
c. EMPLOYER'S NAME OR SCHOOL NAME	c. OTHER ACCIDENT? ☐ YES ☒ NO	c. INSURANCE PLAN NAME OR PROGRAM NAME
d. INSURANCE PLAN NAME OR PROGRAM NAME	10d. RESERVED FOR LOCAL USE	d. IS THERE ANOTHER HEALTH BENEFIT PLAN? ☐ YES ☒ NO If yes, return to and complete item 9 a-d

READ BACK OF FORM BEFORE COMPLETING & SIGNING THIS FORM

12. PATIENT'S OR AUTHORIZED PERSON'S SIGNATURE I authorize the release of any medical or other information necessary to process this claim. I also request payment of government benefits either to myself or to the party who accepts assignment below.

SIGNED _____   DATE _____

13. INSURED'S OR AUTHORIZED PERSON'S SIGNATURE I authorize payment of medical benefits to the undersigned physician or supplier for services described below.

SIGNED _____

14. DATE OF CURRENT: ◄ ILLNESS (1st symptom) INJURY (Accident) PREGNANCY (LMP)	15. IF PATIENT HAS HAD SAME OR SIMILAR ILLNESS, GIVE FIRST DATE MM DD YY	16. DATES PATIENT UNABLE TO WORK IN CURRENT OCCUPATION
MM 10 DD 16 YY CCYY		FROM MM 10 DD 16 YY CCYY TO MM 10 DD 30 YY CCYY

17. NAME OF REFERRING PHYSICIAN OR OTHER SOURCE	17a. I.D. NUMBER OF REFERRING PHYSICIAN	18. HOSPITALIZATION DATES RELATED TO CURRENT SERVICES
Employer		FROM MM DD YY TO MM DD YY

19. RESERVED FOR LOCAL USE	20. OUTSIDE LAB? ☐ YES ☒ NO $ CHARGES

21. DIAGNOSIS OR NATURE OF ILLNESS OR INJURY, (RELATE ITEMS 1,2,3, OR 4 TO ITEM 24E BY LINE)

1. | 850 . ___
2. | 930 . ___
3. | 932 . ___
4. | ___

22. MEDICAID RESUBMISSION CODE	ORIGINAL REF. NO.
23. PRIOR AUTHORIZATION NUMBER	

24. A DATE(S) OF SERVICE From To						B Place of Service	C Type of Service	D PROCEDURES, SERVICES, OR SUPPLIES (Explain Unusual Circumstances) CPT/HCPS MODIFIER	E DIAGNOSIS CODE	F $ CHARGES	G DAYS OR UNITS	H EPSDT Family Plan	I EMG	J COB	K RESERVED FOR LOCAL USE
MM	DD	YY	MM	DD	YY										
10	16	YY	10	16	YY	11		99204	1 2 3	70 00	1				
10	16	YY	10	16	YY	11		70250	1	45 00	1				
10	16	YY	10	16	YY	11		30300	2	85 00	1				
10	16	YY	10	16	YY	11		65205	3	18 00	1				

25. FEDERAL TAX I.D. NUMBER SSN EIN	26. PATIENT'S ACCOUNT NO	27. ACCEPT ASSIGNMENT? (For govt. claims, see back)	28. TOTAL CHARGE	29. AMOUNT PAID	30. BALANCE DUE
11-0987654 ☐ ☒	5509 002	☒ YES ☐ NO	$ 218 00	$	$

31. SIGNATURE OF PHYSICIAN OR SUPPLIER INCLUDING DEGREES OR CREDENTIALS (I certify that the statements on the reverse apply to this bill and are made a part thereof.)	32. NAME AND ADDRESS OF FACILITY WHERE SERVICES WERE RENDERED (If other than home or office)	33. PHYSICIAN'S, SUPPLIERS BILLING NAME, ADDRESS, ZIP CODE & PHONE #
SIGNED *Joanne Jones MD* DATE 10/17/CCYY		JOANNA JONES MD 1029 JONATHAN LANE ANYTOWN USA 12345 765 555 0987
		PIN# P54321 GRP#

(APPROVED BY AMA COUNCIL ON MEDICAL SERVICE 8/88)

PLEASE PRINT OR TYPE

FORM CMS-1500   (12-90)
FORM OWCP-1500   FORM RRB-1500
FORM AMA-OP050591

■ **Figure AD–4** Workers' Compensation Claim

The National Uniform Claim Committee (NUCC) has approved the following changes to the current (12/90) version of the 1500 Health Insurance Claim Form. The changes listed below correspond to the revised 1500 Claim Form (version 08/05).

Location	Change Log
Header	The barcode was removed.
Header	The language "PLEASE DO NOT STAPLE IN THIS AREA" was removed from the left-hand side.
Header	The rectangle with "1500" was added in black ink to the left-hand side.
Header	The title "HEALTH INSURANCE CLAIM FORM" was moved from the lower, right-hand side to the left-hand side.
Header	The language "APPROVED BY NATIONAL UNIFORM CLAIM COMMITTEE 08/05" was added to the left-hand side.
Header	The language "SAMPLE" was added. This language will be removed when the form is approved by OMB.
Box 1	"TRICARE" was added above "CHAMPUS".
Box 1	Under CHAMPVA, "VA File #" was changed to "Member ID#".
Box 17a	The box was split in half length-wise.
Box 17a	This area was shaded. This box will accommodate other ID numbers.
Box 17a	Two vertical lines were added. This field will accommodate a two byte qualifier for other ID numbers.
Box 17b	This field was added.
Box 17b	Two vertical lines were added with the "NPI" label. This field will accommodate the NPI number.
Box 21	The lines after the decimal point in items 1, 2, 3, and 4 were extended to accommodate four bytes.
Box 24	The line with the alpha indicators was removed. The alpha indicators were moved next to the respective titles in the title fields.
Box 24	The line numbers to the left of Box 24 were increased in size and centered with each line.
Box 24	Each of the six lines were split length-wise and shading was added to the top portion of each line. This area is to be used for the reporting of supplemental information.
Box 24	Vertical line separators on each of the six lines have been removed from the shaded area, except for the lines before Boxes 24I and 24J.
Box 24C	"Type of Service" was removed. This field is now titled "EMG".
Box 24D	The field became wider by three bytes.
Box 24D	Shading was added vertically between "CPT/HCPCS" and "MODIFIER".
Box 24D	Vertical lines were added in the unshaded "MODIFIER" section to accommodate four sets of two bytes.
Box 24E	The title was changed from "DIAGNOSIS CODE" to "DIAGNOSIS POINTER".
Box 24E	The field was decreased by three bytes.
Box 24G	This field was increased by one byte.
Box 24H	This field was decreased by one byte.
Box 24I	The title was changed from "EMG" to "ID. QUAL.".

Table AD–2 1500 Health Insurance Claim Form Change Log

Box 24I	A horizontal line was added length-wise across the field separating the shaded and unshaded portions of the field.
Box 24I	The label "NPI" was added in the unshaded portion of the field.
Box 24J	The title was changed from "COB" to "RENDERING PROVIDER ID. #"
Box 24J	A dotted horizontal line was added length-wise across the field separating the shaded and unshaded portions of the field. The NPI number is to be reported in the unshaded field. Another ID number can be reported in the shaded field.
Box 24K	This field, "RESERVED FOR LOCAL USE", was removed.
Box 32	Boxes 32a and 32b were added at the bottom.
Box 32a	This field was added to accommodate reporting of the NPI number and is indicated by the shaded label of "NPI".
Box 32b	This shaded field was added to accommodate the reporting of other ID numbers.
Box 33	Parentheses were added after the title to indicate the location for reporting the telephone number.
Box 33	Boxes 33a and 33b were added at the bottom.
Box 33a	The title of this field was changed from "PIN#" to "a.".
Box 33a	A shaded label of NPI was added to the box to indicate the reporting of the NPI number.
Box 33b	The title was changed from "GRP#" to "b." to accommodate the reporting of other ID numbers.
Box 33b	The field was shaded.
Footer	The language "NUCC Instruction Manual available at: www.nucc.org" was added to the left-hand side.
Footer	The OMB approval numbers were removed and the language "OMB APPROVAL PENDING" was added. The numbers will be added after approval has been received by OMB.
Back	The following language was added in the last line at the bottom of the form: "This address is for comments and/or suggestions only. DO NOT MAIL COMPLETED CLAIM FORMS TO THIS ADDRESS."

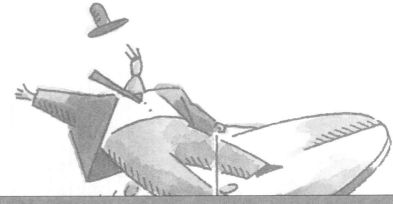

Appendix E

UB-92
(CMS-1450)/UB-04

Table of Contents

UB-92 Form Matrix

Form Locator 1 – Name/Address   Purpose: Directs the claim to the appropriate payer.

1

	Private Insurance	Medicare	Medicaid	Workers' Compensation
Information to Enter	Required.	Required.	Required.	Required.
Enter the name and address, city, state, and zip code of the billing provider. Use the two-digit state abbreviation. Do not use punctuation.				

Form Locator 2 – Unlabeled Field/Workers' Compensation Ratio   Purpose: Not required.

2

3 PATIENT CONTROL NO.

4 TYPE OF BILL

	Private Insurance	Medicare	Medicaid	Workers' Compensation
Information to Enter	Not required.	Not required.	Not required.	Required.
Enter the Workers' Compensation number assigned by the carrier (if known).				

551

Form Locator 3 – Patient Control Number   Purpose: Identifies the patient to the payer.

3 PATIENT CONTROL NO. | 4 TYPE OF BILL

Information to Enter	Private Insurance	Medicare	Medicaid	Workers' Compensation
Enter the patient control number or office account number assigned by the provider.	Required.	Required.	Optional.	Not required

Form Locator 4 – Type of Bill   Purpose: Identifies the patient.

3 PATIENT CONTROL NO. | 4 TYPE OF BILL

Information to Enter	Private Insurance	Medicare	Medicaid	Workers' Compensation
Enter a valid three-digit "Type of Bill" code, which provides specific information about the services rendered. Refer to Appendix C for valid codes.	Required.	Required.	Required.	Required.

Form Locator 5 – Federal Tax Number   Purpose: Number assigned to the provider by the federal government for tax reporting purposes.

5 FED. TAX NO. | 6 STATEMENT COVERS PERIOD FROM THROUGH | 7 COV D. | 8 N-C D. | 9 C-I D. | 10 L-R D. | 11

Information to Enter	Private Insurance	Medicare	Medicaid	Workers' Compensation
Enter the nine-digit Employer Identification Number (EIN) for the provider indicated in Form Locator 1 assigned by the Internal Revenue Service (IRS). Include the hyphen.	Required.	Required.	Optional	Required.

Form Locator 6 – Statement Covers Period   Purpose: Date of service or time-period bill for.

5 FED. TAX NO.	6 STATEMENT COVERS PERIOD FROM / THROUGH	7 COV D.	8 N-C D.	9 C-I D.	10 L-R D.	11

Information to Enter

Enter the beginning and ending date of services, in the MMDDYY format, for the period reflected on the claim.

Private Insurance	Medicare	Medicaid	Workers' Compensation
Required.	Required.	Required.	Required.

Form Locator 7 – Covered Days   Purpose: Number of Medicaid covered days in the billing period.

5 FED. TAX NO.	6 STATEMENT COVERS PERIOD FROM / THROUGH	7 COV D.	8 N-C D.	9 C-I D.	10 L-R D.	11

Information to Enter

Enter the number of inpatient days covered for the billing period noted in Form Locator 6.

Private Insurance	Medicare	Medicaid	Workers' Compensation
Not required.	Not required.	Required.	Not required.

Form Locator 8 – Noncovered Days   Purpose: Number of Medicaid noncovered days in the billing period.

5 FED. TAX NO.	6 STATEMENT COVERS PERIOD FROM / THROUGH	7 COV D.	8 N-C D.	9 C-I D.	10 L-R D.	11

Information to Enter

Enter the number of inpatient days not covered for the billing period noted in Form Locator 6.

Private Insurance	Medicare	Medicaid	Workers' Compensation
Not required.	Not required.	Required.	Not required.

Form Locator 9 – Coinsurance Days Purpose: Number of Medicare coinsurance days in the statement covers period.

5 FED.TAX NO.	6 STATEMENT COVERS PERIOD FROM	THROUGH	7 COV D.	8 N-C D.	9 C-I.D.	10 L-R.D.	11

Information to Enter

Enter the number of covered inpatient hospital days occurring after the 60th day and before the 91st day or the number of covered inpatient SNF days occurring after the 20th day and before the 101st day of the benefit period.

Private Insurance	Medicare	Medicaid	Workers' Compensation
Not required.	Required.	Not required.	Not required.

Form Locator 10 – Lifetime Reserve Days Purpose: Lifetime Reserve Days used during billing period.

5 FED.TAX NO.	6 STATEMENT COVERS PERIOD FROM	THROUGH	7 COV D.	8 N-C D.	9 C-I.D.	10 L-R.D.	11
						(circled)	

Information to Enter

Enter the number of lifetime reserve days used during the billing period noted on the claim.

Private Insurance	Medicare	Medicaid	Workers' Compensation
Not required.	Required.	Not required.	Not required.

Form Locator 11 – Unlabeled Field Purpose: Administratively Necessary Days (AND).

5 FED.TAX NO.	6 STATEMENT COVERS PERIOD FROM	THROUGH	7 COV D.	8 N-C D.	9 C-I.D.	10 L-R.D.	11
							(circled)

Information to Enter

Enter the number of Administratively Necessary Days (AND), use only if specifically requested by payer.

Private Insurance	Medicare	Medicaid	Workers' Compensation
Not required, unless specified by payer.	Not required, unless specified by payer.	Not required, unless specified by payer.	Not required, unless specified by payer.

Form Locator 12 – Patient Name   Purpose: Identifies the patient.

12 PATIENT NAME

Information to Enter	Private Insurance	Medicare	Medicaid	Workers' Compensation
Enter the patient's or injured worker's name (last name, first name, and middle initial). Do not use punctuation, except a "-", for hyphenated names.	Required.	Required.	Required.	Required.

Form Locator 13 – Patient Address   Purpose: Identifies the patient's complete mailing address.

13 PATIENT ADDRESS

Information to Enter	Private Insurance	Medicare	Medicaid	Workers' Compensation
Enter the complete mailing address of the patient or injured worker. Include street name and number, PO box or rural route number, apartment number if applicable, city, state, and zip code. Do not use punctuation, except "#" or "-". Use the two-digit state code and nine-digit zip code.	Required.	Required.	Required.	Required.

Form Locator 14 – Patient Birth Date   Purpose: Identifies the patient.

14 BIRTHDATE	15 SEX	16 M S	17 DATE	ADMISSION 18 HR	19 TYPE	20 SRC	21 D HR	22 STAT

Information to Enter	Private Insurance	Medicare	Medicaid	Workers' Compensation
Enter the month, day, century, and year of birth of the patient or injured (MMDDYYYY). An unknown birth date is not acceptable.	Required.	Required.	Required.	Required.

555

Form Locator 15 – Patient Sex   Purpose: Identifies the patient.

14 BIRTHDATE	15 SEX	16 MS	17 DATE	ADMISSION 18 HR	19 TYPE	20 SRC	21 D HR	22 STAT

Information to Enter

Enter the sex of the patient or injured worker as an "M" for male, an "F" for female, or "U" for unknown.

Private Insurance	Medicare	Medicaid	Workers' Compensation
Required.	Required.	Required.	Required.

Form Locator 16 – Patient Marital Status   Purpose: Indicates the patient's marital status.

14 BIRTHDATE	15 SEX	16 MS	17 DATE	ADMISSION 18 HR	19 TYPE	20 SRC	21 D HR	22 STAT

Information to Enter

Enter the code for the marital status of the patient or injured worker on the day of admission. Enter an "S" for single, an "M" for married, a "D" for divorced, a "W" for widowed, a "P" for Life partner, an "X" for legally separated, and a "U" for unknown.

Private Insurance	Medicare	Medicaid	Workers' Compensation
Required.	Required.	Not required.	Required.

Form Locator 17 – Admission Date   Purpose: Indicates the first date of care.

14 BIRTHDATE	15 SEX	16 MS	17 DATE	ADMISSION 18 HR	19 TYPE	20 SRC	21 D HR	22 STAT

Information to Enter

Enter the original date, in the MMDDYY format, that the patient or injured worker was admitted for inpatient care.

Private Insurance	Medicare	Medicaid	Workers' Compensation
Required.	Required.	Required.	Required.

Form Locator 18 – Admission Hour   Purpose: Indicates the hour during which the patient was admitted.

14 BIRTHDATE	15 SEX	16 M S	17 DATE	ADMISSION 18 HR	19 TYPE	20 SRC	21 D HR	22 STAT

Information to Enter	Private Insurance	Medicare	Medicaid	Workers' Compensation
Enter the admission hour in Military Standard Time, by hour code. For example: • 12:00 – 12:59 midnight = 00 • 05:00 – 05:59 A.M. = 05 • 12:00 – 12:59 noon = 12 • 06:00 – 06:59 P.M. = 18 • Use code 99 if hour is unknown.	Required.	Required.	Required.	Required.

Form Locator 19 – Admission Type   Purpose: Code indicating priority of admission.

14 BIRTHDATE	15 SEX	16 M S	17 DATE	ADMISSION 18 HR	19 TYPE	20 SRC	21 D HR	22 STAT

Information to Enter	Private Insurance	Medicare	Medicaid	Workers' Compensation
Enter the code indicating the priority of this admission. Refer to Appendix C for valid codes.	Required.	Required.	Not required, unless a 1 (emergency) is entered.	Not required for outpatient bills.

Form Locator 20 – Admission Source   Purpose: Indicates where the patient came from prior to admission.

14 BIRTHDATE	15 SEX	16 M S	17 DATE	ADMISSION 18 HR	19 TYPE	20 SRC	21 D HR	22 STAT

Information to Enter	Private Insurance	Medicare	Medicaid	Workers' Compensation
Enter the appropriate admission source code or outpatient registration. Refer to Appendix C for valid codes.	Required.	Required.	Not required.	Required.

557

Form Locator 21 – Discharge Hour   Purpose: Indicates the hour the patient was discharged from inpatient care.

14 BIRTHDATE	15 SEX	16 MS	17 DATE	ADMISSION 18 HR	19 TYPE	20 SRC	21 D HR	22 STAT

Information to Enter

Enter the hour at which the patient or injured worker was discharged from inpatient care, if applicable. Enter the admission hour in Military Standard Time, by hour code.

For example:
- 12:00 – 12:59 midnight = 00
- 05:00 – 05:59 A.M. = 05
- 12:00 – 12:59 noon = 12
- 06:00 – 06:59 P.M. = 18
- Use code 99 if hour is unknown.

Private Insurance	Medicare	Medicaid	Workers' Compensation
Required.	Required.	Required.	Required.

Form Locator 22 – Patient Status   Purpose: Indicates the status of the patient at the end of care period.

14 BIRTHDATE	15 SEX	16 MS	17 DATE	ADMISSION 18 HR	19 TYPE	20 SRC	21 D HR	22 STAT

Information to Enter

Enter the code indicating the status of the patient or injured worker as of the ending service date of the period covered on this bill. Refer to Appendix C for valid codes.

Private Insurance	Medicare	Medicaid	Workers' Compensation
Required.	Required.	Required.	Required.

Form Locator 23 – Medical Record Number   Purpose: Identifies the patient to the institution.

23 MEDICAL RECORD NO.	CONDITION CODES 24	25	26	27	28	29	30	31

Information to Enter

Enter the number assigned by the provider to the patient's or injured worker's medical or health record.

Private Insurance	Medicare	Medicaid	Workers' Compensation
Optional.	Required.	Required.	Optional.

Form Locators 24-30 – Condition Codes   Purpose: Identifies other sources of insurance.

`23 MEDICAL RECORD NO.` | CONDITION CODES | 24 25 26 27 28 29 30 | 31

Information to Enter	Private Insurance	Medicare	Medicaid	Workers' Compensation
Enter the appropriate condition code.	Optional, or as per payer's specifications.	Required.	Required.	Required.

Form Locator 31 – Unlabeled Field   Purpose: Unlabeled field.

`23 MEDICAL RECORD NO.` | CONDITION CODES | 24 25 26 27 28 29 30 | 31

Information to Enter	Private Insurance	Medicare	Medicaid	Workers' Compensation
Not applicable, or enter information as requested by payer.	Not required, or as per payer's specifications.	Not required, or as per payer's specifications.	Not required, or as per payer's specifications.	Not required, or as per payer's specifications.

Form Locators 32-35 – Occurrence Code(s) & Date(s)   Purpose: Indicates a significant event relating to bill.

`32 OCCURRENCE CODE DATE` | `33 OCCURRENCE CODE DATE` | `34 OCCURRENCE CODE DATE` | `35 OCCURRENCE CODE DATE`

Information to Enter	Private Insurance	Medicare	Medicaid	Workers' Compensation
Enter a code and an associated date (in the MMDDYY format) defining a significant event relating to this bill period. Enter a valid occurrence code if applicable.	Required.	Required, if applicable.	Required, if applicable.	Enter a code and date of the work related injury.

559

Form Locator 36 – Occurrence Span Code(s) & Date(s)

Purpose: Identifies a significant event relating to the payment of the claim.

| 36 CODE | OCCURRENCE SPAN FROM THROUGH | 37 A B C |

Information to Enter	Private Insurance	Medicare	Medicaid	Workers' Compensation
Enter the appropriate occurrence code and date span which identifies an event relating to the payment of the claim.	Required.	Required, if applicable.	Required, if applicable.	Required, if applicable.

Form Locator 37 – Transaction Control Number   Purpose: Allows determination of liability and COB.

| 36 CODE | OCCURRENCE SPAN FROM THROUGH | 37 A B C |

Information to Enter	Private Insurance	Medicare	Medicaid	Workers' Compensation
Enter the control number assigned to the original bill by the payer or the payer's intermediary.	Not required.	Required.	Not required.	Not required.

Form Locator 38 – Responsible Party's Name/Address   Purpose: Identifies party responsible for bill payment.

	38

Information to Enter	Private Insurance	Medicare	Medicaid	Workers' Compensation
Enter the name and address, city, state, and zip code of the other party responsible for payment of the bill. Do not use punctuation except a "#" or "-". Use the two-digit state code and nine-digit zip code.	Enter name and address of insurance carrier.	Not required.	Not required.	Enter name and complete mailing address of Workers' Compensation insurance carrier.

Form Locators 39-41 – Value Codes & Amounts
Purpose: Identifies coinsurance, occupancy rate, parent/relative contributions, and other resources applying to the patient's care.

39 CODE	VALUE CODES AMOUNT	40 CODE	VALUE CODES AMOUNT	41 CODE	VALUE CODES AMOUNT
a					
b					
c					
d					

Information to Enter	Private Insurance	Medicare	Medicaid	Workers' Compensation
Enter a valid value code and amount, if applicable. Code 01 indicates the recording of a hospital's most common semi-private rate; code 02 requires $0.00 amount; and code 03 is reserved for national assignment.	Required.	Required.	Required.	Required.

Form Locator 42 – Revenue Code   Purpose: Code that identifies the specific services rendered.

42 REV. CD.	43 DESCRIPTION	44 HCPCS / RATES	45 SERV. DATE	46 SERV. UNITS	47 TOTAL CHARGES	48 NON-COVERED CHARGES	49
1							1

Information to Enter

Enter the applicable revenue code for the services rendered. There are 23 lines available. Refer to Appendix C for valid codes.

Private Insurance	Medicare	Medicaid	Workers' Compensation
Required.	Required.	Required.	Required.

Form Locator 43 – Revenue Description   Purpose: Identifies the specific services rendered.

42 REV. CD.	43 DESCRIPTION	44 HCPCS / RATES	45 SERV. DATE	46 SERV. UNITS	47 TOTAL CHARGES	48 NON-COVERED CHARGES	49
1							1

Information to Enter

Enter the corresponding description or standard abbreviation for each revenue code entered in Form Locator 42 lines 1-23.

Private Insurance	Medicare	Medicaid	Workers' Compensation
Required.	Required.	Optional.	Required.

Form Locator 44 – HCPCS/Rates   Purpose: Identifies the services provided or performed.

42 REV. CD.	43 DESCRIPTION	44 HCPCS / RATES	45 SERV. DATE	46 SERV. UNITS	47 TOTAL CHARGES	48 NON-COVERED CHARGES	49
1							1

Information to Enter

Enter the accommodation rate for inpatient bills and the HCPCS codes applicable to ancillary services and outpatient bills.

Private Insurance	Medicare	Medicaid	Workers' Compensation
Required, for certain conditions.	Required.	Required.	Required, for certain conditions.

Form Locator 45 – Service Dates   Purpose: Identifies the date service was given.

42 REV. CD.	43 DESCRIPTION	44 HCPCS/RATES	45 SERV. DATE	46 SERV. UNITS	47 TOTAL CHARGES	48 NON-COVERED CHARGES	49
1					.	.	1

Private Insurance	Medicare	Medicaid	Workers' Compensation
Information to Enter			
Required.	Required.	Required.	Required.

Enter the date, in the MMDDYY format, that the outpatient service was rendered.

Form Locator 46 – Units of Service   Purpose: Identifies the number of times service was given.

42 REV. CD.	43 DESCRIPTION	44 HCPCS/RATES	45 SERV. DATE	46 SERV. UNITS	47 TOTAL CHARGES	48 NON-COVERED CHARGES	49
1					.	.	1

Private Insurance	Medicare	Medicaid	Workers' Compensation
Information to Enter			
Required.	Required.	Required.	Required.

Enter the total number of covered accommodation days, and ancillary units of service when appropriate.

Form Locator 47 – Total Charges   Purpose: Identifies the total charges by revenue code.

42 REV. CD.	43 DESCRIPTION	44 HCPCS/RATES	45 SERV. DATE	46 SERV. UNITS	47 TOTAL CHARGES	48 NON-COVERED CHARGES	49
1					.	.	1

Private Insurance	Medicare	Medicaid	Workers' Compensation
Information to Enter			
Required.	Required.	Required.	Required.

Enter the total amount related to the revenue codes billed for the statement from and through dates. This amount includes both the covered and noncovered charges.

Form Locator 48 – Noncovered Charges   Purpose: Reflects noncovered charges for the primary payer.

42 REV. CD.	43 DESCRIPTION	44 HCPCS/RATES	45 SERV. DATE	46 SERV. UNITS	47 TOTAL CHARGES	48 NONCOVERED CHARGES	49
1							1

Information to Enter	Private Insurance	Medicare	Medicaid	Workers' Compensation
Enter the total noncovered charges for the primary payer, if applicable, for each service billed.	Required, where applicable.	Required, where applicable.	Required, where applicable.	Not required.

Form Locator 49 – Unlabeled Field   Purpose: Not applicable.

42 REV. CD.	43 DESCRIPTION	44 HCPCS/RATES	45 SERV. DATE	46 SERV. UNITS	47 TOTAL CHARGES	48 NONCOVERED CHARGES	49
1							1

Information to Enter	Private Insurance	Medicare	Medicaid	Workers' Compensation
Not applicable, unless requested by a specific payer.	Not required, unless requested by a specific payer.	Not required, unless requested by a specific payer.	Not required, unless requested by a specific payer.	Not required, unless requested by a specific payer.

Form Locator 50 – Payer Identification   Purpose: Identifies all applicable payers.

50 PAYER	51 PROVIDER NO.	52 REL. INFO	53 ASG. BEN	54 PRIOR PAYMENTS	55 EST. AMOUNT DUE	56
A						
B						
C						
57			DUE FROM PATIENT ▶			

Information to Enter	Private Insurance	Medicare	Medicaid	Workers' Compensation
Enter the name(s) of the payer(s) in priority sequence according to the priority the provider expects to receive payment from these payers. Line A is for the primary payer, line B is for the secondary payer, and line C is for the tertiary payer. All information associated with that specific line (A, B, or C) will be entered on that corresponding line for Form Locators 50-66.	Required.	Required. If Medicare is the payer enter "Medicare."	Required.	Enter the injured worker's identification, Social Security, driver license, or green card number.

Form Locator 51 – Provider Number   Purpose: Further identifies the payer listed in field 50.

50 PAYER	51 PROVIDER NO.	52 REL INFO	53 ASG BEN	54 PRIOR PAYMENTS	55 EST. AMOUNT DUE	56
A						
B						
C						
57			DUE FROM PATIENT ▶			

Information to Enter	Private Insurance	Medicare	Medicaid	Workers' Compensation
Enter the number assigned to the provider by the payer indicated in Form Locator 50, if known.	Required.	Required.	Required.	Required.

Form Locator 52 – Release of Information Certification Indicator
Purpose: Gives the facility permission to release information.

50 PAYER	51 PROVIDER NO.	52 REL INFO	53 ASG BEN	54 PRIOR PAYMENTS	55 EST. AMOUNT DUE	56
A						
B						
C						
57			DUE FROM PATIENT ▶			

Information to Enter	Private Insurance	Medicare	Medicaid	Workers' Compensation
Enter the appropriate code indicating whether the provider has on file a signed statement from the member permitting the provider to release data to other organizations in order to adjudicate the claim. Entering a "Y" indicates that there is a statement on file; an "R" indicates the release is limited or restricted, and an "A" indicates that there is no release on file.	Required.	Required.	Required.	Required.

565

Form Locator 53 – Assignment of Benefits Indicator

Purpose: Informs the payer which diagnosis relates to each procedure.

	52 REL INFO	53 A SG BEN	54 PRIOR PAYMENTS	55 EST. AMOUNT DUE	56
50 PAYER	51 PROVIDER NO.				
A					
B					
C					
57		DUE FROM PATIENT ▶			

Information to Enter	Private Insurance	Medicare	Medicaid	Workers' Compensation
Enter the appropriate code to indicate whether the provider has a signed form authorizing the third-party insurer to pay the provider directly for the service(s) rendered. Entering an "A" indicates that an authorization is on file; an "N" indicates that there is no authorization on file.	Required.	Not required.	Not required.	Required.

Form Locator 54 – Prior Payments

Purpose: Indicates the payment amount received toward this bill.

	52 REL INFO	53 A SG BEN	54 PRIOR PAYMENTS	55 EST. AMOUNT DUE	56
50 PAYER	51 PROVIDER NO.				
A					
B					
C					
57		DUE FROM PATIENT ▶			

Information to Enter	Private Insurance	Medicare	Medicaid	Workers' Compensation
Enter any prior payment amounts the facility has received toward payment of this bill.	Required, if applicable.	Required.	Required.	Not required.

Form Locator 55 – Estimated Amount Due   Purpose: Indicates the estimated amount due from the payer.

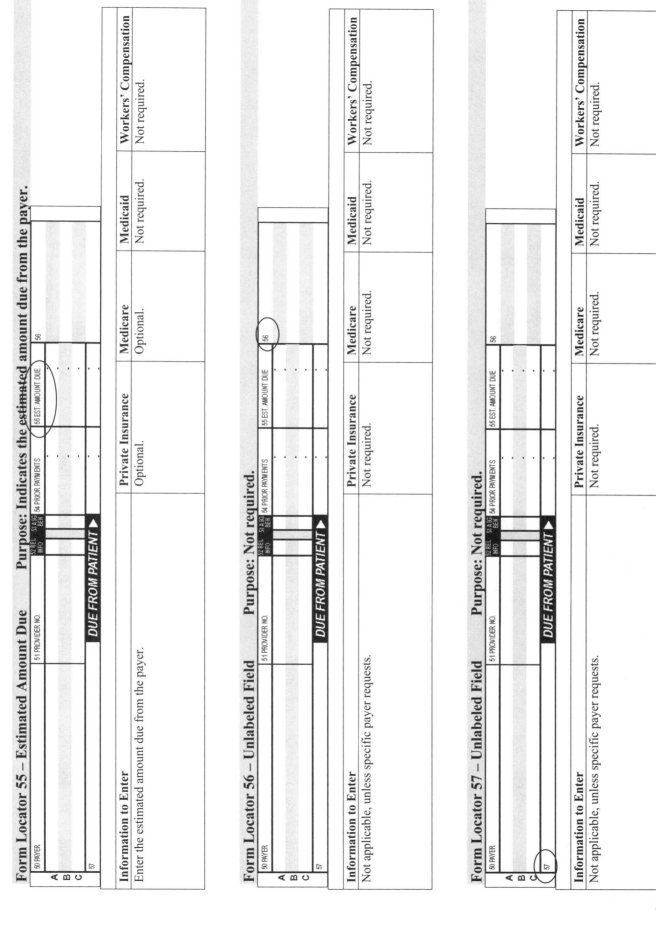

	Private Insurance	Medicare	Medicaid	Workers' Compensation
Information to Enter				
Enter the estimated amount due from the payer.	Optional.	Optional.	Not required.	Not required.

Form Locator 56 – Unlabeled Field   Purpose: Not required.

	Private Insurance	Medicare	Medicaid	Workers' Compensation
Information to Enter				
Not applicable, unless specific payer requests.	Not required.	Not required.	Not required.	Not required.

Form Locator 57 – Unlabeled Field   Purpose: Not required.

	Private Insurance	Medicare	Medicaid	Workers' Compensation
Information to Enter				
Not applicable, unless specific payer requests.	Not required.	Not required.	Not required.	Not required.

Form Locator 58 – Insured's Name   Purpose: Identifies the insured.

58 INSURED'S NAME	59 P. REL	60 CERT. - SSN - HIC. - IDNO.	61 GROUP NAME	62 INSURANCE GROUP NO.
A				A
B				B
C				C

Information to Enter	Private Insurance	Medicare	Medicaid	Workers' Compensation
Enter the insured's name (last, first name and middle initial). Do not use punctuation except a "-" for hyphenated names. Enter information on the lettered line (A, B or C) that corresponds to the line on which information is shown in Form Locator 50.	Required.	Required.	Required.	Not required.

Form Locator 59 – Patient's Relationship to Insured   Purpose: Identifies the patient's relation to insured.

58 INSURED'S NAME	59 P. REL	60 CERT. - SSN - HIC. - IDNO.	61 GROUP NAME	62 INSURANCE GROUP NO.
A				A
B				B
C				C

Information to Enter	Private Insurance	Medicare	Medicaid	Workers' Compensation
Enter the applicable code that indicates the relationship of the patient to the identified insured. Refer to Appendix C for valid codes. Enter information on the same lettered line (A, B or C) that corresponds to the line on which information is shown in Form Locator 58.	Required.	Required.	Required.	Not required.

Form Locator 60 – Certificate/Social Security/Health Insurance Claim Identification Number
Purpose: Identifies the patient to the payer.

58 INSURED'S NAME	59 P. REL	60 CERT. - SSN - HIC. - IDNO.	61 GROUP NAME	62 INSURANCE GROUP NO.
A				A
B				B
C				C

Information to Enter	Private Insurance	Medicare	Medicaid	Workers' Compensation
Enter the insured's identification number assigned by the payer organization. Enter information on the same lettered line (A, B or C) that corresponds to the line on which information is shown in Form Locator 58.	Required.	Enter their Medicare Number.	Enter the Medicaid ID Number.	Enter the patient's WC claim number, if available. If not, enter the employee's policy number or patient's SSN.

Form Locator 61 – Insured Group Name   Purpose: Identifies the plan names of payers.

58 INSURED'S NAME | 59 P. REL | 60 CERT. - SSN - HIC. - ID NO. | 61 GROUP NAME | 62 INSURANCE GROUP NO.

A
B
C

Information to Enter

Enter the group or plan name of the primary, secondary, and tertiary payer through which the coverage is provided to the insured. List in the order of priority as listed in Form Locator 58.

Private Insurance	Medicare	Medicaid	Workers' Compensation
Required.	Required.	Enter, if applicable.	Not required.

Form Locator 62 – Insurance Group Number   Purpose: Identifies the plan numbers of payers.

58 INSURED'S NAME | 59 P. REL | 60 CERT. - SSN - HIC. - ID NO. | 61 GROUP NAME | 62 INSURANCE GROUP NO.

A
B
C

Information to Enter

Enter the identification number or code assigned by the carrier or administrator to identify the group or plan under which the individual is covered.

Private Insurance	Medicare	Medicaid	Workers' Compensation
Required.	Required.	Required.	Not Required.

Form Locator 63 – Treatment Authorization Codes   Purpose: Used to determine eligibility of the current service(s).

63 TREATMENT AUTHORIZATION CODES | 64 ESC | 65 EMPLOYER NAME | 66 EMPLOYER LOCATION

A
B
C

Information to Enter

Enter the number or other indicator that designates the treatment covered by this bill that has been authorized by the payer.

Private Insurance	Medicare	Medicaid	Workers' Compensation
Enter if service(s) provided requires preauthorization.	Enter if service(s) provided requires preauthorization.	Enter if service(s) provided requires preauthorization.	Not required.

Form Locator 64 – Employment Status Code   Purpose: Identifies the insured's employment status.

63 TREATMENT AUTHORIZATION CODES	64 ESC	65 EMPLOYER NAME	66 EMPLOYER LOCATION
A			A
B			B
C			C

	Private Insurance	Medicare	Medicaid	Workers' Compensation
Information to Enter	Required.	Required.	Not required.	Required.

Enter the applicable code which defines the employment status of the individual identified in Form Locator 58. Refer to Appendix C for valid codes.

Form Locator 65 – Employer Name   Purpose: Identifies other sources of insurance. Used to determine the primary source of insurance.

63 TREATMENT AUTHORIZATION CODES	64 ESC	65 EMPLOYER NAME	66 EMPLOYER LOCATION
A			A
B			B
C			C

	Private Insurance	Medicare	Medicaid	Workers' Compensation
Information to Enter	Required.	Not required.	Not required.	Enter the business name of the employer providing Workers' Compensation insurance coverage.

Enter the name of the primary employer that provides the coverage for the insured identified in Form Locator 58 (A, B or C).

Form Locator 66 – Employer Location   Purpose: Indicates employer's address.

63 TREATMENT AUTHORIZATION CODES	64 ESC	65 EMPLOYER NAME	66 EMPLOYER LOCATION
A			A
B			B
C			C

	Private Insurance	Medicare	Medicaid	Workers' Compensation
Information to Enter	Required.	Not required.	Not required.	Enter employer's business address, city, state, and zip code.

Enter the specific location of the employer of the insured or injured individual identified in Form Locator 58.

Form Locator 67 – Principal Diagnosis Code   Purpose: Indicates diagnosis for services performed.

67 PRIN. DIAG. CD.	68 CODE	69 CODE	70 CODE	OTHER DIAG. CODES 71 CODE	72 CODE	73 CODE	74 CODE	75 CODE	76 ADM. DIAG. CD.	77 E-CODE	78

Information to Enter	Private Insurance	Medicare	Medicaid	Workers' Compensation
Enter a valid ICD-9 CM diagnosis code (including fourth and fifth digits if applicable) that describes the principal diagnosis for services rendered.	Required.	Required.	Required.	Required.

Form Locator 68-75 – Other Diagnosis Codes   Purpose: Co-existing diagnoses.

67 PRIN. DIAG. CD.	68 CODE	69 CODE	70 CODE	OTHER DIAG. CODES 71 CODE	72 CODE	73 CODE	74 CODE	75 CODE	76 ADM. DIAG. CD.	77 E-CODE	78

Information to Enter	Private Insurance	Medicare	Medicaid	Workers' Compensation
Enter a valid ICD-9 CM diagnosis code (include fourth and fifth digits if applicable) for any other conditions that co-existed at the time of admission or outpatient service or have subsequently developed, and which have an effect on the treatment. Do not duplicate the principal diagnosis listed in Form Locator 67.	Required.	Required.	Required.	Required.

Form Locator 76 – Admitting Diagnosis Code   Purpose: Indicates the diagnosis at time of admission.

67 PRIN. DIAG. CD.	68 CODE	69 CODE	70 CODE	OTHER DIAG. CODES 71 CODE	72 CODE	73 CODE	74 CODE	75 CODE	76 ADM. DIAG. CD.	77 E-CODE	78

Information to Enter	Private Insurance	Medicare	Medicaid	Workers' Compensation
Enter a valid ICD-9 CM diagnosis code (include fourth and fifth digits if applicable) that describes the diagnosis at the time of admission as stated by the physician.	Not required for outpatient bills.	Not required for outpatient bills.	Not required for outpatient bills.	Not required for outpatient bills.

Form Locator 77 – External Cause of Injury Code (E-Code)   Purpose: Indicates the external cause of injury.

| 67 PRIN. DIAG. CD. | 68 CODE | 69 CODE | 70 CODE | OTHER DIAG. CODES 71 CODE | 72 CODE | 73 CODE | 74 CODE | 75 CODE | 76 ADM. DIAG. CD. | 77 E-CODE | 78 |

Information to Enter	Private Insurance	Medicare	Medicaid	Workers' Compensation
Enter a valid ICD-9 CM diagnosis code (include fourth and fifth digits if applicable) for the external cause of injury, poisoning, or adverse effect.	Required, if applicable.	Not required.	Required, if applicable.	Required, if applicable.

Form Locator 78 – Unlabeled Field   Purpose: Not applicable.

| 67 PRIN. DIAG. CD. | 68 CODE | 69 CODE | 70 CODE | OTHER DIAG. CODES 71 CODE | 72 CODE | 73 CODE | 74 CODE | 75 CODE | 76 ADM. DIAG. CD. | 77 E-CODE | 78 |

Information to Enter	Private Insurance	Medicare	Medicaid	Workers' Compensation
Reserved for national use.	Not required.	Not required.	Not required.	Not required.

Form Locator 79 – Procedure Coding Method Used   Purpose: Identifies the coding system used to fill out the claim.

| 79 PC | 80 | PRINCIPAL PROCEDURE CODE | DATE | 81 | OTHER PROCEDURE CODE | DATE | OTHER PROCEDURE CODE A | DATE | OTHER PROCEDURE CODE B | DATE |
| | | OTHER PROCEDURE CODE C | DATE | | OTHER PROCEDURE CODE D | DATE | OTHER PROCEDURE CODE E | DATE | | |

Information to Enter	Private Insurance	Medicare	Medicaid	Workers' Compensation
Please denote the medical coding system used to complete the claim form. If ICD-9 CM codes are used in Form Locators 80–81, enter a 9.	Required.	Not required.	Enter a 9.	Required.

Form Locator 80 – Principal Procedure Code and Date   Purpose: Indicates the principal surgical procedure.

Private Insurance	Medicare	Medicaid	Workers' Compensation
Required.	Required.	Required.	Required.

Information to Enter
Enter a valid ICD-9 CM code (from Volume 3) and date (in the MMDDYY format) identifying the principal or obstetrical procedure performed during the statement from and through dates. It is a procedure most closely related to the principal diagnosis in Form Locator 67.

Form Locator 81 – Other Procedure Code/Date   Purpose: Other procedure codes and dates.

Private Insurance	Medicare	Medicaid	Workers' Compensation
Required.	Required.	Required.	Required.

Information to Enter
Enter additional ICD-9 CM codes (from Volume 3) and dates (in the MMDDYY format) to identify the significant procedures performed during the period covered by the bill.

Form Locator 82 – Attending Physician Identification Number   Purpose: Identifies the attending physician.

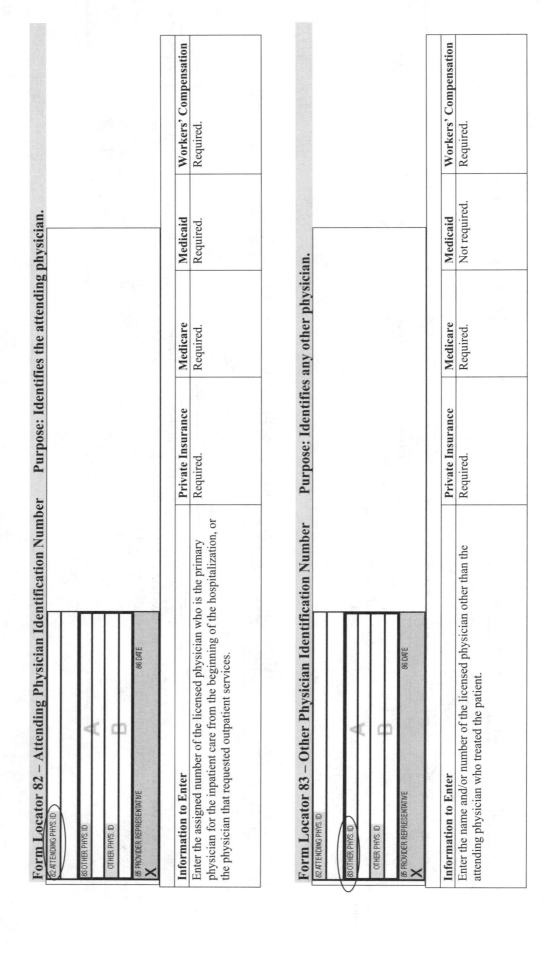

Information to Enter	Private Insurance	Medicare	Medicaid	Workers' Compensation
Enter the assigned number of the licensed physician who is the primary physician for the inpatient care from the beginning of the hospitalization, or the physician that requested outpatient services.	Required.	Required.	Required.	Required.

Form Locator 83 – Other Physician Identification Number   Purpose: Identifies any other physician.

Information to Enter	Private Insurance	Medicare	Medicaid	Workers' Compensation
Enter the name and/or number of the licensed physician other than the attending physician who treated the patient.	Required.	Required.	Not required.	Required.

Form Locator 84 – Remarks Purpose: Indicates any special remarks to be communicated.

a	84 REMARKS
b	
c	
d	

Information to Enter	Private Insurance	Medicare	Medicaid	Workers' Compensation
Enter any additional information to be communicated to the third-party payer.	Required, where applicable.	Required, where applicable.	Required, where applicable.	Required, where applicable.

Form Locator 85 – Provider Representative Purpose: Identifies the person that authorized the billing of the claim.

Information to Enter	Private Insurance	Medicare	Medicaid	Workers' Compensation
Enter the signature of an authorized representative verifying that the physician's certification is in effect. A stamp of the provider's signature is acceptable.	Required.	Required.	Required.	Required.

Form Locator 86 – Date Purpose: Indicates the date bill was signed, or the date the bill was submitted to the payer.

Information to Enter	Private Insurance	Medicare	Medicaid	Workers' Compensation
Enter the date, in the MMDDYY format, the bill was signed, or the date submitted to the payer.	Required.	Required.	Required.	Required.

UB-92 Sample Claims

Figure AE–1 is a completed UB-92 for Abby Addison, who has private insurance through her employer Red Corporation. Abby was treated at Provider Medical Center for hypertension. She was referred to the emergency room by her physician because her blood pressure was highly elevated. She was subsequently admitted at 12:00 P.M. on 05/07/CCYY, and discharged home at 1:00 P.M. on 05/09/CCYY. Rover Insurers Inc. was notified of the admission and authorized the hospital stay. The precertification number is 4762189. The attending physician was Dr. Paul Provider. Her patient control number assigned by the hospital is 028705, and her medical record number is 057820. The total charge for services is $2,903.80.

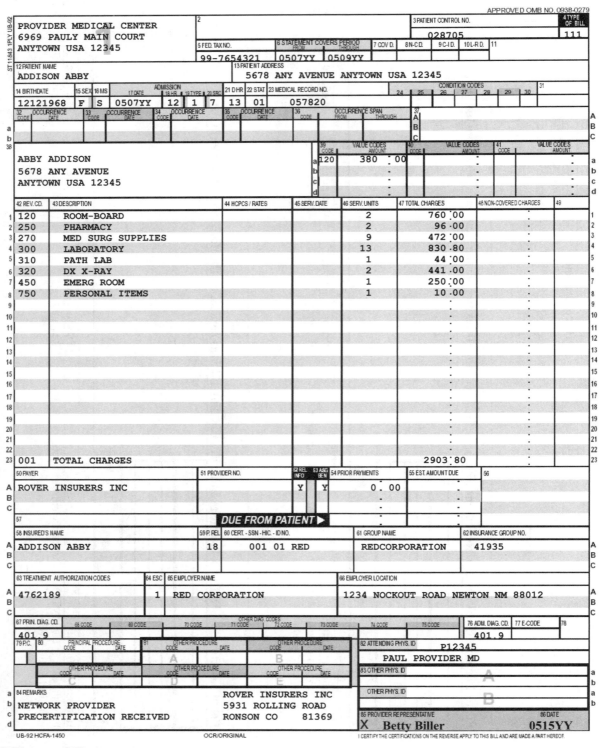

■ Figure AE–1 Private Insurance Claim

Figure AE–2 is a completed UB-92 for Edward Edmunds, who has Medicare coverage. Edward was treated outpatient at Provider Medical Center on 04/05/CCYY, for coronary artery disease. The patient had a combined right heart catherization and transsep- tal left heart catherization through intact septum. The attending physician was Dr. Paul Provider. His patient control number assigned by the hospital is 251321, and his medical record number is 123152. The total charge for services is $1,319.00.

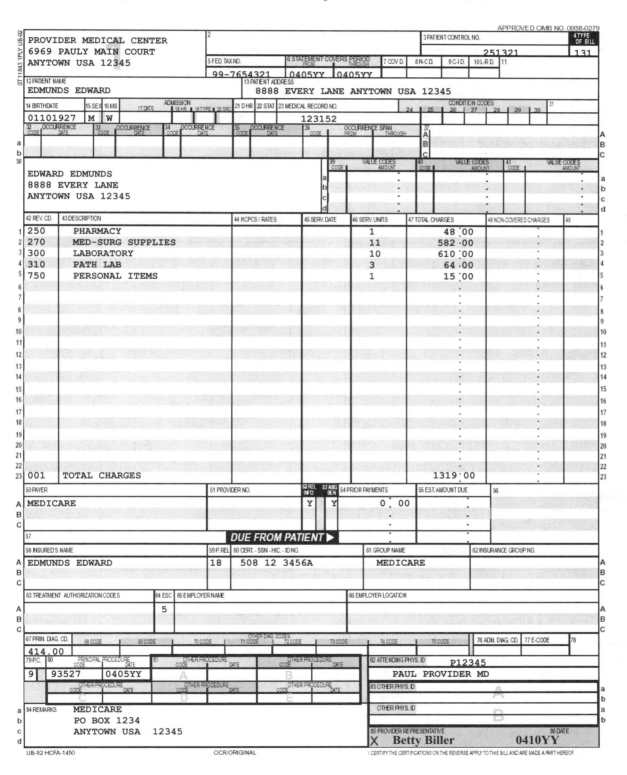

■ **Figure AE–2** Medicare Claim

Figure AE–3 is a completed UB-92 for Daisy Doolittle, who is covered under Medicaid. Daisy was treated outpatient at Provider Medical Center on 08/07/CCYY, for congenital hypothyroidism. The patient had a biopsy of the thyroid, percutaneous core needle. The attending physician was Dr. Paul Provider. Her patient control number assigned by the hospital is 307519, and her medical record number is 915703. The total charge for services is $844.90.

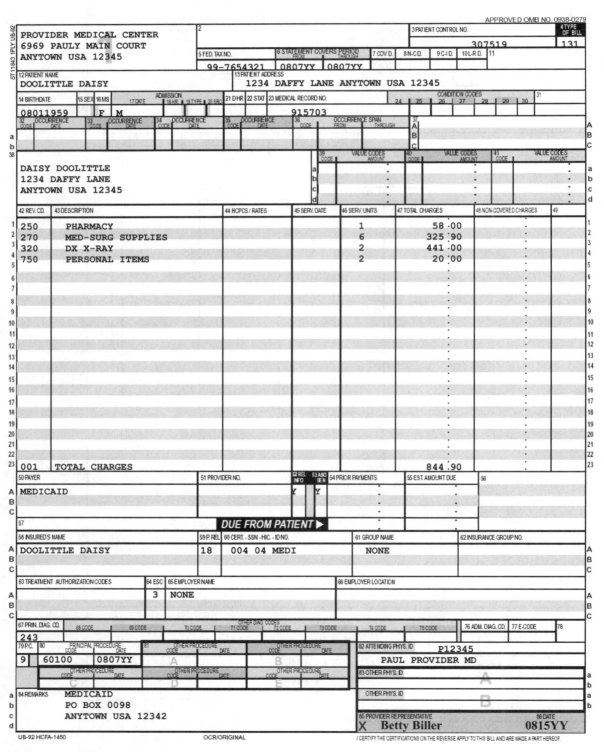

Figure AE–3 Medicaid Claim

Figure AE–4 is a completed UB-92 for Bobby Bumble, who was injured at work and is being treated under his employer's workers' compensation insurance. He was sent to the hospital by his employer because of a slip and fall. Bobby was treated in the emergency room at Provider Medical Center for a concussion, and foreign body in the eyes and nose. He was subsequently admitted at 3:00 P.M. on 10/16/CCYY, and discharged home at 4:00 P.M. on 10/19/CCYY. The attending physician was Dr. Joanna Jones. His patient control number assigned by the hospital is 122709, and his medical record number is 907221. The total charge for services is $2,622.00.

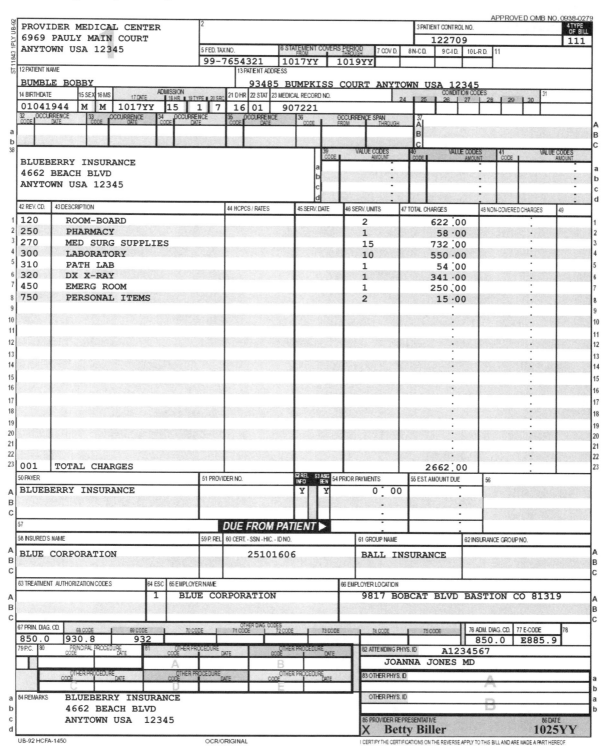

■ **Figure AE–4** Worker's Compensation Claim

UB-92 to UB-04 Crosswalk

The NUBC has recommended that the healthcare industry adopt the following timeline for the transition to the new UB-04. The UB-04 will retain the CMS-1450 designation.

- March 1, 2007 through May 22, 2007: Providers that use paper forms for claim submission will be able to submit either the UB-92 or the UB-04 form.

- May 23, 2007: Discontinued acceptance of the UB-92 form.

These guidelines are recommendations only and the health plan or clearinghouse should be consulted prior to submitting a claim on the revised form.

UB-92 to UB-04 CROSSWALK

	UB-92					**UB-04**					

*FL68,75,80 Size Updated 6/21/05
** FL07, 30 Size Updated 12/15/05

FL	Description	Line	Type	Size	FL	Description	Line	Type	Size	Buffer Space	Notes
FL01	Provider Name	1	AN	25	FL01	Provider Name	1	AN	25		
FL01	Provider Street Address	2	AN	25	FL01	Provider Street Address	2	AN	25		
FL01	Provider City, State, Zip	3	AN	25	FL01	Provider City, State, Zip	3	AN	25		
FL01	Provider Telephone, Fax, Country Code	4	AN	25	FL01	Provider Telephone, Fax, Country Code	4	AN	25		
FL02	Unlabeled Fields	1	AN	20	FL02	Pay-to Name	1	AN	25		New
FL02	Unlabeled Fields	2	AN	30	FL02	Pay-to Address	2	AN	25		New
					FL02	Pay-to City, State	3	AN	25		New
					FL02	Pay-to ID	4	AN	25		New
FL03	Patient Control Number	1	AN	20	FL03a	Patient Control Number		AN	24		
					FL03b	Medical Record Number		AN	24		Moved/New
FL04	Type of Bill	1	AN	3	FL04	Type of Bill	1	AN	4	1	Expanded
FL05	Federal Tax Number	1	AN	4	FL05	Federal Tax Number	1	AN	4		
FL05	Federal Tax Number	2	AN	10	FL05	Federal Tax Number	2	AN	10		
FL06	Statement Covers Period - From/Through	1	N/N	6/6	FL06	Statement Covers Period - From/Through	1	N/N	6/6	1/1	
					FL07	Unlabeled	1	AN	7**		
							2	AN	8**		
FL07	Covered Days	1	N	3		*Eliminated - Substitute new Value Code*					
FL08	Non-covered Days	1	N	4		*Eliminated - Substitute new Value Code*					
FL09	Coinsurance Days	1	N	3		*Eliminated - Substitute new Value Code*					
FL10	Lifetime Reserve Days	1	N	3		*Eliminated - Substitute new Value Code*					
FL11	Unlabeled	1		12		*Eliminated*					
FL11	Unlabeled	2		13		*Eliminated*					
FL12	Patient Name	1	AN	30	FL08	Patient Name - ID	1a	AN	19		New
					FL08	Patient Name	2b	AN	29		
FL13	Patient Address	1	AN	50	FL09	Patient Address - Street	1a	AN	40	1	Discrete
					FL09	Patient Address - City	2b	AN	30	2	Discrete
					FL09	Patient Address - State	2c	AN	2	1	Discrete
					FL09	Patient Address - ZIP	2d	AN	9	1	Discrete
					FL09	Patient Address - Country Code	2e	AN	3		Discrete
FL14	Patient Birthdate	1	N	8	FL10	Patient Birthdate	1	N	8	1	
FL15	Patient Sex	1	AN	1	FL11	Patient Sex	1	AN	1	2	
FL16	Patient Marital Status	1	AN	1		*Eliminated*					
FL17	Admission Date	1	N	6	FL12	Admission Date	1	N	6		
FL18	Admission Hour	1	AN	2	FL13	Admission Hour	1	AN	2	1	
FL19	Type of Admission/Visit	1	AN	1	FL14	Type of Admission/Visit	1	AN	1	2	
FL20	Source of Admission	1	AN	1	FL15	Source of Admission	1	AN	1	1	
FL21	Discharge Hour	1	AN	2	FL16	Discharge Hour	1	AN	2	2	
FL22	Patient Status/Discharge Code	1	AN	2	FL17	Patient Discharge Status	1	AN	2	2	
FL23	Medical/Health Record Number		AN	17		*Moved to FL3b*					
FL24	Condition Codes		AN	2	FL18	Condition Codes		AN	2	1	
FL25	Condition Codes		AN	2	FL19	Condition Codes		AN	2	1	
					FL20	Condition Codes		AN	2	1	

■ **Table AE–2** UB-92 Crosswalk

* FL68,75,80 Size Updated 6/21/05
** FL07, 30 Size Updated 12/15/05

UB-92

FL	Description	Line	Type	Size
FL26	Condition Codes		AN	2
FL27	Condition Codes		AN	2
FL28	Condition Codes		AN	2
FL29	Condition Codes		AN	2
FL30	Condition Codes		AN	2
FL31	Unlabeled	1		5
FL31	Unlabeled	2		6
FL32	Occurrence Code/Date	a	AN/N	2/6
FL32	Occurrence Code/Date	b	AN/N	2/6
FL33	Occurrence Code/Date	a	AN	2/6
FL33	Occurrence Code/Date	b	AN/N	2/6
FL34	Occurrence Code/Date	a	AN	2/6
FL34	Occurrence Code/Date	b	AN/N	2/6
FL35	Occurrence Code/Date	a	AN	2/6
FL35	Occurrence Code/Date	b	AN/N	2/6
FL36	Occurrence Span Code/From/Through	a	AN/N/N	2/6/6
FL36	Occurrence Span Code/From/Through	b	AN/N/N	2/6/6
FL37	ICN/DCN	A	AN	23
FL37	ICN/DCN	B	AN	23
FL37	ICN/DCN	C	AN	23
FL38	Responsible Party Name/Address	1	AN	40
FL38	Responsible Party Name/Address	2	AN	40
FL38	Responsible Party Name/Address	3	AN	40
FL38	Responsible Party Name/Address	4	AN	40
FL38	Responsible Party Name/Address	5	AN	40
FL39	Value Code - Code	a	AN	2
FL39	Value Code - Amount	a	N	9
FL39	Value Code - Code	b	AN	2
FL39	Value Code - Amount	b	N	9
FL39	Value Code - Code	c	AN	2
FL39	Value Code - Amount	c	N	9
FL39	Value Code - Code	d	AN	2
FL39	Value Code - Amount	d	N	9
FL40	Value Code - Code	a	AN	2
FL40	Value Code - Amount	a	N	9
FL40	Value Code - Code	b	AN	2
FL40	Value Code - Amount	b	N	9
FL40	Value Code - Code	c	AN	2
FL40	Value Code - Amount	c	N	9
FL40	Value Code - Code	d	AN	2
FL40	Value Code - Amount	d	N	9
FL41	Value Code - Code	a	AN	2
FL41	Value Code - Amount	a	N	9

UB-04

FL	Description	Line	Type	Size	Buffer Space	Notes
FL21	Condition Codes		AN	2	1	
FL22	Condition Codes		AN	2	1	
FL23	Condition Codes		AN	2	1	
FL24	Condition Codes		AN	2	1	
FL25	Condition Codes		AN	2	1	
FL26	Condition Codes		AN	2	1	New
FL27	Condition Codes		AN	2	1	New
FL28	Condition Codes		AN	2	1	New
FL29	Accident State	1	AN	2	1	New
FL30	Unlabeled	1	AN	12		** No "Xs" on proof
FL30	Unlabeled	2	AN	13		
FL31	Occurrence Code/Date	a	AN/N	2/6	1/1	
FL31	Occurrence Code/Date	b	AN/N	2/6	1/1	
FL32	Occurrence Code/Date	a	AN/N	2/6	1/1	
FL32	Occurrence Code/Date	b	AN/N	2/6	1/1	
FL33	Occurrence Code/Date	a	AN/N	2/6	1/1	
FL33	Occurrence Code/Date	b	AN/N	2/6	1/1	
FL34	Occurrence Code/Date	a	AN/N	2/6	1/1	
FL34	Occurrence Code/Date	b	AN/N	2/6	1/1	
FL35	Occurrence Span Code/From/Through	a	AN/N/N	2/6/6	1/1/1	
FL35	Occurrence Span Code/From/Through	b	AN/N/N	2/6/6	1/1/1	
FL36	Occurrence Span Code/From/Through	a	AN/N/N	2/6/6	1/1/1	New
FL36	Occurrence Span Code/From/Through	b	AN/N/N	2/6/6	1/1/1	New
FL37	Unlabeled	a	AN	8		
FL37	Unlabeled	b	AN	8		
Moved to FL64						Relocated
Moved to FL64						
Moved to FL64						
FL38	Responsible Party Name/Address	1	AN	40	2	
FL38	Responsible Party Name/Address	2	AN	40	2	
FL38	Responsible Party Name/Address	3	AN	40	2	
FL38	Responsible Party Name/Address	4	AN	40	2	
FL38	Responsible Party Name/Address	5	AN	40	2	
FL39	Value Code - Code	a	AN	2	1	
FL39	Value Code - Amount	a	N	9	1	
FL39	Value Code - Code	b	AN	2	1	
FL39	Value Code - Amount	b	N	9	1	
FL39	Value Code - Code	c	AN	2	1	
FL39	Value Code - Amount	c	N	9	1	
FL39	Value Code - Code	d	AN	2	1	
FL39	Value Code - Amount	d	N	9	1	
FL40	Value Code - Code	a	AN	2	1	
FL40	Value Code - Amount	a	N	9	1	
FL40	Value Code - Code	b	AN	2	1	
FL40	Value Code - Amount	b	N	9	1	
FL40	Value Code - Code	c	AN	2	1	
FL40	Value Code - Amount	c	N	9	1	
FL40	Value Code - Code	d	AN	2	1	
FL40	Value Code - Amount	d	N	9	1	
FL41	Value Code - Code	a	AN	2	1	
FL41	Value Code - Amount	a	N	9	1	

* FL68,75,80 Size Updated 6/21/05
** FL07, 30 Size Updated 12/15/05

	UB-92					UB-04				Buffer	
FL	Description	Line	Type	Size		FL	Description	Line	Type	Size	Space Notes
FL41	Value Code - Code	b	AN	2		FL41	Value Code - Code	b	AN	2	1
FL41	Value Code - Amount	b	N	9		FL41	Value Code - Amount	b	N	9	1
FL41	Value Code - Code	c	AN	2		FL41	Value Code - Code	c	AN	2	1
FL41	Value Code - Amount	c	N	9		FL41	Value Code - Amount	c	N	9	1
FL41	Value Code - Code	d	AN	2		FL41	Value Code - Code	d	AN	2	1
FL41	Value Code - Amount	d	N	9		FL41	Value Code - Amount	d	N	9	1
FL42	Revenue Code	1-23	N	4		FL42	Revenue Code	1-23	N	4	0.5
FL43	Revenue Code Description	1-23	AN	24		FL43	Revenue Code Description	1-22	AN	24	0.5
						FL43-44	PAGE ___ OF ___ CREATION DATE	23	N/N	3/3	0.5 New
FL44	HCPCS/Rates/HIPPS Rate Codes	1-23	AN/N/AN	9		FL44	HCPCS/Rates/HIPPS Rate Codes	1-22	AN/N/AN	14	0.5 Expanded size
FL45	Service Date	1-23	N	6		FL45	Service Date	1-22	N	6	0.5
						FL45	Creation Date	23	N	6	0.5 New
FL46	Units of Service	1-23	N	7		FL46	Units of Service	1-22	N	7	0.5
FL47	Total Charges	1-23	N	10		FL47	Total Charges	1-23	N	9	0.5 Removed sign field
FL48	Non-Covered Charges	1-23	N	10		FL48	Non-Covered Charges	1-23	N	9	0.5 Removed sign field
FL49	Unlabeled	1-23	AN	4		FL49	Unlabeled	1-23	AN	2	0.5
FL50	Payer - Primary	A	AN	25		FL50	Payer Name - Primary	A	AN	23	
FL50	Payer - Secondary	B	AN	25		FL50	Payer Name - Secondary	B	AN	23	
FL50	Payer - Tertiary	C	AN	25		FL50	Payer Name - Tertiary	C	AN	23	
FL51	Provider Number	A	AN	13		FL51	Health Plan ID	A	AN	15	
FL51	Provider Number	B	AN	13		FL51	Health Plan ID	B	AN	15	
FL51	Provider Number	C	AN	13		FL51	Health Plan ID	C	AN	15	
FL52	Release of Information - Primary	A	AN	1		FL52	Release of Information - Primary	A	AN	1	1
FL52	Release of Information - Secondary	B	AN	1		FL52	Release of Information - Secondary	B	AN	1	1
FI52	Release of Information - Tertiary	C	AN	1		FL52	Release of Information - Tertiary	C	AN	1	1
FL53	Assignment of Benefits - Primary	A	AN	1		FL53	Assignment of Benefits - Primary	A	AN	1	1
FL53	Assignment of Benefits - Secondary	B	AN	1		FL53	Assignment of Benefits - Secondary	B	AN	1	1
FL53	Assignment of Benefits - Tertiary	C	AN	1		FL53	Assignment of Benefits - Tertiary	C	AN	1	1
FL54	Prior Payments - Primary	A	N	10		FL54	Prior Payments - Primary	A	N	10	1
FL54	Prior Payments - Secondary	B	N	10		FL54	Prior Payments - Secondary	B	N	10	1
FL54	Prior Payments - Tertiary	C	N	10		FL54	Prior Payments - Tertiary	C	N	10	1
FL54	Prior Payments - Patient	4	N	10			Eliminated Patient Prior Payments				
FL55	Estimated Amount Due - Primary	A	N	10		FL55	Estimated Amount Due - Primary	A	N	10	1
FL55	Estimated Amount Due - Secondary	B	N	10		FL55	Estimated Amount Due - Secondary	B	N	10	1
FL55	Estimated Amount Due - Tertiary	C	N	10		FL55	Estimated Amount Due - Tertiary	C	N	10	1
FL55	Estimated Amount Due - Patient	4	N	10			Eliminated Due from Patient				
FL56	Unlabeled	1		13		FL56	NPI	1	AN	15	
FL56	Unlabeled	2		14		FL57	Other Provider ID - Primary	A	AN	15	
						FL57	Other Provider ID - Secondary	B	AN	15	
						FL57	Other Provider ID - Tertiary	C	AN	15	
FL57	Unlabeled	1		27			Deleted from UB-04				
FL58	Insured's Name - Primary	A	AN	25		FL58	Insured's Name - Primary	A	AN	25	1
FL58	Insured's Name - Secondary	B	AN	25		FL58	Insured's Name - Secondary	B	AN	25	1
FL58	Insured's Name - Tertiary	C	AN	25		FL58	Insured's Name - Tertiary	C	AN	25	1
FL59	Patient's Relationship - Primary	A	AN	2		FL59	Patient's Relationship - Primary	A	AN	2	1
FL59	Patient's Relationship - Secondary	B	AN	2		FL59	Patient's Relationship - Secondary	B	AN	2	1

*FL68,75,80 Size Updated 6/21/05
**FL07, 30 Size Updated 12/15/05

	UB-92						**UB-04**				Buffer	
FL	**Description**	**Line**	**Type**	**Size**		**FL**	**Description**	**Line**	**Type**	**Size**	**Space**	**Notes**
FL59	Patient's Relationship -Tertiary	C	AN	2		FL59	Patient's Relationship - Tertiary	C	AN	2	1	
FL60	CERT./ SSN/ HIC/ ID NO. - Primary	A	AN	19		FL60	Insured's Unique ID - Primary	A	AN	20		
FL60	CERT./ SSN/ HIC/ ID NO.- Secondary	B	AN	19		FL60	Insured's Unique ID - Secondary	B	AN	20		
FL60	CERT./ SSN/ HIC/ ID NO. - Tertiary	C	AN	19		FL60	Insured's Unique ID - Tertiary	C	AN	20		
FL61	Insurance Group Name - Primary	A	AN	14		FL61	Insurance Group Name - Primary	A	AN	14	1	
FL61	Insurance Group Name -Secondary	B	AN	14		FL61	Insurance Group Name -Secondary	B	AN	14	1	
FL61	Insurance Group Name - Tertiary	C	AN	14		FL61	Insurance Group Name - Tertiary	C	AN	14	1	
FL62	Insurance Group Number - Primary	A	AN	17		FL62	Insurance Group Number - Primary	A	AN	17	1	
FL62	Insurance Group Number - Secondary	B	AN	17		FL62	Insurance Group Number - Secondary	B	AN	17	1	
FL62	Insurance Group Number - Tertiary	C	AN	17		FL62	Insurance Group Number - Tertiary	C	AN	17	1	
FL63	Treatment Authorization Code - Primary	A	AN	18		FL63	Treatment Authorization Code - Primary	A	AN	30	1	
FL63	Treatment Authorization Code - Secondary	B	AN	18		FL63	Treatment Authorization Code - Secondary	B	AN	30	1	
FL63	Treatment Authorization Code - Tertiary	C	AN	18		FL63	Treatment Authorization Code - Tertiary	C	AN	30	1	
						FL64	Document Control Number	A	AN	26		
						FL64	Document Control Number	B	AN	26		
						FL64	Document Control Number	C	AN	26		
FL64	Employment Status Code - Primary	A	N	1			*Deleted from UB-04*					
FL64	Employment Status Code - Secondary	B	N	1			*Deleted from UB-04*					
FL64	Employment Status Code - Tertiary	C	N	1			*Deleted from UB-04*					
FL65	Employer Name - Primary	A	N	24		FL65	Employer Name - Primary	A	AN	25		
FL65	Employer Name - Secondary	B	N	24		FL65	Employer Name - Secondary	B	AN	25		
FL65	Employer Name - Tertiary	C	N	24		FL65	Employer Name - Tertiary	C	AN	25		
FL66	Employer Location - Primary	A	AN	35			*Deleted from UB-04*					
FL66	Employer Location - Secondary	B	AN	35			*Deleted from UB-04*					
FL66	Employer Locations -Tertiary	C	AN	35			*Deleted from UB-04*					
						FL66	DX Version Qualifier		AN	1		New Denotes ICD v.
FL67	Principal Diagnosis Code	1	AN	6		FL67	Principal Diagnosis Code		AN	8		Expanded field
FL68	Other Diagnoses	1	AN	6		FL67A	Other Diagnosis		AN	8		Expanded field
FL69	Other Diagnoses	1	AN	6		FL67B	Other Diagnosis		AN	8		Expanded field
FL70	Other Diagnoses	1	AN	6		FL67C	Other Diagnosis		AN	8		Expanded field
FL71	Other Diagnoses	1	AN	6		FL67D	Other Diagnosis		AN	8		Expanded field
FL72	Other Diagnoses	1	AN	6		FL67E	Other Diagnosis		AN	8		Expanded field
FL73	Other Diagnoses	1	AN	6		FL67F	Other Diagnosis		AN	8		Expanded field
FL74	Other Diagnoses	1	AN	6		FL67G	Other Diagnosis		AN	8		Expanded field
FL75	Other Diagnoses	1	AN	6		FL67H	Other Diagnosis		AN	8		Expanded field
						FL67I	Other Diagnosis		AN	8		New
						FL67J	Other Diagnosis		AN	8		New
						FL67K	Other Diagnosis		AN	8		New
						FL67L	Other Diagnosis		AN	8		New
						FL67M	Other Diagnosis		AN	8		New
						FL67N	Other Diagnosis		AN	8		New
						FL67O	Other Diagnosis		AN	8		New
						FL67P	Other Diagnosis		AN	8		New
						FL67Q	Other Diagnosis		AN	8		New
						FL68	Unlabeled	1a	AN	8*		
						FL68	Unlabeled	1b	AN	9*		
FL76	Admitting Diagnosis/Patient's Reason for Visit	1	AN	6		FL69	Admitting Diagnosis Code	1	AN	7		Expanded by 1
						FL70	Patient's Reason for Visit Code	A	AN	7		Distinct FL
						FL70	Patient's Reason for Visit Code	B	AN	7		Distinct FL
						FL70	Patient's Reason for Visit Code	C	AN	7		Distinct FL

UB-92						UB-04					

*FL68,75,80 Size Updated 6/21/05
**FL07, 30 Size Updated 12/15/05

FL	Description	Line	Type	Size		FL	Description	Line	Type	Size	Buffer Space	Notes
						FL71	PPS Code	1	AN	3	2	New
FL77	External Cause of Injury Code	1	AN	6		FL72	External Cause of Injury Code	1a	AN	8		
						FL72	External Cause of Injury Code	1b	AN	8		New
						FL72	External Cause of Injury Code	1c	AN	8		New
FL78	Unlabeled					FL73	Unlabeled	1	AN	9		
FL79	Procedure Coding Method Used	1	N	1			*Deleted from UB-04*					Deleted
FL80	Principal Procedure Code/Date	1	N/N	6/6		FL74	Principal Procedure Code/Date		N/N	7/6	1/1	Expanded by 1
FL81	Other Procedure Code/Date	A	N/N	6/6		FL74a	Other Procedure Code/Date		N/N	7/6	1/1	Expanded by 1
FL81	Other Procedure Code/Date	B	N/N	6/6		FL74b	Other Procedure Code/Date		N/N	7/6	1/1	Expanded by 1
FL81	Other Procedure Code/Date	C	N/N	6/6		FL74c	Other Procedure Code/Date		N/N	7/6	1/1	Expanded by 1
FL81	Other Procedure Code/Date	D	N/N	6/6		FL74d	Other Procedure Code/Date		N/N	7/6	1/1	Expanded by 1
FL81	Other Procedure Code/Date	E	N/N	6/6		FL74e	Other Procedure Code/Date		N/N	7/6	1/1	Expanded by 1
						FL75	Unlabeled	1	AN	4*	0*	
						FL75	Unlabeled	2	AN	4	1	
						FL75	Unlabeled	3	AN	4	1	
						FL75	Unlabeled	4	AN	4	1	
FL82	Attending Physician ID	a	AN	23		FL76	Attending - NPI/QUAL/ID	1	AN/AN/AN	11/2/9		New Layout
FL82	Attending Physician ID	b	AN	32		FL76	Attending - Last/First	2	AN/AN	16/12		New Layout
FL83A	Other Physician ID	a	AN	25		FL77	Operating - NPI/QUAL/ID	1	AN/AN/AN	11/2/9		New Layout
FL83A	Other Physician ID	b	AN	32		FL77	Operating - Last/First	2	AN/AN	16/12		New Layout
FL83B	Other Physician ID	a	AN	25		FL78	Other ID - QUAL/NPI/QUAL/ID	1	AN/AN/ AN/AN	2/11/2/9		New Layout
FL83B	Other Physician ID	b	AN	32		FL78	Other ID - Last/First	2	AN/AN	16/12		New Layout
						FL79	Other ID - QUAL/NPI/QUAL/ID	1	AN/AN/ AN/AN	2/11/2/9		New
						FL79	Other ID - Last/First	2	AN/AN	16/12		New
FL84	Remarks	1	AN	43		FL80	Remarks	1	AN	19*		Reduced Field Size
FL84	Remarks	2	AN	48		FL80	Remarks	2	AN	24*		Reduced Field Size
FL84	Remarks	3	AN	48		FL80	Remarks	3	AN	24*		Reduced Field Size
FL84	Remarks	4	AN	48		FL80	Remarks	4	AN	24*		Reduced Field Size
						FL81	Code-Code - QUAL/CODE/VALUE	a	AN/AN/AN	2/10/12		New
						FL81	Code-Code - QUAL/CODE/VALUE	b	AN/AN/AN	2/10/12		New
						FL81	Code-Code - QUAL/CODE/VALUE	c	AN/AN/AN	2/10/12		New
						FL81	Code-Code - QUAL/CODE/VALUE	d	AN/AN/AN	2/10/12		New
FL85	Provider Rep. Signature	1	AN	22			*Deleted from UB-04*					
FL86	Date Bill Submitted	1	Date	6			*Deleted from UB-04; See FL45, line 23*					

Glossary

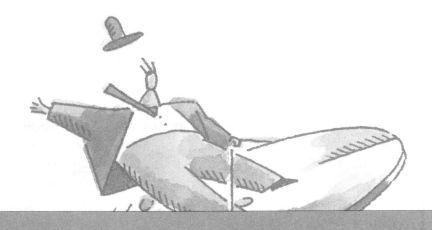

1500 Health Insurance Claim Form—An insurance claim form approved by the National Uniform Claim Committee (NUCC) in November 2005. It will replace the CMS-1500.

Accident—An unintentional injury that has a specific time, date, and place.

Accounting Control Summary—A weekly or monthly report form that shows each day's charges, payments, and adjustments for the period indicated.

Accounts Payable—Money paid out, usually for goods or services.

Accounts Receivable—Money being received by a business.

Acknowledgment Report—Reports generated by an insurance carrier indicating claims that were received electronically.

Active Member Roster—Lists those patients whose HMO coverage has continued into the next month.

Actively at Work—A provision that states that a person must be at work (or actively engaged in their normal activities, if a dependent) on the date coverage becomes effective. If he or she is not at work or actively engaged in their normal activities, the contract does not become effective until the employee or dependent returns to work.

Adjustments—Changes that can either increase or decrease the remaining balance.

Advance Beneficiary Notice (ABN)—A written notice a provider gives a Medicare beneficiary before rendering services, which informs a patient that a particular procedure may not be considered medically necessary by Medicare, and that if payment is denied by Medicare, the patient will be responsible for paying for the procedure.

Aggregate Deductible—A deductible that requires all major medical deductibles applied for all family members be added together to attain the family limit.

Air Ambulance—A helicopter or other flight vehicle used to transport severely injured or ill persons to a hospital.

Allowable Expense—Any necessary, reasonable, and customary item of medical or dental expense, at least partly covered under at least one of the plans covering the patient.

Allowed Amount—What the insurance company considers to be a reasonable charge for the procedure performed, often less than the amount which the doctor bills.

Alphabetical Filing—Filing medical charts alphabetically by the first letter of the patient's last name.

Alter—Change or amend the information contained in a record or chart.

Ambulatory Patient Classifications (APCs)—Similar to DRGs but are for patients who receive services on an outpatient basis.

Assignment of Benefits Form—A form requesting all insurance payments to be directed to the provider holding the assignment.

Audits—Performed to prevent and detect fraud.

Authorized Treatment Record Form—A form used to track the usage of preauthorized services rendered by a provider's office.

Balance Billing—Sending an additional bill to another party for payment of any remaining amounts on a claim.

Bankruptcy—The act whereby a debtor announces they no longer have the ability to pay creditors and asks relief from the federal courts.

Base Call Charge—The amount automatically charged for an ambulance to respond to a call even if the patient is not subsequently transported.

Basic Benefits—Benefits that are usually paid at 100% and are paid before major medical benefits are paid.

Benefit Period—A period that begins on the first day of admission to the hospital and ends 60 days after the patient has been discharged from the hospital.

Benign—Localized growth that does not spread (metastasize) and is not usually terminal.

Bilateral Procedures—Surgeries that involve a pair of similar body parts (i.e., breasts, eyes).

Binding Machine—Binds several pages of a document together, often with a strip down the left–hand side of the document.

Biofeedback—Training a person to consciously control automatic, internal body functions.

Block Procedures—Multiple surgical procedures performed during the same operative session, in the same operative area.

Body—The place in a correspondence where you present the purpose of the communication.

Bonding—The process by which an employer can be indemnified for the loss of money or other property sustained through dishonest acts of a "bonded" employee.

Brightness Control—A knob that changes the brightness of the image on the screen.

Calculator—A machine that computes numbers.

Cancer in Situ—Means that the malignant growth is still localized in one area and has not spread.

Capitation—A monthly payment made to a provider in exchange for providing the healthcare needs of a member.

Carrier—Private insurance company that processes Medicare's Part B claims.

Carryover Provision—Any amounts that the patient pays toward their deductible in the last three months of the year will carry over and will be applied toward the next year's deductible.

Categorically Needy—People who usually make less than the poverty level every month.

Center for Medicare and Medicaid Services (CMS)—The organization that oversees the Medicare and Medicaid programs.

Central Processing Unit (CPU)—The rectangular box that houses the memory and functional components of the computer.

Certified Mail—A package or envelope that must be signed for on delivery.

Chemotherapy Drugs—Drugs administered to help fight cancer and other serious diseases.

Children's Chart—A medical file specifically for children.

Claim—A bill for services rendered by a provider.

Claim Attachment—Any document providing additional medical information to the claims payer that cannot be accommodated within the standard billing form.

Claims Register—A database that lists all claims created by a practice. This database can usually be sorted by date, doctor, or patient name.

Claims Submission Report—A report that lists all claims that have been fully completed and are being submitted to the insurance carrier by the provider's office.

Claims Audit—An analysis of claims payments made to a healthcare provider to determine whether the claims were allowable and whether the provider was paid the appropriate amount for services rendered.

Clarity in Writing—Exactness of language.

Clean Claims—Claims that have all the necessary information to enable them to be processed quickly.

Closed-Ended Question—A question that limits or restricts a response, usually to a yes or no answer or other brief response.

CMS-1500 Claim Form—A standardized form for use as a "universal" form for billing professional services.

COD—Cash on delivery shipping service.

Coherence in Writing—Information that flows logically from one idea to the next.

Coinsurance—The portion of covered expenses the member pays, and the portion the plan pays after any deductible amounts are met.

Collate—To place copies in order.

Complaints—Verbal expressions of dissatisfaction with a provider or services.

Complimentary Close—Where you bring your letter to an end in a short polite manner, and always begins with a capital letter and ends with a comma.

Computer Disk Drive—A place for the storage of information.

Computer Monitor—The screen that is connected to the printer.

Concurrent Care—When two doctors are seeing a patient at the same time for two unrelated medical conditions.

Concurrent Review—The process for monitoring the use and delivery of medical services.

Condition Code—A two-digit code used to identify conditions relating to this bill that may affect payer processing.

Consultation—At the request of another physician, a specialist may request diagnostic services and make therapeutic recommendations.

Contrast Control—A knob that turns the contrast up and down between varying fields.

Controlled Drugs—Drugs that are more tightly controlled by federal mandates as a result of their addictive, experimental, toxic, or other highly volatile properties. There are four classifications ranging from the least controlled to the most controlled.

Conversion Factor—A numerical factor used to multiply or divide to arrive at a sum.

Coordination of Benefits (COB)—A process that occurs when two or more plans provide coverage on the same person. Coordination between the two plans is necessary to allow for payment of 100% of the allowable expense.

Copayment—An amount that the member pays at each visit.

Correction Fluid—A liquid that covers over the writing on paper.

Correspondence—Written communication between two people.

Cover Letter—An introductory letter to your résumé.

CT Scans (Computed Tomography)—365-degree pictures of specific body areas.

Cumulative Trial Balance—A list that shows each patient alphabetically and shows any charges, payments, or adjustments to the patient's account.

Current Procedural Terminology (CPT®)—A listing of descriptive terms and identifying codes for reporting medical services and procedures performed by physicians.

Cursor—The small-lighted symbol on the monitor screen that indicates where you are in the program or document.

Custodial Care—Care that is primarily for the purpose of meeting the personal daily needs of the patient and could be provided by personnel without medical care skills or training.

Customer Service—To service the customer or patient.

Daily Journal—*See* Day Sheet.

Day Sheet (also known as a Daily Journal)—A daily balance sheet that shows the patient's name, the individual fee charged for the day, any payments made, and the current balance.

Death Benefits—Compensation to the family of a deceased employee for the loss of income that the deceased employee would have provided to the family.

Deductible—The amount that the patient must pay before the insurance pays their benefits.

Defendant—The person being sued.

Deposit Slip—An overview and balance of monies being deposited.

Diagnosis-Related Group (DRG)—Under DRG, a flat rate payment is made based on the patient's diagnosis instead of the hospital's itemized billing.

Diagnostic Testing Report—A transcribed interpretation, "reading," of a laboratory or radiology test.

Diagnostic X-Rays—Flat or two-dimensional pictures of a particular body part or organ.

Dialysis—A maintenance procedure used for end-stage renal disease when the kidneys cease functioning.

Disenrollment—When a patient transfers their care from a provider.

Doctor's First Report of Injury/Illness—The doctor must file this report regardless of the type of workers' compensation claim or benefits. This form requests basic information on the date, time, and location of the injury/illness and treatment, the patient's subjective complaints and objective findings, the diagnosis, and the treatment rendered.

Downcoding—When an insurance carrier changes a code to a similar code that has a lower level of service.

Dunning Notice—A statement or sentence reminding the recipient to make a payment on their account.

Durable Medical Equipment—Equipment that can withstand repeated use, is primarily and customarily used to serve a medical purpose, is generally not useful to a person in the absence of an illness or injury, and is appropriate for use in the home.

Durable Medical Equipment Regional Carriers (DMERCs)—One of four regional Medicare carriers responsible for the processing of Durable Medical Equipment claims.

Early and Periodic Screening, Diagnosis, and Treatment (EPSDT)—A preventive screening program designed for the early detection and treatment of medical problems in welfare children.

Effectiveness in Writing—Being able to evoke the type of response you want your reader to have, whether you want the reader to subscribe to a magazine or to purchase a product or service.

Electronic Claims—Claims that are routinely submitted electronically to insurance carriers.

Electronic Claim Submission—A process whereby insurance claims are submitted via computerized data (either by data diskette or modem) directly from the provider to the insurance company.

Electronic Prescriptions—Prescriptions that are entered into the provider's computer, then electronically sent to the computer at the patient's pharmacy.

Eligibility—The qualifications which make a person eligible for coverage.

Eligibility Card—A card that shows that a recipient may be eligible for Medicaid.

Eligibility Roster—A list of patients who have chosen the provider as their Primary Care Provider.

Emancipation—A legal process whereby a minor child assumes legal responsibility for himself, and the child's parent or legal guardian is no longer legally responsible for the child.

Embezzlement—The act of an employee illegally taking funds from a company for which they work.

Emergency—Defined as existing when delay in treatment of the patient would lead to a significantg increase in the threat to life or body part.

Empathy—Being able to participate in another person's feelings or perceptions.

Enclosures—Anything that you are sending along with the letter, such as x-rays or forms.

Encounter Form—A form used to record both clinical and financial information about the patient; and is frequently used as a billing and routing document.

End-Stage Renal Disease (ESRD)—A condition that occurs when a person's kidneys fail to function.

Enteral Therapy—The administration of nutritional products directly into the small intestines.

Eponyms—Illnesses or conditions named after a person.

Errors and Omissions Insurance—This insurance covers damages caused by mistakes (errors) or damages caused by something an employee failed to do (omissions).

Evaluation and Management Codes—Codes that designate procedures used to evaluate the patient's condition and to assist the patient in managing that condition.

Exclusive Provider Organization (EPO)—A plan in which the patient must select a Primary Care Provider and can use only physicians who are part of the network or who are referred by the PCP.

Explanation of Benefits (EOB)—A letter from a payer indicating how a member's benefits have been applied in response to the submission of a claim.

External Audit—Considered a retrospective review because it is performed after a claim has been submitted for payment and after the claim has been processed by the insurance carrier.

External Auditor—Someone hired by an insurance company or governmental organization such as Medicare or Medicaid to perform an audit.

Facsimile Machine (more commonly referred to as the fax machine)—A machine that transmits pictures over the phone lines by transmitting a series of dot messages.

Family Deductible—A deductible that requires a specified number of family members to satisfy their individual deductible. Once the required number of family members meets their individual deductible, the family deductible is then considered met for the remaining family members. There are two types of family deductibles: aggregate and nonaggregate.

Fee Schedule—A list of predetermined charges for medical services and supplies.

Fee-for-Service—*See* Indemnity Insurance Plan.

Follow-up Days—Days immediately following a surgical procedure in which a doctor must monitor a patient's condition in regard to that particular procedure.

Fraud—Intentional misrepresentation of a fact with the intent to deprive a person of property or legal rights.

Generic Drug—A nonproprietary drug not protected by trademark and whose name is usually descriptive of the drug's chemical structure.

Grievances—Written complaints made by a member regarding dissatisfaction with a provider or services.

Group Plan—A group insurance plan is a plan under which members of a structured group insure themselves against potential losses in the event of death, disability, and the need for medical treatments that may occur. This form of coverage allows coordination of benefits.

Guarantor—A person that undertakes the responsibility for payment of a debt.

Hard Drive—Provides space (memory) for information to be stored within the computer itself.

Heading—Contains the return address, date, and a reference line and other notations if applicable.

Health Care Procedure Coding System (HCPCS)—An index used for billing injections, medication, supplies, and durable medical equipment.

Health Insurance Portability and Accountability Act (HIPAA)—A law dealing with the portability issues referring to persons being covered by insurance when they transfer from one job to another.

Health Maintenance Organizations (HMOs)—Organizations or companies that provide both the coverage for care and the care itself. Members pay a set amount every month and the HMO agrees to provide all their care, or to pay for the covered care they cannot provide.

Home Services—Visits performed by a provider in the patient's home.

Hospital Inpatient Services—The evaluation and management of a patient provided in a hospital setting.

ICD-9-CM—A statistical coding of medical diagnoses and procedures.

Immunosuppressive Drugs—Drugs for the suppressions of the immune system.

Incomplete Data Master List—A complete listing of patients whose patient charts do not have properly filled out or completed forms.

Indemnity Insurance Plan (also known as Fee-for-Service)—A principle of insurance that provides medical coverage when a loss occurs, and restores the insured party to the approximate financial condition that they had before the loss occurred.

Independent Physician Associations (IPAs)—Groups of providers who have banded together for the sole purpose of signing a contract with an MCP.

Individual Practice Organizations (IPO)—A legal entity of a network of private practice physicians, who have organized to negotiate contracts with insurance companies and HMOs.

In-Network Providers—Providers who agree to provide services at a reduced amount in exchange for the referrals from an insurance carrier within a PPO.

Innovation—The act of introducing something new.

Inside Address—The address to which the letter is being sent.

Insurance Claims Register—Lists all claims that have been fully completed and are being submitted to the insurance carrier by the provider's office.

Insurance Coverage Form—A form used by many practices to verify insurance coverage and document this information.

Insurance Tracer—A form or letter sent to the insurance carrier to inquire about the disposition of a previously submitted claim.

Intermediaries—Private insurance companies that process Medicare's Part A claims.

Internal Audit—Considered prospective reviews because they are performed before a claim is submitted for payment.

International Classification of Diseases—9th Revision Clinical Modification (ICD-9-CM)—An indexing of diseases and conditions.

Job Stress—The harmful physical and emotional responses that occur when the requirements of the job do not match the capabilities, resources, or needs of the worker.

Keyboard—The primary means of communicating with your computer.

Laboratory Examinations—The analyzing of body substances to determine their chemical or tissue type makeup.

Legend—A label inscribed as follows: "Caution: Federal (United States) law prohibits dispensing without a prescription."

Legend Drug—A drug requiring a prescription. The "legend" always appears on the label.

Lien—A legal document that expresses claim on the property of another for payment of a debt.

Lifetime Maximum—The lifetime maximum is the total dollar payments the insurance carrier will make toward the lifetime care of a patient.

Limiting Charges—Under Federal law, balance billing by nonparticipating physicians is strictly limited to no more than 15% above Medicare's approved amount.

Listening—Making an effort to hear.

Main Terms—Identifying names that are the keys by which the ICD-9-CM is structured. They usually list the type of disease or condition rather than where in the body the disease or condition is located.

Maintaining Records—Keeping the information in a record updated and filing the chart or record in a manner that makes it easy to locate if you should need it at a later date.

Malignant—Means that the cancer or growth is growing. Malignant growths will spread throughout the body until they kill the patient.

Malignant Primary—Means that the growth is growing at the point of origin of the neoplasm.

Malignant Secondary—Means that the site where the growth is growing is not where the disease originated. It has spread to this location from the primary site.

Managed Care—A system for organizing the delivery of health services so that the cost of care is reduced and the quality of care is maintained or improved.

Management Service Organization (MSO)—A separate corporation set up to provide management services to a medical group for a fee.

Mandatory Program—Requires the patient to obtain an SSO for special procedures, or there is an automatic reduction or denial of benefits.

Medicaid—A healthcare program established under Title XIX of the Social Security Act to provide the needy with access to medical care.

Medicaid Remittance Advice—Provides information about claims that were paid, adjusted, voided, and denied.

Medical Dictionary—Lists medical terms and their definitions, synonyms, illustrations, and supplemental information.

Medical Necessity Denials—The most common reason for denial of claims by Medicare; these are services that are considered not medically necessary.

Medical Service Order—A form that states that the patient is being referred to the provider in regards to a work-related injury and that the employer is responsible for coverage of services.

Medical-Legal Evaluation—An evaluation that provides medical evidence for the purpose of proving or disproving medical issues in a contested workers' compensation claim.

Medically Needy—A patient whose high medical expenses and inadequate healthcare coverage (often as a result of catastrophic illnesses) have left them at risk of being indigent.

Medically Oriented Equipment—Equipment that is primarily and customarily used for medical purposes.

Medicare—The Federal Health Insurance Benefit Plan for the aged and disabled.

Medicare Abuse—Abuse does not require the proof of intent to defraud the Medicare system in order to be assessed. It appears quite similar to fraud except that it is not possible to establish that abusive acts were committed knowingly, willfully, and intentionally.

Medicare Fraud—The intentional misrepresentation of information that could result in an unauthorized benefit.

Medicare Health Insurance Claim Number (HICN)—A unique identification number assigned to Medicare beneficiaries that normally consists of a Social Security number followed by a letter of the alphabet and possibly another letter or number (i.e., 123-45-6789A).

Medicare HMO—An HMO that has contracted with the federal government under the Medicare Advantage program (formerly called Medicare + Choice) to provide health benefits to persons eligible for Medicare that choose to enroll in the HMO, instead of receiving their benefits and care through the traditional fee-for-service Medicare program.

Medicare Redetermination Notice (MRN)—The redetermination letter issued by the Appeals Department that contains all the information necessary to request the next level of appeal.

Medicare Remittance Notice (MRN)—An explanation of benefits issued to providers (who accept Medicare assignment) for claims submitted to Medicare for a certain period of time.

Medicare Secondary Payer (MSP)—Medicare pays secondary to employer-sponsored group insurance, individual policies carried by the employee, workers' compensation insurance, Black Lung benefits, automobile or no-fault insurance, and third-party liability.

Medicare Summary Notice (MSN)—An explanation of benefits sent to the Medicare beneficiary, detailing the processing of claims submitted for payment.

Medicare Supplements (also known as Medigap Policies)—Separate plans written exclusively for Medicare participants that pay for amounts that Medicare does not pay.

Medications—Drugs used to treat diseases, symptoms, or discomforts.

Medigap Policies—*See* Medicare Supplements.

Memo—Short for memorandum, it is a letter intended for distribution within a company.

Mental and Nervous Expenses—Claims submitted for psychiatric services, marriage and family counseling, and drug and alcohol treatment.

Modifiers—Two-digit codes that can be added to CPT® codes to denote unusual circumstances. These modifiers more fully describe the procedure that was performed.

Multiline Phones—More than one telephone line into an office.

Multiple Procedures—More than one surgical procedure performed during the same operative session.

National Provider Identifiers (NPI)—A standard unique health identifier for providers; it consists of nine numbers plus a check-digit in the 10th position.

Neoplasm—A growth (tumor) that results from abnormal cell activity.

New Member Roster—Lists those patients who have signed up for HMO coverage and have chosen the provider as their PCP. This list also shows those existing patients who have recently chosen this provider as their PCP.

Nonaggregate Deductible—A deductible that requires a specified number of individual deductibles be satisfied before the family limit is met.

Noncompliance—Not following the instructions given by the provider.

Nondisability—Minor injuries that will not require the patient to be kept from his job.

Nonlegend Drug—A drug that does not require a prescription.

Nonparticipating Providers—Providers who treat Medicare patients but who decide whether to accept assignment on a case-by-case basis.

Notice of Non-Coverage—A Letter that must be provided to all Medicare HMO members at the time of discharge from an inpatient facility. It advises them of their right to an immediate professional review on a proposed discharge.

Nuclear Medicine—Combine use of radioactive elements and x-rays to image an organ or body.

Occupational Therapy—A type of physical therapy, the objective of which is to either restore normal movement, or, in the case of paralysis, to teach the patient alternative ways of dealing with his or her handicap to meet the demands of everyday living.

Occurrence Code—A code and associated date defining a significant event relating to this bill that may affect payer processing.

Occurrence Span Codes—A code and the related dates that identify an event relating to the payment of the claim. These codes identify occurrences that happened over a span of time.

Office Visits—The evaluation and management of a patient's condition in a physician's office, clinic or outpatient department of a hospital.

Open-Ended Question—A question that cannot be answered with a yes, no, or other brief response.

Opening—A subpart of the body of a letter, that attracts attention and develops interest.

Operative Report—A transcribed report describing the surgical procedure performed.

Optical Character Recognition (OCR)—An automated scanning process that reads the information on claim forms.

Order of Benefit Determinations (OBD)—The 13 rules determining the order of insurance benefit payment.

Orthotics—Devices used to straighten or correct a deformity or disability.

Out-of-Network Providers—Providers that do not agree to provide services at a reduced amount in exchange for the referrals from an insurance carrier within a PPO.

Overinsurance—A situation that occurs when a person is covered under two or more policies and is eligible to collect an accumulation of benefits that will actually exceed the amount charged by the provider.

Over-the-Counter Drug (OTC)—A drug that may be purchased without a prescription. Also known as a nonlegend drug.

Parenteral Therapy—Therapy that involves administering substances to a patient via a tube inserted into a vein (i.e., medications or nutritional supplements).

Part A—Medicare's basic plan or hospital insurance.

Part B—Medicare's medical (supplementary, voluntary) insurance that covers physician services, outpatient hospital services, home health care, outpatient speech and physical therapy, and durable medical equipment.

Part C—Medicare's advantage portion which includes coverage in an HMO, PPO, and so on.

Part D—Medicare's prescription drug component (effective 2006).

Participating Providers—Providers who agree not to practice "balance billing," or charging patients for more than the Medicare allowed amount.

Patient Aging Report—Allows the medical biller to categorize a patient account's outstanding balance by the length of time the charges have been due.

Patient Claim Form—A form for billing professional services that are provided by self-funded plans.

Patient History Form—A form that helps identify previous incidents of illness that may be important in treating a patient's present condition.

Patient Information Sheet—A form used to collect general information regarding the patient.

Patient Ledger Card (also known as a Statement of Account)—A card used to indicate a chronologic record of all services rendered to a patient.

Patient Receipt—A written acknowledgment that a specific sum of money has been received.

Patient Statement—An individual summary (either by patient or by family) that lists all the services, charges, payments, adjustments, and balance due that occurred during the month.

Payer of Last Resort—All third parties including Medicare, TRICARE, Workers' Compensation, and private insurance carriers must pay before Medicaid pays.

Pediatric Chart—A patient file for a child.

Pended—Held for further information.

Permanent Disability—A situation that usually commences after temporary disability when it is determined that the patient will not be able to return to work. This means that nothing more can be done and the patient will have the disability for the rest of his or her life.

Petty Cash Count Slip—This is used to keep track of the amount of money kept in petty cash.

Petty Cash Fund—A fund that is used for giving change to customers who are making cash payments and for buying miscellaneous small supplies.

Petty Cash Receipt—A form that is used whenever money is removed from the petty cash fund indicating how much money was removed and who received it.

Pharmaceuticals—Drugs.

Physical Medicine—The manipulation and physical therapy associated with the nonsurgical care and treatment of the patient.

Physical Therapy—The science of physical or corrective rehabilitation or treatment of abnormal conditions of the musculoskeletal system through the use of heat, light, water, electricity, sound, massage, and active, passive, or restrictive exercise.

Physician Hospital Organization (PHO)—An organization of physicians and hospitals that bands together for the purpose of obtaining contracts from payer organizations.

Physician's Final Report—The report notifying the WC carrier that no further treatment is needed (or that no further treatment will significantly alter the patient's condition) and that the patient has been discharged. The report should indicate that the patient has been discharged, the level of the patient's permanent disability, if any, and the balance due on the patient's account.

Physician's Current Procedure Terminology (CPT®)—A systematic listing for coding the procedures or services performed by a physician or provider.

Physician's Desk Reference (PDR)—A book used to determine whether a pharmaceutical product is a prescription or nonprescription drug.

Place of Service Code—A numerical code to indicate the location where the service was rendered.

Post—To list items such as payments or charges in a log.

Power Switch—A control that turns the computer or the monitor on or off.

Preadmission Testing—Testing done before the patient enters the hospital for surgery.

Preauthorization—To gain approval of the services that are to be performed, and often to obtain an understanding of whether or not the insurance carrier will provide coverage for those services.

Precertify—To get preapproval for admission on elective, nonemergency hospitalization.

Preexisting Conditions—Conditions that existed before a patient is covered under a contract.

Preferred Provider Organizations (PPOs)—A plan in which the insurance carrier contracts with providers to join their "network." These providers agree to provide services at a reduced amount in exchange for the referrals from the carrier, and the carrier agrees to reimburse network providers at a higher percentage than providers outside the network.

Preventive Medicine—Routine, well care provided when there is not an active illness or disease.

Primary Care Provider (PCP)—The provider a patient has chosen for their primary medical care.

Primary Plan—The plan that determines and pays its benefits first without regard to the existence of any other coverage.

Professional Courtesy—When a doctor renders medical services to another professional, such as a doctor, pharmacist, or nurse, or to a relative.

Prompt Payment Laws—Laws that dictate how quickly an insurance company must pay a clean claim once it is received.

Proprietary Drug—A drug that is patented or controlled by a manufacturer. The manufacturer copyrights the trade or brand name. This is not the same as the generic name, which identifies the drug's chemical composition.

Prospective Review—Determines the need and appropriateness of the recommended care.

Prosthetic Devices—Devices designed to replace a missing body part or to restore some function to a paralyzed body part.

Provider—The person or entity that provides healthcare services. This can be a doctor, chiropractor, hospital, emergency facility, x-ray technician, or any certified professional who is licensed to provide healthcare services.

Provider Identification Number (PIN)—A number assigned to providers/suppliers in Medicare Part B for the practice location(s) where they provide services to beneficiaries.

Psychiatric Services—Treatment for psychotic and neurotic disorders, organic brain dysfunction, alcoholism, and chemical dependency.

Radiation Oncology Services—The use of radiation to treat a condition.

Reference Book—A source of information to which a reader is referred.

Rehabilitation Benefit—A benefit provided to retrain an injured employee in a physical ability which will help them to seek future employment.

Reinsurance—An insurance policy that protects the company against catastrophic medical costs levied against their plan, either by a single employee or by all employees as a whole.

Relative Value Study (RVS)—A listing of procedures and their appropriate codes, along with a unit value that has been assigned to the procedure.

Release of Information Form—A form used to allow the provider to request additional information from other providers of service or to share information with an insurance carrier.

Request for Additional Information Form—A form designed to ask for information or records from various sources.

Resource-Based Relative Value Scale (RBRVS)—A standardized physician's payment schedule. Payments for services are determined by the resource costs needed to provide them.

Respondeat Superior—An employer who is liable for harms caused by an employee while that employee is acting within the scope of their employment.

Résumé—A summary of employment experience and qualifications.

Retrospective Review—The process used to determine after discharge whether the hospitalization and treatment were medically necessary and covered by the terms of the benefit program.

Return Receipt Requested—On delivery, a receipt is issued and mailed back to the sender of the package. This allows the sender to have proof of the delivery and the name of the person who signed for it.

Revenue Codes—A code that identifies a specific accommodation, ancillary service, or billing calculation.

Salutation—A form of greeting the letter recipient. It normally begins with the word "Dear" and always includes the person's last name.

Second Opinion—A consultation designed as a benefit to the patient by confirming the need for a surgery.

Second Surgical Opinion Consultation (SSO)—Used to eliminate elective surgical procedures that are classified as unnecessary.

Secondary Plan—The plan that pays after the primary plan has paid its benefits.

Self-Funded Plan—A company that insures itself and its own workers.

Self-Insurance—A plan in which employers place monthly premium amounts into an escrow account and pay all medical claims from this account.

Share of Cost—The amount the patient is responsible for paying for services rendered.

Signature—The name of the person writing the latter or for whom the letter has been written.

Signature Card—A card that shows the person authorized to make changes, the dates they are authorized for, and the scope of the changes they are allowed to make.

Skilled Nursing Facility (SNF)—Facility primarily engaged in providing skilled nursing care and related services for residents who require medical or nursing care; or rehabilitation services for the rehabilitation of injured, disabled, or sick persons.

Skip—A person who has received services without payment and has moved and left no forwarding address.

SOAP Notes—Medical documentation of patient complaint(s) and treatment, which must be consistent, concise, and comprehensive. They should be documented in such a way as to show everything there is to know about the current status of the patient.

Social Health Maintenance Organization (S/HMO)—An organization that provides the full range of Medicare benefits offered by standard HMO, plus additional services.

Source of Admission Code—A one-digit code indicating how the patient was referred to the facility.

Speech Therapy—Therapy for the purpose of improving speech and verbal communication skills.

Standing Appointment—Any appointment that happens on a regular basis.

State Insurance Commissioner—This person is responsible for overseeing the insurance companies and their practices within the state.

Statement of Account—*See* Patient Ledger Card.

Statute of Limitations—The maximum time that a debt can be collected from the time it has been incurred.

Stoploss—An attempt to limit payments by an insured person, or a group/IPA in the case of a catastrophic illness or injury to a member.

Subclassifications—Secondary classifications under a main classification.

Subjective Findings—Those findings that cannot be discerned by anyone other than the patient.

Subpoena—A demand to appear at a certain time and place to give testimony on a certain matter.

Subpoena Duces Tecum—Requires production of books, records, papers, or other tangible evidence.

Summary—A brief statement of information covered.

Superbills—These are billing forms used by many providers of service and suppliers. This form services as a charging slip to expedite the process of medical insurance reimbursement.

Temporary Disability—A situation in which the patient is not able to perform his or her job requirements until he or she recovers from the injury involved.

Terminated Member Roster—Lists those members whose coverage has been terminated or who have chosen to terminate this provider as their PCP.

Therapeutic Injections—Injections required in the treatment of an illness or disease.

Tickler File—Often expanding file folder that helps you remember items that need to occur on a specific date.

Transitional Thought—Seques into the topic of the next paragraph.

Treating Physician (TP)—Initially establishes the employee's eligibility for workers' compensation benefits and provides care and treatment to the injured employee.

Triage—The screening of patients to determine their priority for treatment when there are more patients than medical personnel and resources available.

Triage Reports—Reports generated at the scene of accidents, in emergency rooms, and in urgent care clinics.

TRICARE—The Department of Defense's healthcare program for members of the uniformed services and their families and survivors, and retired members and their families.

Type of Admission Code—A two-digit code indicating the priority of the patient when they entered the hospital.

UB-04—A billing form approved by the NUCC in February 2005 that will replace the UB-92.

Ultrasonography—A picture created by bouncing sound waves off the desired structure.

Uniform Bill—1992 (UB-92)—A form used by hospitals or other hospital-type facilities for inpatient and outpatient billing.

Unique Physician Identification Number (UPIN)—A number for identifying the physician ordering or referring services.

Unlisted Codes—The codes that end in "99" and are listed at the end of each CPT® section and subsection.

Unnecessary Surgery—Surgery that is recommended as an elective procedure when an alternative method of treatment may be preferable.

Usual, Customary, and Reasonable (UCR)—Under UCR, each procedure that is performed is given a number value (called a relative unit value) based on how difficult the procedure is to perform, the overhead involved, and the chance of incurring a malpractice lawsuit.

Utilization Review (UR)—A process whereby insurance carriers review the treatment of a patient and determine whether or not the costs will be covered.

V Code—The V code listing is a supplementary listing of factors that affect the health status of the patient.

Value Code—A code and the related dollar amount that identifies data of a monetary nature that is necessary for processing the claim.

Van Transportation Units—Specially equipped vans that can handle wheelchairs and patients who are unable to get in and out of a regular vehicle.

Verification—Repeating information and asking if you have understood it correctly.

Vocational Rehabilitation—Retraining in a different job field when the injured employee is unable to return to their former position.

Voluntary Program—Encourages participants to have an SSO, but there is no automatic reduction of benefits if the patient does not comply.

Withhold—The HMO may retain a portion of the monthly capitation amount to protect the HMO from inadequate patient care or financial management by the PCP.

Workers' Compensation (WC)—A separate medical and disability reimbursement program that provides 100% coverage for job-related injuries, illnesses, or conditions arising out of and in the course of employment.

Credits

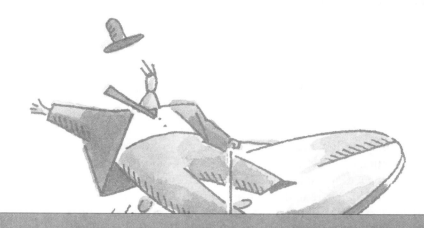

CHAPTER 15 **Pages 424, 429, 454:** Courtesy of ICDC Publishing, Inc.

APPENDIX B **Pages 465–467:** Courtesy of ICDC Publishing, Inc. **Pages 468–470:** Courtesy of Department of Industrial Relations, CA. **Pages 471–480:** Courtesy of ICDC Publishing, Inc. **Page 481:** Courtesy of Centers for Medicare and Medicaid Services. **Page 482:** Courtesy of National Uniform Billing Committee. **Pages 483–487:** Courtesy of ICDC Publishing, Inc. **Page 488 (top and bottom):** Courtesy of ICDC Publishing, Inc. **Pages 489, 491:** Courtesy of ICDC Publishing, Inc. **Pages 490:** © 2006 Jupiterimages Corporation.

APPENDIX C **Pages 493–495:** Courtesy of ICDC Publishing, Inc. **Page 496:** Courtesy of American Medical Association. **Pages 497–500:** Courtesy of Centers for Medicare and Medicaid Services. **Pages 501–515:** Courtesy of National Uniform Billing Committee. **Pages 516–522:** Courtesy of ICDC Publishing, Inc.

APPENDIX D **Pages 524–542, 543–545, 547–549:** Courtesy of Centers for Medicare and Medicaid Services.

APPENDIX E **Pages 551–579, 581–585:** Courtesy of National Uniform Billing Committee.

Index

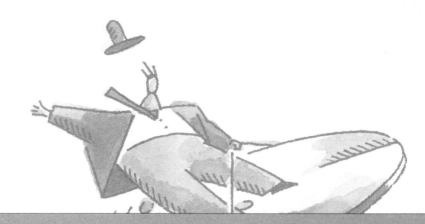

M

Mail, 392
Main
  procedure, 267
  term, 248
Maintenance procedure, 284
Major medical benefits, 63
Major medical plans, 230
Malignant, 250
  CA in situ, 250
  lesion, 252
  primary, 250
  secondary, 250
Managed care, 125, 163
  carriers, 176
  insurers, 347
  organizations, 163
Managed care plans (MCPs). *See* MCP
Management Service Organization (MSO), 166
Mandatory program, 74
Manual
  files, 406
  systems, 196
Manufacturer, 224
Manufacturer's index (white), 224
Marriage, Family, and Child Counselor (MFCC), 284, 460
Master of Social Work (MSW), 284, 460
Maternal and Child Health Services, 125
Maternity
  bundling, 315
  care, 315
  cases, 278
  counseling, 278
  expenses, 278
  procedure, 315
  procedure code, 278
MCPs, 167
  Chief Medical Officer, 177
  initiated disenrollment, 179
  policy and procedure manual, 173
  responsibilities, 186
Medicaid, 126
  agency, 132
  as secondary payer, 130
  beneficiary, 128
  benefits, 128
  billing guidelines, 133
  claim forms, 130
  claims, 129, 326
  covered services, 128
  eligibility, 128
  identification number, 132
  patients, 132
Medicaid-allowed amount, 130
Medicaid Remittance Advice (MRA), 129
Medical
  advice, 19
  and surgical supplies, 229
  assistants, 4
  billers, 29, 58, 174, 302, 317, 346, 358, 398, 405, 412, 424
  billing, 358
  bills, 4, 316
  charting, 32
  coding, 4
  dictionaries, 222
  documentation rules, 32
  emergency, 5

equipment provider, 5
equipments, 229, 348
ethics, 16
evidence, 146
group, 179
history reports, 46, 358
insurance reimbursement, 302
issues, 146
justification, 132
necessity denials, 114
offices, 30, 196, 211, 316
office setting, 4
practice, 196
provider, 143
reference book, 223
reports, 358
review panel, 172
service order, 146
services, 233, 319
supply items, 229
team, 4
technology, 163
treatment plans, 30
Medical charts, 29
  storing, 34
Medical doctor (MD), 106, 460
Medical-legal evaluations, 146
Medically
  needy, 128
  oriented equipment, 230
Medical Management Incentive Program, 172
Medical records, 30, 147, 348, 358
  complexity of, 37
  confidentiality of, 10
  librarians, 246
  number, 336
  retention of, 34
  storing, 35
Medical technologist (MT), 460
Medical while hospitalized (MWH), 269
Medicare, 102
  abuse, 124
  advance notice, 326
  allowance, 112
  and medicaid programs, 302
  appeals process, 120
  approved amount, 111
  assignment, 112
  beneficiaries, 104
  benefits, 103
  billing guidelines, 126
  billing notices, 107
  carrier, 320
  carrier claim, 107
  claims, 112, 234, 326, 544, 577
  coverage, 102
  denials, 117
  eligibility, 102
  fraud and abuse, 122
  guidelines, 102, 118
  health insurance card, 105
  health insurance claim number, 106
  HMO, 125
  limitations, 315
  limiting charge, 184
  notice, 320
  number, 107
  of medicaid remittance advice, 200